THE THORAX

Second Edition,
Revised and Expanded
(in three parts)

PART B: APPLIED PHYSIOLOGY

THE THORAX

*Second Edition,
Revised and Expanded
(in three parts)*

PART B: APPLIED PHYSIOLOGY

Edited by

Charis Roussos
*National and Kapodistrian
University of Athens Medical School
Athens, Greece*

*McGill University
Montreal, Quebec, Canada*

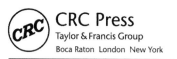

CRC Press
Taylor & Francis Group
Boca Raton London New York

CRC Press is an imprint of the
Taylor & Francis Group, an **informa** business

First published 1995 by Marcel Dekker, Inc.

Published 2019 by CRC Press
Taylor & Francis Group
6000 Broken Sound Parkway NW, Suite 300
Boca Raton, FL 33487-2742

© 1995 by Taylor & Francis Group, LLC
CRC Press is an imprint of Taylor & Francis Group, an Informa business

First issued in paperback 2019

No claim to original U.S. Government works

ISBN 13: 978-0-367-44894-3 (pbk)
ISBN 13: 978-0-8247-9600-6 (hbk)

**Visit the Taylor & Francis Web site at
http://www.taylorandfrancis.com**

**and the CRC Press Web site at
http://www.crcpress.com**

Library of Congress Cataloging-in-Publication Data

The thorax / edited by Charis Roussos. — 2nd ed., rev. and expanded.
    p.   cm. — (Lung biology in health and disease ; v. 85)
    Contents: pt. A. Physiology — pt. B. Applied physiology — pt. C. Disease.
    ISBN 0-8247-9504-0 (pt. A : alk. paper). — ISBN 0-8247-9600-4 (pt. B : alk. paper).
— ISBN 0-8247-9601-2 (pt. C : alk. paper).
    1. Chest—Diseases. 2. Chest—Muscles. 3. Chest—Physiology. I. Roussos, Charis.
II. Series.
    [DNLM: 1. Thoracic Diseases. 2. Thorax. 3. Respiration.   W1 LU62 v.85 1995 /
WF 970T4877 1995]
RC941.T48   1995
617.5'4—dc20
DNLM/DLC
for Library of Congress   95-32396
                                                                                    CIP

To Ludwig A. Engel,
an example of scientific excellence;
a superb teacher;
an unending source of creativity in research;
a model of strength;
a prototype of dedication and courage;
and our friend.

INTRODUCTION

Although Galen is credited with recognizing that the thorax played some role in moving air in and out of the lungs, it was much later that the function of the thorax was established:

> The lungs do not move naturally of their own motion, but they follow the motion of the thorax and the diaphragm. The lungs are not expanded because they are filled with air, but they are filled with the air because they are expanded.

> *Franciscus Sylvius de la Boe*
> *Opera Medica—1681*

Later physiologists such as the French N. P. Adelon described the thorax as a "cavity situated below the neck but above the abdomen, which contains the heart and the lungs and acts with regard to the latter as a bellows to fill them with air" (Physiologie de l'homme—1831).

It is noteworthy that not until the post-World War II era did a significant research focus on the thorax develop. This occurred essentially because of the compelling need to learn about the mechanics of breathing. Yet, in 1951, Wallace O. Fenn concluded in a review article titled "Mechanics of Respiration" that "At best an outline of the mechanical problems of breathing has been stretched and some possible methods of attack have been suggested for future addition to our knowledge of the subject" (Am. J. Med. 1951; 10).

Exactly 10 years ago Volume 29 of this series of monographs appeared. Charis Roussos and Peter T. Macklem were the editors and its title was *The Thorax*. In the Foreword, E. J. Moran Campbell wrote: "The bibliographies in this book attest to the growth of interest (in the mechanics of breathing) in the last quarter century." The book was in two parts and it included 47 chapters. The average number of references per chapter numbered 50.

This new volume, edited by Charis Roussos, clearly attests to the work that has been done since the first edition. It includes 91 chapters contributed by over 100 authors, and the references number in the thousands. One could say that this three-part book is an encyclopedia of the thorax.

No one, of course, questions that life is inherently tied to the respiratory function that brings oxygen to the tissues. "In some animals air reaches the lung by buccal deglutition that literally pushes it into the lungs as food reaches the stomach. However, in humans, it is because of the action of the thorax that air alternatively enters and exits the lung" (Adelon). In this volume, all the mechanisms of this action in health and disease are described and analyzed in great detail. The editor and the authors have accomplished an extraordinary amount of work to complete this truly landmark book. I am greatly appreciative that they gave me the opportunity to include it in the "Lung Biology in Health and Disease" series.

Claude Lenfant, M.D.

FOREWORD

The second edition of *The Thorax* is a remarkable achievement. I cannot think of an aspect of the respiratory muscles that is not covered. History, anatomy, kinematics, statics, dynamics, energetics, biochemistry, cell and molecular biology, pharmacology, psychophysics, imaging, morphology, patient symptoms, and physical signs are all dealt with—and more. This eclectic approach reflects the current fad in biological research to break a system down into its components, whether they be molecules, forces, strains, vectors, or sensations. The spectacular successes of molecular biology and genetics indicate without a shadow of reservation how successful modern science has been.

Yet reductionism in science, in spite of its successes, has always conflicted with the science that deals with how all the component parts work when they are integrated into a single functioning unit. How the whole works, rather than how each component functions in isolation, also plays a prominent part in *The Thorax*. Indeed, this volume presents a nice balance between reductionist and integrative approaches.

Such a balance is tricky these days. So much of science is molecular that integrative approaches are getting short shrift. Yet understanding of what molecules do in isolation is unlikely to impart understanding (let alone wisdom) of how diseases make human beings sick. Although this book has retained a nice balance, it seems that many of us have been completely seduced by the appeal of molecular science.

Academic clinical department heads appear to have caved into science funding policy so that nowadays a requirement for a full-time position in a subspecialty division is usually expertise in molecular and/or cellular biology.

This is hardly ideal for the teaching and practice of medicine. The science of medicine is above all a study of how molecules and cells within the body function as integrated units; of how disorders can be explained and understood, not as dysfunctions of single molecules or cells but as abnormalities of the *interactions* between many molecules and many cells. *The Thorax* provides state-of-the-art information on interactions and, because it does so, will provide invaluable information to a generation of doctors and scientists who have not been taught how to integrate the individual components of cells, organs, or whole organisms and who, without that knowledge, cannot understand function.

Although the modern physician may have difficulty in coping with the function and dysfunction of whole organisms, it seems likely that the next scientific revolution will be precisely in this area. How complex systems which are never in equilibrium function can now be studied rigorously. Complexity has already given remarkable new insights into Darwinian evolution. The idea that survival of the fittest is limited to systems that can adapt meaningfully means that systems in equilibrium are destined to become extinct because they lack the mechanism for adaptation. Similarly, chaotic systems cannot adapt meaningfully. Thus only systems that function at the edge of order and chaos can survive. Evolution means that all that is living in our universe—ourselves, flora, fauna, and indeed all biological systems—are systems that are neither in equilibrium nor chaotic, but that teeter on the brink between the two.

Teetering on the brink suggests that complex systems may become too ordered or too chaotic. If survival depends on remaining at the border between equilibrium and chaos, then disease is a situation that pushes us into one camp or the other. What determines whether a system is in equilibrium, is chaotic, or functions normally? The answer to this question is profoundly important for the practice of medicine.

Feed-forward systems are important for adaptation; the number of interactions between the nodes of a system is an important determinant of whether the system is chaotic or not; negative feedback loops are essential for homeostasis; sensitivity to initial conditions may determine if a particular environmental insult causes disease or not. These are the parameters that need to be critically examined to determine if a biological system is becoming abnormal because it is approaching equilibrium or because it is becoming chaotic.

The study of complexity is certain to bring remarkable new insights into the mechanisms of disease and new therapeutic interventions. I predict that it will have a profound effect on the practice of medicine—at least as great as the great scientific revolution produced by molecular biology. Nowhere is this more likely to be true than in respiration. The ventilatory mechanisms controlling acid–base balance, oxygen delivery, and CO_2 elimination and which involve complex interactions between receptors, spinal, brainstem, and cortical neural controllers and pathways, respiratory muscles, lungs, and chest wall is obviously a complex system functioning close to, but not in, equilibrium, capable of beneficial adaptations to changing environmental conditions. Thus, understanding of chaotic, complex, and equilibrated systems of respiration is likely to lead to the next major advances in understanding the thorax and the diseases that plague it.

Because it provides an excellent balance between integrative and cellular/molecular approaches, the present volume is well positioned to be an important stepping stone to the newest biology. It gives the basis for understanding respiratory complexity. It should be an essential building block in the construction of the bridge between present-day understanding of disease and the exciting new approaches that students of complexity will bring.

Peter T. Macklem

PREFACE TO THE SECOND EDITION

The first edition of *The Thorax*, published about 10 years ago, was confined to two volumes. Since then, the literature relating to the chest wall has expanded quite rapidly, as indicated by the enormous increase in the size of the reference sections at the end of each chapter. Hence, the second edition consists of three volumes and contains almost double the number of pages of the first edition.

The goal of *The Thorax*, Second Edition, is to provide a comprehensive, authoritative, and contemporary discussion of the physiology (Part A) and pathophysiology (Part B) of the chest wall as well as an overview of the diagnostic and therapeutic modalities (Part C). It also identifies those areas of the field that need further research and investigation. This book will be an invaluable aid to clinical investigators by providing answers to the basic questions and helping them gain a better understanding of clinical problems, areas of controversy, and lacunae of knowledge. Hopefully, this will stimulate further research efforts.

The Thorax, Second Edition, was completed with the help of over 125 authors. As in the first edition, contributors were selected based on their knowledge of and expertise in their respective fields. Thus, whether clinicians or scientists, they are at the forefront of their disciplines, and are undoubtedly in the best position to analyze and summarize information and debate controversial issues. The geographical diversity of contributors is striking—Argentina, Australia, Belgium, Canada, England, Finland, France, Greece, Italy, Sweden, and the United States—and reflects the international interest in advancing our knowledge of the function and dysfunction of the chest wall. I believe that these contributors have given the book a lively flavor, making it very up-to-date and comprehensive, while putting the future of the field in both realistic and exciting perspective.

The first volume, Part A, updates information on the striated muscles and briefly and lucidly relates it to the respiratory muscles. Thus, Chapters 1–12 lead smoothly to the complex subsequent chapters on mechanics and energetics (Chapters 13–25) and control (Chapters 26–34) of respiratory muscles. The second volume, Part B, deals extensively with the methods of measurement of chest wall function. It points out to researchers areas that need further investigation and illustrates to clinicians the pitfalls and limitations of each method (Chapters 35–44). This volume also discusses the relation between the chest wall and commonplace activities or conditions such as speech, dyspnea, exercise, diving, and anesthesia, to mention a few (Chapters 45–60). Thus the significant role that the thorax plays in various physiological and pathological conditions is explained. The third volume, Part C, focuses on disease states. Chapters 61–65 deal with the methods of diagnosis by which to establish the normality or dysfunction of the chest wall. These chapters try to offer as much practical information to the clinician as possible. Chapters 66–76 describe the pathophysiology of the respiratory muscles and the chest wall as a whole in various clinical conditions. Finally, Chapters 77–91 describe the therapeutic approaches necessary to improve the function of the ventilatory pump in various disease states. Some overlap between the chapters was encouraged, which allowed for an uninterrupted flow of thoughts and helped to achieve the detailed coverage of the topics.

The book would have been impossible to produce without the help of all the distinguished authors to whom I am profoundly indebted, not only for their contributions but for their support when I began my new position at the University of Athens Medical School. During this interesting period of creativity, they helped mature my thinking through animated discussions. I am grateful to Miss M. Titcomb for her excellent secretarial assistance and cooperation, and I thank my colleagues in Evangelismos Hospital of Athens for creating an environment that, despite the sometimes insurmountable administrative difficulties, has been conducive to scholarly work. Finally, I am most grateful to my family—Alexandra, Konstantinos, and Katerina—for their forbearance during these interesting years, for sharing my excitement, and for supporting me during periods of fatigue.

Charis Roussos

PREFACE TO THE FIRST EDITION

It is only somewhat belatedly that chest physicians have begun to focus their attention on the chest wall. Physiologists have continued their interest since at least the time of Hippocrates, but physicians have mostly avoided the role of the chest wall except when it was obviously involved in diseases such as flail chest, kyphoscoliosis, or neuromuscular disorders.

However, just as hypertension can lead to congestive heart failure, the chest wall can also malfunction due to disorders that are external to it. Lung disease can put such a load on the chest wall muscles and low cardiac output states can sufficiently impair their supply, that they may fail to develop the respiratory pressure swings required for normal alveolar ventilation. It is this growing awareness that is leading chest physicians to become more interested in the chest wall aspect of respiratory disease. Furthermore, chest wall disorders offer new possibilities for treatment, even though the external disorders cannot be effectively reversed. Indeed, a substantial number of chest physicians think that the most crippling aspects of respiratory disease, namely, shortness of breath and hypercapnic respiratory failure, arise from disordered chest wall function and not from the lung.

Thus this book attempts to gather the essence of this timely topic: the function and dysfunction of the chest wall. It is meant to provide a comprehensive view of the physiology and pathophysiology of the chest wall with an overview of the various therapeutic modalities presently available. In its own right, this book is not simply a resumé of current information, but contains several chapters of original scientific contribution. Our aim is not only to describe the burgeoning wealth of information which has accumulated, but also to emphasize what remains unsolved, thereby stimulating further research in this domain.

We are also attempting, as implied by the title, to restore the original meaning of the word "thorax." Most chest physicians equate "thorax" with rib cage. As one of us points out, this is not in accord with its original meaning in ancient Greek. At that time, "thorax" meant "chest wall" and this is how we use the term in this book. We hope our readers will also restore the original meaning to the word "thorax."

During the period needed to produce this book, the infusion of new knowledge continued unabated and new concepts evolved, rendering this work an editorial challenge, but also, we hope, a gratifying scientific contribution.

Charis Roussos
Peter T. Macklem

PROLOGUE
THE THORAX THROUGH
HISTORY INTO MEDICINE

The *Gould Medical Dictionary* defines the term "thorax" as

> The chest. The portion of the trunk above the diaphragm and below the neck. The framework of bones and soft tissues bounded by the diaphragm below; the ribs and the sternum in the front; the ribs and the thoracic portion of the vertebral column behind; above, by the structures in the lower part of the neck; and containing the heart enclosed in pericardium, the lungs invested by the pleura and mediastinal structures.

Clearly, in this definition, the thorax is equivalent to the chest that is also defined in Gould as "the earliest form of container for storing clothes, documents, valuables and other possessions."

It is obvious from the above description that, in the English medical literature, the concept of the term thorax is that of a container along with its contents, i.e., a chest. The Greek word thorax, though, did not always have this meaning. Its conceptual transformation as it passed from Greek into English exemplifies some interesting problems in the history of medicine: for one, how common words are transformed into medical terms, and also how knowledge is transferred from one language to another.

As French (1978) points out in his scholarly review "The Thorax in History," early scholars encountered many difficulties in the transmission of anatomical knowledge from one language to another. The original language presented a

technical term which was made clear by the descriptive content, but no corresponding term of sufficient accuracy existed in the language receiving the word. The
scholars then had to invent an analogous term which reflected at the same time their
understanding of the function of the organ. This problem, as it relates to the history
of medicine, is illustrated by the various translations of the term thorax into many
different languages—like *clibanus* (oven), a term denoting the rigidity of the thorax
as a heat-containing structure holding the heat-producing heart (from a Latin
translation of Galen's work, *On the Usefulness of Parts*) or like chest (container)
in English.

   It is my intention, in this historical search, to credit to the term thorax its
original meaning, thus to justify its usage in the title of the present monograph. I
will try to trace the word from its earliest beginnings, even before it entered the
Greek language, and follow it in its long journey through many centuries of Greek
history and cultural evolution. At the crossroads of culture and medicine, I will
follow the word as it became a medical term, up to the point where it acquired its
present meaning. The search for these roots is aided by the memories of this journey
to be found in the nonmedical usage of the word thorax in modern Greek language.

   Etymologically, thorax is a word probably of Sanskritic origin and it entered
the Greek language very early. It is believed to be derived from the words *dharaka*,
dhara, *dharahma*, which mean receptacle or vessel and also holding, supporting,
life-bearing, containing, maintaining, and protecting. In its transition into the Greek
language, thorax retained protection as its primary meaning. Thus, thorax came to
signify a wall-like device placed externally around vulnerable parts of the body, of
a ship or a city for the purpose of their fortification and therefore protection
(Herodotus, Book I).

   The use of the word thorax to mean the protective wall of the life-supporting
organs of the body, that is, the heart, lungs, and intestines, dates back at least as
far as the epic poems of Homer, written in the 8th century B.C. Homer wrote in
the *Iliad* about a war between the Trojans and the Greeks which allegedly took
place in 1180 B.C. In his vivid descriptions, he referred to the thorax, meaning a
leather or copper cover which protected the chest of soldiers. Thorax meant corset,
ciurass, breastplate to the Homeric Greeks.

   As Greek culture became more sophisticated and advanced and blacksmiths
improved and expanded their skills, we find descriptions of more elaborate thoraces.
Unlike those of the Homeric Greeks, these later thoraces did not stop at the waistline
but covered the whole trunk. Alcaeus, a lyric poet of the 7th century B.C., referred
to thoraces using the descriptive adjectives of "complex and elaborate." In another
poem he referred to the price of the thorax, implying that the thorax was no longer
the simple copper or leather armor of the soldier, but a piece of equipment that
reflected the wealth and status of its bearer. There are abundant descriptions of
thoraces as armor by other ancient Greek authors too. Herodotus talked about
laminated and squamous (scale-bearing) thoraces (Herodotus, Books II and IX),
and Pausanias of a thorax consisting of a coat of mail or chain mail.

The 5th century witnessed significant progress and evolution in the Greek culture. It ushered in the classical period of ancient Greece and saw giants of philosophy, art, and science. The Ionian philosophy, based on observation, reached a peak and man started to observe and study his own body very carefully. This meant that he needed new words to name the new concepts and the parts of the body according to their function. Around this time the meaning of thorax undergoes a two-step transformation.

In the first phase, the armor—the thorax—which had until now protected the internal organs from the anterior like a wall, becomes incorporated into the new knowledge of the body structure and function. In this process it moves into the interior and gives its name to the anatomy of the very body structures it used to cover, thus becoming the chest wall. The change in the meaning of the word is reflected in one of the plays of Aristophanes, one of the wittiest Greek writers, who used the word thorax in a pun. In his play *Wasps*, he described a duel and commented on the strength of the "thorax" of the winner. When one of the listeners remarked that fighters were not allowed to wear "thoraces" in this type of a duel, the narrator explained that "thorax" meant the chest wall of the fighter, not his breastplate.

In the second phase we witness a further transformation of the term. As the medical interest during this period gravitates toward the internal organs, the anatomical thorax is losing its exclusive meaning as a wall and by generalization it comes to signify both the wall and the cavity enclosed by this wall. In other words, the conceptualization of the structure termed "thorax" is shifting toward that of a chest. The limits, though, of this chest remain ambiguous, as the meaning of thorax as armor remains vivid in the memory of Greek scientists and philosophers.

Each author defines the boundaries of the thorax according to the shield wall he is referring to (it is interesting to note that the same ambiguity about the precise demarcation of the boundaries of the chest wall is to be found among scientists even to the present day). Evidence of this new evolution of the meaning of the word thorax is to be found in both the writings of Plato, who used the word with its colloquial meaning, and the scientific works of Hippocrates and Aristotle.

Plato in *Timaeus* described the hierarchy of the functions of the human body and related them to the hierarchy of values of human life. In his description of the body, he mentioned that the "cavity of the Thorax" is divided into the upper part over the diaphragm, which contains the heart, and the lower part below the diaphragm, which contains the intestines.

The official entrance of the term into medicine came with Hippocrates, the Father of Medicine. For him the boundaries of the bodily thorax coincided with those of the armor thorax. In his book *The Art*, he describes the thorax as the cavity in which the liver is covered, that is, the trunk.

Aristotle was one of the most germinal minds of antiquity and he became the founder of the scientific thinking of the Western world. It is interesting to note the ambiguity that exists in his writings vis-à-vis the definition of thorax. In his work *Problems*, he differentiates between thorax and abdomen as he refers to the three regions of the body, that is, the head, the thorax (chest), and the stomach. In his *History of Animals*, in the same chapter, he uses the term thorax interchangeably to define both the chest and the trunk. So we first read that the thorax (chest) has a back and a front . . . next after the thorax in front is the belly, and further down he says that the penis is situated externally at the base of the thorax (trunk). In *Parts of Animals*, the thorax is described as extending from the head to the "residual vent."

Medicine as the science we know today started with Galen, the famous Greek physician, the founder of experimental physiology. Using vivisections and dissections as the Egyptians had done centuries before him, he gained a fine knowledge of anatomy and physiology. Galen was a rigorous scientist and, as he was forced to make up medical terminology from common words, he was very careful to define his new terms precisely. An example of this is the definition of thorax. In his *The Usefulness of Parts* we read "all that cavity bounded by the ribs on both sides, extending to the sternum and the diaphragm in front and curving down to the spine in the rear is customarily called Thorax by the physician." It is worth noting how similar this definition is to the one in the *Gould Medical Dictionary*.

Thorax has never become exclusively a medical term in the Greek language, thus it never lost its primary meaning of fortified protective wall. Through the centuries we find the term thorax used figuratively to mean armor or breastplate in the Hellenic Greek of the New Testament. In Paul, we read about the thorax (breastplate) of love and faith. In the contemporary common Greek language thorax means fortified wall [hence the medical term *pneumothorax*, meaning a wall of air around the lungs] and the verb "thorakizo" or "to install a thorax" means to apply external fortification around ships, cars, etc. in the form of armor.

We have now reached the modern era and we find the term thorax once more at the crossroads of history and medicine, at least in the conscience of a Greek scientist, the editor of the present monograph. As it was pointed out in the present search, thorax has maintained the meaning of a protective fortified wall for 30 centuries of Greek culture and history. In medicine the term thorax gradually lost its original meaning when the concept of the chest wall as a vital organ failed to be recognized, thus rendering its symbol "the thorax" void of meaning. Currently, though, we observe new developments in respiratory physiology and medicine with the chest wall becoming the subject of rigorous scientific research. History and medicine thus have met, as "thorax," the old symbol of the fortified wall, is acquiring substance again. Medicine is restoring to the chest wall its appropriate significance. The editor is attempting to do so by giving the title *The Thorax* to the present monograph, the subject matter of which is precisely the chest wall, restoring thus the original meaning to this ancient term.

References

Alcaeus 15, *Codicus Atheneaus*, 1123.560, 11.374, 4.136.
Aristophanes, *Wasps*, 1194.
Aristotle, *History of Animals*, Book I, 493a, 10 and 493a, 25.
Aristotle, *Parts of Animals*, Book IV, 686b, 5.
Aristotle, *Problems*, Book XXXIII, 962a, 35.
French, R. K. (1978). The thorax in history. *Thorax* 33.
Galen, *On the Usefulness of Parts*, Book VI, 300.
Blakiston's Gould Medical Dictionary.
Herodotus, Book I, 181.
Herodotus, Book II, 182.
Herodotus, Book IX, 22.
Hippocrates, *The Art*, Book X, 10.
Homer, *Iliad*, 4.133, 5.99, 11.234, 15.529.
Paul, *Ephesians* 6.14.
Pausanias, Book I, 21.6.
Plato, *Timaeus*, 69.E.

Charis Roussos

CONTRIBUTORS TO PART B: APPLIED PHYSIOLOGY

Murray D. Altose, M.D.   Professor, Department of Medicine, Case Western Reserve University School of Medicine, Cleveland, Ohio

Apostolos Armaganidis, M.D.   Assistant Professor, Critical Care Department, University of Athens, Evangelismos Hospital, Athens, Greece

Michel Aubier, M.D., Ph.D.   Professor and Research Director, Department of Pneumology, Université de Paris, Paris, France

François Bellemare   Assistant Professor, Department of Anesthesia, University of Montreal, Hôtel-Dieu Hospital, Montreal, Quebec, Canada

Jorge Boczkowski, M.D., Ph.D.   Established Investigator, Institut National de la Santé et de la Recherche Médicale, Faculté Xavier Bichat, Paris, France

Demosthenes Bouros, M. D., F.C.C.P.   Associate Professor, Department of Thoracic Medicine and Clinical Pharmacology, University of Crete Medical School, Heraklion, Greece

T. Douglas Bradley Associate Professor, Department of Medicine, University of Toronto, Toronto, Ontario, Canada

A. Charles Bryan, B.S., M.B., Ph.D., F.R.C.P.(C) Emeritus Professor of Pediatrics, Critical Care and Respiratory Research, Hospital for Sick Children, Toronto, Ontario, Canada

E. J. Moran Campbell, M.D., Ph.D., F.R.C.P., F.R.S.(C). Professor, Department of Medicine, McMaster University, Hamilton, Ontario, Canada

Thomas L. Clanton, Ph.D. Associate Professor, Pulmonary and Critical Care Division, Department of Internal Medicine, Ohio State University, Columbus, Ohio

Marc Decramer, M.D., Ph.D. Professor, Respiratory Division, Department of Medicine, University Hospitals, Katholieke Universiteit Leuven, Leuven, Belgium

Ludwig A. Engel, M.B.B.S., Ph.D., F.R.A.C.P. Head, Thoracic Medicine Unit, Westmead Hospital, Sydney, Australia

Sandra J. England, Ph.D. Associate Professor, Department of Pediatrics, UMDNJ-Robert Wood Johnson Medical School, New Brunswick, New Jersey

Marc Estenne, M.D., Ph.D. Professor of Medicine, Chest Service, Erasme University Hospital, Brussels, Belgium

Gaspar A. Farkas, Ph.D. Associate Professor, Department of Physical Therapy and Exercise Science, State University of New York at Buffalo, Buffalo, New York

Marc Estenne, M.D., Ph.D. Associate Professor, Department of Physical Therapy and Exercise Science, State University of New York at Buffalo, Buffalo, New York

Henry E. Fessler, M.D. Assistant Professor, Pulmonary and Critical Care Medicine, The Johns Hopkins Medical Institutions, Baltimore, Maryland

Simon C. Gandevia, B.Sc. (Med), Ph.D., M.D., D.Sc., F.R.A.C.P. Principal Research Fellow, Prince of Wales Medical Research Institute and University of New South Wales, Sydney, New South Wales, Australia

Claude Gaultier, M.D., Ph.D. Professor, Laboratory of Physiology, Hôpital Antoine Beclere, Paris, France

Malcolm Green, B.M., B.Ch., B.Sc., M.A., D.M., F.R.C.P. Consultant Physician, Royal Brompton Hospital and Director, Respiratory Muscle Laboratory, National Heart and Lung Institute, London, England

Frederic G. Hoppin, Jr., M.D. Professor of Medicine, Department of Physiology, Brown University Medical School, Providence, Rhode Island

Rolf D. Hubmayr, M.D. Professor of Medicine; Director, Thoracic Research Unit, Pulmonary and Critical Care Medicine, Mayo Clinic, Rochester, Minnesota

Mark David Inman, M.D., Ph.D. Postdoctoral Research Fellow, Department of Medicine, McMaster University, Hamilton, Ontario, Canada

Yves Jammes, M.D., D.Sc. Professor of Physiology and Chairman, Laboratoire de Physiopathologie Respiratoire, Faculty of Medicine, Institut Jean Roche, Marseille, France

Norman L. Jones, M.D., F.R.C.P., F.R.C.P.C. Professor Emeritus, Department of Medicine, McMaster University, Hamilton, Ontario, Canada

John B. Jordanoglou, M.D., Ph.D. Professor and Director, Department of Respiratory Medicine, Athens University Medical School, Athens, Greece

Kieran J. Killian, M.D., F.R.C.P.C., F.R.C.P.I. Professor, Division of Respirology, Department of Medicine, McMaster University, Hamilton, Ontario, Canada

Peter T. Macklem, O.C., M.D., F.R.S.(C) Scientific Director, Respiratory Health Network of Centres of Excellence, and Professor of Medicine, McGill University, Montreal, Quebec, Canada

Sheldon Magder, M.D., F.R.C.P.(C) Associate Professor, Director, Division of Critical Care, Department of Medicine, Royal Victoria Hospital, McGill University, Montreal, Quebec, Canada

F. Dennis McCool, M.D. Associate Professor of Medicine, Brown University Medical School, Providence; and Medical Director of Respiratory Care, Memorial Hospital of Rhode Island, Pawtucket, Rhode Island

D. K. McKenzie, B.Sc. (Med), M.B., B.S., Ph.D. Associate Professor, Department of Respiratory Medicine, Prince of Wales Medical Research Institute, Sydney, New South Wales, Australia

John Moxham, M.D., F.R.C.P. Professor, Department of Thoracic Medicine, King's College School of Medicine and Dentistry, London, England

Manuel Paiva, Ph.D.   Professor, Biomedical Physics Laboratory, Université Libre de Bruxelles, Brussels, Belgium

Solbert Permutt, M.D.   Professor, Pulmonary and Critical Care Division, Department of Medicine, The Johns Hopkins Medical Institutions, Baltimore, Maryland

Kai Rehder, M.D.   Emeritus Professor, Department of Anesthesiology, Mayo Clinic, Rochester, Minnesota

Dudley F. Rochester, M.D.   Professor Emeritus, Pulmonary and Critical Care Division, Department of Medicine, University of Virginia Health Sciences Center, Charlottesville, Virginia

Charis Roussos, M.D., M.Sc., Ph.D., M.R.S., F.R.C.P.(C)   Professor of Medicine, Critical Care Department and Thoracic Unit, National and Kapodistrian University of Athens Medical School, Athens, Greece; and Professor of Medicine, McGill University, Montreal, Quebec, Canada

Nikos Siafakas, M.D., Ph.D.   Professor, Department of Thoracic Medicine, University of Crete Medical School, Heraklion, Greece

George E. Tzelepis   Associate Director, Critical Care Division, Onassis Cardiosurgical Center, Athens, Greece

David O. Warner, M.D.   Associate Professor, Department of Anesthesiology, Mayo Clinic, Rochester, Minnesota

Robert A. Wise, M.D.   Associate Professor, Pulmonary and Critical Care Medicine, Johns Hopkins University School of Medicine, Baltimore, Maryland

Ailiang Xie, M.D.   Research Fellow, Institute of Medical Science, University of Toronto, Toronto, Ontario, Canada

Luciano Zocchi, M.D.   Assistant Professor, First Institute of Human Physiology, University of Milan, Milan, Italy

CONTENTS OF PART B: APPLIED PHYSIOLOGY

PART IV METHODS OF MEASUREMENT

A cumulative index appears in Part C

CONTENTS OF PART A: PHYSIOLOGY

CONTENTS OF PART C: DISEASE

Part IV

METHODS OF MEASUREMENT

35

Electrical Assessment of Respiratory Muscles

D. K. McKENZIE

Prince of Wales Medical Research Institute
Sydney, New South Wales, Australia

SIMON C. GANDEVIA

Prince of Wales Medical Research Institute
University of New South Wales
Sydney, New South Wales, Australia

Accurate neurophysiological assessment of the respiratory muscles has been hampered by a number of technical problems, especially in conscious humans. In an ideal situation, force, muscle fiber length, and speed of contraction can be measured, the muscles can be stimulated electrically, and the electromyogram can be recorded with minimal far-field interference from surrounding muscles and minimal recording artefact. The latter may be produced by changes in the relationship of the electrodes to the muscle or variation in conductivity of surrounding tissues. The respiratory muscles include the diaphragm, which is largely inaccessible to noninvasive recording techniques, although the phrenic nerves can be stimulated. The intercostal and abdominal muscles present technical difficulties whether studied individually or together because they are layered, and the latter are innervated by multiple ventral roots. Finally, there is no reliable method to derive absolute muscle force produced by any of the individual muscles involved in the generation of respiratory pressures.

This chapter outlines a number of pitfalls in the electrical assessment of respiratory muscles and highlights those studies and methods that have attempted to address these problems. It deals almost exclusively with studies of human subjects and discusses some of the more exciting approaches that have emerged in recent years.

I. Phrenic Nerve Stimulation

Phrenic nerve stimulation is not a new art. Caldani is said to have achieved this in 1786, shortly after Galvani's report of "animal magnetism." In 1866 Samson described the successful use of "galvanism of the phrenic nerve" to resuscitate a 4-year-old who became apneic during chloroform anaesthesia (for a more complete historical review, see Glenn and Phelps, 1985; Editorial, 1950). Interest in the possibility of electrophrenic respiration was rekindled during the epidemic of poliomyelitis in the late 1940s (Sarnoff et al., 1948), and this research led ultimately to the development of pacemakers for the phrenic nerves (for review, see Glenn and Phelps, 1985).

Accurate assessment of phrenic nerve function is now an important part of the investigation of patients with neuromuscular disease because other tests of respiratory muscle strength lack sensitivity and specificity. The pressure-volume characteristics of normal lungs are such that a decline in vital capacity will be detected only with severe weakness of inspiratory muscles. Moreover, measures of maximal static inspiratory pressure (MIP) and maximal transdiaphragmatic pressure (P_{di}) show a very wide distribution in normal subjects (see Sec. IV). Phrenic nerve stimulation is also an important research tool (for discussion, see NHLBI Workshop, 1990).

The phrenic nerve is accessible for stimulation as it descends over the anterior surface of scalenus anterior. The optimal site for cathodal stimulation is at or below the level of the cricoid cartilage. Above this level it is possible to miss the contribution from the 5th cervical ventral root, which joins the nerve obliquely. As the point of stimulation is moved lower in the neck, more of the brachial plexus is excited and unpleasantly strong contractions of the arm may occur.

For routine clinical studies, transcutaneous stimulation is adequate using a "pen" electrode with a hemispheric cathode 3–4 mm in diameter. Such an electrode was described by Sarnoff and colleagues, although they subsequently recommended a "thimble" electrode (Sarnoff and Sarnoff, 1950). The electrode is placed just posterior to sternomastoid at the level of the cricoid cartilage and pushed medially towards the groove between scalenus anterior and medius. Single stimuli delivered at 0.5–1.0 Hz, and gradually increasing in intensity, will elicit twitch responses of the diaphragm, best monitored by observing compound muscle action potentials (CMAPs) in the diaphragmatic electromyogram (EMG, see below). These must be viewed on a storage-type oscilloscope or monitor with a time resolution of at least 5 ms/cm (Fig. 1). When a definite CMAP is observed, the stimulus intensity is held constant at a submaximal level while the electrode is moved to the site that produces the largest CMAP. The voltage (or current) is then increased to maximal levels when there is no increase in CMAP amplitude. Intensities should be increased at least another 20% to be sure of activating all large phrenic motor axons (i.e., "supramaximal" stimulation). The site and type of the anode are relatively unimportant, and various methods have been described. A standard Ag-AgCl ECG electrode placed just below the medial third of the clavicle is satisfactory. Other investigators have used a standard bipolar stimulating electrode (with saline-soaked felt tips, 5 mm diam, e.g., Mier et al., 1987).

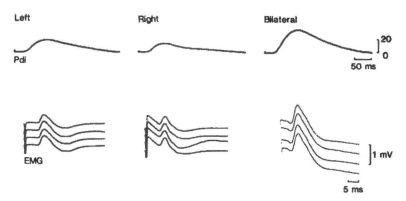

Figure 1   Changes in transdiaphragmatic pressure (P_{di}) evoked by supramaximal stimulation of the left phrenic nerve (left), right phrenic nerve (middle) and both nerves (right). Each trace represents the average of four responses. Individual CMAPs are shown below. Calibration for P_{di} is 20 cm H_2O. (Reprinted from McKenzie et al., 1988.)

For prolonged studies, especially those requiring bilateral stimulation, the cathodes can be mounted on a micromanipulator-like stage within a neck brace (Gandevia and McKenzie, 1985) or wire electrodes used. An alternative approach is to use needle or hook-wire electrodes, which are more comfortable for the subject. This approach was first described by MacLean and Mattioni (1981), who used a standard monopolar needle electrode. For studies involving strong contractions of inspiratory muscles, including the neck muscles, hook-wires are more stable (Hubmayr et al., 1989; McKenzie et al., 1992). Insulated stainless steel wire (75 μm diam), bared of insulation for 3–5 mm, is hooked over the bevel of a 25 SWG hypodermic needle, which is removed after insertion. The anode can be a similar wire inserted subcutaneously at the same level anterior to sternocleidomastoid. Such an arrangement of electrodes can provide stable stimulating conditions for several hours during prolonged experiments involving repeated maximal inspiratory efforts. Maximal CMAPs are obtained with stimulus intensities of 10–50 V (about one-tenth that for surface stimulation) and spread of current to the brachial plexus and cervical cutaneous nerves is greatly reduced or even eliminated. With this more selective stimulation it is important to avoid placing the cathode too high in the neck or the contribution of 5th cervical root will be missed.

II. Recording the Diaphragmatic Electromyogram

A. Direct (Intramuscular) Recordings

The first recordings of diaphragmatic EMG were made with various types of needle electrodes inserted via the pleural space usually over the lower costal margin between the anterior and midaxillary lines (Tokizane et al., 1951; Draper et al., 1957; Taylor,

1960). This method overcomes many of the problems of indirect surface recordings (Campbell, 1958; see also below) but did not achieve widespread popularity because of the risks of pneumothorax. In a detailed study of the influence of changes in lung volume on the amplitude of EMG recordings from a variety of electrode arrangements, Gandevia and McKenzie (1986) used pairs of fine hook-wire electrodes (75 μm) inserted into costal diaphragm via a hypodermic needle (a method described by Bigland and Lippold, 1954; see also Basmajian and Stecko, 1962). Recordings free of distortion were obtained at lung volumes between 0.5 L below functional residual capacity (FRC) and half-inspiratory capacity, but the amplitude of maximal CMAPs decreased at volumes above and below this range due to movement of the electrodes or changes in conductivity (Fig. 2).

Hook wires are more stable than monopolar or concentric needle electrodes, which need to be held in place, but stability cannot be relied upon during strong contractions or large muscle movements. Concentric needle electrodes offer the advantage of selectivity (down to several single low-threshold motor units), whereas the hook-wire electrodes provide a multiunit recording (unless specially tailored).

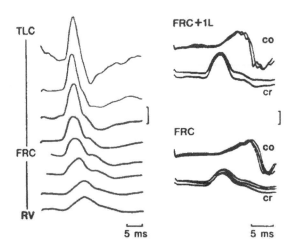

Figure 2 Left: Maximal compound muscle action potentials (CMAPs) recorded via esophageal electrodes and produced by supramaximal stimulation of left phrenic nerve at different lung volumes. This series of successive responses was recorded during a single relaxed expiration. Size of maximal CMAPs decreased approximately fivefold from volumes near TLC to volumes near RV. Note also the changes in shape of the CMAPs. Right: In same subject (separate experiment), effect of a 1-liter inspiration on maximal CMAPs recorded simultaneously from esophageal electrodes (cr) and costal needle electrodes (co). There was an increase in size of maximal crural CMAPs, but there was no change in peak-to-peak amplitude or area of maximal costal CMAPs. Note longer latency to costal recording site, which reflects, in part, increased conduction distance to that site (see Fig. 3). Vertical calibration in both panels, 1 mV. (Reprinted from Gandeva and McKenzie, 1986.)

Another approach to direct recording of diaphragmatic EMG has been described in detail (Bolton et al., 1992; see also Koepke et al., 1958). Bolton and colleagues recorded from the intercartilaginous portion of the muscle along the anterior costal margin. This site is below the pleural reflection and eliminates the risk of pneumothorax and reduces pleuritic pain.

B. Esophageal Electrodes

To circumvent the inherent problems of needle and chest-wall electrodes, Petit et al. (1960) and Agostoni et al. (1960) introduced recording from the crural fibers of diaphragm via esophageal electrodes. The former group used stainless steel spheres (0.6 cm diam) attached to insulated copper wires and introduced orally to the level of the gastroesophageal junction (1–2 cm apart) and described the persistence of diaphragmatic activity in early expiration. The latter group placed silver electrodes inside a perforated polyvinyl tube.

Esophageal electrodes became widely used, and modifications of the technique were reported. A double transnasal catheter with integrated platinum wire electrodes enabled simultaneous recording of P_{di} and crural EMG (Onal et al., 1981). A Swan Ganz catheter with cardiac pacing electrodes, shortened by 10 cm, is readily modified into a gastroesophageal catheter. With appropriate placement of standard respiratory balloons, the two large lumina of the catheter provide measures of gastric pressure (distal port) and esophageal pressure (proximal port) with adequate frequency response (McKenzie and Gandevia, 1985), while the pacing electrodes can record crural EMG (with interelectrode distances of 1, 6, or 7 cm). The narrow lumen normally used to inflate the balloon at the tip can be used to inflate a third respiratory balloon to "anchor" the catheter at the gastroesophageal junction when a small weight (10–20 g) is attached to the proximal end of the catheter near the nares (Melissinas et al., 1981). This reduces the tendency for the catheter to move down with peristaltic waves or up with increases in abdominal pressure, but slightly increases discomfort during prolonged studies. The optimal distance between this stabilizing balloon and the distal recording electrode is about 1 cm for the right crus and 2 cm for the left crus (McKenzie and Gandevia, 1985).

A voluminous literature emerged with descriptions of EMG responses to loading and changes in posture and relationships between changes in P_{di} and diaphragmatic EMG recorded with esophageal electrodes. Unfortunately, much of this literature is flawed by artefactual changes in recording conditions for diaphragmatic EMG with changes in lung volume, chest wall shape, and diaphragmatic shape. This was in spite of warnings as early as 1960 that recording conditions might not be stable (Agostoni et al., 1960). Dubois and colleagues (1963) noted that the electrodes could move and that "quantitative interpretation of the results . . . requires a great carefulness."

In a detailed study of these recording artefacts, the size of maximal diaphragmatic CMAPs produced by supramaximal stimulation of the phrenic nerve was found to vary systematically with changes in diaphragmatic position (Gandevia and McKenzie, 1986). As lung volume increased from near residual volume (RV) to near total lung capacity (TLC), the size of the CMAP increased about fivefold on average (Fig. 2). It also increased as the diaphragm descended during "isovolume" maneuvers at different lung volumes. When isovolume maneuvers were performed at the extremes of the lung volume range, the amplitude of CMAPs could vary more than 10-fold. Radiographic studies showed that the electrodes maintained a close relationship to the crural fibers, so it was postulated that the changes in recording conditions were due to widening of the hiatus as the diaphragm moved cephalad (see also Agostoni and Torri, 1962), changes in the volume conductivity around the electrode (De Lisa and Brozovitch, 1983), and the effect of changes in muscle length (e.g., Kim et al., 1985).

Several methods have been proposed in an attempt to overcome the problems associated with esophageal recordings of diaphragmatic EMG. McKenzie and Gandevia (1986) used the amplitude of CMAPs produced by supramaximal single stimuli delivered to one (or both) phrenic nerves as a "calibration" signal to normalize quantitative measures of ongoing EMG activity. Others have proposed normalization of EMG to the maximal activity achieved by static voluntary effort at that lung volume (or thoracoabdominal configuration). This method is limited because the geometric relationship between the electrodes and the crural fibers changes with increasing effort (Bellemare and Bigland-Ritchie, 1984; McKenzie and Gandevia, 1985) and because the exact extent of voluntary activation of the diaphragm during attempted maximal effort is variable in many subjects (Allen et al., 1993).

A different approach to the problem was taken by Daubenspeck and colleagues (1989), who used an array of eight electrodes providing seven sequential pairs over a distance of 7.2 cm along the catheter. They derived a summed measure of diaphragmatic EMG activity, which was relatively resistant to changes in lung volume (threefold change in CMAP amplitude between RV and TLC but only 20% change over 2 L around FRC). Thus, despite changes in catheter position, it is possible to determine the optimal "leading-off" surface (e.g., Sinderby et al., 1993).

C. Chest Wall Electrodes

Surface electrodes placed on the chest wall have been used frequently to provide quantitative recordings of diaphragmatic EMG in spite of early warnings from Campbell (1958) about interference from overlying muscles. These recordings are adequate for quantitation when the diaphragm is the only muscle contracting, such as in patients with quadriplegia (e.g., Sharp et al., 1993). Diaphragmatic CMAPs can be recorded during relaxation, breathing, and other maneuvers, but the amplitude may vary with lung volume and respiratory maneuver (Bellemare and Bigland-Ritchie, 1984; Gandevia and McKenzie, 1985; Gandevia and McKenzie, 1986).

The extent of this problem is critically dependent on the site of placement of electrodes on the chest wall and has been quantitated precisely by Lansing and Savelle (1989). Quantitative recordings of moving time averages of EMG with chest wall electrodes are of no value in many situations because the activity is dominated by the most superficial muscles, including both layers of intercostal muscle, and in some sites by overlying abdominal and other chest wall muscles.

III. Artefact Suppression and Spectral Analysis

In addition to the technical problems described above, analysis of EMG signals from the diaphragm and chest wall musculature is complicated by motion artefact and the electrocardiogram (ECG). Motion artefact has significant power only at very low frequencies (usually below 10 Hz) and can be removed by appropriate analogue or digital filtering. The ECG has frequency components throughout the frequency spectrum of surface recordings of diaphragmatic EMG, although the bulk of the power is in the lower frequency range (Schweitzer et al., 1979).

A. Suppression of ECG "Artefact"

A variety of methods has been proposed to suppress or eliminate the contribution of ECG to EMG recordings, ranging from simple "clipping" to sophisticated computer subtraction methods. However, all methods have limitations.

Clipping the top of the QRS complex is unsatisfactory because it leaves the bulk of the complex and may introduce new artefactual harmonics to the frequency spectrum (Schweitzer et al., 1979). Others have attempted to remove the ECG by blocking the EMG signal for the duration of the QRS complex and replacing it with the EMG activity recorded immediately prior to the QRS complex and held in a sample/hold circuit (Moriette et al., 1985). However, this method leaves the remainder of the ECG complex, which includes most of the low-frequency power.

It is possible with computerized processing to subtract an ECG complex obtained during relaxation from the EMG signal recording during contraction. However, it is likely that the ECG signal will vary with effort due to changes in both heart rate and recording conditions, and this introduces further artefact.

The simplest and most accurate recordings are analyzed as epochs triggered by the QRS complex with a suitable delay (beyond the T wave) and completed before the next QRS complex. Such recordings have been used in spectral analysis of human diaphragmatic EMG (Schweitzer et al., 1979; Gross et al., 1979). Time integrals of these epochs may be corrected for changes in recording conditions by taking into account changes in the amplitude of CMAPs produced by supramaximal phrenic nerve stimulation (McKenzie and Gandevia, 1986).

B. Power Spectral Analysis

Computerized methods have been increasingly applied to analyze respiratory muscle EMG signals in the hope that they may provide useful measures of both respiratory center output and evidence of incipient respiratory muscle fatigue. Measurement of the ratio of spectral power at high frequencies to power at low frequencies was popular because it can be obtained using two bandpass filters (e.g., 30–50 Hz and 130–250 Hz). For computerized methods using fast Fourier transforms, the centroid frequency has been proposed as a useful index.

The frequency power spectrum of EMG signals depends principally on the conduction velocity of the myoelectric potential along the muscle membrane and the frequency of firing, recruitment pattern, and synchronization of motor units (for review see De Luca, 1984). Membrane conduction velocity is proportional to fiber diameter, inversely proportional to fiber length (Okada, 1987), and influenced by temperature and metabolic changes in the extracellular fluid. Contractions of increasing force progressively recruit larger motor units while the firing frequency of active units increases toward maximal values. Fatigue induced by sustained static efforts is associated with both a slowing of membrane conduction velocity (e.g., Lindström et al., 1970; Krantz et al., 1983) and a reduction in motor unit firing frequencies (Bigland-Ritchie et al., 1982). Thus there is a shift of power to lower frequencies (Kogi and Hakamada, 1962; for review, see Sato, 1982).

However, the value of spectral analysis of EMG in assessment of muscle activation and fatigue remains controversial. A number of technical factors are known to have important influences. For example, the upper limit to the frequency spectrum for EMG is set by the interelectrode distance, and the spectrum is influenced by the signal-to-noise ratio, which (usually) increases with the strength of contraction. Changes in muscle length and velocity also alter spectral densities, as do changes in the distance between the recording electrodes and the muscle. The latter influence will contribute to the centroid frequency being lower for chest wall compared with esophageal recordings of diaphragmatic EMG (e.g., Sharp et al., 1993). In summary, attempts are succeeding in improving the quality of diaphragmatic surface EMG so that more accurate descriptions of muscle fiber conduction velocity can be derived (Sinderby et al., 1993).

The spectral shift with fatigue induced by strong contractions is likely to be an epiphenomenon influenced by many independent factors. For example, the slowing of membrane conduction is critically dependent on the fatigue protocol and may not occur in some forms of fatiguing work. Moreover, some discrepancies have been observed between changes in spectral power and the force-generating capacity, membrane conduction velocity and metabolic profile of muscle during the development of and recovery from fatigue (e.g., Miller et al., 1987; Béliveau et al., 1991). These problems, coupled with the difficulties in obtaining artefact-free recordings of diaphragmatic EMG (see above), suggest that spectral analysis currently has a limited role in evaluation of diaphragm function. However, future technical developments may lead to reassessment of this view.

IV. Clinical Studies of Phrenic Nerve and Diaphragm Function

Accurate assessment of phrenic nerve and diaphragm function in patients with neuromuscular disease or trauma relies on electrical assessment using the methods described above (see Secs. I and II). The phrenic nerve terminal motor latency (conduction time) is determined by measurement of the time from stimulus onset to the onset of the CMAP. For these studies, accurate placement of recording electrodes is essential to reveal an essentially biphasic potential with a clear onset of activity for easy measurement (Figs. 1 and 2). In theory, this is achieved by placing one electrode over the motor point of the stimulated muscle and one remotely on the tendon. For the diaphragm the motor point is approximately halfway from the costal (or vertebral) attachment and the central tendon (see Sec. II). Standardized sites for electrode placement are also necessary because the conduction distance (and therefore latency) to different regions of the diaphragm varies substantially (Fig. 3). Conduction times also increase as a function of the subject's height and age. These relationships can provide accurate prediction equations for normal conduction times to any region of the diaphragm (McKenzie and Gandevia, 1985).

Prolonged or absent conduction times have been documented in a variety of neuropathies, demyelinating diseases, trauma (e.g., postsurgical), and compression from mediastinal and hilar tumors (Fig. 4). A characteristic decrement in CMAP amplitude with repetitive stimulation can be found in myasthenia gravis (for review, see Mier, 1990).

The mechanical function of the diaphragm can also be assessed at the time of stimulation by recording the twitch response in transdiaphragmatic pressure. The responses to left, right, and simultaneous bilateral stimulation should be recorded (Figs. 1 and 4). The response to bilateral stimulation is generally greater than the sum of the responses of the left and right hemidiaphragms, due to excessive shortening of muscle fibers in the latter situation because the unstimulated hemidiaphragm acts as an in-series elastic element. The twitch responses to stimulation of the left phrenic nerve average about 12 cm H_2O, while those of the right are usually slightly smaller (about 8 cm H_2O). The response to bilateral stimulation has a wide normal range with reported values varying from 9 to 45 cm H_2O, but the majority of normal subjects have values between 20 and 30 cm H_2O. To date there has been little systematic investigation of the reasons for this wide normal range. One obvious factor is twitch potentiation, by which the amplitude of a relaxed twitch is augmented as much as twofold by an antecedent brief maximal tetanic (or voluntary) contraction (Sandow, 1965; Manning and Stull, 1982). While there is less potentiation for the diaphragm than limb muscles (McKenzie et al., 1992), this aspect of routine testing should be

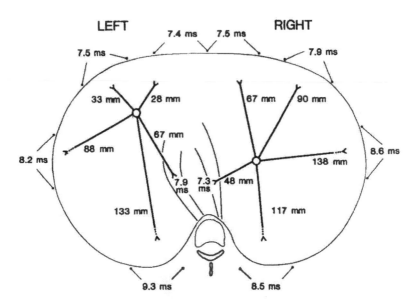

Figure 3 Schematic illustration of conduction distance from the entry point of each phrenic nerve into diaphragmatic pleura to the motor point of diaphragmatic muscle fibers adjacent to each of the EMG recording sites. For costal regions, it was assumed that the motor point was halfway between costal attachment and central tendon. Mean values of measurements in three cadavers are shown. Lines drawn for lateral and posterior sites are not to scale because of curvature of diaphragm. Length of phrenic nerves from cricoid cartilage to the nerve's entry point into diaphragmatic pleura (right: 312 ± 22 mm; left: 364 ± 13 mm) was added to each distance to derive total conduction distance. Mean values for conduction time along phrenic nerves obtained at each site in three subjects are also shown. Conduction time of phrenic nerves to the various EMG recording sites correlated with total conduction distance to those sites (r = 0.94).

standardized. Abdominal binders have been used to increase the twitch response to phrenic nerve stimulation, but their effect may be due simply to lengthening of the diaphragmatic muscle fibers (Mier et al., 1990).

The maximal P_{di} produced by maximal quasi-static voluntary effort also varies widely between normal individuals and between different maneuvers involving the diaphragm (inspiratory or Mueller, expulsive with glottis open, and "combined" inspiratory-expulsive). Maximal P_{di} is least with the former and greatest with the latter, with normal values ranging almost an order of magnitude (from 50 to 300 cm H_2O) (Laporta and Grassino, 1985).

The variation between maneuvers is not a function of the extent of voluntary drive to the diaphragm, which can be maximal in all three types (Bellemare and Bigland-Ritchie, 1984; Gandevia and McKenzie, 1985; Gandevia et al., 1990). It can be explained by the fact that neither the expulsive nor the inspiratory maneuver

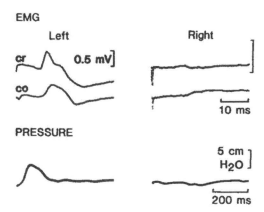

Figure 4 Clinical study of a patient with right phrenic palsy. A CMAP with an appropriate latency is just visible on the right with both esophageal (cr = crural) and chest wall (co = costal) electrodes, although no pressure response was detected.

is truly isometric, with lengthening of muscle fibers in the former situation and shortening in the latter (Gandevia et al., 1992).

Some of the variation between subjects is almost certainly due to variable central activation of the diaphragm (Allen et al., 1993). This can be documented by the technique of twitch interpolation (Merton, 1954) in which bilateral phrenic stimulation is applied during graded voluntary efforts up to maximal. The presence of a twitch response during "maximal" efforts indicates suboptimal activation of the phrenic motoneuron pool. Extrapolation of the inverse relationship between voluntary effort and twitch response (Fig. 5) can provide an estimate of the theoretical maximal voluntary P_{di} (Bellemare and Bigland-Ritchie, 1984), but the validity of this extrapolation has not been established.

V. Other Respiratory Muscles

Compared with the extensive literature on electrical assessment of the diaphragm, there is less information on the clinical assessment of other respiratory muscles. However, a number of research studies have provided methodological details for the investigation of most respiratory muscles.

A. Intercostal Muscles

The electrical activity of human intercostal muscles has been recorded during normal, augmented, and loaded breathing and during hyperinflation. Assessment of their mechanical function has been restricted largely to animal studies because of the difficulties in obtaining measurements of force and length changes. Depending

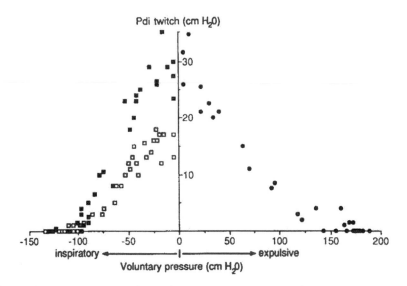

Figure 5 Data from one subject during voluntary inspiratory efforts [esophageal pressure (inspiratory) plotted to the left, i.e., negative] and expulsive efforts [gastric pressure (expulsive) plotted to the right, i.e., positive]. Inspiratory efforts were evaluated with unilateral (open square) and bilateral stimulation of the phrenic nerves (closed square). Expulsive efforts were studied with bilateral stimulation. Stimuli were delivered at supramaximal levels. The vertical axis shows the transdiaphragmatic twitch pressure (P_{di} twitch), which was approximately double with bilateral compared with unilateral phrenic stimulation. For both maneuvers (performed near FRC) the P_{di} twitch could be extinguished during some attempted maximal efforts. (From Gandevia et al., 1990.)

on the site of placement, surface electrodes may record activity in both the internal and external layers and any overlying muscle (obliquus abdominis, pectoralis, latissimus dorsi, etc.). Needle electrodes must be used with caution to avoid the risk of pneumothorax (e.g., see Taylor, 1960).

The first detailed electromyographic study of the intercostal muscles appears to have been conducted by Campbell (1955a), although there are a number of earlier contributions (for review, see Taylor, 1960). He used both surface electrodes and concentric needles to map the activity in various intercostal spaces during spontaneous and augmented breathing, expiratory efforts, and changes in posture. Taylor (1960) explored the activity in the different layers of intercostal muscle using specially constructed bifilar needle electrodes. In more recent years De Troyer and colleagues used concentric electrodes to make detailed studies of the actions of intercostal muscles (e.g., Sampson and De Troyer, 1982) and triangularis sterni (Fig. 6), an expiratory agonist in the standing posture (Estenne et al., 1988). The use of hook-wire electrodes increases the risk of pneumothorax because the electrode tips trail the hypodermic needle point. However, Watson and Whitelaw (1987)

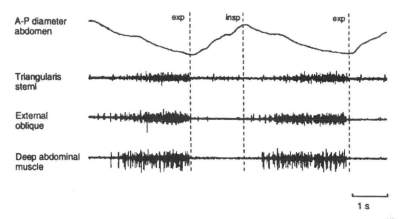

Figure 6 EMG activity of the triangularis sterni, the external oblique, and the deeper abdominal muscle layer recorded via needle electrodes in a subject breathing quietly in the standing posture. The three muscles contract only during expiration. (Adapted from Estenne et al., 1988.)

provide a detailed description of a safe method, which they used to record single motor unit activity in intercostal muscles (see also Whitelaw and Watson, 1992).

For clinical studies, some of the lower intercostal nerves can be stimulated transcutaneously via a probe electrode, and muscle activity can be recorded with surface, needle, or hook-wire electrodes (Pradhan and Taly, 1989; Macefield and Gandevia, 1992). Thus, it is possible to obtain a measure of intercostal nerve terminal motor conduction time in these intercostal spaces. Intercostal motor conduction velocity can be obtained with two pairs of recording electrodes in the 6th intercostal space and stimulation of the 6th intercostal nerve in the triangle of auscultation (medial to the inferior angle of the scapula, bordered by trapezius, latissimus dorsi, and rhomboideus major). Responses to stimulation at two proximal sites in the 6th interspace can also be recorded from abdominal muscles so that conduction velocity can be derived (Pradhan and Taly, 1989). In some studies high-voltage stimulators over the spine have been used to stimulate the proximal segments of the ventral roots of several intercostal nerves (Lance et al., 1988; McKenzie et al., 1990). With stimulus intensities up to 750 V (50 or 100 μs duration) maximal CMAPs can be obtained in up to six intercostal spaces by placing the stimulating electrodes over the corresponding vertebrae.

B. Abdominal Muscles

The abdominal muscles are the major expiratory muscles and also play an important mechanical role in opposing descent of the diaphragm, thereby driving the ribcage along its passive inspiratory pathway by the elevation of abdominal pressure. In patients with severe airflow obstruction and hyperinflation, contraction of the abdominal muscles in late expiration passively lengthens the diaphragm to a more advantageous position on its length-tension relationship.

Electrical assessment of the abdominal muscles presents problems in recording EMG from the different layers and in stimulation of the muscle(s). Independent stimulation of the recti and oblique muscles can be achieved with large surface area electrodes (e.g., Mier et al., 1985; Gandevia et al., 1990), but a large stimulus artefact is generated in recordings of EMG. For gross studies of EMG activity, surface electrodes placed over rectus abdominus and external oblique provide adequate recordings (e.g., Campbell and Green, 1955). More detailed studies of the individual muscles require intramuscular electrodes (Fig. 6), and accurate placement may be assisted by ultrasonography (Strohl et al., 1981).

C. Scalenes and Accessory Muscles

The scalene muscles are obligatory inspiratory muscles and are accessible (at least partly) for both surface (e.g., Campbell, 1955b) and intramuscular recordings (e.g., Raper et al., 1966). These early studies documented activity during quiet breathing and progressive recruitment during inhalation to TLC and hyperpnea. More recent studies have documented reflex responses to brief airway occlusion (Plassman et al., 1987) and variations in maximal activity during different voluntary respiratory and postural efforts (Gandevia et al., 1990).

The sternocleidomastoid is a true "accessory" inspiratory muscle, which is superficial and can be stimulated readily via its accessory nerve supply. Its postural and respiratory activities have been documented in a number of studies (Campbell, 1955b; Vitti et al., 1973; Adams et al., 1989; Gandevia et al., 1990). Moxham and colleagues (1980) devised a means of measuring rotational torque of the head as an index of force development and produced force-frequency curves for a number of respiratory and nonrespiratory muscles. A number of other trunk muscles may display respiratory rhythms under various circumstances (e.g., pectoralis, trapezius, erector spinae, quadratus lumborum) (see Tokizane et al., 1951).

VI. Newer Methods of Assessment

The development of high voltage (up to 1500 V, 50–100 μs decay) stimulators for use in human subjects (Merton and Morton, 1980) has enabled investigation of central motor pathways to respiratory and other muscles. Transient changes in magnetic fields can also be used to achieve transcranial stimulation. Both forms of stimulation of the human motor cortex produce descending volleys including both direct and indirect (transsynaptic) activation of corticofugal axons (Burke et al., 1990, 1993). For most muscles the net influence at the motoneuronal level is excitatory and greatly augmented by weak voluntary effort (for review, see Rothwell et al., 1991).

Motor cortical stimulation has been used to document short-latency responses in human diaphragm (Gandevia and Rothwell, 1987; see also Maskill et al., 1991), intercostal and trunk muscles (Gandevia and Plassman, 1988), and neck muscles (Gandevia and Applegate, 1988) (Fig. 7). Used in conjunction with spinal stimulation, it was demonstrated that the central conduction from motor cortex to the C5 spinal segment is similar for diaphragm and deltoid (Gandevia and Rothwell, 1987) (Fig. 8).

Magnetic stimulation has also been employed to stimulate the proximal nerve roots including those to the diaphragm (Similowski et al., 1989). However, even with maximal coil output, it is not always possible to obtain a maximal twitch of the diaphragm. Submaximal stimulation produces interpretational difficulties, if only because any change in axonal excitability will change the size of the motor volley.

Two approaches that can provide direct evidence of motor cortical involvement in volitional breathing have been described recently. Guz and colleagues used positron emission tomography to image brain blood flow and documented increases during large inspirations bilaterally in the primary motor cortex, in the right premotor area, and in the cerebellum (Colebatch et al., 1991). Macefield and Gandevia (1991) recorded clear premotor cerebral potentials from scalp electrodes (*Bereitschaftspotentials*) commencing 1.2 s before the onset of brisk, voluntary inhalations and exhalations. Motor potentials not present during quiet breathing

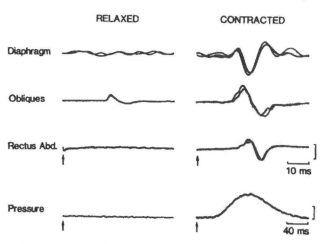

Figure 7 EMG responses (CMAPs) to transcranial stimulation of the motor cortex from three trunk muscles (upper three traces) during relaxation (left) and weak voluntary effort (right). Twitch pressure responses are shown below (gastric pressure). Note the augmentation of response when the average resting membrane potentials of the motoneuron pools are reduced by voluntary effort.

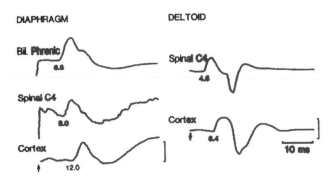

Figure 8 Data obtained during a single study to show the rapid central conduction time from cortex to phrenic motoneurons. CMAPs for the diaphragm were recorded via esophageal electrodes (left) and for the anterior deltoid (right) via closely spaced surface electrodes. All stimuli were delivered during weak inspiratory efforts at FRC. All responses are averages of 4–10 stimuli. The difference between the latency for cortical and spinal stimulation is an estimate of the minimal central conduction time for the descending volley evoked by the cortical stimulus. Latency measurements are indicated in milliseconds. The central conduction time was 4.0 ms for the diaphragm and 3.9 ms for the deltoid. Cortical stimuli were delivered at the vertex and lateral to it for activation of the diaphragm and deltoid, respectively; spinal stimuli were delivered via a cathode at C4 (see text). Vertical calibrations: left, 1 mV; right 1.5 mV. (Reprinted from Gandevia and Rothwell, 1986.)

were also detected during voluntary breathing about 25 ms before the onset of EMG activity (Fig. 9).

The adaptation of some of these newer methods for clinical studies can provide information about the level and extent of central or peripheral deficits in respiratory output.

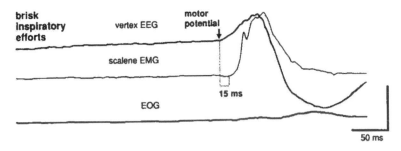

Figure 9 Average records ($n = 50$) from one subject performing brisk nasal inhalations to illustrate the temporal relation between the cortical motor potential and the onset of EMG. Vertical calibrations: rectified EMG, 6 μV; EEG, 100 μV. The displacement of the EEG trace above the EMG trace represents the absolute premotor negativity that developed prior to the motor potential. (Adapted from Macefield and Gandevia, 1991.)

Acknowledgments

The authors' work is supported by the National Health and Medical Research Council (of Australia) and the Asthma Foundation of New South Wales. The authors are grateful to Gabrielle Allen for comments on the text.

References

Adams, L., Datta, A. K., and Guz, A. (1989). Synchronization of motor unit firing during different respiratory and postural tasks in human sternocleidomastoid muscle. *J. Physiol.* (London), 413:213–231.

Agostoni, E., Sant'Ambrogio, G., and Del Portillo Carrasco, H. (1960). Electromyography of the diaphragm in man and transdiaphragmatic pressure. *J. Appl. Physiol.*, 15:1093–1097.

Agostoni, E., and Torri, G. (1962). Diaphragm contraction as a limiting factor to maximum expiration. *J. Appl. Physiol.*, 17:427.

Allen, G. M., McKenzie, D. K., Gandevia, S. C., and Bass, S. (1993). Reduced voluntary drive to breathe in asthmatic subjects. *Respir. Physiol.*, 93:29–40.

Basmajian, J. V., and Stecko, G. (1962). A new bipolar electrode for electromyography. *J. Appl. Physiol.*, 17:849–851.

Béliveau, L., Helal, J.-N., Gaillard, E., Van Hoecke, J., Atlan, G., and Bouissou, P. (1991). EMG spectral shift- and ^{31}P-NMR-determined intracellular pH in fatigued human biceps brachii muscle. *Neurology*, 41:1998–2001.

Bellemare, F., and Bigland-Ritchie, B. (1984). Assessment of human diaphragm strength and activation using phrenic nerve stimulation. *Respir. Physiol.*, 58:263–267.

Bigland-Ritchie, B., Johansson, R., Lippold, O. C. J., and Wood, J. J. (1982). Changes of single motor unit firing rates during sustained maximal voluntary contractions. *J. Physiol.* (London), 328:27–28.

Bigland, B., and Lippold, O. C. J. (1954). Motor unit activity in the voluntary contraction of human muscle. *J. Physiol.* (London), 123:322–335.

Bolton, C. F., Grand'Maison, F., Parkes, A., and Shkrum, M. (1992). Needle electromyography of the diaphragm. *Muscle Nerve*, 15:678–681.

Burke, D., Hicks, R., Gandevia, S. C., Stephen, J., Woodforth, I., and Crawford, M. (1993). Direct comparison of corticospinal volleys in human subjects to transcranial magnetic and electrical stimulation. *J. Physiol.* (London), 470:383–393.

Burke, D., Hicks, R., and Stephen, J. P. H. (1990). Corticospinal volleys evoked by anodal and cathodal stimulation of the human motor cortex. *J. Physiol.* (London), 425:283–299.

Campbell, E. J. M. (1955a). An electromyographic examination of the role of the intercostal muscles in breathing in man. *J. Physiol.* (London), 129:12–26.

Campbell, E. J. M. (1955b). The role of the scalene and sternomastoid muscles in breathing in normal subjects. An electromyographic study. *J. Anat.*, 89:378–386.

Campbell, E. J. M. (1958). *The Respiratory Muscles*. London, Lloyd-Luke.

Campbell, E. J. M., and Green, J. H. (1955). The behaviour of the abdominal muscles and the intra-abdominal pressure during quiet breathing and increased pulmonary ventilation. A study in man. *J. Physiol.* (London), 127:423–426.

Colebatch, J. G., Adams, L., Murphy, K., Martin, A., Lammertsma, A. A., Tochon-Danguy, H. J., Clark, J. C., Friston, K. J., and Guz, A. (1991). Regional cerebral blood flow during volitional breathing in man. *J. Physiol.* (London), 443:91–103.

Daubenspeck, J. A., Leiter, J. C., McGovern, J. F., Knuth, S. L., and Kobylarz, E. J. (1989). Diaphragmatic electromyography using a multiple electrode array. *J. Appl. Physiol.*, 67:1525–1534.

De Lisa, J. A., and Brozovitch, F. V. (1983). Volume conduction in electromyography: experimental and theoretical review. *Electromyogr. Clin. Neurophysiol.*, 23:651–673.

De Luca, C. J. (1984). Myoelectrical manifestations of localized muscular fatigue in humans. *Crit. Rev. Biomed. Eng.*, 11:251–279.

Draper, M. H., Ladefoged, P., and Whitteridge, D. (1957). Expiratory muscles involved in speech. *J. Physiol.* (London), 138:17–18P.

Dubois, P., Damoiseau, J., Deroanne, R., Troquet, J., Delhez, L., and Petit, J. M. (1963). Contrôle radiographique de la position des électrodes exploratrices de l'activité électrique du diaphragm par voie œsophagienne chez l'homme conscient. *Acta Tuberculosea et Pneumologica Belgica*, 54:456–462.

Editorial (1950). From "animal magnetism" to electrophrenic respiration. *N. Engl. J. Med.*, 242:340–341.

Estenne, M., Ninane, V., and De Troyer, A. (1988). Triangularis sterni muscle use during eupnea in humans: effect of posture. *Respir. Physiol.*, 74:151–162.

Gandevia, S. C., and Applegate, C. (1988). Activation of neck muscles from the human motor cortex. *Brain*, 111:801–814.

Gandevia, S. C., Gorman, R. B., McKenzie, D. K., and Southon, F. C. G. (1992). Dynamic changes in human diaphragm length: maximal inspiratory and expulsive efforts studied with sequential radiography. *J. Physiol.* (London), 457:167–176.

Gandevia, S. C., and McKenzie, D. K. (1985). Activation of the human diaphragm during maximal static efforts. *J. Physiol.* (London), 367:45–56.

Gandevia, S. C., and McKenzie, D. K. (1986). Human diaphragmatic EMG: changes with lung volume and posture during supramaximal phrenic stimulation. *J. Appl. Physiol.*, 60:1420–1428.

Gandevia, S. C., McKenzie, D. K., and Plassman, B. L. (1990). Activation of human respiratory muscles during different voluntary manoeuvres. *J. Physiol.* (London), 428:387–403.

Gandevia, S. C., and Plassman, B. L. (1988). Responses in human intercostal and truncal muscles to motor cortical and spinal stimulation. *Respir. Physiol.*, 73:325–338.

Gandevia, S. C., and Rothwell, J. C. (1987). Activation of the human diaphragm from the motor cortex. *J. Physiol.* (London), 384:109–118.

Glenn, W. W. L., and Phelps, M. L. (1985). Diaphragm pacing by electrical stimulation of the phrenic nerve. *Neurosurgery*, 17:974–984.

Gross, D., Grassino, A., Ross, W. R. D., and Macklem, P. T. (1979). Electromyogram pattern of diaphragmatic fatigue. *J. Appl. Physiol.*, 46:1–7.

Hubmayr, R. D., Litchy, W. J., Gay, P. C., and Nelson, S. B. (1989). Transdiaphragmatic twitch pressure. Effects of lung volume and chest wall shape. *Am. Rev. Respir. Dis.*, 139:647–652.

Kim, M. J., Druz, W. S., and Sharp, J. T. (1985). Effect of muscle length on electromyogram in a canine diaphragm strip preparation. *J. Appl. Physiol.*, 58:1602–1607.

Koepke, G. H., Smith, E. M., Murphy, A. J., and Dickinson, D. G. (1958). Sequence of action of the diaphragm and intercostal muscles during respiration: I. Inspiration. *Arch. Phys. Med. Rehabil.*, 39:426–430.

Kogi, K., and Hakamada, T. (1962). Frequency analysis of the surface electromyogram in muscle fatigue. *J. Sci. Labour*, 38:519–528.

Krantz, H., Williams, A. M., Cassel, J., Caddy, D. J., and Silberstein, R. B. (1983). Factors determining the frequency content of the electromyogram. *J. Appl. Physiol.*, 55:329–399.

Lance, J. W., Drummond, P. D., Gandevia, S. C., and Morris (1988). Harlequin syndrome: the sudden onset of unilateral flushing and sweating. *J. Neurol. Neurosurg. Psychiatry*, 15:635–642.

Lansing, R., and Savelle, J. (1989). Chest surface recording of diaphragm potentials in man. *Electroencephalogr. Clin. Neurophysiol.*, 72:59–68.

Laporta, D., and Grassino, A. (1985). Assessment of transdiaphragmatic pressure in humans. *J. Appl. Physiol.*, 58:1469–1476.

Lindström, L., Magnusson, R., and Petersén, I. (1970). Muscular fatigue and action potential conduction velocity changes studied with frequency analysis of EMG signals. *Electromyography*, 10:341–355.

Macefield, G., and Gandevia, S. C. (1991). The cortical drive to human respiratory muscles in the awake state assessed by premotor cerebral potentials. *J. Physiol.* (London), 439:545–558.

Macefield, G., and Gandevia, S. C. (1992). Peripheral and central delays in the cortical projections from human truncal muscles: rapid central transmission of proprioceptive input from the hand but not the trunk. *Brain*, 115:123–135.

MacLean, I. C., and Mattioni, T. A. (1981). Phrenic nerve conduction studies: a new technique and its application in quadriplegic patients. *Arch. Phys. Med. Rehabil.*, 62:70–73.

Manning, D. R., and Stull, J. T. (1982). Myosin light chain phosphorylation-dephosphorylation in mammalian skeletal muscle. *Am. J. Physiol.*, 242:C234–C241.

Maskill, D., Murphy, K., Mier, A., Owen, M., and Guz, A. (1991). Motor cortical representation of the diaphragm in man. *J. Physiol.* (London), 443:105–121.

McKenzie, D. K., Bigland-Ritchie, B., Gorman, R. B., and Gandevia, S. C. (1992). Central and peripheral fatigue of human diaphragm and limb muscles assessed by twitch interpolation. *J. Physiol.* (London), 454:643–656.

McKenzie, D. K., and Gandevia, S. C. (1985). Phrenic nerve conduction times and twitch pressures of the human diaphragm. *J. Appl. Physiol.*, 58:1496–1504.

McKenzie, D. K., and Gandevia, S. C. (1986). Changes in human diaphragmatic electromyogram with positive pressure breathing. *Neurosci. Lett.*, 70:86–90.

McKenzie, D. K., Plassman, B. L., and Gandevia, S. C. (1988). Maximal activation of the human diaphragm but not inspiratory intercostals during static respiratory efforts. *Neurosci. Lett.*, 89:63–68.

Melissinos, C. G., Bruce, E. N., Goldman, M. D., Elliott, E., and Mead, J. (1981). Pattern of diaphragmatic activity during forced expiratory vital capacity. *J. Appl. Physiol.*, 51:1515–1525.

Merton, P. A. (1954). Voluntary strength and fatigue. *J. Physiol.* (London), 123:553–564.

Merton, P. A., and Morton, H. B. (1980). Stimulation of the cerebral cortex in the intact human subject. *Nature*, 285:227.

Mier, A. (1990). Respiratory muscle weakness. *Respir. Med.*, 84:351–359.

Mier, A., Brophy, C., Estenne, M., Moxham, J., Green, M., and De Troyer, A., (1985). Action of abdominal muscles on rib cage in humans. *J. Appl. Physiol.*, 58:1438–1443.

Mier, A., Brophy, C., Moxham, J., and Green, M. (1987). Phrenic nerve stimulation in normal subjects and in patients with diaphragmatic weakness. *Thorax*, 42:885–888.

Mier, A., Brophy, C., Moxham, J., and Green, M. (1990). Influence of lung volume and rib cage configuration on transdiaphragmatic pressure during phrenic nerve stimulation in man. *Respir. Physiol.*, 80:193–202.

Miller, R. G., Giannini, D., Milner-Brown, H. S., Layzer, R. B., Koretsky, A. P., Hooper, D., and Weiner, M. W. (1987). Effects of fatiguing exercise on high-energy phosphates, force, and EMG: evidence for three phases of recovery. *Muscle Nerve*, 10:810–821.

Moriette, G., Van Reempts, P., Moore, M., Cates, D., and Rigatto, H. (1985). The effect of rebreathing CO_2 on ventilation and diaphragmatic electromyography in newborn infants. *Respir. Physiol.*, 62:387–397.

Moxham, J., Wiles, C. M., Newhan, D., and Edwards, R. H. T. (1980). Sternomastoid muscle function and fatigue in man. *Clin. Sci.*, 59:463–468.

NHLBI Workshop. Respiratory muscle fatigue: report of the respiratory muscle fatigue workshop group. (1990) *Am. Rev. Respir. Dis.*, 142:474–480.

Okada, M. (1987). Effect of muscle length on surface EMG wave forms in isometric contractions. *Eur. J. Appl. Physiol.*, 56:482–486.

Õnal, E., Lopata, M., Ginzburg, A. S., and O'Connor, T. D. (1981). Diaphragmatic EMG and transdiaphragmatic pressure measurements with a single catheter. *Am. Rev. Respir. Dis.*, 124:563–565.

Petit, J. M., Milic-Emili, G., and Délhéz, L. (1960). Role of the diaphragm in breathing in conscious normal man: an electromyographic study. *J. Appl. Physiol.*, 15:1101–1106.

Plassman, B., Lansing, R. W., and Foti, K. (1987). Inspiratory muscle responses to airway occlusion during learned breathing movements. *J. Neurophysiol.*, 57:274–288.

Pradhan, S., and Taly, A. (1989). Intercostal nerve conduction study in man. *J. Neurol. Neurosurg. Psychiatry*, 52:763–766.

Raper, A. J., Thompson, W. T., Shapiro, W., and Patterson, J. L. (1966). Scalene and sternomastoid muscle function. *J. Appl. Physiol.*, 21:497–502.

Rothwell, J. C., Thompson, P. D., Day, B. L., Boyd, S., and Marsden, C. D. (1991). Stimulation of the human motor cortex through the scalp. *Exp. Physiol.*, 76:159–200.

Sampson, M. G., and De Troyer, A. (1982). Role of intercostal muscles in the rib cage distortions produced by inspiratory loads. *J. Appl. Physiol.*, 52:517–523.

Sandow, A. (1965). Excitation-contraction coupling in skeletal muscle. *Pharmacol. Rev.*, 17:265–320.

Sarnoff, S. J., Hardenbergh, E., and Whittenberger, J. L. (1948). Electrophrenic respiration. *Science*, 108:482.

Sarnoff, L. C., and Sarnoff, S. J. (1950). The thimble electrode. A device for the rapid localization of motor points. *Arch. Phys. Med.*, 31:448–450.

Sato, H. (1982). Functional characteristics of human skeletal muscle revealed by spectral analysis of the surface electromyogram. *Electromyogr. Clin. Neurophysiol.*, 22:459–516.

Schweitzer, T. W., Fitzgerald, J. W., Bowden, J. A., and Lynn-Davies, P. (1979). Spectral analysis of human inspiratory diaphragmatic electromyograms. *J. Appl. Physiol.*, 46:152–165.

Sharp, J. T., Hammond, M. D., Aranda, A. U., and Rocha, R. D. (1993). Comparison of diaphragm EMG centroid frequencies—esophageal versus chest surface leads. *Am. Rev. Respir. Dis.*, 147:764–767.

Similowski, T., Fleury, B., Launois, S., Cathala, H. P., Bouche, P., and Derenne, J. P. (1989). Cervical magnetic stimulation: a new painless method for bilateral phrenic nerve stimulation in conscious humans. *J. Appl. Physiol.*, 67:1311–1318.

Sinderby, C., Lindström, L., and Grassino, A. E. (1993?). Inter-electrode distance filtering function in measurements of diaphragmatic EMG. *Am. Rev. Respir. Dis.*, 147:A697.

Strohl, K. P., Mead, J., Banzett, R. B., Loring, S. H., and Kosch, P. C. (1981). Regional differences in abdominal muscle activity during various maneuvers in humans. *J. Appl. Physiol.*, 51:1471–1476.

Taylor, A. (1960). The contribution of the intercostal muscles to the effort of respiration in man. *J. Physiol.* (London), 151:390–402.

Tokizane, T., Kawamata, K., and Tokizane, H. (1951). Electromyographic studies on the human respiratory muscles. *Jap. J. Physiol.*, 2:232–247.

Vitti, M., Fujiwara, M., Basmajian, J. V., and Iida, M. (1973). The integrated roles of longus colli and sternocleidomastoid muscles: an electromyographic study. *Ant. Rec.*, 177:471–484.

Watson, T. W. J., and Whitelaw, W. A. (1987). Voluntary hyperventilation changes recruitment order of parasternal intercostal motor units. *J. Appl. Physiol.*, 62:187–193.

Whitelaw, W. A., and Watson, T. W. J. (1992). Spike trains from single motor units in human parasternal intercostal muscles. *Respir. Physiol.*, 88:289–298.

36

Noninvasive Methods for Measuring Ventilation

F. DENNIS McCOOL

Brown University Medical School
Providence
Memorial Hospital of Rhode Island
Pawtucket, Rhode Island

I. Introduction

Accurate measurement of pulmonary ventilation requires the use of devices such as masks or mouthpieces coupled to the airway opening. These devices may alter ventilation, and their encumbrance is frequently inconvenient. It would be desirable for some purposes to have measurements that are noninvasive and nonencumbering. Devices that sense respiratory excursions at the body surface can do this, although at some cost of accuracy. Konno and Mead (1967) extensively evaluated a "two-degree-of-freedom" model of chest wall motion. They measured anteroposterior dimensions of the rib cage and abdomen and summed the two signals to obtain tidal volume. Ventilation could be estimated to within 10% of actual ventilation during quiet breathing and exercise when a given posture was maintained. Smith and Mead (1986) later described a third degree of freedom of chest wall motion; axial displacements of the chest wall due to postural movements of the spine and pelvis could cause large displacements of the rib cage and abdomen. This third degree of freedom can be assessed from the distance between the xiphisternal junction and pubic symphysis, and this approach provides a reasonable degree of accuracy with measurements of ventilation in freely moving subjects.

This chapter will briefly comment upon the devices used to assess thoracoabdominal motion and then review the rationale for and limitations of the two- and three-degree-of-freedom models of chest wall motion as well as their applications for use in the laboratory and in the field.

II. Devices Used to Measure Chest Wall Motion

A number of devices have been used to measure motion of the rib cage and abdomen including mercury in rubber strain gauges, pneumobelts, magnetometers, and respiratory inductive plethysmograph (RIP) belts (Wade, 1954; Bendixen et al., 1964; Shapiro and Cohen, 1965; Konno and Mead, 1967; Mead et al., 1967; Grimby et al., 1968; Gilbert et al., 1971, 1972; Sharp et al., 1975, 1977; Stagg et al., 1978; Sackner et al., 1980a; Zimmerman et al., 1983). In practice, magnetometers and RIP belts are primarily used.

Respiratory magnetometers consist of tuned pairs of electromagnetic coils, one transmitting and the other receiving a specific high-frequency AC electromagnetic field. To measure the anteroposterior diameter of the rib cage, one coil is usually placed over the sternum at the level of the 4th intercostal space and the other over the spine at the same level. To measure the anteroposterior diameter of the abdomen, another pair is usually placed on the abdomen at the level of the umbilicus and over the spine at the same level. Over the operational range of distances, the output voltage is linearly related to the distance between the pair provided the axes of the magnetometers remain parallel to each other. As rotation of the axes may change the voltage, the transducer and receiver coils must be secured to the skin in a parallel fashion and rotation due to motion of underlying soft tissue must be minimized. A potential limitation of their use is in environments that contain large metal structures or electric motors. Such devices produce extraneous electromagnetic fields and consequently affect the magnetometer voltage output. Magnetometer coils have been used in diverse environments such as under water (Reid et al., 1986) and under conditions of microgravity (Edyvean et al., 1991).

The RIP belts consist of two loops of wire, which are coiled and sewed into an elastic belt. To measure changes in cross-sectional areas of the rib cage and abdomen, one belt is secured around the midthorax and a second belt is placed around the midabdomen. Care must be taken in securing them to prevent axial slippage of the belts along the body surface. The abdominal belt should also be positioned to be clear of the lateral lower rib cage. The voltage change from the belts turns out to be linearly related to changes of the enclosed cross-sectional area. When the RIP belts are operated in the DC-coupled mode, they can detect shifts in chest wall dimensions, e.g., a change of FRC. However, the AC-coupled mode is preferred for measurements of tidal volume. Magnetometers, on the other hand, are stable enough for measuring both changes in FRC and tidal volume in a given posture.

III. Two-Degree-of-Freedom Model

A. Rationale

The movable components of the thoracic cavity are taken to be the anterior and lateral walls of the rib cage and the diaphragm. The first rib and adjacent structures of the neck are relatively immobile. Changes in volume of the thoracic cavity then will be reflected by displacements of the rib cage and diaphragm. Displacement (motion) of the rib cage can be directly assessed. Diaphragm displacement cannot be measured directly, but since the abdominal contents are essentially incompressible, caudal motion of the diaphragm relative to the pelvis and the volume it displaces is reflected by outward movement of the anterolateral abdominal wall. The two-degree-of-freedom model (Konno and Mead, 1967) holds that the volume displacement of the respiratory system is equal to the sum of the volume displacements of the rib cage and abdomen,

$$V_T = \alpha \Delta RC + \beta \Delta Ab \qquad (1)$$

where ΔRC and ΔAb represent displacements of the rib cage and abdomen, respectively, and α and β are volume-motion coefficients. With this method, ventilation can be estimated to within 10% of the minute ventilation measured at the mouth as long as the subject is confined to one body position.

Two different approaches primarily used for determining the necessary volume-motion coefficients of the rib cage and abdomen are the isovolume technique and the multiple linear regression technique. In the isovolume technique, the subject first performs an isovolume maneuver, shifting volume back and forth between the rib cage and abdominal compartments while holding the glottis closed so that there is no net volume change of the system. As V_T is zero, Eq. (1) can be rearranged to give

$$RC = -(\beta/\alpha)Ab \qquad (2)$$

On a plot of the RC vs. Ab signals, the slope of the isovolume line is the ratio β/α. Second, the subject breathes quietly. From the measurement of V_T, ΔRC, ΔAb, and the ratio β/α, Eq. (1) can then be solved for the absolute values of a and b. In practice, the gains of the rib cage and abdomen signals are often adjusted such that the slope of the isovolume line is 1, thereby making the rib cage and abdomen displacements equal for any volume change; the two signals can then be directly summed to give volume. The isovolume method is based on the assumptions that displacements of the surfaces of the rib cage and abdomen are representatively sampled at the measured location and are similar during isovolume efforts and spontaneous breathing. Since volume-motion coefficients change with posture (Zimmerman, 1988; Paek et al., 1990), the isovolume calibration must be repeated in each body position.

Alternatively, computer-assisted regression techniques are used to determine volume-motion coefficients by solving a matrix of multiple simultaneous equations of changes in chest wall dimensions and lung volume. Stagg et al. (1981) used this method to calculate volume-motion coefficients for AP measurements of the rib cage and abdomen. Multiple linear regression was performed on multiple samples of lung volume, rib cage, and abdominal signals during a single breath. An advantage of this technique is that no special calibration maneuver is required to generate volume-motion coefficients.

B. Limitations

A limitation of any approach that uses chest wall motion to assess ventilation is that the overall volume change of the chest wall being measured includes not only changes in lung volume, but also blood volume shifts into and out of the thoracoabdominal cavity. This may occur when the respiratory system is subjected to large pressure changes, or with changes in posture (e.g., between supine and upright position). In contrast, vascular shifts between the rib cage and abdomen are isovolume for the chest wall and do not affect measurements of tidal volume. Although blood volume shifts related to changes in posture may have an effect on measurements of tidal volume, in practice they do not pose a severe limitation because they usually do not occur within the time frame of a breath.

Another limitation to using measurements of body surface motion is related to distortion that may occur within the rib cage or abdomen (e.g., between the upper and lower rib cage or between the lower transverse and AP rib cage). Indeed, several investigators have described such distortion of the rib cage during inspiration in both healthy subjects (Robertson et al., 1980; Sackner et al., 1980a; D'Angelo, 1981; Crawford et al., 1983; McCool et al., 1985) and patients (Danon et al., 1979; Ringel et al., 1983; McCool et al., 1987). For distortion within the lower rib cage, measurements of cross-sectional area should reflect volume displacements more accurately than measurements of AP diameters alone. Robertson et al. (1980) confirmed this assertion by demonstrating that the addition of measurements of rib cage and abdomen transverse dimensions improved estimates of lung volume changes over those obtained from AP measurements alone. In this context, the RIP belts have the advantage over a single pair of AP magnetometers of responding well to changes in cross-sectional area.

A major limitation of the two-variable approach, however, is due to changes in spinal flexion that may accompany changes in posture. In this context, there are two major reasons why the two-degree-of-freedom model fails. The first error is due to the substantial displacement of the summed rib cage and abdomen signals that occurs with isovolume spinal flexion and extension or pelvic rotation (Smith and Mead, 1986) (Fig. 1). These shifts are a consequence of conservation of volume. As one of the thoracoabdominal boundaries is pushed in, another must be pushed out. Paek et al. (1990) found that the increase in chest wall

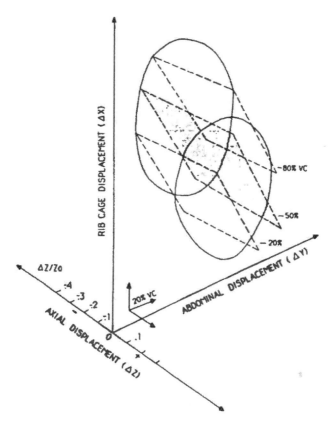

Figure 1 Konno Mead isovolume lines performed over a range of spinal flexion and extension. These lines are shifted dramatically as the axial dimension is changed. (From Smith and Mead, 1986.)

dimensions with isovolume bending was primarily attributable to an increment of the rib cage compartment (Fig. 2). As one bends forwards, the abdominal contents displace the diaphragm cephalad, and this in turn expands the rib cage. This inspiratory movement of the rib cage may be mediated through the insertional forces of the passively stretched diaphragm on the rib cage (Loring and Mead, 1982) or through the zone of apposition of the diaphragm to the rib cage (Mead, 1979).

The second error is due to posturally induced changes in volume-motion coefficients. With isovolume spinal flexion, the rib cage comes down with respect to the pelvis and the axial dimension of the anterior abdominal wall becomes smaller. Therefore less abdominal cavity is bordered by the anterior abdominal wall. With a smaller anterior abdominal wall surface to displace, a given volume displacement of the abdominal compartment would be accompanied by a greater

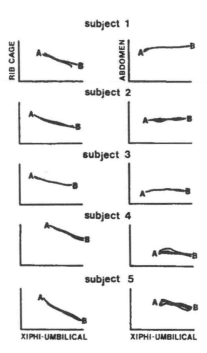

Figure 2 Changes in rib cage, abdomen, and xiphiumbilical distance during isovolume spinal flexion and extension maneuvers. A is fully flexed and B is fully upright. The rib cage dimension increased in all subjects, whereas there was little change in the abdominal signal with spinal flexion. (From Paek et al., 1990.)

outward displacement of the anterior abdominal wall and the abdominal volume-motion coefficient should be reduced. This prediction was confirmed by Paek et al. (1990) (Fig. 3) and by Zimmerman et al. (1983), who noted a smaller abdominal coefficient when seated than when standing. The effects of spinal flexion on the rib cage volume-motion coefficient were variable in these studies. With Zimmerman et al. (1983), it increased in six subjects and was unchanged in the remaining three.

To quantify the first error, Smith and Mead (1986) demonstrated changes in the summed rib cage and abdomen signals during isovolume bending, which were as great as 50% of the magnitude seen in a vital capacity maneuver. Paek et al. (1990) similarly found that the error related to displacement of the rib cage averaged 28% of vital capacity (range of 12–43%) (Fig. 4). The magnitude of the second error (resulting from applying the volume-motion coefficients derived in one posture to the changes in the rib cage and abdomen while breathing in another posture) has also been evaluated. Paek et al. (1990) derived rib cage and abdomen volume-motion coefficients in the fully upright posture and applied them to the changes in rib cage and abdomen while breathing in the bent posture. V_T was overestimated by an

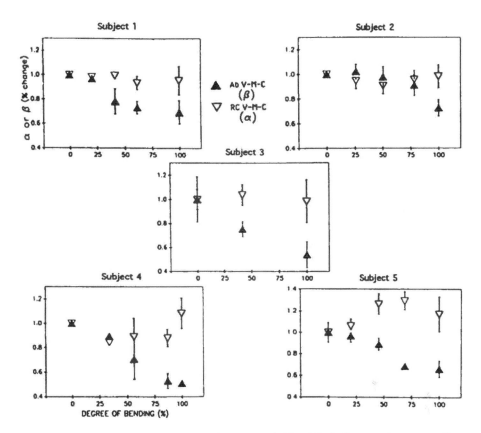

Figure 3 As the degree of bending increases (xiphiumbilical distance decreases), the abdominal volume-motion coefficient (▲) decreases and the rib cage volume-motion coefficient (▽) is generally unchanged. (From Paek et al., 1990.)

average of approximately 14%. This was similar to that reported by Zimmerman et al. (1983) (10–12%) when misapplying the upright volume-motion coefficients to breathing in the seated posture. Conversely, the misapplication of volume-motion coefficients determined for the bent posture resulted in an underestimation of V_T in the upright posture that averaged 8% (Fig. 5).

These errors limit the utility of the two-degree-of-freedom model, with the displacement error being the greater in magnitude. The two errors may be additive or subtractive. For example, if one inhales while bending, the volume-motion coefficients derived in the upright posture will overestimate the abdominal volume contribution. As the rib cage becomes larger with bending, the displacement error is also inspiratory in sign. With this breathing strategy, overestimates may be as great as 50–60% of the vital capacity (Fig. 6).

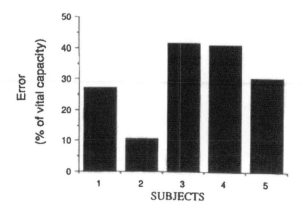

Figure 4 The error related to isovolume changes in rib cage and abdomen dimensions that occur with bending. (From Paek et al., 1990.)

IV. Three-Degree-of-Freedom Model

A. Rationale

Following up on the observation that isovolume axial displacements of the chest wall with changes in spinal attitude can cause large changes in the other dimensions of the chest wall, Smith and Mead (1986) demonstrated that this variable could be monitored by using an additional magnetometer pair that sensed the distance between the xiphoid and the pubic symphysis (Xi). They proposed a three-degree-of-freedom model of movement of the chest wall,

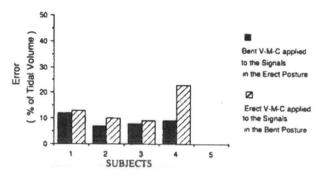

Figure 5 The error related to the misapplication of volume motion coefficients derived in one position to another. (From Paek et al., 1990.)

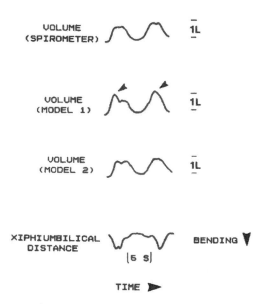

VOLUME (SPIROMETER) — 1L

VOLUME (MODEL 1) — 1L

VOLUME (MODEL 2) — 1L

XIPHIUMBILICAL DISTANCE — BENDING ▼

|5 s|

TIME ▶

Figure 6 Comparison of spirometric volume and volume estimated by the two- and three-degree-of-freedom models (1 and 2, respectively). As the subject inhales while bending (decrease in xiphiumbilical distance), model 1 overestimates tidal volume. (From Paek et al., 1990.)

$$V_T = \alpha \Delta RC + \beta \Delta Ab + \gamma \Delta Xi \qquad (3)$$

where γ is a volume-motion coefficient, and predicted that the addition of the Xi variable to the standard two-degree-of-freedom model should improve volume estimates. Indeed, McCool et al. (1986) showed that the addition of the third independent variable enhances the accuracy with which volume is estimated from body surface motion in those maneuvers that incorporate changes in spinal attitude (e.g., standing-sitting, lifting, and walking) (Fig. 7).

Whereas Smith and Mead (1986) had previously assessed changes in the axial dimension by measuring the xiphipubic distance, Paek et al. (1990) chose to place the magnetometer coils over the umbilicus rather than the pubis since it is a more convenient location to utilize in freely moving subjects. Furthermore, the soft tissue artefacts related to rotation of the pubic magnetometer could be minimized by attaching the umbilical magnetometer coil to a flexible plastic ruler and inverting the coil into the umbilicus. When the magnetometer is fixed in such a fashion, the signal from the xiphiumbilical magnetometer pair was directly proportional to the signal from a xiphipubic magnetometer pair.

The rib cage, abdomen, and xiphiumbilical signals can be calibrated to measure changes in volume by using the following sequence: subjects first will breathe on a spirometer circuit or through a pneumotachograph to generate

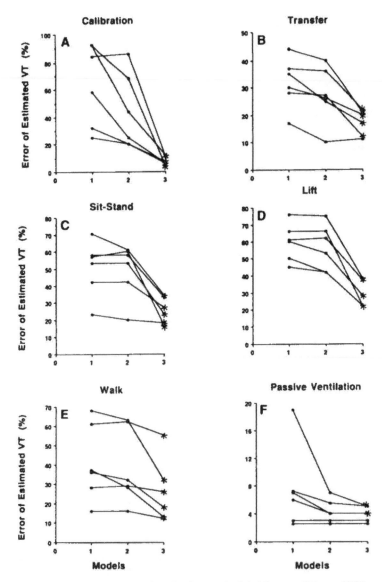

Figure 7 Percent error of estimated tidal volume calculated for one- ($V_T = \alpha\Delta RC$), two- ($V_T = \alpha\Delta RC + \beta\Delta Ab$), and three- ($V_T = \alpha\Delta RC + \beta\Delta Ab + \gamma\Delta Xi$) degree-of-freedom models during a variety of maneuvers that involve changes in posture. The calibration maneuver consists of taking deep and shallow breaths using primarily the rib cage and then the abdomen as one flexes and extends the spine. An asterisk (*) indicates significant ($p < 0.01$) improvement when comparing models 2 and 3. (From McCool et al., 1986.)

simultaneous tidal volume and chest wall motion signals. Tidal volume, RC, Ab, and Xi signals are then recorded as the subject performs a calibration manuever that incorporates flexing and extending the spine while taking deep and shallow breaths. This maneuver should provide data for 20–25 breaths of different sizes performed at different degrees of spinal flexion. The end-expiration and end-inspiration points of the spirometric volume tracing and the corresponding changes in chest wall dimensions are then extracted from the sampled data. Multiple linear regression is next performed on the spirometric tidal volumes and the changes in chest wall dimensions to calculate the volume-motion coefficients. The computer-assisted multiple linear regression technique used is similar to that proposed by Stagg et al. (1978). However, a more complex calibration maneuver than the stereotypical breathing pattern used by Stagg et al. (1978) is required because of the changes in spinal flexion that are encountered when subjects are allowed to change body position. Indeed, coefficients obtained from a calibration maneuver with diverse body motions more accurately predicted ventilation than did the volume-motion coefficients taken from a maneuver in which the chest wall moved with two degrees of freedom (McCool et al., 1986). In an attempt to improve the signal-to-noise ratio by increasing the average range of volume between points, McCool et al. (1986) only sampled points at end-inspiration and end-expiration rather than frequently during a single breath. This provides an acceptable number of data points when multiple breaths are studied.

B. Limitations

The three-degree-of-freedom model, as given in Eq. (3), is still limited in accuracy to about 15% of actual ventilation in individuals who are doing freely moving postural tasks such as bending and lifting or sitting and standing. The error related to posturally induced isovolume shifts of the rib cage and abdomen dimensions is already incorporated in this model, but in theory the model could be improved further if the effects of spinal flexion on the volume-motion coefficients were incorporated.

The most pronounced effect of spinal flexion is on the abdominal volume-motion coefficient (β) (Zimmerman et al., 1983; Paek et al., 1990). With bending, β decreases as the xiphiumbilical distance decreases (Fig. 2). To incorporate this dependency, we rewrote Eq. (3) with the abdominal volume-motion coefficient ($B_u + \epsilon Xi$), where B_u is the value of B obtained in the upright position, ϵ is the linear slope of the relationship of B with Xi, and Xi is the departure of the xiphiumbilical distance from that measured in the upright position (Paek et al., 1990):

$$V_T = \alpha \Delta RC + (B_u + \epsilon Xi)\Delta Ab + \gamma \Delta Xi \tag{4}$$

Equation (4) represents a three-variable model, which now reflects the dependence of β on the xiphiumbilical distance in addition to the factor correcting for the displacement error. Volume estimates made using this model, however, did not improve accuracy in most subjects (Table 1) (Paek et al., 1990). The lack of significant improvement may reflect a relatively small error related to the changes in β. Other factors that might further improve this model but have not been tested include (1) using a curvilinear model to characterize the posturally induced changes of β, (2) correction for posturally dependent changes of α, and (3) assessing other degrees of freedom with which the system moves, e.g., measurements of upper rib cage or of upper, lower, or transverse abdomen. The extra variables, however, add to the complexity of monitoring and calibrating and may not significantly improve the estimates over what is currently achieved.

C. Estimation of Minute Ventilation

The three-degree-of-freedom model has been tested in the laboratory during maneuvers designed to encompass various body postures and a host of activities, including those commonly used by workers in industry (Paek and McCool, 1992). During such maneuvers, the mean values of tidal volume (V_T) were generally within 3% of spirometric values with R^2 values greater than 0.84, the mean values of

Table 1 R^2 Values for Estimated and Spirometric Tidal Volumes

Subject No.	Model No.		
	1	2	3
		Light Lifting	
1	0.60	0.89[a]	0.90[b]
2	0.84	0.94[a]	0.95[c]
3	0.85	0.85[b]	0.86[b]
4	0.75	0.93[a]	0.94[c]
5	0.76	0.82[a]	0.82[b]
Mean ± SD	0.76 ± 0.10	0.88 ± 0.05	0.89 ± 0.055
		Heavy Lifting	
1	0.49	0.90[a]	0.90[b]
2	0.85	0.87[a]	0.87[b]
3	0.79	0.87[a]	0.87[b]
4	0.83	0.93[a]	0.93[c]
5	0.67	0.75[a]	0.72[b]
Mean ± SD	0.72 ± 0.15	0.86 ± 0.07	0.86 ± 0.08

Model 1, $V_T = \alpha\Delta RC + \beta\Delta Ab$; Model 2, $V_T = \alpha\Delta RC + \beta\Delta Ab + \gamma\Delta x$;
Model 3, $V_T = \alpha\Delta RC + (\beta_u + \epsilon xi)\Delta Ab + \gamma\Delta x$.
[a] $p < 0.01$.
[b] $p > 0.05$.
[c] $p < 0.05$.
Source: Paek et al., 1990.

inspiratory time (T_I) were within 7% with R^2 values greater than 0.79, and the values for ventilation ($\dot{V}_E$) within 20% (Tables 2 and 3; Fig. 8). Within these limitations, the three-variable model of body surface motion can be very useful for assessing breathing patterns and ventilation in freely ranging subjects in the laboratory. It is more accurate than the two-degree-of-freedom model during activities that incorporate changes in spinal attitude or body position ($R^2 = 0.97 \pm 0.15$ for the three-degree-of-freedom model and $R^2 = 0.83 \pm 0.15$ for the two-degree-of-freedom model for estimated vs. actual volume). When body position is unchanged, however, the two models have comparable accuracy (McCool et al., 1986).

V. Applications

Noninvasive measures of ventilation have been used as a means of (1) evaluating issues of ventilatory control such as the effects of respiratory apparatus on ventilation and (2) evaluating breathing in an ambulatory environment. The latter application may be of potential benefit in assessing an individual's exposure to indoor or outdoor airborne contaminants, e.g., in the workplace.

A. Mouthpiece Dependency of Breathing Pattern

Noninvasive measurements make it possible to compare breathing in the presence or absence of a mouthpiece. The effects of a mouthpiece on breathing pattern have been studied during quiet breathing (Gilbert et al., 1972; Askanazi et al., 1980; Sackner et

Table 2 Coefficient of Determination Values for Correlation Between Body Surface Displacement and Spirometric Measurements

Activity	Parameter	Mean $\pm$ SD	Range
Cycling	V_T	0.97 $\pm$ 0.02	−0.92−0.98
	T_I	0.88 $\pm$ 0.01	−0.66−0.97
	f	0.98 $\pm$ 0.02	−0.94−0.99
Arm cranking	V_T	0.93 $\pm$ 0.07	−0.67−0.98
	T_I	0.79 $\pm$ 0.14	−0.47−0.98
	f	0.98 $\pm$ 0.01	−0.96−0.99
Pulling	V_T	0.91 $\pm$ 0.05	−0.62−0.97
	T_I	0.81 $\pm$ 0.06	−0.75−0.94
	f	0.93 $\pm$ 0.06	−0.86−0.99
Lifting	V_T	0.84 $\pm$ 0.12	−0.82−0.96
	T_I	0.85 $\pm$ 0.06	−0.71−0.87
	f	0.96 $\pm$ 0.04	−0.82−0.97

R^2 values were obtained by pooling data over all runs. V_T, tidal volume; T_I inspiratory time; f, breathing frequency.
Source: Paek and McCool, 1992.

Table 3 Percentage Difference Between Body Surface
Displacement and Spirometric Measurements

Activity	Parameter	Mean ± SD[a]	Range[b]
Cycling	V_T	1.98 ± 1.71	−5.65− 7.96
	T_I	4.13 ± 3.12	−2.82−13.72
	f	0.16 ± 0.31	−0.33− 1.97
Arm cranking	V_T	2.88 ± 3.08	−9.57− 6.40
	T_I	5.38 ± 3.86	−4.55−15.36
	f	0.23 ± 0.42	−1.57− 0.21
Pulling	V_T	2.04 ± 5.08	−6.78− 4.51
	T_I	6.28 ± 4.38	−4.55−15.36
	f	0.28 ± 0.18	−1.57− 0.21
Lifting	V_T	2.88 ± 1.72	−4.81− 9.25
	T_I	4.85 ± 2.83	−1.66−15.81
	f	0.27 ± 0.40	−0.50− 0.61

[a]Mean ± SD of the absolute values of the difference.
[b]Range of the actual difference.
V_T, tidal volume; T_I inspiratory time; f, breathing frequency.
Source: Paek and McCool, 1992.

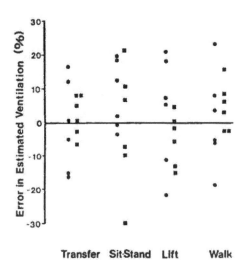

Transfer Sit·Stand Lift   Walk

Figure 8 Differences between minute ventilation determined by spirometry and that
determined by the three-degree-of-freedom model for each individual doing different
maneuvers. (From McCool et al., 1986.)

al., 1980b; Dolfin et al., 1982; Perez and Tobin, 1985; Rodenstein et al. 1985), cycle ergometry (Sackner et al., 1980a), and CO_2 rebreathing (Gilbert et al., 1971; Newton, 1983; Weissman 1984). Generally using a mouthpiece and noseclip will increase V_T and $\dot{V}_E$ with variable effects on breathing frequency (Gilbert et al., 1972; Dolfin et al., 1983; Perez and Tobin, 1985; Rodenstein et al., 1985). Studies during exercise on a cycle or treadmill show more varied effects; tidal volume is either increased (Sackner et al., 1980a) or decreased (Stark et al., 1988). In order to evaluate other typical physical tasks that may be encountered in daily settings, Paek and McCool (1992) studied activities such as lifting and transferring light and heavy objects in addition to cycling. They also found an increase in V_T ($34 \pm 26\%$) and a decrease in breathing frequency ($10 \pm 27\%$) when breathing through a mouthpiece similar in sign and magnitude to that previously reported (Table 4). The increase in tidal volume more than offset the reduction of breathing frequency such that minute ventilation was greater (17%) during the on-mouthpiece period. Thus the respiratory apparatus used to measure ventilation will itself decrease breathing frequency and increase tidal volume and ventilation over a range of tasks and task intensities.

The mouthpiece effect on tidal volume and ventilation is less at the higher levels of ventilation (Paek and McCool, 1992). The attenuation of the mouthpiece effect on V_T may reflect the alinearity of the ventilation–tidal volume relationship previously described during exercise (Hey et al., 1966). As exercise intensity and minute ventilation are increased, tidal volume increases linearly to approximately a tidal volume of one-half vital capacity. Further increases in ventilation are primarily due to an increase in breathing frequency. Thus at the higher levels of exercise, V_T plateaus at a high value that is only slightly augmented by a mouthpiece.

Table 4 Percent Changes in Breathing Pattern and Ventilation During Use of a Mouthpiece

Parameter	Mean ± SD	Range
V_T	$34.0^a \pm 25.6$	$-25.5 - 92.4$
f	$-10.2^b \pm 26.7$	$-52.5 - 108.2$
$\dot{V}_E$	$16.5^a \pm 28.0$	$-41.9 - 153.8$
T_I	$19.2^b \pm 30.1$	$-50.3 - 89.0$
T_T	$20.4^a \pm 32.6$	$-52.0 - 110.5$
T_I/T_T	-0.1 ± 7.4	$-17.5 - 19.2$

[a] $p < 0.01$ when compared with on- and off-mouthpiece periods by paired t-test.
[b] $p < 0.05$ when compared with on- and off-mouthpiece periods by paired t-test.
V_T, tidal volume; f, breathing frequency; $\dot{V}_E$ minute ventilation; T_I, inspiratory time; T_T, total time; T_I/T_T, duty cycle.
Source: Paek and McCool, 1992.

Respiratory drive (V_T/T_I) is increased by the mouthpiece, whereas respiratory timing (T_I/T_T, ratio of inspiratory time to total breath time or duty cycle) is generally unchanged. What increases drive is unclear. Some studies suggest that nasal or oral receptors are irritated by the noseclip or mouthpiece (Dolfin et al., 1983), whereas others suggest that mouth breathing itself, not the irritation, is the responsible mechanism (Hirsch et al., 1982; Perez and Tobin, 1985; Rodenstein et al., 1985).

B. Assessing Ventilation in the Field

Until recently, there has been no simple noninvasive method for measuring ventilation in freely mobile subjects. Measurements of airflow at the mouth are impractical in ambulatory subjects and in themselves alter ventilation. The feasibility of using body surface motion to measure ventilation in the field was demonstrated by McCool and Paek (1993). They used the three-degree-of-freedom model to make measurements of ventilation in nine subjects performing auto body work. By comparison with simultaneous spirometric tracings, they established that ventilation could be measured on average to within 15% of actual ventilation as subjects performed various activities such as sanding and spray painting (Table 5). This method could also detect transients in ventilation as activity increased. They concluded that ventilation can be measured with accuracy from body surface displacements in freely moving subjects outside the laboratory.

An older approach to measuring ventilation in the field has entailed the

Table 5 Mean Values of Minute Ventilation Obtained During 5-Minute Monitoring Periods

Subject	$\dot{V}_E$ (actual) (liters/min)	$\dot{V}_E$ (BSD) (liters/min)	R_2	Error (%)
1	13.1	14.7	0.86	12
2	12.4	10.6	0.93	14
3	19.3	21.6	0.88	13
4	18.9	22.9	0.83	21
5	11.6	13.2	0.88	14
6	19.3	19.2	0.81	14
7	12.1	12.3	0.85	0
8	6.1	8.3	0.83	2
9	13.1	14.5	0.95	36
Mean	15.3	14.0	0.87	14

Error is percentage of change of $\dot{V}_E$ (BSD) compared with $\dot{V}_E$ (actual) from pneumotachograph. $\dot{V}E$ (BSD), minute venilation derived from body surface displacements.
Source: McCool and Paek, 1993.

monitoring of heart rate (HR) (Shamoo et al., 1990; Samet et al., 1993). Since changes in heart rate parallel changes in metabolic rate and thus ventilation, HR can be used as a surrogate of $\dot{V}_E$ providing that the relationship between heart rate and ventilation is known for each individual. This relationship is usually determined either during treadmill exercise or cycle ergometry.

A potential limitation to this approach, however, is the use of a mouthpiece to measure ventilation when characterizing the $\dot{V}_E$-HR relationship. McCool and Paek (1993) found that a mouthpiece strikingly increased ventilation at a given heart rate (Fig. 9). The mechanism for this is unknown. It is unlikely that the increased resistance imposed by a mouthpiece increases energy consumption sufficiently to explain the increase in ventilation since the mouthpiece is usually attached to large-caliber, low-resistance tubes. Moreover, the deadspace of a mouthpiece cannot fully explain the increase in ventilation for a given heart rate; Sackner et al. (1980b) observed that ventilation increased even after eliminating the deadspace effect. Furthermore, the observation that a mouthpiece produces a nearly parallel shift of the $\dot{V}_E$-HR relationship argues against the deadspace mechanism (Table 6); since the deadspace ventilation is a smaller fraction of the total ventilation at the higher levels of exercise, the deadspace effect should be less as exercise progresses, thereby decreasing the slope of the $\dot{V}_E$-HR relationship. Alternatively, irritation of nasal or oral receptors by the mouthpiece or noseclips (Dolfin et al., 1983) may account for the generalized increase in ventilation throughout exercise. To circumvent this problem, body surface displacements rather than a mouthpiece can be used to measure ventilation during the $\dot{V}_E$-HR calibration procedure.

Other factors that affect the $\dot{V}_E$-HR calibration curves and therefore limit their applicability include (1) the lower ranges of resting heart rates found in the field, which require extrapolation of the $\dot{V}_E$-HR relationship to lower ranges of heart rates than those obtained in the lab, and (2) the uncoupling of heart rate from ventilation

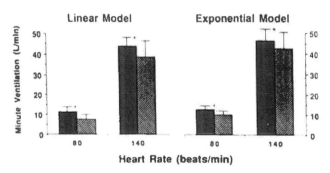

Figure 9 Minute ventilation calculated using the three-degree-of-freedom model while subjects were exercising on a cycle ergometer. Ventilation is overestimated during mouthpiece breathing with both low- and high-intensity exercise (low and high heart rate ranges). (From McCool and Paek, 1993.)

Table 6 Individual Relationships Between Minute Ventilation and Heart Rate During Progressive Work Load Cycling for Field Study Subjects

Subject	On-mouthpiece		Off-mouthpiece	
	Slope	R^2	Slope	R^2
1	0.44	0.87	0.43	0.83
2	0.39	0.85	0.44	0.96
3	0.54	0.89	0.61	0.90
4	0.71	0.94	0.70	0.94
5	0.73	0.89	0.68	0.91
6	0.60	0.92	0.52	0.91
7	0.38	0.93	0.25	0.78
8	0.32	0.92	0.27	0.95
9	0.30	0.93	0.22	0.73
Mean ± SD	0.49 ± 0.16	0.90 ± 0.03	0.46 ± 0.18	0.88 ± 0.08

Source: McCool and Paek, 1993.

such as occurs with voluntary increases in $\dot{V}_E$ or in patients who take cardiac medication such as beta blockers.

Developing methods of measuring ventilation in the field has important implications for risk assessment of air contaminants. The amount of a pollutant absorbed by or deposited in an exposed individual over a specific time period is referred to as dose. The inhaled dose, in turn, depends upon ventilation, ambient exposure conditions, and exposure duration (Brain and Valberg, 1979; Valberg et al., 1985). For the average adult human, minute ventilation may increase to over 100 liters per minute during brief heavy exercise, thereby increasing the rate of delivery of an inhaled toxin more than 10-fold when compared to rest. However, the number of particles deposited in the lung not only depends upon the number of particles delivered (Horvath, 1981), but also on the fraction of particles deposited. This is a function of complex interaction among variables such as velocity and residence time, which in turn depend upon V_T, f, and T_I (Bennett et al., 1985; Brain et al., 1988; Morgan et al., 1984; Heyder et al., 1986). The use of noninvasive means to assess ventilation has advantages over devices that use a mouthpiece since it will not alter breathing patterns and will free the airway for more natural entrainment patterns of particles and gases.

VI. Conclusions

Ventilation can be usefully assessed from measurements of body surface motion. The most commonly used method views the volume change of the system with two degrees of freedom—those of the rib cage and of the abdomen—but this model becomes severely limited when changes in posture occur. This limitation can be overcome in part by adding a third degree of freedom—that of the motion of the chest wall in the axial dimension. These noninvasive measures of ventilation have been used to assess the effects of respiratory apparatus, such as a mouthpiece or noseclips, on ventilation at rest and with exercise and on the utility of heart rate as a predictor of $\dot{V}_E$ in the field. Adapting current technology to measure chest wall dimensions in the field for prolonged periods of time would allow accurate assessments of $\dot{V}_E$ during environmental exposures to particles and gases both at home or in the workplace.

References

Askanazi, J., Silverberg, P. A., Foster, R. J., Hyman, A. I., Milic-Emili, J., and Kinney, J. M. (1980). Effect of respiratory apparatus on breathing pattern. *J. Appl. Physiol.*, 48:192–196.

Bendixon, H. H., Smith, G. M., and Mead, J. (1964). Pattern of ventilation in young adults. *J. Appl. Physiol.*, 19:195–198.

Bennett, W. D., Messina, M. S., and Smaldone, C. (1985). Effect of exercise on deposition and subsequent retention of inhaled particles. *J. Appl. Physiol.*, 59:1046–1054.

Brain, J. D., Skornik, W. A., Spaulding, G. L., and Harbison, M. (1988). The effects of exercise on inhalation of particles and gases. In *Variations in Susceptibility to Inhaled Pollutants. Identification, Mechanisms and Policy Implications*. Edited by J. D. Brain, B. D. Beck, A. J. Warren, and R. A. Shaikh. Baltimore, MD, Johns Hopkins University Press.

Brain, J. D., and Valberg, P. A. (1979). Deposition of aerosol in the respiratory tract. *Am. Rev. Respir. Dis.*, 120:1325–1373.

Crawford, A. B. H., Dodd, D., and Engel, L. A. (1983). Changes in rib cage shape during quiet breathing, hyperventilation and single inspiration. *Respir. Physiol.*, 54:197–209.

D'Angelo, E. (1981). Cranio-caudal rib cage distortion with increasing inspiratory airflow in man. *Respir. Physiol.*, 44:215–237.

Danon, J., Druz, W. S., Goldberg, N. B., and Sharp, J. T. (1979). Function of the isolated paced diaphragm and the cervical assessory muscles in C_1 quadriplegics. *Am. Rev. Respir. Dis.*, 119:909–919.

Dolfin, T., Duffy, P., Wilkes, D., England, S., and Bryan, H. (1983). Effects of a face mask and pneumotachograph on breathing in sleeping infants. *Am. Rev. Respir. Dis.*, 128:977–979.

Edyvean, J., Estenne, M., Paiva, M., and Engel, L. A. (1991). Lung and chest wall mechanics in microgravity. *J. Appl. Physiol.*, 71(5):1956–1966.

Gilbert, R., Auchincloss, J. H., Jr., Baule, G., Peppi, D., and Long, D. (1971). Breathing pattern during CO_2 inhalation obtained from motion of the chest and abdomen. *Respir. Physiol.*, 13:238–252.

Gilbert, R., Auchincloss, J. H., Jr., Brodsky, J., and Boden, W. (1972). Changes in tidal volume, frequency, and ventilation induced by their measurement. *J. Appl. Physiol.*, 33:252–254.

Grimby, G., Bunn, J., and Mead, J. (1968). Relative contribution of rib cage and abdomen to ventilation during exercise. *J. Appl. Physiol.*, 24:159–165.

Heyder, J., Gebhart, J., Rudolf, G., Schiller, C. F., and Stahlhofen, W. (1986). Deposition of particles in the human respiratory tract in the size range 0.005–15 μm. *J. Aerosol. Sci.*, 17:811–825.

Hey, E. N., Lloyd, B. B., Cunningham, D. J. C., Jukes, M. G. M., and Bolten, D. P. G. (1966). Effects of various respiratory stimuli on the depth and frequency of breathing in man. *Respir. Physiol.*, 1:193–205.

Hirsch, J. A., and Bishop, B. (1982). Human breathing patterns on mouthpiece or face mask during air, CO_2, or low O_2. *J. Appl. Physiol.*, 53:1281–1290.

Horvath, S. M. (1981). Impact of air quality in exercise performance. *Exerc. Sport Sci. Rev.*, 9:265–296.

Konno, K., and Mead, J. (1967). Measurement of the separate volume changes of rib cage and abdomen during breathing. *J. Appl. Physiol.* 22:407–422.

Loring, S. H., and Mead, J. (1982). Action of the diaphragm on the rib cage inferred from a force-balance analysis. *J. Appl. Physiol.*, 53:756–760.

McCool, F. D., and Paek, D. (1993). Measurements of ventilation in freely ranging subjects. *Health Effects Inst. Res. Rep.*, 59:1–17.

McCool, F. D., Kelly, K. B., Loring, S. H., Greaves, I. A., and Mead, J. (1986). Estimates of ventilation from body surface measurements in unrestrained subjects. *J. Appl. Physiol.*, 61:1114–1119.

McCool, F. D., Loring, S. H., and Mead, J. (1985). Rib cage distortion during voluntary and involuntary breathing acts. *J. Appl. Physiol.* 58:1703–1712.

McCool, F. D., Pichorko, B. M., Slutsky, A. S., Sarkarati, M., Rossier, A., and Brown, R. (1986). Changes in lung volume and rib cage configuarion with abdominal binding in quadriplegia. *J. Appl. Physiol.*, 60(4):1198–1202.

Mead, J. (1979). Functional significance of the area of apposition of diaphragm to rib cage. *Am. Rev. Respir. Dis.*, 119:31–32.

Mead, J., Peterson, J., Grimby, G., and Mead, J. (1967). Pulmonary ventilation measured from body surface movements. *Science*, 196:1383–1384.

Morgan, W. K. C., Ahamd, D., Chamberlain, M. J., Clague, H. W., Pearson, M. G., and Vinitski, S. (1984). The effect of exercise on the deposition of an inhaled aerosol. *Respir. Physiol.*, 56:327–338.

Newton, P. E., Mamilton, L. H., and Foster, H. V. (1983). Measurement of ventilation using digitally filtered transthoracic impedance. *J. Appl. Physiol.*, 4:1161–1166.

Paek, K., Kelly, K. B., and McCool, F. D. (1990). Postural effects on measurements of tidal volume from body surface displacements. *J. Appl. Physiol.*, 68:2482–2487.

Paek, D., and McCool, F. D. (1992). Breathing patterns during varied activities. *J. Appl. Physiol.*, 73:887–893.

Perez, W., and Tobin, M. J. (1985). Separation of factors responsible for change in breathing pattern induced by instrumentation. *J. Appl. Physiol.* 59:1515–1520.

Reid, M. B., Loring, S. H., Banzett, R. B., and Mead, J. (1986). Passive mechanics of upright human chest wall during immersion from hips to neck. 60(5):1561–1570.

Ringel, E. R., Loring, S. H., McFadden, E. R., and Ingram, R. D., Jr. (1983). Chest wall configurational changes before and during acute obstructive episodes in asthma. *Am. Rev. Respir. Dis.*, 128:607–610.

Robertson, C. H., Jr., Bradley, M. E., and Homer, L. D. (1980). Comparison of two and four magnetometer methods of measuring ventilation. *J. Appl. Physiol.*, 49:355–362.

Rodenstein, D. O., Mercenier, C., and Stanescu, D. C. (1985). Influence of respiratory route on the resting breathing pattern in humans. *Am. Rev. Respir. Dis.*, 131:163–166.

Sackner, J. D., Nixon, A. N., Davis, B., Atkins, N., and Sackner, M. A. (1980a). Non-invasive measurement of ventilation during exercise using a respiratory inductive plethysmograph. *Am. Rev. Respir. Dis.*, 122:867–871.

Sackner, J. D., Nixon, A. N., Davis, B., Atkins, N., and Sackner, M. A. (1980b). Effects of breathing through external deadspace on ventilation at rest and during exercise. *J. Appl. Physiol.*, 122:933–940.

Samet, J. M., Lambert, W. E., James, D. S., Mermier, C. M., and Chick, T. W. (1993). Assessment of heart rate as a predictor of ventilation. *Health Effects Inst. Res. Rep.*, 59:19–55.

Shamoo, D. A., Trim, S. G., Little, D.E., Linn, W. S., and Hackney, J. D. (1990). Improved quantitation of air pollution dose rates by improved estimation of ventilation rate. In *Total Exposure Assessment Methodology: A New Horizon*. Proceedings of the EPA/AWMA Specialty Conference, November 1989, Las Vegas, NV. Pittsburgh, PA, Air and Waste Management Association.

Shapiro, A., and Cohen, H. (1965). The use of mercury capillary length gauges for the measurement of the volume of thoracic and diaphragmatic components of human reppsiration: a theoretical analysis and a practical method. *Trans. NY Acad. Sci.*, 27:634–649.

Sharp, J. T., Goldberg, N. B., Druz, W. S., and Danon, J. (1975). Relative contributions of rib cage and abdomen to breathing in normal subjects. *J. Appl. Physiol.*, 39:608–618.

Sharp, J. T., Goldberg, N. B., Druz, W. S., and Fishman, H. C. (1977). Thoracoabdominal motion in chronic obstructive pulmonary disease. *Am. Rev. Respir. Dis.*, 115:47–56.

Smith, J. C., and Mead, J. (1986). Three degree of freedom description of movement of the human chest wall. *J. Appl. Physiol.*, 60:928–934.

Stark, G. P., Hodous, T. K., and Hankinson, J. L. (1988). The use of inductive plethysmography in the study of the ventilatory effects of respirator wear. *Am. Ind. Hyg. Assoc. J.*, 49:401–408.

Stagg, D., Goldman, M., and Davis, J. N. (1978). Computer-aided measurement of breath volume and time components using magnetometers. *J. Appl. Physiol.*, 44:623–633.

Valberg, P. A., Wolff, R. K., and Mauderly, J. L. (1985). Redistribution of retained particles: effect of hyperpnea. *Am. Rev. Respir. Dis.*, 131:273–280.

Wade, D. L. (1954). Movements of the thoracic cage and diaphragm in respiration. *J. Physiol.*, 124:193.

Weissman, C. J., Askanazi, J., Milic-Emili, J., and Kinney, J. M. (1984). Effect of respiratory apparatus on respiration. *J. Appl. Physiol.*, 57:475–480.

Zimmerman, P. V., Connellan, S. L., Middleton, H. C., Tobona, M. V., Goldman, M. D., and Pride, N. (1983). Postural changes in rib cage and abdominal volume-motion coefficients and their effect on calibration of a respiratory inductance plethysmograph. *Am. Rev. Respir. Dis.*, 127:209–214.

37

Rib Motion in Health and Disease

JOHN B. JORDANOGLOU

Athens University Medical School
Athens, Greece

I. Historical Review

The movement of air through the lungs has been recognized since the Egyptian-Babylonian era of medicine as necessary for human life. The mechanism by which the air passes through the lungs was not mentioned until Galen (A.D. 138–201), who postulated "for in inspiration without obstruction, the animal inhales the air by means of the diaphragm alone, until the time when, should its inspiration meet with resistance, it brings into use the intercostal muscles besides the diaphragm." This is probably the first published work on the mode of pumping action of the chest wall–lungs system. Furthermore, Galen mentioned that the ribs move upwards and outwards (Duchenne, 1866).

These ideas about the function of the chest wall remained essentially the same until the fifteenth century when Leonardo da Vinci (1452–1519) wrote in his notes that a rib during inspiration rotates around an axis located in the posterior part of the rib. He also described in simple terms the relationship between the magnitude of the spatial vector and the size of the rotating radius for a certain angle of elevation. Moreover, he described the analysis in right angles of the spatial vector to the sagittal and the vertical components. These ideas are actually the fundamental concepts of the analysis of the movement of the rib rotating around the neck axis. Later, Andreas Vesalius (1514–1564) gave an excellent demonstration that the contracting diaphragm pulled the ribs in which it is inserted outwards and upwards (Duchenne, 1866).

These concepts about rib movement and its effect on the dilatation of the thoracic cavity remained basically the same until the nineteenth century. In 1831 Magendie became aware of the rotational movement of the ribs and of the effect that the radius at several points on the rib had on the amount of rib movement. Hutchinson (1852) considered the rotation of the ribs around two axes: an anteroposterior axis giving rise to the change of the lateral diameter, and a transverse axis producing the change of the sagittal diameter. Duchenne (1866), in his famous experiments with electrical stimulation of the phrenic nerve of living humans, observed that the diaphragmatic ribs are elevated and moved outwards, and, furthermore, "while the transverse diameter of the base of the thorax was enlarged its anteroposterior diameter equally increased, but almost imperceptibly." Moreover, Duchenne stated "that under action of the high frequency induction current . . . simultaneously the rib moved outward by a sort of a rotatory motion on its ends." Also, he postulated, "it is indeed known that all the ribs are elevated and separated from each other outwardly and that the more they become horizontal, the further the sternum is pushed forward and upward."

Landerer (1881) described the movement of the ribs around the neck axis. Briefly, he maintained that the amount of movement of the ribs at several points depends on the position of the neck axis as related to the sagittal plane and on the so-called radius vector, i.e., the orthogonal distance of the points from the neck axis. Moreover, he showed in cadavers that the lower ribs (8th–10th) may move backwards during inspiration.

In 1892 Thane wrote that the chief movement of the ribs generally is a rotation around an axis "directed obliquely outwards and backwards, as well as mostly somewhat downwards, passing through the costocentral articulation and the neck of the rib, and a little in front of the costotransverse joint." The change of the horizontal chest diameter during inspiration was explained by the single rotation of the rib around this axis, the neck axis. Later, in 1909, Keith described at least two types of rib movements:

> one representative of the upper costal mechanism and the other of the lower or diaphragmative mechanism. . . . Two movements of the ribs are recognised, one round an axis corresponding to the spinal articulation of the rib, and another round the spine-sternal articulation. The first movement gives increase to the back-to-front diameter, the other to the side-to-side. . . . The results of a movement of the lower ribs—or better, of the action of the diaphragmatic mechanism—is to increase the transverse and back-to-front diameter of the lower thorax and the vertical diameter of the whole cavity.

Fick (1911) postulated that ribs may move around the neck axis, which he described as the line between two fixed points on each rib: the center of the head of the rib and the center of the costotransverse joint. This line corresponds to the long axis of the neck of the rib. Fick considered this to be the only axis of movement of the rib. In the 8th, 9th, and 10th ribs, the transverse process of the vertebra lies under the tubercle of the rib, so that movement of the neck of the rib around a vertical axis (backwards or forwards) is not completely impossible. The movement of these lower ribs is essentially the same as that of the upper ribs, but they show significantly greater passive mobility compared to the upper ribs due to greater slackness of the ligaments. The two neck axes of a costal ring are not a straight line, converging in front.

This oblique position of the axes of rotation is of fundamental importance to the change of the shape of the thorax during breathing. This was recognized by Trendelenburg in 1779 but forgotten again until Helmholtz mentioned it in 1856. Fick also analyzed the rotatory movement of the ribs around the neck axis. In the same year Luciani (1911) postulated that ribs rotate around an axis passing along the neck of the rib. Hoover (1922) distinguished two parts of the thoracic cage where the mechanism of the respiratory rib excursion differed. He believed that the upper part consisted of the sternum and the upper five ribs moving round one axis passing through the head of the ribs and the transverse process of the vertebrae. The lower part of the cage consisted of the 6th to the 10th ribs, the movement of which was around a vertical axis. In 1935 Steindler postulated that the ribs move around one axis, namely, "the line running through the centre of the costal heads and through the tubercles of the ribs." According to this theory the mobility in the costovertebral articulations has only one degree of freedom because of the double articulation. During the rotatory movement, the points on each rib describe concentric arcs around the axis. The axis of the movement of the ribs is oblique in relation to the cardinal planes of the chest. The degree of obliqueness of this axis changes with the position of the transverse process of the vertebrae and with the angle of inclination of the ribs with the horizontal plane. The axis of movement of the ribs is almost entirely in the frontal plane in the upper dorsal vertebrae, while in the lower ribs this axis assumes a more sagittal position. Consequently, the upper ribs move forward while the lower ribs outward. The greatest amount of inward and outward excursion is between the 5th and 8th ribs.

Fraser and Robbins (1937) proposed two types of rib movements: around an axis corresponding to the rib-vertebral articulations and around an anteroposterior axis. Werenskiold (1938) postulated that the ribs rotate around the neck axis and that in the upper ribs the costal movement expands the thorax sagitally while in the lower ribs it does so transversely because of the oblique position of the neck axis. Moreover, he maintained that the lower ribs move backwards, presumably around a vertical axis. Barlow in *Buchanan's Manual of Anatomy* (1949) postulated that the 2nd to 6th ribs rotate around the costovertebral axis, while the 7th to 10th ribs rotate around both the costovertebral and the costosternal axes. Furthermore, he thought that the lower ribs (7th–10th) may move around a vertical axis as well. In 1950, in *Gray's Anatomy* it was maintained that the ribs move around two axes: the neck axis and the anteroposterior or vertebrosternal axis. In Cunningham's

Textbook of Anatomy (1951) it is maintained that the rib moves around one axis, the costovertebral axis, which has an outward, backward, and slightly downward direction, except for the 1st vertebra, in which the axis is directed upward, and the 2nd, in which it is transverse. Because of the downward inclination of the ribs and the obliqueness of the rib-neck axis, the raising of the rib in inspiration causes the sternal end of the rib to move upwards, forwards, and laterally. The change of the transverse diameter is large in the middle ribs, in which the obliqueness of the costovertebral axis is more marked, while in the upper ribs, in which the neck axis is less oblique, the transverse diameter shows only a slight change or remains unaltered. However, the transverse diameter may change because of movement of the ribs around a costosternal axis.

Grant in 1952 maintained that the 2nd to 7th costal arches rotate around the costovertebral joints. During this movement in inspiration, the sternal ends and middle parts of the ribs are raised and the lower borders are everted. Consequently, the sagittal and the transverse chest diameters are increased. The vertebrosternal ribs cannot be forced backwards because of the position of the transverse processes behind the ribs (see also Grant and Basmajian, 1965). The vertebrochondral ribs (8th–10th) glide backwards and upwards during inspiration. They cannot rotate. This movement of the 8th to 10th ribs is favored by the shape and the position of the costotransverse facets (flat and face anterosuperiorly). Grant wrote that this movement of the lower ribs "resembles a pair of curved spreading calipers opening" and causes the increase of the transverse diameter of the lower part of the thorax and the upper part of the abdomen.

Fulton (1955) considered rib movement to consist of rotation around one axis: the rib-neck axis. During inspiration, the elevation of the ribs around this axis results in an increase of the sagittal thoracic diameter, while in the lower ribs (6th–10th) this movement produces an increase of the transverse diameter as well. Fulton mentioned that the eversion of the ribs during inspiration is another cause of the increase of the transverse diameter. He postulated this eversion to be a secondary effect of the rotation of the ribs. Furthermore, he cited the inclination angle of the ribs as a factor contributing to the change of the chest diameters.

Campbell (1958) modified the description of Keith about the movements of the chest in the following way: the movement of the operculum is around the neck axis, producing a slight change in the sagittal chest diameter. During quiet breathing there is no movement of this region. The next region includes the vertebrosternal ribs (2nd–6th). These ribs move around two axes: the neck axis and the axis that passes through the angle of the rib and the costosternal joint. Elevation of the downward- and forward-sloped rib around the neck axis produces an increase in the sagittal chest diameter. This is the "pump-handle" movement. The transverse diameter changes because of the movement of the rib around the anteroposterior axis because the middle of the rib lies below this axis. This is the "bucket-handle" movement. In the region of the vertebrochondral ribs (7th–10th), the axes of movement are essentially the same as those in the upper ribs.

In 1959 Last considered that all the ribs rotate around the neck axis, while the lower ribs (7th–10th) may move around an anteroposterior axis in addition to the movement around the costovertebral axis. Last also mentioned the obliqueness of the ribs (angle of inclination) as contributing to the change of the horizontal thoracic diameters.

Von Hayek (1960), considering the motion of the rib around the neck axis, stated: "since ribs and vertebrae are interconnected by two joints, motion is only possible about a single axis which passes through the head of the rib and the costal tubercle (Tuberculum costae); this is the axis of the neck of the rib." Von Hayek cited Felix's (1928) statement about the neck axis that "it [the neck axis] alone determines the type of movement of the ribs." However, he believed, on the basis of the morphology of the articular surfaces of the transverse joint, that "other motion in addition to that about the costal neck are possible in these joints." That is, von Hayek accepted that the upper ribs (2nd–5th) rotate around the neck axis, while in the lower ribs (7th–10th) the tubercle glides backward and upward on the transverse process during inspiration. Finally, he stated that

> a movement about the costal neck axis which is so important for the upper ribs can therefore be excluded as principal movements for the lower ribs (6th–12th). If one wishes to designate the inspiratory movements of the ribs chiefly as movements about an axis, there is only an approximate antero-posterior axis which passes through the head of the rib.

Carlson (1961) believed that the movement of the 6th to 10th ribs produces an increase of the transverse diameter as well, but did not mention any axis of movement. Sinclair postulated in 1961 that the upper costotransverse joints allow the tubercle of the rib to rotate and not to slide on the transverse process, while the lower joints permit not only rotation but also slight gliding movements. He cited the rotatory movement of the ribs around the rib-neck axis and around a sagittal axis, which passes through the head of the rib and the chondrosternal joint.

Agostoni (1964) postulated that the ribs move around their neck axis. Because of the angle formed by the two axes of a costal ring, decussating in front, the part of the rib undergoing the largest movement is placed more ventrally in the upper ribs and more laterally in the lower ribs. Therefore, the change in diameter is predominantly dorsoventral in the upper part and lateral in the lower part of the thorax. Moreover, because of the rotation of the ribs around one axis, the greatest movement should occur at the point where the radial distance from the neck axis is greatest. In 1965 Ganong stated that "the ribs pivot as if hinged at the back, so that when the external intercostals contract, they elevate the lower ribs. This pushes the sternum outward and increases the anteroposterior diameter of the chest. The transverse diameter is actually changed little if at all."

Since that time, most manuals of anatomy and physiology espouse the same ideas about costal motion, with the exception of some authors who refer to our work. However, the "pump-handle" and "bucket-handle" theories of movement persist.

II. Purpose of the Study

The above review of previous work shows clearly that there is little agreement between authors about rib movement during a tidal inspiratory effort. Some authors have accepted the monoaxial movement of the rib around the rib-neck axis, while others have adopted the multiaxial movement around two or even three axes. Others believe the axis of movement of the upper ribs to be different from that of the lower ribs.

Moreover, several authors have implicated certain factors as affecting the amount of inspiratory change of thoracic diameter during the monoaxial or multiaxial motion of the ribs. However, there is no sound theory relating chest expansion to inspiratory excursion of the ribs.

In order to determine the types of rib movement, a specially designed instrument has been used. A theoretical analysis of the rotational motion of the rib and of the factors that influence the change of thoracic diameter was developed and tested on a mechanical analogue of the rib-vertebra system. This instrument was also used on living subjects for analysis of inspiratory costal motion. Finally, the effect of the curvature of the dorsal region of the spinal column on the inspiratory change of the chest diameter has been examined using a computer method developed for this purpose.

III. Analysis of the Rotational Motion of the Rib

According to the concept of the rotational movement of the rib around the neck axis, any point Z on the rib draws the arc ZeZi on its plane of rotation (B) during inspiration (Fig. 1). The chord of the arc represents the vector S. The plane of rotation B is perpendicular to the axis of rotation at the point O, and so vector S is at right angles with the neck axis (Figs. 1–3). The orthogonal distance of point Z of the rib from the neck axis at point O is the rotating radius R. The length of the radius depends on the site of the point on the rib (Fig. 3).

The amount of rotation of any costal point around the neck axis on the plane of rotation (B) is shown by the angle $\hat{b}$. The relation of the magnitude of vector S to radius R and elevation angle $\hat{b}$ is given by the Eq. (1):

$$S = R \times 2 \sin\frac{\hat{b}}{2} \tag{1}$$

It becomes obvious that the magnitude of vector S increases proportionally with the increase of the radius and of angle $\hat{b}$ (Fig. 4).

Vector S, being oblique within the rectangular system of the chest, may initially be analyzed on the plane of rotation (B) to two component vectors at right angles, S_1 and S_2 (Fig. 2). The rectangular system of the chest consists of the

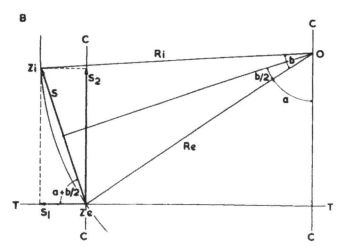

Figure 1 Diagram corresponding to a left rib seen laterally from the left side while the chest is upright. The plane of the paper is the plane of rotation B. The lines CC and TT represent the lines of perpendicular intersection of the homonymous planes (C and T) with plane B. Point O is the point on the neck axis at which plane B meets the axis at right angles. The angle between vectors S and S_1 is equal to $\hat{a} + \hat{b}/2$

cardinal planes of the chest (sagittal G, transverse T, and frontal F), which meet at right angles at the costal point Z (Fig. 2). The lines of intersection of these planes are the sagittal (g), the transverse (t), and the vertical (v) diameters of the thorax (Fig. 2).

The analysis of vector S to its components S_1 and S_2 is affected not only by the size of elevation angle $\hat{b}$ but also by the inclination angle $\hat{a}$ of the rib at the point Z at the expiratory position (Figs. 1,2). Angle $\hat{a}$ is formed on the plane of rotation B by the radius R at the expiratory position and the line of the perpendicular intersection of planes B and C (Figs. 1,2). Plane C is the vertical plane on which the neck axis lies (Fig. 2). The component vector S_1 is horizontal, lying on the line of intersection of planes B and T, and the S_2 component lies on the line of intersection of planes B and C (Fig. 2). Analysis of vectors S_1 and S_2 to the final component vectors, parallel to the diameters of the chest, depends on the position of the rib-neck axis in relation to the rectangular system of the thorax, i.e., on the size of the angles $\hat{d}$ and $\hat{h}$ (Fig. 2). Angle $\hat{d}$ is formed on plane C by the neck axis itself and the vertical diameter v of the chest (Figs. 2,5). Angle $\hat{h}$ is formed by the sagittal diameter g of the chest and the line of intersection of vertical plane C with transverse plane T (Figs. 2,5). The sizes of angles $\hat{d}$ and $\hat{h}$ are not constant, but change with the position of the vertebra in relation to the planes of the chest. The change in length of the sagittal (g), transverse (t), and vertical (v) chest diameters at a point along the rib during inspiration is given by the final component vectors Sg, St, and Sv, respectively:

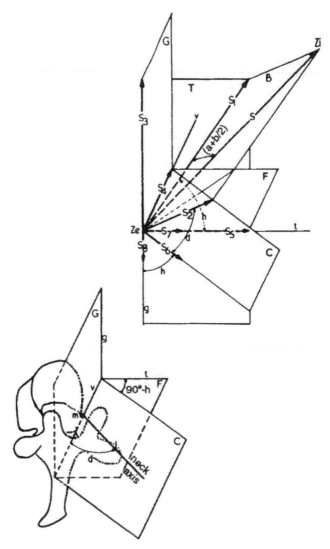

Figure 2 A dorsal vertebra and point Z on the corresponding right rib are seen obliquely from above, behind, and laterally from the left side. The neck axis directed downwards, outwards, and backwards lies on plane C. The plane of the paper is the transverse plane T. The planes G, F, and C of the vertebra are parallel to the homonymous planes at point Z of the rib. The angle between vectors S_1 and S_5 as well as between vectors S_8 and S_6 is equal to angle h of the neck axis. The angle between vectors S_2 and S_6 on plane C is equal to angle d of the neck axis. The angle between the horizontal component S_1 and vector S on plane B is equal to a + b/2.

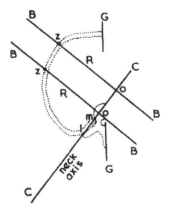

Figure 3 A left rib with the left half of the corresponding dorsal vertebra seen from above. The lines GG, CC, and BB represent the homonymous planes (G, C, B) seen from above. Points 1 and m lie on plane C and define the neck axis. The planes of rotation B meet the neck axis at points o at right angles. Radius R is the orthogonal distance between point o on the neck axis and point Z on the rib.

$$S_g = S_3 - S_8 \tag{2}$$
$$S_t = S_5 + S_7 \tag{3}$$
$$S_v = S_4 \tag{4}$$

and

$$\frac{Sg}{S} = \cos(\hat{a}+\hat{b}/2)\sin \hat{h} - \sin(\hat{a}+\hat{b}/2)\cos \hat{d} \cos \hat{h} \tag{5}$$

$$\frac{St}{S} = \cos(\hat{a}+\hat{b}/2)\cos \hat{h} + \sin(\hat{a}+\hat{b}/2)\cos \hat{d} \sin \hat{h} \tag{6}$$

$$\frac{Sv}{S} = \sin(\hat{a}+\hat{b}/2)\sin \hat{d} \tag{7}$$

Positive vectors represent increase and negative vectors decrease of the thoracic diameter in the inspiratory phase (Fig. 2).

The above theoretical analysis shows that the S vectors are perpendicular to the rib-neck axis and that the quantitative change of the chest diameter along the ribs during inspiration is affected by (1) the radial distance of the points on the rib from the neck axis, (2) the angle of inclination of the rib at the considered points, (3) the angle of elevation of the rib, (4) the horizontal deviation of the neck axis from the sagittal diameter, and (5) the deviation of the neck axis from the vertical diameter (Jordanoglou, 1967, 1970).

The effects of angles â and b̂ of the rib, at a costal point, and of angles d̂ and ĥ of the rib-neck axis on the ratios Sg/S, St/S, and Sv/S are shown in the

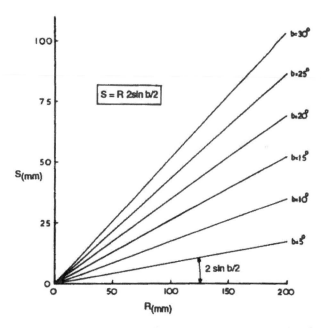

Figure 4 Relationship between the magnitude of vector S (mm) and radius R (mm) at several angles of elevation of the rib.

diagrammatic presentation of Eqs. (5)–(7) (Figs. 6–8) (unpublished data). The transposition of the rib-neck axis from the downward, backward, and outward positions to the transverse position (increase of angles $\hat{d}$ and $\hat{h}$) is accompanied by an increase in the Sg/S ratio (Fig. 6). When the neck axis is lying on the frontal plane ($\hat{h} = 90$), the ratio Sg/S is not affected by the downward or upward

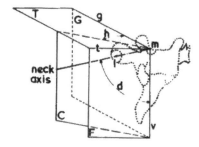

Figure 5 A dorsal vertebra seen from the front and the right lateral side. Points m and l define the neck axis of the rib. Planes G, C, and F have a common line of intersection, the vertical (v) chest diameter. These three planes are at right angles with the transverse plane T. The neck axis and angle $\hat{d}$ lie on plane C, while angle $\hat{h}$ lies on plane T.

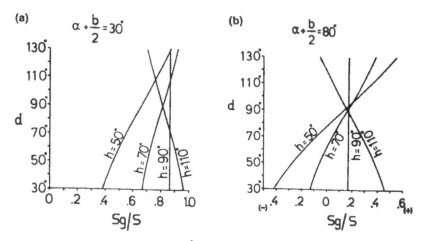

Figure 6 Relationship between angle $\hat{d}$ of the rib-neck axis and the ratio Sg/S at several values of the horizontal angle $\hat{h}$ of the neck axis. The increase of angle $\hat{a} + \hat{b}/2$ shifts the effect of the angles $\hat{d}$ and $\hat{h}$ to the left (see text).

displacement of the transverse process of the vertebra ($90° > \hat{d} > 90°$). However, with an anteriorward and lateralward transposition of the neck axis ($\hat{h} > 90°$), the Sg/S ratio becomes smaller with the upward displacement of the axis (increase of angle $\hat{d}$). When the rib tends to a horizontal end-inspiratory position (increase of the angle $\hat{a} + \hat{b}/2$), the above-mentioned changes of angles $\hat{d}$ and $\hat{h}$ of the neck axis are followed by smaller increments of or even a decrease in the sagittal diameter (smaller positive or increasing negative values of the Sg/S ratio). The St/S ratio is diminished during inspiration as a result of the displacement of the rib-neck axis from a downward, backward, and outward to an upward, forward, and outward position ($\hat{d} < 90° \rightarrow \hat{d} > 90°$, $\hat{h} < 90° \rightarrow \hat{h} > 90°$) (Fig. 7). At an end-inspiratory, nearly horizontal position of the rib, the effect of the position of the rib-neck axis on the St/S ratio is enhanced. The Sv/S ratio is increased by the upward transposition of the neck axis to the horizontal plane (transverse plane T) ($\hat{d} < 90° \rightarrow \hat{d} = 90°$), where this ratio has its maximum value (Fig. 8). If the neck axis is displaced further upwards ($\hat{d} > 90°$), the Sv/S ratio becomes smaller. This effect of angle $\hat{d}$ of the neck axis on the Sv/S ratio is intensified by the increase of the inclination angle of the rib at the end-inspiratory position.

It is apparent that the position of the rib-neck axis as well as of the costal body is dynamic since the angles $\hat{d}$, $\hat{h}$, and $\hat{a}$ change with the degree of the curvature of the dorsal spinal column in healthy subjects and in patients. Consequently, at a given rotational movement of the rib during inspiration, the change of the thoracic diameter is dependent on the transposition of the dorsal vertebrae around the sagittal, transverse, or vertical thoracic diameter in relation to the cardinal planes of the chest.

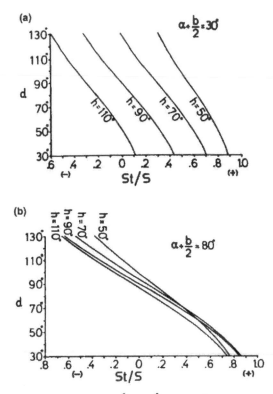

Figure 7 Relationship between angles d̂ and ĥ of the rib-neck axis and the ratio St/S. Angle â + b̂/2 changes the slope of the relationship (see text).

IV. Instrumentation

A. Theoretical Considerations

The direction of the S vectors along a rib can be determined in relation to the rectangular system of the chest. The spatial vector S has a certain position lying on an oblique plane A, perpendicular to the frontal plane (F) and in between the transverse (T) and the sagittal (G) planes (Fig. 9) (Jordanoglou 1967, 1969) This plane A meets the transverse (T) and the sagittal (G) planes of the thorax along the sagittal (g) diameter (Fig. 9). It is evident that there is only one position of the plane A within the rectangular system of the chest at which the spatial vector S may lie on this plane. Consequently, the direction of the spatial vector S can be defined if the position of the plane A within the cardinal planes of the chest and the position of the vector S on the plane A are determined. This is achieved by measuring the angles ϑ and $\hat{\varphi}$. (Fig. 9). The position of vector S on plane A is determined by the angle $\hat{\varphi}$. This angle lies on plane A (Fig. 9). Since vector S has an oblique direction in relation to the rectangular

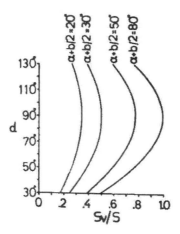

Figure 8 Diagram showing the effect of angle $\hat{d}$ of the rib-neck axis on the Sv/S ratio. The maximum value of Sv/S for any angle $\hat{a} + \hat{b}/2$ corresponds to $\hat{d} = 90°$.

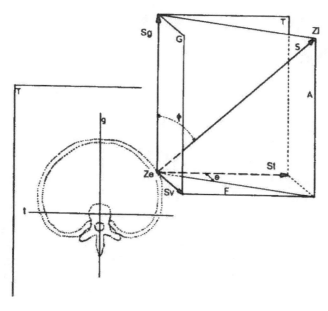

Figure 9 A costal ring seen from above. The plane of the paper is the transverse plane T of the chest. The planes of the rectangular system are parallel to the planes of the chest. Planes G and F are perpendicular to plane T. The line of the perpendicular intersection of planes G and F is the vertical diameter (v) of the chest. Plane A is perpendicular to plane F. Angle $\hat{\vartheta}$ lies on plane F. Angle $\hat{\varphi}$ and vector S lie on plane A (see text).

system of the chest, it may be divided into three components: sagittal (Sg), transverse (St), and vertical (Sv) (Fig. 9). These component vectors represent the change in length of the corresponding thoracic diameters at a certain point along the rib that covers the distance S during inspiration. The ratios of these component vectors to the initial vector S at any point Z along the rib is as follows:

$$\frac{Sg}{S} = \cos \hat{\varphi} \tag{8}$$

$$\frac{St}{S} = \sin \hat{\varphi} \cos \hat{\vartheta} \tag{9}$$

$$\frac{Sv}{S} = \sin \hat{\varphi} \sin \hat{\vartheta} \tag{10}$$

The ratio Sg/S, St/S, and Sv/S as well as the magnitude of the vector S can be determined by using a specially designed instrument, called the ALDI (angular linear displacement indicator), that measures angular and linear displacement simultaneously (Figs. 10,11) (Jordanoglou and Smith, 1970).

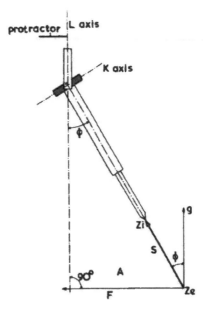

Figure 10 Point Z belongs to a left rib of a supine chest with its operculum towards the left side of the diagram and seen laterally from the right side. The plane of the paper is plane A. Line F is the line of the perpendicular intersection of plane F with plane A. The ALDI instrument is in a position of alignment with vector S. Angle $\hat{\varphi}$ between vector S and the sagittal diameter g is equal to angle $\hat{\varphi}$ between diameter g and the long axis of the transducer.

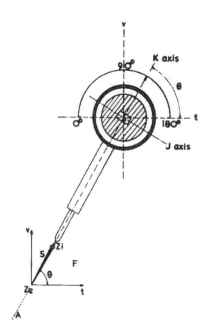

Figure 11 Point corresponding to a left rib seen from above with the chest supine and the operculum in the direction of the v diameter. The plane of the paper is plane F of the g, t, v rectangular system of the thorax. The plane of the protractor of the ALDI is parallel to plane F but lies higher. Vector S has an oblique direction upward towards the center of the ALDI instruments, which is in position of alignment with vector S. Angle $\hat{\vartheta}$ on plane F is equal to angle ϑ on the protractor. Vector S, the long axis of the transducer, and the K axis of the ALDI lie on the same plane A, which is perpendicular to plane F.

The idea of this instrument was to set up a mechanical system parallel to the rectangular system of the chest that could be aligned with the vector S at any costal point during inspiration. At the position of alignment of the instrument with vector S, the amount of displacement of the rib and the magnitude of the change of the chest diameter at that point can be measured.

B. Function of the ALDI Instrument

The function of this instrument is to measure the magnitude of vector S and angles $\hat{\varphi}$ and $\hat{\vartheta}$ from which the component vectors Sg, St, Sv can be calculated. Plane F of the rectangular system of the mechanical analogue is horizontal, so that it is parallel to the carriage of the ALDI instrument (Fig. 12). The 90° diameter of the protractor of ALDI is set parallel to the vertical diameter (v) of the supine chest (Fig. 11). The endpoint of the shaft of the transducer of ALDI touches point Z on a rib and follows it freely to its excursion from position e to position i. The position of alignment of

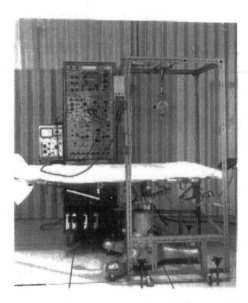

Figure 12   Photograph of set-up for measuring ratios Sg/S, St/S, and Sv/S and the S vectors in living subjects. The subject lies supine on the adjustable table. The framework of the ALDI instrument is set parallel to the rectangular system of the chest so that the carriage of the ALDI is parallel to the frontal plane of the chest. This carriage permits the ALDI instrument to move parallel to the transverse, vertical, and sagittal diameters of the chest.

vector S on the costal point with the long axis of the transducer is achieved when at a certain angle $\hat{\vartheta}$ on the protractor of ALDI the output from the K potentiometer remains zero and the output from the J potentiometer shows a constant deviation from the zero line at the beginning and the end of vector S (Fig. 10). In this position, the magnitude of vector S is equal to the movement of the shaft of the transducer, while the direction of vector S is shown by angle $\hat{\vartheta}$ on the protractor as the constant deviation of the pointer from the 0° or 180° mark (transverse diameter, t) and by the angle $\hat{\varphi}$ as the deviation of the transducer from the sagittal diameter (g) (zero line) on plane A. Angle $\hat{\varphi}$ and the magnitude of vector S are indicated on the recording paper by the output from the J potentiometer and from the transducer, respectively.

V.   Verification of Vector Analysis of Rib Movement

The vector analysis of rib movement was verified using the mechanical analogue of the rib-vertebra system (Fig. 13) (unpublished data). Using this analogue, the angles of the rib-neck axis $(\hat{d}, \hat{h})$, the inclination $(\hat{a})$ and elevation $(\hat{b})$ angles, and the radius R of a "costal" point can be predetermined. At various combinations of the angles $\hat{d}$, $\hat{h}$, $\hat{a}$, and $\hat{b}$ and of radius R on the mechanical analogue, the inspiratory excursion of the "costal" point (vector S) and its component vectors Sg, St, and Sv

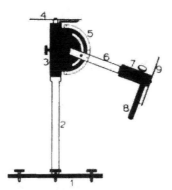

Figure 13 Diagram of the mechanical analogue of the rib-vertebra system. (1) Base of the analogue corresponding to transverse plane T of the subject in the standing position. (2) Metallic rod representing the vertical diameter. (3) Joint permitting rod 6 to turn around rod 2 (angle ĥ measured on protractor) or to move on a vertical plane (5), which is a protractor on which angle d̂ is measured. (6) Rod representing the neck axis around which metallic bar 8 rotates at the joint 7. The angle of elevation is measured on the protractor (9). Bar 8 corresponds to a radius R.

were measured with the ALDI instrument. The magnitudes of these vectors were also calculated from Eq. (5)–(7). The results are shown in Table 1. The values of vector S and of ratios Sg/S, St/S, and Sv/S calculated from the theoretical equations were shown to be equal to those obtained using the ALDI instrument. It may therefore be concluded that the theory of rotation of the ribs around the neck axis is valid. Furthermore, it was shown that, in the mechanical analogue, the S vectors

Table 1 Results for the Ratios Sg/S, St/S, Sv/S, and S Vectors Measured on the Mechanical Analogue by Using the ALDI Instrument and Calculated from Eqs. (5)–(7) and (1).

Sg/S		St/S		Sv/S		S (mm)	
Theory	ALDI	Theory	ALDI	Theory	ALDI	Theory	ALDI
0.47	0.46	0.08	0.08	0.82	0.83	18.53	18.39
±0.09	±0.09	±0.32	±0.32	±0.07	±0.07	± 6.35	± 6.31
$r = 0.998$		$r = 0.998$		$r = 0.998$		$r = 0.999$	
$p = 0.000$		$p = 0.000$		$p = 0.000$		$p = 0.000$	

Values are mean (±1 SD) from 11 measurements on the mechanical analogue at a constant R and at several combinations of the angles (â + b̂/2), d̂, and ĥ. The ratios Sg/S, St/S, and Sv/S and vector S were measured using the ALDI instrument at the predetermined values of the angles â, b̂, ĥ, and d̂ and of R and calculated from Eqs. (5)–(7) and (1). Predetermined values: $â = 50°–70°$, $b̂ = 5°–10°$, $ĥ = 60°–120°$, $d̂ = 47.5°–110°$, $R = 180$ mm.

were parallel one to another and perpendicular to the axis of the rotational movement of the "costal" point, whatever the position of the axis was within the rectangular system.

VI. Measurement of Costal Movement of Living Subjects

The subject lay supine with the thorax naked on an adjustable table set horizontal by the aid of a level. With the chest in this position, the frontal plane (F) was horizontal, while the sagittal (G) and the transverse (T) thoracic planes and plane A were vertical. The framework was horizontal and placed, in relation to the subject, parallel to the chest diameter with its center corresponding roughly to the middle of the sternum (Fig. 12) (Jordanoglou, 1969).

A small plastic pad was placed on each of the costal points and on the pad the endpoint of the shaft of the transducer. The pad was held on the rib with one hand, while the other hand of the investigator held the ALDI from the semicircular ring (Fig. 14). The subject breathed tidally while the ALDI, at different distances

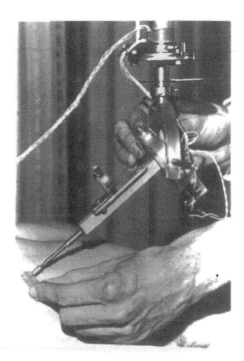

Figure 14 Photograph of the ALDI instrument applied on a point of a rib of a living subject in the position of alignment (see text).

from the chest wall, moved parallel to the transverse and vertical chest diameters as well as around the axis L of the ALDI until the "position of alignment" was achieved.

At the position of alignment the in-and-out movement of the shaft of the transducer (magnitude of vector S) and the angle $\hat{\varphi}$ were recorded while the angle $\hat{\vartheta}$ was read on the protractor of the ALDI. Recordings obtained at the position of alignment of the transducer with vector S on a point of several ribs are shown in Figure 15. Fifty-three ribs were examined in nine normal subjects (7 males and 2

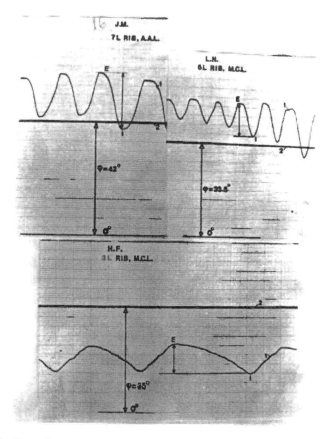

Figure 15   Recordings from a normal subject (J.M.) and two patients suffering from kyphoscoliosis (L.N.) and ankylosing spondylitis (H.F.). These recordings were taken when the transducer was aligned with the spatial vector S at a point on a rib. The wavy line represents the fluctuating output from the transducer. The difference between the expiratory (E) and the inspiratory (I) level of this line is the magnitude of the costal excursion at this point. The straight line shows the constant output from the J potentiometer. The distance between this line and the reference line (0° line) indicates the size of the angle $\hat{\varphi}$ at this point. The output from the potentiometer K is shown on the oscilloscope screen.

females) and 35 ribs in six patients (5 males and 1 female) suffering from kyphoscoliosis (3) and ankylosing spondylitis (3). The age of the normal subjects was between 20 and 33 year, while the age range of the patients was 16–56 years. Measurements were made at two or three points along the rib (2nd–9th) for one to six tidal breaths and in the lower end of sternum in six normal subjects, two patients with ankylosing spondylitis, and two patients with kyphoscoliosis. The results of the measurements of the inspiratory excursion of the ribs (vector S) and of the ratios Sg/S, St/S, and Sv/S in normal subjects and patients are shown in Tables 2 and 3 (Fig. 16). In normal subjects and in all patients the spatial vectors were parallel to each other along every rib, upper or lower (2nd–9th). Furthermore, in all the subjects studied except the patients with kyphoscoliosis, the vectors had an oblique direction anteriorwards, lateralwards, and upwards during inspiration and symmetrical in both hemithoraxes. The findings indicate that all of the ribs rotate around one axis only, which must be the rib-neck axis, since they are hinged to the transverse process of the vertebrae.

However, in some normal subjects or patients with predominant diaphragmatic respiration, it was noticed that the spatial vectors along the rib were parallel to each other to a certain inspiratory level. Beyond this level, towards the upper limit of the inspiratory capacity, the direction of the vectors showed a sharp deviation from the parallel position. The inspiratory level at which this deviation appeared showed

Table 2 Results from Normal Subjects and Patients with Ankylosing Spondylitis

Subjects	Sg/S		St/S		Sv/S		S (cm)	
	R	L	R	L	R	L	R	L
	Ribs							
Normal (N = 9)	0.80	0.80	0.30	0.31	0.49	0.50	1.11	1.09
	±0.07	±0.06	±0.09	±0.09	±0.09	±0.08	±0.43	±0.37
	n = 27	n = 26	n = 27	n = 26	n = 27	n = 26	n = 75	n = 88
	Lower end of sternum							
	0.86		0.00		0.48		0.76	
	Ribs							
Patients (N = 3)	0.89	0.86	0.19	0.24	0.41	0.43	0.56	0.51
	±0.04	±0.05	±0.08	±0.07	±0.05	±0.09	±0.18	±0.17
	n = 4	n = 11	n = 4	n = 11	n = 4	n = 11	n = 10	n = 30
	Lower end of sternum							
	0.93		0.00		0.38		0.58	

Values for the ratios Sg/S, St/S, Sv/S and for the vectors S are the mean ($\pm$ 1 SD) from all the ribs (2nd–9th), the costal points, and the tidal breaths, separately for the right (R) and the left hemithorax (L). N: Number of subjects, n: number of measurements (see text).

Table 3 Results from Three Patients with Kyphoscoliosis

Kyphoscoliosis	Rib	Sg/S	St/S	Sv/S	S (cm)
Predominant kyphotic element	4R	0.72	−0.04	0.69	0.38
	4L	0.71	−0.01	0.71	0.47
	7R	0.73	−0.01	0.68	0.40
	7L	0.77	0.00	0.64	0.30
	sternum lower end	0.77	0.00	0.64	0.55
Convexity towards left side	3R	0.94	0.21	0.27	1.10
	3L	0.78	0.31	0.55	1.00
	5R	0.93	0.23	0.29	0.60
	5L	0.77	0.17	0.61	1.03
	7R	0.71	0.42	0.57	0.63
	7L	0.84	0.18	0.50	0.45
	sternum lower end	0.68	0.00	0.73	0.55
Convexity towards right side	4R	0.94	−0.27	0.20	0.50
	4L	0.72	0.44	0.54	0.52
	5R	0.93	−0.31	0.20	0.55
	5L	0.69	0.44	0.57	0.68
	7R	0.87	−0.42	0.23	0.42
	7L	0.66	0.50	0.56	0.45

Values for the ratios Sg/S, St/S, Sv/S and for the vectors S are the mean from 2–3 points along the rib and from 1–3 tidal breaths (see text).

individual variation and depended on the velocity of the inspiratory excursion: with smooth inspiratory efforts the deviation appeared in higher inspiratory levels than with fast efforts. Presumably, this sudden change in the direction of the vectors along the rib was due to elastic deformity of the rib-vertebra system. The inspiratory excursion of the ribs (vector S) in ankylosing spondylitis and kyphoscoliosis is much shorter than in normal subjects. In patients with kyphoscoliosis the movement of the rib is rotational around the rib-neck axis. In these cases, the vertebrae are tilted so that the plane of the spatial vectors, and so the rib-neck axis, are shifted in relation to the rectangular system of the chest. In one patient with kyphoscoliosis and the kyphotic element predominant, the change in the transverse diameter was zero. In a patient with convexity towards the left side, the increase of the transverse diameter in the left hemithorax was smaller than in the right. The opposite happens in a patient with the convexity to the right side, in whom the transverse diameter is decreased in the right hemithorax and increased in the left. In this case, the

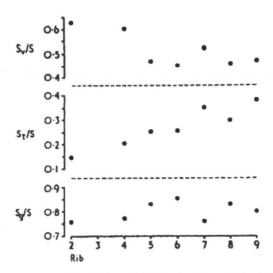

Figure 16   Mean values of Sg/S, St/S, and Sv/S ratios from all ribs (2nd–9th, except the 3rd) in normal subjects. It is evident that the St/S ratio is increased from the 2nd to the 9th rib. Below the 4th rib, the Sv/S ratio is decreased and the Sg/S ratio increased. These changes remain nearly constant from the 5th to the 9th rib.

sternum moves to the left side, while in all the other patients and in normal subjects the sternum moves forwards and upwards on the sagittal diameter during the inspiratory efforts.

VII.   Determination of the Dynamic Position of the Rib-Neck Axis and of the Inclination of the Ribs in Living Subjects

Since the rib rotates around the rib-neck axis, it is possible to calculate angles $\hat{d}$, $\hat{h}$, $(\hat{a} + \hat{b}/2)$ in living subjects if the ratios Sg/S, St/S, and Sv/S and the projection of the angle $\hat{d}$ on the frontal plane F (angle $\hat{d}F$) are known (Jordanoglou et al., 1972). Angle $\hat{d}F$ is related to angles $\hat{d}$ and $\hat{h}$ of the neck axis by:

$$\tan \hat{d}F = \tan \hat{d} \sin \hat{h} \qquad (11)$$

The diagrammatic representation of Eq. (11) is shown in Figure 17 (J. Jordanoglou, unpublished data). Angle $\hat{d}F$ was measured on an x-ray film of the dorsal region of the spinal column taken on the frontal plane of a body in the supine position. The vertical line through the middle of the vertebra and the line passing through the middle of the costocentral and the costotransverse articulations are the sides of angle $\hat{d}F$. The ratios Sg/S, St/S, and Sv/S were measured by the ALDI instrument as previously described. Then a computerized process was followed.

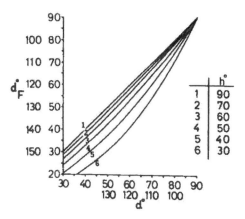

Figure 17 Diagrammatic representation of the tan $\hat{d}F$ = tan$\hat{d}$ sin$\hat{h}$ [Eq. (11)]. It is shown that for angle $\hat{d}F$ between 60° and 120°, the error of angle $\hat{d}$ is less than 5° for angle $\hat{h}$ 60°–90°.

The angle $(\hat{a} + \hat{b}/2)_1$ was calculated from angle $\hat{d}F$ and the Sv/S ratio according to Eq. (7). Angle $\hat{h}_1$ was computed from ratios Sg/S and St/S and angles $(\hat{a} + \hat{b}/2)_1$, and $\hat{d}F$. Angle $\hat{d}$ was then computed using Eq. (11) from angles $\hat{h}_1$ and $\hat{d}F$. This was the first loop. The second loop started from angle $\hat{d}_1$ and Sv/S for the calculation of $(\hat{a} + \hat{b}/2)_2$. Angle $\hat{h}_2$ was computed from ratios Sg/S and St/S and angles $(\hat{a} + \hat{b}/2)_2$ and $\hat{d}_1$. Angle $\hat{d}_2$ was computed from angles $\hat{d}_1$ and $\hat{h}_2$. By the end of each loop the computed angles $\hat{a} + \hat{b}/2$, $\hat{d}$, and $\hat{h}$ were used for the calculation of the ratios Sg/S, St/S, and Sv/S, which thereafter were compared to the measured values by the ALDI instrument. After a number of loops, the calculated ratios were equal to the measured ones. At that point, the computed angles $\hat{d}$, $\hat{h}$, and $\hat{a} + \hat{b}/2$ represented the dynamic angles at the considered position of the chest within the rectangular system.

   This method was used on the mechanical analogue of the rib-vertebra system and on living subjects. In the mechanical analogue the angles $\hat{d}$, $\hat{h}$, and $\hat{a} + \hat{b}/2$ were prede- termined in 10 combinations, for every one of which the ratios Sg/S, St/S, and Sv/S were measured using the ALDI instrument and the angle $\hat{d}F$ on an x-ray film. Angles $\hat{d}$, $\hat{h}$, and $\hat{a} + \hat{b}/2$ computed by the method of reiterated looping differed from the predetermined ones by less than $2.3°$ for angle $\hat{d}$, $3.2°$ for angle $\hat{a} + \hat{b}/2$, and $6.5°$ for angle $\hat{h}$ (unpublished data).

   This method was applied in five normal subjects lying supine on an adjustable table to measure the ratios Sg/S, St/S, and Sv/S with the ALDI instrument. At the same position of the body, angle $\hat{d}F$ was measured on the x-ray film as previously described (Table 4) (Fig. 18) (unpublished data). The results showed that (1) angle $\hat{d}F$ is very close to angle $\hat{d}$, (2) angles $\hat{d}$, $\hat{h}$, and $\hat{a} + \hat{b}/2$ were nearly the same in both hemithoraxes, (3) angle, $\hat{a} + \hat{b}/2$ remained nearly the same in all of the ribs (2nd–9th), (4) angle $\hat{h}$ increased and angle $\hat{d}$ decreased from the 2nd to the 9th rib,

Table 4 Values of Dynamic Angles $\hat{d}$, $\hat{h}$, and $\hat{a} + \hat{b}/2$ (in degrees) at the Supine Position of the Body Computed by the Reiterated Looping Method

Normal Subjects	Rib	$\hat{dF}$	$\hat{d}$	$\hat{h}$	$\hat{a} + \hat{b}/2$
1	2R	112.5	110.7	65.5	42.9
	2L	107.5	106.3	68.5	41.8
	7R	95	94.6	67.3	34.1
	7L	91	91	66.5	40.3
2	4R	106	105.1	71	37.1
	4L	110	108	63	22
	7R	97.5	97	69.5	30.7
	7L	107.0	105.6	66	30.2
3	5R	97	97	61.5	27
	7R	98	97.8	67.5	30.8
4	2R	131	121.8	49	50.1
	2L	129	121.6	45	50.8
	6R	72	72	88	39.2
	6L	74	74	87	33.6
5	2R	112	108.5	56	42.5
	2L	105	103.7	67	25.4
	5R	85	85	83	35.9
	5L	88.5	88.5	79	27.8
	7R	72	72	83	38.3
	7L	75	75	78	31.5
	9R	56	56	88	38.8
	9L	64	64.9	73	31

Calculated Sg/S, St/S, Sv/S ratios from the computed angles $\hat{d}$, $\hat{h}$, $\hat{a} + \hat{b}/2$ differed from measured ones (by ALDI) by less than 0.5%.

and (5) there was a distinct difference between the computed angle and the angle measured statically on anatomical preparation of the dorsal vertebrae (Table 5).

This difference between the anatomical and the dynamic values of angle $\hat{h}$ is due to the transposition of each dorsal vertebra and so of the rib-neck axis mainly around a transverse axis (or even sagittal and/or vertical axis) in living subjects. The transposition of the thoracic vertebrae significantly affects not only angle $\hat{h}$ but also the angles $\hat{d}$ and $\hat{a} + \hat{b}/2$.

This method of calculating angles $\hat{d}$, $\hat{h}$, and $\hat{a} + \hat{b}/2$ from ratios Sg/S, St/S, and Sv/S and angle $\hat{dF}$ may be used in clinical practice if it is necessary to follow up patients with deformities or injuries of the spinal column or of the thoracic wall.

VIII. Summary

A review of references about rib movement shows that there is no agreement about which axes are used in the movement of the different ribs or about how rib movement

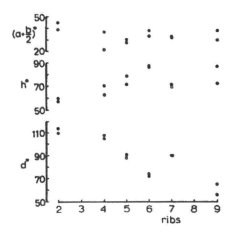

Figure 18 Diagram showing the mean values of angles d̂, ĥ and â + b̂/2 in five normal subjects lying supine measured by the method of reiterated computing from the ratios Sg/S, St/S, and Sv/S and the angle dF. It is evident that angle â + b̂/2 remains nearly constant in all of the ribs, angle ĥ increases, while angle d̂ decreases from the 2nd to the 9th rib. (●) Right side; (○) left side.

is related to the change in length of the thoracic diameters. Costal movement is defined in living subjects by determining the spatial vectors along the ribs produced during inspiration. The determination of these spatial vectors is achieved by an instrument specially designed for this purpose, which can be aligned with the rectangular system of the chest and with the spatial vectors of the ribs. This ALDI instrument permits simultaneous recording of linear and angular displacements. Its

Table 5 Value of the Angle Formed by the Transverse Process of the Dorsal Vertebra and the Sagittal Diameter[a] and of the Angle ĥ[b] (in degrees)

Thoracic vertebra	Trendelenburg, 1779	Meissner, 1857	Volkmann, 1876	Fick, 1911	v. Hayek, 1960	Dynamic angle ĥ on living subjects lying supine, 1975
2	55	34	64	55	70	47–67
4	38	25	55.5	50	50	67
5	41	24	54	48	45	62–81
6	42.5	22.5	54.5	48	45	88
7	43.3	21	54.5	44	45	71
9	47	19	46	40	45	81

[a]Measured statically in anatomical preparations.
[b]Measured dynamically.

function is checked experimentally using a mechanical analogue simulating the rib-vertebra system.

On the basis of the rotational movement of the ribs around the neck axis, a theoretical analysis was developed showing the factors affecting the amount of costal movement and the change in length of the chest diameter during smooth inspiration. These factors are the radial distance of the point of the rib from the neck axis, the elevation angle of the rib, the inclination angle of the rib at the considered point, and the angles that the neck axis forms with the sagittal and vertical diameters. This theory was validated by measuring the vector S and the ratios Sg/S, St/S, and Sv/S using the ALDI instrument at several predetermined values of angles $\hat{d}$, $\hat{h}$, and $\hat{a}$ + $\hat{b}$/2 and of the radius R. The calculated values of these ratios from theoretical equations coincided with the ones measured using the ALDI instrument.

Rib movement was studied on 53 ribs in 9 normal subjects and 35 ribs in 6 patients suffering from kyphoscoliosis and ankylosing spondylitis. It was shown that all of the ribs (2nd–9th) in normal subjects during smooth inspiration rotated around their own rib-neck axes and not around other axes that have been postulated. The direction of the inspiratory movement of the ribs was oblique, upwards, outwards, and forwards and was symmetrical in both hemithoraxes. In patients with ankylosing spondylitis and kyphoscoliosis, rib movement was no different from that of normal subjects. In such patients, rib movement was restricted as compared with that in normal subjects. Moreover, in kyphoscoliosis, the vertebrae were tilted so that the neck axis and consequently the plane of rotation of the ribs relative to the three cardinal planes of the chest was shifted.

A computerized reiterative method permitted the calculation of the angles of the neck axis $(\hat{d},\hat{h})$ and of the inclination of the rib $(\hat{a} + \hat{b}/2)$ within the rectangular system of the chest from the ratios Sg/S, St/S, and Sv/S measured using the ALDI instrument and from the projection of the angle $\hat{d}$ on the frontal plane $(\hat{d}F)$ on an x-ray film of the dorsal region of the spinal column. This method was tested on a mechanical analogue and used with living subjects for calculating the dynamic values of these angles. The dynamic values of the angles $\hat{d}$, $\hat{h}$, and $\hat{a}$ +$\hat{b}$/2 were dependent on the relative position of the dorsal vertebrae within the cardinal chest planes, i.e., on the curvature of the dorsal region of the spinal column at several positions of the body. The dynamic angles $\hat{d}$ and $\hat{h}$ of the dorsal vertebrae are different from the static angles measured in anatomical preparations.

The methodology used for the measurement of Sg/S, St/S, and Sv/S and of the dynamic values of angles $\hat{d}$, $\hat{h}$, and $\hat{a}$ + $\hat{b}$/2 may be of clinical use in the investigation of patients suffering from disease or injuries of the thoracic cage or of the spinal column.

Acknowledgment

I am grateful to M. Melea for her excellent secretarial work.

References

Agostoni, E. (1964). Action of respiratory muscles. In *Handbook of Physiology-Respiration*. Vol. I. Edited by W. O. Fenn, H. Rahn. Washington D.C., American Physiological Society.

Barlow, T. E. (1949). *Buchanan's Manual of Anatomy*. Edited by F. W. Jones. 8th ed. London, Bailliere, Tindall and Cox.

Campbell, E. J. M., (1958). *The Respiratory Muscles and the Mechanics of Breathing*. London, Lloyd-Luke.

Carlson, L. D., (1961). Anatomy and physics of respiration. In *Medical Physiology and Biophysics*. 18th ed. Edited by T. C. Ruch and J. F. Fulton. Philadelphia, W.B. Saunders Co.

Cunningham, D. J. (1951). *Textbook of Anatomy*. 9th ed. Edited by J. C. Brash. London, Geoffrey Cumberlege, Oxford University Press.

Da Vinci, L. (1452–1519). Quaderni d' Anatomia I. Publicati da Vangensten, Fonahn, Hopstock.

Duchenne, G. B. (1949). *Physiology of Motion, Demonstrated by Means of Electrical Stimulation and Clinical Observation and Applied to the study of Paralysis and Deformities*. Translated by E. B. Kaplan. Philadelphia, J.B. Lippincott Co.

Felix, W. (1928). Topographische Anatomie des Brustkorbes, der Lunge und der Pleura. In *Sauerbruch's Chirurgie der Brustorganne*. Bd. I. Berlin.

Fick, R. (1911). *Handbuch der Anatomie und Mechanik der Gelenke*. Jena,.

Fraser, J. E., and Robbin, R. H. (1937). *Manual of Practical Anatomy*. London, Bailliere, Tindall and Cox.

Fulton, J. F. (1955). *A Textbook of Physiology*. 17th ed. Philadelphia, W.B. Saunders Co.

Galen, (1962). *Galen on Anatomical Procedures*. Translated by W. L. H. Duckworth. Edited by M. C. Lyons and B. Towers. Cambridge, Cambridge University Press.

Ganong, W. F. (1965). *Review of Medical Physiology*. Oxford, Blackwell Scientific Publications.

Grant, J. C. B. (1952). *A Method of Anatomy, Descriptive and Deductive*. 5th ed. London, Bailliere, Tindall and Cox Ltd.

Grant, J. C. B., and Basmajian, J. V. (1965). *Grant's Method of Anatomy*. 7th ed. Edinburgh, E. and S. Livingstone Ltd.

Gray, H. (1950). *Anatomy of the Human Body*. 25th ed. Edited by C. Mayo Goss. Philadelphia, Lea and Febiger.

Hayek, von H. (1960). *The Human Lung*. Translated by V. E. Krahl. New York, Hafner Publishing Co., Inc.

Hoover, C. F. (1922). The function and integration of the intercostal muscles. *Arch. Int. Med.*, 30:I.

Jordanoglou, J. (1967). Rib movement and its effect on thoracic dimensions in health and disease. Ph.D. thesis, London University.

Jordanoglou, J. (1969). Rib movement in health, kyphoscoliosis and ankylosing spondylitis. *Thorax*, 24:407–414.

Jordanoglou, J. (1970). Vector analysis of rib movement. *Respir. Physiol.*, 10:109–120.

Jordanoglou, J., and Smith, L. (1970). A new instrument for measuring rib movement. *J. Appl. Physiol.*, 28:501–504.

Jordanoglou, J., Kontos, J., and Gardikas, C. (1972). Relative position of the rib within the chest and its determination on living subjects with the aid of a computer program. *Respir. Physiol.*, 16:41.

Hutchinson, J. (1852). Thorax. In *Todd's Cyclop. Anat. Physiol.* Vol. IV. London Longman, Brown, Green, Longmans and Roberts, p. 1017.

Keith, A. (1909). The mechanism of respiration in man. In *Further Advances in Phyiology*. Edited by L. Hill, London, E. Arnold.

Landerer, A. (1881). Ueber die Athembewegungen des Thorax. Leipzig, Verlag von Veit and Co.

Last, R. J. (1959). *Anatomy Regional and Applied*. 2nd ed. London, J. and A. Churchill Ltd.

Luciani, L. (1911). *Human Physiology. Circulation and Respiration*. Vol. I. Translated by F. A. Welby, edited by M. Camis. London, MacMillan and Co. Ltd.

Magendie, F. (1931). *Elementary Compendium of Physiology for the Use of Students.* Translated by E. Milligan. Edinburgh.

Sinclair, D. (1961). *An Introduction to Functional Anatomy.* 2nd ed. Oxford, Blackwell Scientific Publication.

Steindler, A. (1935). *Mechanics of Normal and Pathological Locomotion in Man.* London, Bailliere, Tindall and Cox.

Thane, G. D. (1892). Arthrology, myology. In *Quain's Elements of Anatomy.* Vol. II. 10th ed. Edited by E. A. Schafer and G. D. Thane. Longmans, Green and Co.

Vesalius, A. First public Anatomy at Bologna. An eyewitness report by Baldasar Heseler together with his notes on Matthaeus Curtius' lectures on Anatomia Mundini. Edited with introduction, translation into English and notes by R. Eriksson.

Werenskiold, B. (1938). *Ueber Bau und Funktion der Rippenhockergelenke.* Oslo, Skrifter Utgitt Av Det Norske Videnskaps-Akademi.

38

Pressures Developed by the Respiratory Muscles

MARC DECRAMER

Katholieke Universiteit Leuven
Leuven, Belgium

PETER T. MACKLEM

Respiratory Health Network of
  Centres of Excellence
McGill University
Montreal, Quebec, Canada

I. Introduction

In a mechanical apparatus such as the respiratory system, where motion is transduced into volume, forces are expressed in terms of pressure. Contraction of respiratory muscles essentially causes pressures in the respiratory system to change, and consequently lung volume to alter. Pressures thus produce the mechanical outcome of respiratory muscle contraction and are, in combination with volume and flow, commonly used to estimate the mechanical properties of the respiratory system (1,2). Several pressures may be measured. First, the pressure across the whole respiratory system, transrespiratory pressure (P_{rs}), is measured as the pressure at the airway opening (P_{ao}) relative to that at the surface of the body. The former is measured through measurement of mouth pressures (3–13), nasal pressure, or nasopharyngeal pressure (11,14).

Second, one can measure the pressure difference across the chest wall (P_{cw}). This is accomplished in practice by measurement of pleural pressure, usually measured by means of esophageal pressure (P_{es}) relative to body surface pressure (15–21). Transpulmonary pressure (P_L) is the difference between airway opening pressure and pleural pressure (P_{pl}) and reflects the mechanical properties of the lung. Third, abdominal pressure (P_{ab}) is the pressure within the abdominal cavity and is usually measured by means of gastric pressure (P_{ga}) (22–25) or less commonly as rectal pressure (26,27). Finally, the difference between P_{ab} and P_{pl} is called transdiaphragmatic pressure (P_{di}) and gives the pressure difference across the diaphragm (22,24). These pressures are schematically represented in Figure 1.

In general, these pressures give the mechanical outcome of respiratory muscle contraction as a whole. Measurement of the pressure developed by individual respiratory muscles with the exception of the diaphragm is less straightforward, because it involves assumptions or data on how the different muscles mechanically interact with one another. The present chapter will primarily focus on the measurements of pressures in normal humans and patients.

II. Methodology

Pressures are now generally measured using differential pressure transducers. Several devices are used to transmit pressure to the transducer, including balloon-catheter systems, liquid-filled catheters, needles, etc. Alternatively, pressures may be measured in situ with minitransducers. In addition, pressures may also be inferred

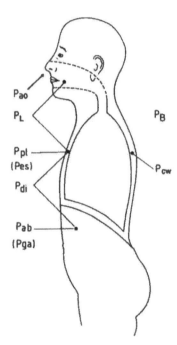

Figure 1 Schematic diagram illustrating the relevant pressures. P_{ao} = airway opening pressure; P_L = transpulmonary pressure; P_{pl} = pleural pressure; P_{es} = esophageal pressure; P_{di} = transdiaphragmatic pressure; P_{ab} = abdominal pressure; P_{ga} = gastric pressure; P_{cw} = transthoracic pressure; P_B = barometric pressure.

from indirect measurements. Each of these procedures is associated with particular methodological problems which are briefly discussed here.

A. Balloon-Catheter Systems

In respiratory physiology it is customary to measure surface pressures by means of balloon-catheter systems (16,17,28). Pressures usually measured with this system are P_{es} and P_{ga}. Each of these pressure measurements is susceptible to particular potential artifacts. When an esophageal or gastric balloon is put in place it should be empty to minimize risks of tears. The chances that the balloon will become wrapped and folded around the enclosed catheter are substantial. Therefore, it is a recommended procedure to fill the balloon fully to untwist it while it is in place and then to withdraw air from it until it is at the desired volume.

Esophageal Pressure

Measurement of P_{pl} by means of P_{es} was introduced by Luciani (1878) (29) and Buytendijk (1949) (15) and further developed by Mead and Milic-Emili (1,18,20) and Fry (28). Several factors potentially affect the measurement.

Balloon Volume

The effects of the volume of air in the balloon on the pressure recorded were extensively studied by Milic-Emili (2,18). In general, care must be taken to perform measurements in the range of volume in which the rubber remains unstretched, but with increasing balloon volume distortion of the measured pressure is increased due to the elastance of the esophagus. The use of esophageal pressure to estimate pleural pressure assumes that there is no pressure difference across the wall of the esophagus. However, if the esophagus is distended by a large balloon volume, esophageal elastance results in a finite pressure difference where esophageal pressure is more positive than pleural pressure. Therefore, a minimal balloon volume is desirable. However, the balloon volume must not be so small that the pressure within the balloon is less than the pressure outside it. In order for the balloon catheter system to be accurate, there must be no pressure difference across either the balloon or the esophageal wall.

Furthermore, along the length of the balloon there may be substantial pressure differences where the esophagus abuts the posterior surface of the heart. The effect of the heart on esophageal pressure will almost certainly be to increase it. A small bubble in a long balloon will automatically migrate to the point along the length of the balloon where the pressure is most negative. This concept results in conflicting demands for accuracy.

Short balloons require smaller volumes of air so that the pressure difference across them is zero. However, the possibility that the pressure they measure will be affected by the heart increases. Longer balloons will tend to avoid cardiac artifacts but require larger volumes, which will increase the effects of esophageal elastance.

There is no agreement about optimal balloon length. The recommended length is 10 cm if the balloon is extremely compliant and if an accurate estimate of P_{pl} is required. However, if one is only interested in changes in P_{pl}, 5-cm-long balloons are adequate.

Measurements are usually made with minimal balloon volume, which is usually about 0.4–0.6 ml for esophageal pressure measurement for a 5-cm-long balloon. In measurement of positive pressures more air in the balloon may be required depending upon the compressibility of air and the volume displacement coefficient of the balloon-catheter system.

Balloon Dimensions and Position

Balloon perimeter is usually chosen to be equal to or slightly smaller than esophageal perimeter (3.2–3.5 cm) (2,30). Balloon length is usually chosen to be 5 cm. The simplest way to verify balloon position is by using a dynamic occlusion test (Fig. 2). During an occluded inspiratory effort, the change in transpulmonary pressure is zero because there is only a neligible change in lung volume. If the measured esophageal pressure accurately reflects the average change in pleural pressure, it will not change relative to mouth pressure (2,30). Consequently, the balloon should be positioned in a site where no change in transpulmonary pressure during an occluded effort is present. This corresponds to the midesophagus. This method has been studied in humans in different body positions (30), in anesthetized humans (31), in chronic obstructive pulmonary disease (COPD) patients in acute respiratory failure (32), and in neonates (33). In COPD patients in whom transmission of alveolar pressure to the mouth is problematic, this method cannot be used, since the method basically assumes that mouth pressure correctly reflects alveolar pressure. When the balloon records positive pressures, as during forced expiration, the compliance of the balloon-catheter-transducer system (volume-displacement coefficient) must be sufficiently low so that the air in the balloon is not totally displaced.

Catheter Dimensions

Catheter dimensions are important as well, since they mainly determine the frequency characteristics of the balloon-catheter system. Ideally the catheter has an internal diameter of 1.4 mm (PE 200) and a length of 100 cm. Such a system usually has a flat frequency response up to 10 Hz, which is adequate for most respiratory maneuvers (34). Better frequency characteristics may be required in neonates or when measurements at high frequencies are performed (35).

Abdominal Pressure

Abdominal pressure is usually determined through measurement of gastric pressure with balloons similar to those used for measurement of esophageal pressure. The balloon is filled with 1 ml of air, since usually positive pressure variations are being measured. Balloons float on top of the stomach bubble, and if the air-liquid interface

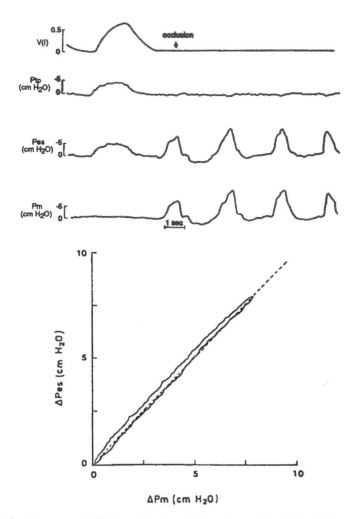

Figure 2 (Upper panel) Volume (V), transpulmonary pressure (P_{tp}), esophageal pressure (P_{es}), and mouth pressure (P_m) during a dynamic occlusion test. (Lower panel) P_{es} vs. P_m for the first occluded inspiratory effort in upper panel. (From Ref. 30.)

moves vertically during breathing the balloon may move up and down a hydrostatic gradient and record pressures unrelated to elastic, frictional, or inertial factors. The magnitude of this artifact has never been quantified. Pressure changes in the abdomen are generally considered to be uniform (25), although under some conditions marked inhomogeneity of abdominal pressure swings may be present (23). The latter inhomogeneity, although conceptually important, is only of limited significance in clinical measurement of gastric pressure since with coordinated respiratory muscle contractions abdominal pressure swings are fairly homogeneous (27). Regional differences can be of clinical importance, however, in the diagnosis of unilateral diaphragmatic paralysis, when inspiratory differences in subcostal displacement and pressure can be observed and palpated.

B. Liquid-Filled Catheters

The disadvantage of this method is the difficulty in obtaining absolute pressures, whereas its advantage is the better frequency response such that smaller catheters may be used. Consequently, the method is frequently used in neonates (36,37). Coates et al. (38) also demonstrated the validity of liquid-filled catheters for the measurement of esophageal pressure in preterm neonates with important chest wall distortion.

C. Minitransducers

These devices placed in the esophagus are commonly used by gastroenterologists (39) to record esophageal pressure waves. They are not usually used by respirologists. Measurement of transdiaphragmatic pressure was performed by these devices (40), as well as measurement of esophageal pressure in supine anesthetized humans (41). Minitransducers were also used to measure intramuscular pressure in the diaphragm (42) and in the parasternal intercostals (43). In the parasternal intercostals intramuscular pressure was related to the tension developed by these muscles, whereas in the diaphragm pleural and abdominal pressures applied to the muscle were the main determinants of intramuscular pressure. Presently available techniques, however, do not allow intramuscular pressure measurements to be made in humans. Transducer-tipped catheters have the advantage over balloons in that they measure pressure at a highly specified local site. Unlike balloons, they do not choose a site where local artifacts, which tend to lead to an overestimate in pressure (e.g., the esophagus), are minimized.

D. Inferring Pressures

Several methods have been developed that do not actually measure pressure, but infer it with a reasonable degree of accuracy. Alveolar pressure may be inferred from pressure changes measured inside a constant volume whole body plethysmograph. Pressures have also been inferred from observed pressure-displacement curves and estimated from model predictions (44–46). First, Macklem et al. (44) developed a model of inspiratory muscle mechanics taking into account the previously demonstrated difference between the actions of the costal and crural diaphragms on the rib cage (47,48). This model separated P_{di} into two hypothetical pressures: $P_{di,cos}$ and $P_{di,cru}$. The model, however, views the rib cage as a unitary structure, not being deformable such that pressures acting on the rib cage would be additive. Since subsequent experimental work refuted this thesis (46,49), Macklem's group developed a new model taking into account rib cage distortability (46).

The mechanical and electrical analogs are shown in Figures 3 and 4, respectively. The rib cage is divided into two compartments: a lung-apposed part, the pulmonary rib cage, and a diaphragm-apposed part, the abdominal rib cage. Pressure balance equations across the latter model allow the inference of another pressure with physiological meaning: P_{link}, or the pressure linking the two parts of the rib cage. Second, within the framework of the same model analysis, observation of the relationship between gastric pressure and rib cage cross-sectional area allows the determination of the insertional component of transdiaphragmatic pressure. Indeed, during relaxation the relationship between rib cage dimensions, measured in the area of apposition and gastric pressure, gives the relaxation characteristics of the abdominal rib cage, since these rib cage dimensions are determined by P_{ab}. Indeed, under these circumstances the diaphragm is not contracting and only the effects of P_{ab} on the rib cage are present. With diaphragmatic contraction and an inspiration in which there is no rib cage distortion and $P_{link} = 0$, both the insertional component and the appositional component of its action move the abdominal rib cage. Assuming that the appositional component equals the effects of gastric pressure during relaxation, an assumption being entirely reasonable, the difference between

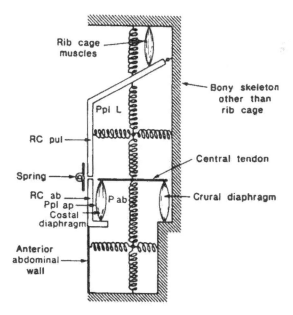

Figure 3 Mechanical model of the rib cage showing rib cage muscles, elastic properties of the respiratory system, and agencies acting to displace and distort rib cage. $P_{pl,L}$ = pressure at the inner surface of the rib cage; RCpul = lung-apposed rib cage; RCab = abdomen-apposed rib cage; $P_{pl,ap}$ = pleural pressure in the zone of apposition. (From Ref. 46.)

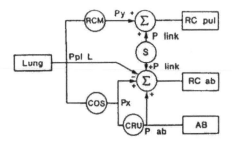

Figure 4 Hydraulic or electric analog of mechanical model represented in Figure 3. RCM = rib cage muscles; COS = costal diaphragm; CRU = crural diaphragm; AB = abdomen; S = spring linking the two rib cage compartments. Circles containing Σ represent summing junctions. Other circles represent pressure or voltage generators. Rectangles represent structures that are displaced. (From Ref. 46.)

the rib cage dimensions and gastric pressure relationship in the two conditions gives the insertional component of transdiaphragmatic pressure. This procedure is illustrated in Figure 5.

Recently, a new method for inference of pressure has been applied to the quadriceps (50), the biceps brachii (51), the adductor pollicis (52), the erector spinae (53), and the diaphragm (54). The method consists in recording the pressure signal produced by muscular contraction by means of a microphone. The technique is called phonomyography. The origin of the sound signal produced during

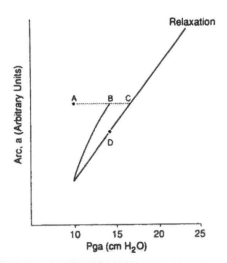

Figure 5 Relationship between gastric pressure P_{ga} and $A_{rc,a}$ during relaxation and during inspiration while actively maintaining an undistorted rib cage. The insertional component of P_{di} is given by distance BC. (From Ref. 46.)

contraction is still unclear, although the signal appears to be related with force oscillation, rather than with absolute force. The integrated myography signal is related to the force produced during maximal voluntary contraction in a linear or quadratic fashion.

During stimulation it decreased with increasing stimulation frequency, while force increased, signaling that the measured signal is no unequivocal measure of the tension or force developed. During phrenic nerve stimulation a linear relationship between twitch P_{di} and the integrated phonomyogram was present (54) (Fig. 6), suggesting that the technique has the potential to provide a noninvasive measure of P_{di}. More study is needed to validate the latter concept.

Efforts also have been made to infer pleural pressure from a noninvasive measurement—surface inductive plethysmography (55,56). This is based on the presumptive relationship between suprasternal fossa retraction and the fall in pleural pressure during inspiration. The method is promising, potentially interesting, but requires more extensive validation to be used routinely.

III. Pressure Measurements During Quiet and Supratidal Breathing

A. Pleural Pressure

During inspiration from the equilibrium volume of the respiratory system, pleural pressure falls, and its magnitude reflects the effort made by the inspiratory muscles. During quiet breathing in humans the combined action of inspiratory muscles is responsible for the fall in pleural pressure. It is difficult to distinguish the

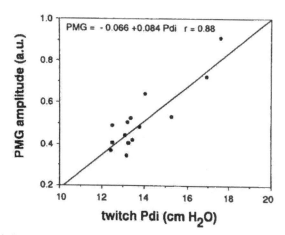

Figure 6 Relationship between integrated phonomyogram signal and twitch P_{di} in normal subjects. (From Ref. 54.)

diaphragmatic contribution from the contribution of other inspiratory muscles such as the parasternal intercostals and the scalenes (57).

When expiration is active so that the end-expiratory V_L is below functional residual capacity (FRC), expiratory muscle relaxation at the onset of inspiration may contribute to the fall in pleural pressure. This occurs in supine anesthetized dogs and in normal humans during exercise and CO_2 rebreathing (58–61). Often a phase lag between inspiratory and expiratory muscle activation is present such that the fall in pleural pressure is achieved in two distinct phases. The initial fall in pleural pressure then represents the contribution of expiratory muscles, whereas the fall later on in inspiration represents the contribution of inspiratory muscles. A tracing illustrating these events is shown in Figure 7. We recently demonstrated in supine anesthetized dogs that aminophylline administration clearly enhanced this first phase of inspiration and, hence, the contribution of expiratory muscles (60).

The fall in pleural pressure during inspiration may be used as an index of the effort produced by the respiratory muscles during breathing by calculating the product of the mean fall in pleural pressure and the fractional duration of inspiration (T_I/T_{TOT}). This is called a pressure-time product and is related to the load on the respiratory muscles during inspiration (62–64). It may also allow quantification of the load during incremental exercise testing (65). It should be realized, however, that this measure is very imprecise because it only takes into account the pressures developed by the respiratory system to inflate the lungs and ignores those required to displace the abdomen and the rib cage as well as the pressure required to produce the chest wall distortion that occurs even during quiet breathing and to a much greater extent during hyperventilation.

B. Gastric Pressure

During quiet inspiration gastric pressure increases due to diaphragmatic contraction. This has at least two immediate consequences. First, the inspiratory rise in gastric

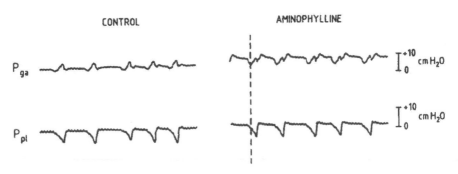

Figure 7   Tracing showing P_{ga} and P_{pl} during breathing before (left) and after administration of aminophylline. Dashed line indicates the onset of the second phase of inspiration.

pressure is expected to be dependent upon diaphragmatic action, and hence its magnitude is expected to be reduced with reduced diaphragmatic function. This is the case (66). In patients and dogs with diaphragm paralysis, gastric pressure falls during inspiration (67–70). In patients with unilateral diaphragm paralysis inspiratory gastric pressure swings are on average clearly reduced such that the inspiratory rise in gastric pressure is abolished (71). However, in these circumstances there should be substantial gradients in P_{ab} (23,72). These have been detected clinically (but not quantified) as a visual asymmetry between subcostal abdominal displacements, which are less on the ipsilateral side with a decrease in palpable increase in P_{ab} during inspiration on that side.

In supine anesthetized dogs and in humans during exercise and CO_2 breathing (61,73), the rise in gastric pressure is often preceded by a fall (Fig. 7). This fall represents the relaxation of abdominal muscles and may be used to quantify the latter.

C. Transdiaphragmatic Pressure

The measurement of P_{di} by Agostoni and Rahn (22) was a major scientific breakthrough in respiratory mechanics. The P_{di} swing during tidal breathing represents the force exerted by the diaphragm during tidal breathing. As a consequence, this swing is usually zero in patients with bilateral diaphragm paralysis (74). The ratio of P_{di} developed during a breath to maximal P_{di} reflects the force reserve of the diaphragm. If this ratio exceeds 40% with a duty cycle of 0.4–0.5, diaphragmatic fatigue ensues (75). Roussos and Macklem (75) were the first to propose a tension-time index for the diaphragm that would delimit a degree of effort above which the diaphragm would become fatigued and below which it would not. This was done rigorously in the sense that the physiological conditions under which the tension-time index [equivalent to the one later published by Bellemare and Grassino (62)] was valid were specified.

Patients with COPD might be close to their fatigue threshold because of a reduced force reserve (63). As a consequence they might approach their fatigue threshold during quiet breathing (76). Pourriat et al. (77) demonstrated that the ratio P_{di}/P_{dimax} had some value in predicting weaning outcome. Values below 0.35 were predictive of successful weaning, whereas values above 0.45 were indicative of weaning failure.

D. Pleural Pressure–Gastric Pressure Diagram

This diagram is based upon the fact that P_{ab} drives the relaxed chest wall while pleural pressure is responsible for lung volume changes. During relaxation, therefore, $P_{ab} = V_L/C_W$ and $P_L = V_L/C_L$. The slope of the relationship during relaxation is therefore $P_L/P_{ab} = C_W/C_L$. To the extent that this slope is greater during quiet breathing than during relaxation, the measured change in P_{ab} is insufficient to account for the chest wall displacement. This pressure, therefore, must come from another source, namely, the inspiratory muscles of the rib cage, which do not produce an increase in P_{ab}. Indeed, in contrast to the diaphragm, these muscles when contracting in isolation produce a decrease in P_{ab}. Therefore the greater the ratio $-P_{pl}/P_{ab}$ during inspiration, the greater the contribution of the inspiratory rib cage muscles. There are, however, specific limitations in the use of this relationship (78).

This diagram has been used extensively to infer the relative contributions of the diaphragm and the rib cage muscles to respiratory efforts (78–80). Originally it was claimed that the diagram allowed quantification of the contribution of the diaphragm and the intercostal/accessory muscles, respectively. This is not the case for a variety of reasons. First, an implicit assumption in the original analysis is that the diaphragm displaced the rib cage along its passive P_{ab}-rib cage volume or V_{rc} relationship. If so, Müller's maneuver performed solely with the diaphragm should produce an equal inflating force on both rib cage and abdomen so that neither compartment would be displaced. Macklem et al. (78), however, showed that a Müller's maneuver without chest wall configuration change required activation of the rib cage muscles. Furthermore, diaphragmatic contraction alone causes important rib cage distortion (46,49). Second, during diaphragmatic contraction part of the P_{di} developed acts on the rib cage such that the rib cage muscles do not generate all of the pressure acting on the rib cage (46,81,82). Third, the complexity of diaphragmatic anatomy and action (23,44,46–48) also renders the analysis overly simple.

Although original assumptions underlying the analysis have now been largely refuted, plotting P_{pl} vs. P_{ga} during respiratory maneuvers is still a very useful approach in analyzing the contributions of the diaphragm and the rib cage muscles. The procedure is briefly as follows. First, the relationship between P_L and P_{ga} is obtained during a relaxed expiration from total lung capacity (TLC) to FRC. At FRC with the diaphragm relaxed, $P_L = 5$ cm H_2O, $P_{pl} = -5$ cm H_2O, and $P_{ga} = \sim 5$ cm H_2O. The difference between the two is 10 cm H_2O, which Agostini and Rahn (22) attributed to hydrostatic effects and the pressure across the wall of the stomach. They assumed, as have most others since, that at upright FRC, $P_{di} = 0$. Once the relationship between P_L and P_{ga} is established during relaxation, P_{pl} and P_{ga} are recorded during respiratory maneuvers and referred to this relaxation line (Fig. 8). A loop shifting to the left in this diagram indicates a breath with a relatively important contribution of the rib cage muscles, whereas a loop shifting to the right signals recruitment of the diaphragm. Quiet breathing in upright humans occurs close to the relaxation line. The information obtained in this P_{pl}–P_{ga} diagram is similar to the information obtained in a Konno-Mead diagram, which plots rib cage dimensions vs. abdominal dimensions (83). However, inferring contributions of specific muscle groups from the latter diagram is not straightforward because of the complexity of muscle action on the rib cage and because inspiratory rib cage muscle and abdominal muscle recruitment have the same actions on the relative displacements of rib cage and abdomen, whereas they have opposite effects on P_{ga}.

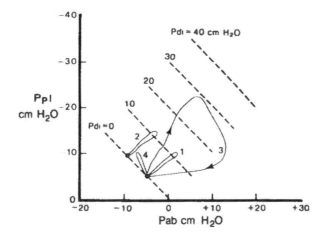

Figure 8 Pleural pressure–abdominal pressure relationships for a variety of different breaths. Loop 1 = quiet breathing; loop 2 = breath starting from an increased end-expiratory lung volume; loop 3 = breath starting with recruitment of rib cage muscles, followed by diaphragmatic recruitment; loop 4 = breath predominantly taken with intercostal muscles. Relaxation line coincides with the loop during quiet breathing. (From Ref. 79.)

Similarly, the displacement of the end-expiratory position in these diagrams provides information on recruitment of expiratory muscles. Indeed, with expiratory muscle recruitment both end-expiratory P_{pl} and P_{ga} increase, and P_{di} increases due to passive stretching of the diaphragm. Such patterns have been observed in humans during exercise (84).

E. Occlusion Pressures

Measurement of the mouth pressure developed 100 ms after airway occlusion has been used as a measurement of ventilatory drive (85,86). Although it is independent of the mechanical properties of the lung, it is highly dependent on the contractile state of the inspiratory muscles, their degree, and velocity of shortening, all of which are uncontrolled variables. Furthermore, if inspiration starts from below the equilibrium lung volume, relaxation of the expiratory muscles alone will result in a value of $P_{0.1}$, which depends upon the ratio of the difference between FRC and the volume at the beginning of inspiration and respiratory system compliance. In this instance $P_{0.1}$ represents expiratory, not inspiratory, drive. In addition, the measurement is dependent upon the transmission of alveolar pressure to the mouth (32,87). However, it is a better estimate of ventilatory drive than, e.g., minute ventilation. In normal subjects it is about 1 cm H_2O, whereas in patients with acute respiratory failure values as high as 10 cm H_2O have been obtained (88).

Similarly, P_{di} 100 ms after occlusion may be measured, reflecting the neural drive to the diaphragm (88). This index is evidently influenced by diaphragmatic shortening, velocity of shortening, and strength as well. Nevertheless, occlusion pressures have been shown to be useful in predicting weaning outcome. In one study, weaning from mechanical ventilation was successful in 78% of the patients with $P_{0.1} < 4.2$ cm H_2O, whereas 89% of cases with $P_{0.1}$ above this limit failed to wean (89). Similar results were obtained in two other studies in which patients with $P_{0.1}$ below 6 cm H_2O were weaned, whereas those with values above this limit failed to wean (90,91). This predictive value of $P_{0.1}$ was, however, not found in all studies (77).

IV. Pressure Measurements During Maximal Voluntary Contraction

A. Mouth Pressure

It is customary in clinical practice to measure respiratory muscle strength as maximal inspiratory mouth pressure P_{Imax} and maximal expiratory pressure P_{Emax}. The technique that is currently used as the standard technique is the one described by Black and Hyatt (3). Briefly, the patient performs maximal inspiratory or expiratory maneuvers in a seated position, with a noseclip on, by blowing into or sucking from a small metal cylinder. One end of the cylinder has a circular rubber mouthpiece in which the patient purses his lips to prevent perioral air leakage. The other end has a small orifice (2-mm diam, 15-mm length), serving as an air leak to minimize the contribution of the facial muscles to the pressure generated and to keep the glottis open.

P_{Imax} is generally measured at residual volume (RV), while P_{Emax} is measured at total lung capacity (TLC). Several studies have reported values in normal subjects (3–10). In general, P_{Emax} was found to be greater than P_{Imax} and pressures were generally greater in men than in women. Indeed, in the above-mentioned studies in females P_{Emax} ranged from 61 to 70% and P_{Imax} from 62 to 75% of the value obtained in males. In addition, in most studies maximal pressures declined with age (3,5,9,10). McElvaney et al. (92), however, failed to demonstrate such age decline.

Although, as outlined above, maximal pressures are usually measured at the extremes of lung volume, this technique has at least one major disadvantage. At these lung volumes the pressure measured is also influenced by the recoil pressure of the total respiratory system. Accordingly, P_{Imax} measured at RV is the sum of the pressure actively developed by the inspiratory muscles and the outward recoil pressure present at this lung volume. Similarly, P_{Emax} measured at TLC is determined by the pressure developed by expiratory muscles and by the inward recoil pressure of the total respiratory system present at this lung volume (5,7,10). Therefore, it may be recommended to measure these pressures at FRC, a volume at which the recoil pressure of the total respiratory system is zero (7).

Maximal pressure is usually defined as the pressure sustained for at least 1 s and not as peak pressure (3). Peak pressure may be considerably greater than sustained pressure (93). The maximum is taken of a variable number of attempts, ranging from 3 to 10. Although intraindividual variability is relatively small (6–9%) (3,5,8), intersubject variability is usually large, possibly due to submaximal efforts and lack of coordination or to true between-subject variability. This intersubject variability limits the clinical usefulness of these maximal pressures.

Maximal pressures are usually reduced in patients with COPD due to hyperinflation and generalized muscle weakness (94,95). Both are responsible for the reduction in P_{Imax}, while the latter is responsible for the reduction in P_{Emax}. Respiratory muscle strength is also clearly reduced in interstitial lung disease (96,97) and neuromuscular disease (98,99). Hypercapnic respiratory failure develops in patients with neuromuscular disease when respiratory muscle strength is reduced to 30% of predicted, and intubation is usually necessary when P_{Imax} is reduced below 20 cm H_2O (100).

Similarly, in patients receiving mechanical ventilation a P_{Imax} value of 20–30 cm H_2O was found to be indicative of weaning failure (101), and during diaphragm fatigue it was shown to fall (102). The measurement of P_{Imax}, however, in intubated patients is problematic. Marini et al. (103) proposed to measure the pressure developed during airway occlusion with a one-way valve allowing exhalation only. Maximal pressure was obtained within 25 s. This technique, however, was shown to be largely investigator dependent (104).

A final problem related to the measurement of maximal mouth pressure is that these measurements are clearly effort dependent and, consequently, that very low pressures do not necessarily reflect weak muscles but may be related to poor coordination or submaximal effort. This seriously limits the clinical usefulness of these tests and opens the question of tests independent of patient cooperation.

B. Pleural Pressure

Respiratory muscle strength may also be measured by means of the pleural pressure generated during a maximal inspiratory or expiratory maneuver. In order to reflect the pressures developed by the respiratory muscles, the difference between pleural pressure during relaxation and that during muscular contraction at the same lung volume should be measured. P_{plmin} or minimal pleural pressure generated during a maximal inspiratory maneuver against an occluded airway is classically used as a measure of inspiratory muscle strength (105).

This method has the advantage of not being susceptible to artifacts caused by the cheeks and closure of the glottis, while it has the disadvantage of being invasive in the sense that it requires placement of an esophageal balloon. Alternatively, esophageal pressure may also be measured during a maximal sniff maneuver (11,106).

Similarly, measurement of maximal esophageal pressure during a forceful cough has been proposed as an estimate of expiratory muscle strength (107,108).

C. Nasopharyngeal Pressure

Recently, nasopharyngeal pressures and mouth pressures measured by means of balloon-catheter systems have been used as a measure of respiratory muscle strength (11–14). Mouth and nasopharyngeal pressures were shown to correlate well with sniff esophageal pressure in normal subjects and patients with muscle weakness. Consequently, these pressures may provide less invasive ways to estimate respiratory muscle strength, although validation of this approach in patients with COPD still needs to be performed (14). A limited study by Mulvey et al. (14) indicates that sniff nasopharyngeal pressures are of limited value in patients with abnormal lung mechanics.

Nasopharyngeal pressure during a sniff clearly reflects the flow-resistive pressure drop across the nose, whereas esophageal pressure relative to airway opening pressure is the negative of transpulmonary pressure. If the two are equal, this is because during a sniff most of the transpulmonary pressure drop occurs across the nose. This is unlikely to be the case in airways obstruction.

D. Transdiaphragmatic Pressure

The methods described above assess global respiratory muscle function, while measurement of P_{di} allows more specific assessment of diaphragmatic function. Since the diaphragm is the major inspiratory muscle, such specific assessment is expected to be useful. Nevertheless, several methodological problems remain associated with this measurement. First, a great deal of confusion has been present about the best maneuver to perform measurement of P_{di}. Agreement is apparently reached about the fact that a maximal inspiratory maneuver, Müller's maneuver, is inappropriate (78,109–111). The issue of the best maneuver for measurement of P_{di} has systematically been studied by Laporta and Grassino (112). They assessed five different maneuvers in 35 subjects (10 normals, 12 COPD, 13 restrictive lung disease) in search of the optimal technique to obtain maximal and reproducible results. The best maneuver appeared to be a combined Müller-expulsive maneuver with visual feedback. This is a two-step maneuver in which the patient first performs an expulsive maneuver, then superimposes a Müller's maneuver, with visual feedback of P_{es} and P_{ga} on the oscilloscope to maximize P_{di} by achieving both a positive P_{ga} and a negative P_{es}. This maneuver yielded the highest P_{di}, was most reproducible, and was easily mastered by the subjects.

Several reasons that the combined Müller-expulsive maneuver with feedback provides the best P_{di} measurement have been proposed. Laporta and Grassino (112) speculated that diaphragmatic activation was greater during this maneuver than during Müller's or expulsive maneuvers alone. This is supported by the data of Hershenson et al. (110), who found that twitch stimulation of the phrenic nerve elicited a response when superimposed on Müller's maneuver, but not when performed during a combined maneuver. An alternative or additional explanation may be the occurrence of diaphragm fiber lengthening during the combined maneuver (113). A pure diaphragmatic Müller's maneuver is not isometric, and both the velocity of shortening and the shorter fiber length result in a smaller P_{di}.

An alternative maneuver is a maximal sniff. During a sniff the nose acts as a Starling resistor or flow-limiting segment and values similar to the values during inspiratory efforts against an occluded airway are obtained (114). The maneuver was shown to produce greater P_{di} than Müller's maneuver, with a smaller variability and a greater reproducibility. As mentioned above, during the sniff maneuver esophageal pressure may also be measured (106). Sniffs are often considered to be more natural and therefore easier to perform by patients.

Evidently, the fact that measurement of P_{di} in general requires placement of two balloons remains a major drawback in the assessment of diaphragmatic strength. Its dependence upon patient cooperation (see below) further limits the clinical usefulness of the measurement of sniff P_{di}.

E. Relaxation Rate

Muscle fatigue is known to be associated with a slower relaxation rate. Consequently, this measurement has been used to attempt to detect the presence of diaphragmatic fatigue in normal subjects subjected to inspiratory loads (115–117). These studies showed that diaphragmatic fatigue was associated with a reduced relaxation rate. Relaxation rate is quantified either as the maximal relaxation rate at the onset of relaxation or as the time constant of the monoexponential decay in the second half of relaxation.

Recently this technique has been applied to clinical situations (14,118–120). In intubated patients the nose is replaced by a Starling resistor placed at the end of the endotracheal tube. Goldstone et al. (121) demonstrated that the maximal relaxation rate (MRR) was reduced in patients who failed to wean from mechanical ventilation. The usefulness of this measurement may be limited by the fact that MRR is effort dependent (122). This can be avoided by normalizing from the P_{di} achieved ($dP_{di}/dt/P_{di}$). Mak and Spiro reported a similar technique assessing the relaxation rate of the sternocleidomastoid muscle during single-pulse stimulation (123). This technique has the advantage of being independent of patient cooperation. Although MRR appears a simple and promising test of respiratory muscle function applicable to an intensive care situation, its precise place in respiratory muscle assessment still needs to be determined. Recovery of MRR with fatigue is usually less than 30 min, suggesting that this test measures high-frequency fatigue rather than the potentially more clinically relevant low-frequency fatigue.

V. Pressure Measurements During Supramaximal Stimulation

Previous tests depended upon patient cooperation, which seriously limited their clinical applicability, particularly in ill patients and patients admitted to the intensive care unit. In recent years the pressure developed by respiratory muscles has also been measured during supramaximal stimulation. In essence the phrenic nerves are stimulated so that the test is essentially a test of diaphragmatic function. Usually P_{di} is measured during stimulation, but alternatively P_{pl} may be measured, or mouth pressure. The latter measurement has the definite advantage of being noninvasive, its drawback, however, being the time constant of the equilibration between alveolar pressure and mouth pressure. This is not a problem in intubated patients. Stimulation can be electrical or magnetic, the latter having been developed more recently.

A. Electrical Stimulation

Electrical stimulation of the phrenic nerves represents the classical technique to assess diaphragmatic contraction nonvoluntarily. The nerve is stimulated at the posterior border of the sternocleidomastoid muscle at the level of the cricoid cartilage. This point corresponds to the most superficial position of the nerve. Stimulations may be performed transcutaneously with surface electrodes (117,124, 125) or percutaneously with needle (117) or wire electrodes (126). Transcutaneous stimulation is simple but may require a greater current to overcome the resistance of the skin and, hence, may be more painful. Trains of stimuli to provide tetani are painful and cannot be used routinely. Single supramaximal shocks, however, are easily tolerated. Patients find swallowing an esophageal balloon more unpleasant than single phrenic shocks. Needle electrode stimulation may traumatize nerves or vessels. In addition to P_{di}, phrenic nerve conduction time and the amplitude of the compound action potential may also be measured (125,127,128). From the twitch P_{di} one can obtain peak twitch tension, time-to-peak tension, dP/dt, and the relaxation characteristics of the diaphragm.

To assess diaphragmatic contractility, stimulation must be performed bilaterally, usually at FRC with the patient seated or supine while the airway is occluded. Abdominal binding may be performed in order to limit diaphragmatic shortening during stimulation. Supramaximal stimulation is usually determined by the diaphragm mass action potential. This should be measured with surface electrodes placed in interspaces 6–8 over the area of apposition bilaterally and the current increased until the amplitude of the compound mass action potential is maximal and independent of further increase in current. Some investigators have used tetanizing stimulation frequencies (125,129), but this is painful and consequently of limited use in patients. Normally twitch stimulations are performed. When applied unilaterally, twitches are not useful in assessing twitch P_{di} values (127,130). Twitches obtained during bilateral stimulation range from 31 to 48 cm H_2O, the highest values being obtained with the abdomen bound (117,124–126,131). Above FRC twitch P_{di} decreases linearly with increases in lung volume (126,132,133).

An important further development of phrenic nerve stimulation is the twitch occlusion technique (124,128,134). In this method twitches are superimposed on progressively increasing diaphragmatic contractions. With greater diaphragmatic contraction, and hence greater P_{di}, twitch response diminishes. When a twitch response is no longer discernible, diaphragm activation is assumed to be maximal (Fig. 9). An inverse relationship between P_{di} and twitch response is thus present, and P_{dimax} can be determined by extrapolation of the observed relationship between P_{di} twitch response and P_{dimax} (Fig. 9). The method thus allows assessment of diaphragmatic activation during P_{di} measurement. The same method can be applied with measurement of mouth pressure instead of P_{di}.

B. Magnetic Stimulation

Recently two new techniques of phrenic nerve stimulation have been developed. First, a technique to stimulate the cervical roots of the phrenic nerves was described (135). A magnetic coil encased in a 9-cm-diameter plate is placed with the center

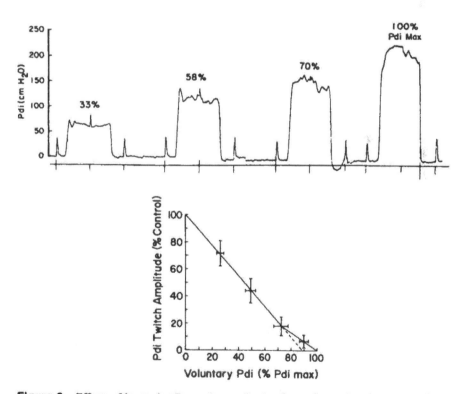

Figure 9 Effects of increasing P_{di} on the amplitude of superimposed twitch contractions. As P_{di} increased from 33 to 100% of maximum, the magnitude of the superimposed twitch diminished and in fact was absent at P_{di} 100% (upper panel). The relationship between P_{di} twitch and P_{di} is inversely linear (lower panel). The approach can thus be used to determine maximal P_{di} by extrapolation. (From Ref. 124.)

of the plate over the spinous process of C_7 (Fig. 10, upper panel). An electrical current applied to the coil generates an electrical field in a plane parallel to the coil, which in turn generates electrical currents surrounding the phrenic nerves. Adequate stimulation of the phrenic nerves can be obtained by positioning the coil (Fig. 10, lower panel). The stimulation is entirely painless, which is an important advantage. Disadvantageous, however, is the lack of specificity (136) presumably caused by simultaneous stimulation of the neck accessory muscles. This results in a greater

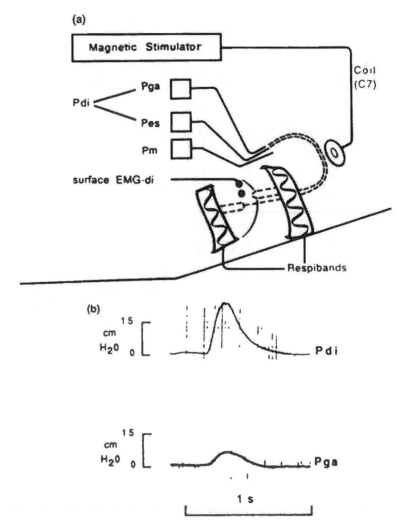

Figure 10   (Upper panel) Diagram illustrating position of electrodes for cervical magnetic stimulation. (Lower panel) P_{di} twitch and P_{ga} twitch obtained. (From Ref. 135.)

P_{di} than during electrical stimulation due reduced abdominal displacement and decreased shortening of diaphragmatic fibers.

Second, stimulation may also be performed through stimulation of the motor cortex. This is done with a magnetic coil similar to the coil used for cervical stimulation, but applied over the skull (137) (Fig. 11). Specificity of stimulation depends upon the design, shape, and positioning of the coil. Stimulation is entirely painless, but maximal stimulation requires background activity in the phrenic motor neurons to be present. Although the technique appears very promising in studying subjects whose cooperation is limited, more study is needed to determine its place in the assessment of respiratory muscle function. Particularly, studies on the potential hazards of magnetic stimulation must be conducted before it can become a technique routinely used in clinical medicine.

VI. Summary

Pressure is commonly used as an estimate of the mechanical outcome of respiratory muscle contraction. It is measured with a variety of techniques, including air-filled balloons, liquid-filled catheters, needles, and minitransducers. Pressure can also be inferred indirectly from displacements or from model analyses. Pressure measure-

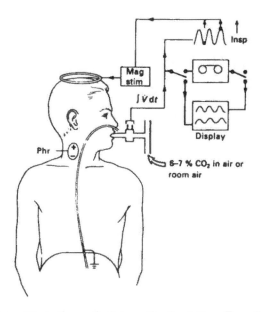

Figure 11   Diagram illustrating cortical magnetic stimulation. (From Ref. 127.)

ments during tidal breathing are used to infer the relative contributions of different respiratory muscles to respiratory efforts. Pleural pressure, gastric pressure, and transdiaphragmatic pressure are used to this aim. Pressures measured 100 ms after airway occlusion are used to assess ventilatory drive. Pressures measured during maximal voluntary contraction are classically used to determine respiratory muscle strength. Mouth pressures and transdiaphragmatic pressures are most widely used for this purpose. Aside from the technical problems involved in these measurements, they are all dependent upon patient cooperation and thus give variable results. This problem is absent when applying an external, well-controlled supramaximal stimulus. Bilateral phrenic nerve twitches are likely to become the standard method of assessment of diaphragmatic function in addition to sniff transdiaphragmatic pressures. The latter maneuver also requires patient cooperation but seems to be easier for most patients to perform. The disadvantage of electrical stimulation is that it is somewhat painful. Further development of magnetic stimulation, which is entirely painless, may solve this problem. Magnetic stimulation, however, provides less specific phrenic stimulation whether applied cervically or transcranially.

References

1. Mead, J., and Milic-Emili, J. (1964). Theory and methodology in respiratory mechanics with glossary of symbols. In *Handbook of Physiology*. Vol. I. Edited by W. O. Fenn and H. Rahn. Washington, D.C., American Physiological Society, pp. 363–376.
2. Milic-Emili, J. (1984). Measurement of pressures in respiratory physiology. In *Techniques in the Life Sciences, Techniques in Respiratory Physiology*. Edited by A. B. Otis. Shannon, Ireland, Elsevier Scientific Publishers, pp. 1–22.
3. Black, L. F., and Hyatt, R. E. (1969). Maximal respiratory pressures: normal values and relationship to age and sex. *Am. Rev. Respir. Dis.*, 99:696–702.
4. Cooke, C. D., Mead, J., and Orzalesi, M. M. (1964). Static volume-pressure characteristics of the respiratory system during maximal efforts. *J. Appl. Physiol.*, 95:1016–1022.
5. Rinqvist, T. (1966). The ventilatory capacity in healthy adults: an analysis of causal factors with special reference to the respiratory forces. *Scand. J. Clin. Lab. Invest.*, 18 (suppl):1–111.
6. Leech, J. A., Ghezzo, H., Stevens, D., and Blecklake, M. R. (1983). Respiratory pressures and function in young adults. *Am. Rev. Respir. Dis.*, 128:17–23.
7. Rochester, D., and Arora, N. S. (1983). Respiratory muscle failure. *Med. Clin. North. Am.*, 67:573–598.
8. Wilson, D. O., Cooke, N. T., Edwards, R. H. T., and Spiro, S. G. (1984). Predicted normal values for maximal respiratory pressures in caucasian adults and children. *Thorax*, 39:535–538.
9. Vincken, W., Ghezzo, H., and Cosio, M. G. (1987). Maximal static respiratory pressures in adults: normal values and their relationship to determinants of respiratory function. *Bull. Eur. Physiopathol. Resp.*, 23:435–439.
10. Decramer, M., Demedts, M., Rochette, F., and Billiet, L. (1980). Maximal transrespiratory pressures in obstructive lung disease. *Bull. Eur. Physiopathol. Resp.*, 16:479–490.
11. Koulouris, N. G., Mulvey, D. A., Laroche, C. M., Sawicka, E. H., Green, M., and Moxham, J. (1989). The measurement of inspiratory muscle strength by sniff esophageal, nasopharyngeal, and mouth pressures. *Am. Rev. Respir. Dis.*, 139:641–646.
12. Héritiér, F., Perret, C., and Fitting, J. W. (1991). Maximal sniff mouth pressure compared with maximal inspiratory pressure in acute respiratory failure. *Chest*, 100:175–178.

13. Wanke, T., Schenz, G., Zwick, H., Popp, W., Ritschka, L., and Flicker, M. (1990). Dependence of maximal sniff generated mouth and transdiaphragmatic pressures on lung volume. *Thorax*, 45:352–355.
14. Mulvey, D. A., Elliott, M. W., Koulouris, N. G., Carroll, M. P., Moxham, J., and Green, M. (1991). Sniff esophageal and nasopharyngeal pressures and maximal relaxation rates in patients with respiratory dysfunction. *Am. Rev. Respir. Dis.*, 143:950–953.
15. Buytendijk, H. J. (1949). Oesophagusdruk en longelasticiteit. Dissertation, University of Groningen.
16. Mead, J., McIlroy, M. B., Selverstone, N. J., and Kriete, B. C. (1955). Measurement of intraesophageal pressure. *J. Appl. Physiol.*, 7:491–495.
17. Mead, J., and Gaensler, E. A. (1959). Esophageal and pleural pressures in man, upright and supine. *J. Appl. Physiol.*, 14:81–83.
18. Milic-Emili, J., and Petit, J. M. (1959). Relationship between endoesophageal and intrathoracic pressure variations in dog. *J. Appl. Physiol.*, 14:535–537.
19. Milic-Emili, J., Mead, J., Turner, J. M., and Glauser, E. M. (1964). Improved technique for estimating pleural pressure from esophageal balloons. *J. Appl. Physiol.*, 19:207–211.
20. Milic-Emili, J., Mead, J., and Turner, J. M. (1964). Topography of esophageal pressure as a function of posture in man. *J. Appl. Physiol.*, 19:212–216.
21. Milic Emili, J., Henderson, J. A. M., Dolovich, M. B., Trop, D., and Keneko, K. (1966). Regional distribution of inspired gas in the lung. *J. Appl. Physiol.*, 21:749–759.
22. Agostini, E., and Rahn, H. (1960). Abdominal and thoracic pressures at different lung volumes. *J. Appl. Physiol.*, 5:1087–1092.
23. Decramer, M., De Troyer, A., Kelly, S., Zocchi, L., and Macklem, P. T. (1984). Regional differences in abdominal pressure swings in dogs. *J. Appl. Physiol.*, 57:1682–1687.
24. Agostino, E., and Mead, J. (1964). Statics of the respiratory system. In *Handbook of Physiology*. Vol I. Edited by W. O. Fenn and H. Rahn. Washington D.C., American Physiological Society, pp. 387–409.
25. Duomarco, J. L., and Rimini, R. (1947). La presion intra-abdominal en el Hombre. Buenos Aires, El Atheneo.
26. Rushmer, R. F. (1946). The nature of intraperitoneal and intrarectal pressures. *Am. J. Physiol.*, 147:242–249.
27. Mead, J., Yoshino, K., Kikushi, G., Barnas, G. M., and Loring, S. H. (1990). Abdominal pressure transmission in humans during slow breathing maneuvers. *J. Appl. Physiol.*, 68:1850–1853.
28. Schilder, D. P., Hyatt, R. E., and Fry, D. L. (1959). An improved balloon system for measuring intraesophageal pressure. *J. Appl. Physiol.*, 14:1057–1058.
29. Luciani, L. (1878). Delle oscillazioni della pressione intratoracica e intraaddominale. *Arch. Sci. Med.*, 2:177–224.
30. Baydur, A., Behrakis, P. K., Zin, W. A., Jaeger, M., and Milic-Emili, J. (1982). A simple method for assessing the validity of the esophageal balloon technique. *Am. Rev. Respir. Dis.*, 126:788–791.
31. Higgs, B. D., Behrakis, P. K., Bevan, D. R., and Milic-Emili, J. (1983). A simple method for assessing the validity of esophageal balloon technique in anesthetized subjects. *Anesthesiology*, 59:340–343.
32. Murciano, D., Aubier, M., Bussi, S., Derenne, J. P., Pariente, R., and Milic-Emili, J. (1982). Comparison of esophageal, tracheal, and mouth occlusion pressure in patients with chronic obstructive pulmonary disease during acute respiratory failure. *Am. Rev. Respir. Dis.*, 126:837–841.
33. Beardsmore, C. S., Helms, P., Stocks, J., Hatch, D. J., and Silverman, M. (1980). Improved esophageal balloon technique for use in infants. *J. Appl. Physiol.*, 49:735–742.
34. McCall, C. B., Hyatt, R. E., Noble, F. W., and Fry, D. L. (1957). Harmonic content of certain respiratory flow phenomena of normal individuals. *J. Appl. Physiol.*, 10:215–218.
35. Nagels, J., Landser, F. J., Van der Linden, L., Clément, J., and van de Woestijne, K. P.

(1980). Mechanical properties of the lungs and chest wall during spontaneous breathing. *J. Appl. Physiol.*, 49:408–416.

36. Asher, M. I., Coates, A. L., Collinge, J. M., and Milic-Emili, J. (1982). Measurement of pleural pressure in neonates. *J. Appl. Physiol.*, 52:491–494.

37. LeSouëf, P. N., Lopes, J. M., England, S. J., Bryan, M. H., and Bryan, A. C. (1983). Influence of chest wall distortion on esophageal pressure. *J. Appl. Physiol.*, 55:353–358.

38. Coates, A. L., Davis, G. M., Vallinis, P., and Outerbridge, E. W. (1989). Liquid-filled esophageal catheter for measuring pleural pressure in preterm neonates. *J. Appl. Physiol.*, 67:889–893.

39. Akkermans, L. M. A. (1991). Esophageal manometry. Microtransducers. *Dig. Dis. Sci.*, 36:14S–16S.

40. Gilbert, R., Peppi, D., and Auchinloss, J. H., Jr. (1979). Measurement of transdiaphragmatic pressure with a single gastric-esophageal probe. *J. Appl. Physiol.*, 47:628–630.

41. Chartrand, D. A., Jodoin, C., and Couture, J. (1991). Measurement of pleural pressure with oesophageal catheter-tip micromanometer in anaesthetized humans. *Can. J. Anaesth.*, 38:518–521.

42. Decramer, M., Jiang, T. X., and Reid, M. B. (1990). Respiratory changes in diaphragmatic intramuscular pressure. *J. Appl. Physiol.*, 68:35–43.

43. Leenaerts, P., and Decramer, M. (1990). Respiratory changes in parasternal intercostal intramuscular pressure. *J. Appl. Physiol.*, 68:868–875.

44. Macklem, P. T., Macklem, D. M., and De Troyer, A. (1983). A model of inspiratory muscle mechanics. *J. Appl. Physiol.*, 55:547–557.

45. Decramer, M., De Troyer, A., Kelly, S., and Macklem, P. T. (1984). Mechanical arrangement of costal and crural diaphragms in dogs. *J. Appl. Physiol.*, 56:1484–1490.

46. Ward, M. E., Ward, J. W., and Macklem, P. T. (1992). Analysis of human chest wall motion using a two-compartment rib cage model. *J. Appl. Physiol.*, 72:1338–1347.

47. De Troyer, A., Sampson, M., Sigrist, S., and Macklem, P. T. (1981). The diaphragm: two muscles. *Science*, 213:199–202.

48. De Troyer, A., Sampson, M., Sigrist, S., and Macklem, P. T. (1982). Action of costal and crural parts of the diaphragm on the rib cage in dog. *J. Appl. Physiol.*, 53:30–39.

49. Jiang, T. X., Demedts, M., and Decramer, M. (1988). Mechanical coupling of upper and lower canine rib cages and its functional significance. *J. Appl. Physiol.*, 64:620–626.

50. Stokes, M. J., and Dalton, P. A. (1991). Acoustic myographic activity increases linearly up to maximal voluntary isometric force in human quadriceps muscle. *J. Neurol. Sci.*, 101:163–167.

51. Maton, B., Petitjean, M., and Cnockeart, J. C. (1990). Phonomyogram and electromyogram relationships with isometric force reinvestigated in man. *Eur. J. Appl. Physiol. Occup. Physiol.*, 60:194–201.

52. Stokes, M. J., and Casper, R. G. (1992). Muscle sounds during voluntary and stimulated contractions of the human adductor pollicis muscle. *J. Appl. Physiol.*, 72:1908–1913.

53. Stokes, I. A. F., Moffroid, M. S., Rush, S., and Hauge, L. D. (1988). Comparison of acoustic and electrical signals from erectores spinae muscles. *Muscle Nerve*, 11:331–336.

54. Similowski, T., Petitjean, M. B., Maton, B., Monod, H., and Derenne, J. P. (1992). Phonomyogram of the diaphragm during phrenic stimulation and sniff test. *Am. Rev. Respir. Dis.*, 145:A255.

55. Tobin, M. J., Jenouri, G. A., Watson, H., and Sackner, M. A. (1983). Noninvasive measurement of pleural pressure by surface inductive plethysmography. *J. Appl. Physiol.*, 55:267–275.

56. Moavero, N. E., Lipton, D. S., Jenouri, G. A., Pine, J., Schneider, A., and Sachner, M. A. (1984). Non-invasive semi-quantitative measurements of tidal pressure-volume and flow relations of lung in COPD patients. *Bull. Eur. Physiopathol. Resp.* 20:333–339.

57. De Troyer, A., and Estenne, M. (1984). Coordination between rib cage muscles and diaphragm during quiet breathing in humans. *J. Appl. Physiol.*, 57:899–906.

58. De Troyer, A., and Ninane, V. (1986). Triangularis sterni: a primary muscle of breathing in the dog. *J. Appl. Physiol.*, 60:14–21.

59. Krayer, S., Decramer, M., Vettermann, J., Ritman, E. L., and Rehder, K. (1988). Volume quantification of chest wall motion in dogs. *J. Appl. Physiol.*, 65:2213–2220.
60. Decramer, M., Deschepper, K., Jiang, T. X., and Derom, E. (1991). Effects of aminophylline on respiratory muscle interaction. *Am. Rev. Respir. Dis.*, 144:797–802.
61. Pardy, R. L., Hussain, S. N., and Macklem, P. T. (1984). The ventilatory pump in exercise. *Clin. Chest Med.*, 5:35–49.
62. Bellemare, F., and Grassino, A. (1982). Effect of pressure and timing of contraction on human diaphragm. *J. Appl. Physiol.*, 53:1190–1195.
63. Rochester, D. F. (1991). Respiratory muscle weakness, pattern of breathing, and CO_2 retention in chronic obstructive pulmonary disease. *Am. Rev. Respir. Dis.*, 143:901–903.
64. Bégin, P., and Grassino, A. (1991). Inspiratory muscle dysfunction and chronic hypercapnia in chronic obstructive disease. *Am. Rev. Respir. Dis.*, 143:905–912.
65. Wanke, T., Formanek, D., Schenz, G., Popp, W., Gatol, H., and Zwick, H. (1991). Mechanical load on ventilatory muscles during an incremental cycle ergometer test. *Eur. Respir. J.*, 4:385–392.
66. Hillman, D. R., and Finucane, K. E. (1988). Respiratory pressure partitioning during quiet inspiration in unilateral and bilateral diaphragmatic weakness. *Am. Rev. Respir. Dis.*, 137:1401–1405.
67. Decramer, M., Jiang, T. X., and Demedts, M. (1987). Effects of acute hyperinflation on inspiratory muscle use. *J. Appl. Physiol.*, 63:1493–1498.
68. Kelly, S., Zin, W. A., Decramer, M., and De Troyer, A. (1984). Salutary effect of inspiratory fall in abdominal pressure during diaphragm paralysis. *J. Appl. Physiol.*, 56:1320–1324.
69. De Troyer, A., and Kelly, S. (1982). Chest wall mechanics in dogs with acute diaphragm paralysis. *J. Appl. Physiol.*, 53:373–379.
70. Newsom-Davis, J., Goldman, M., Loh, L., and Casson, M. (1976). Diaphragm function and alveolar hypoventilation. *Q. J. Med.*, 45:87–100.
71. Lisboa, C., Paré, P. D., Pertuzé, J., Contreras, G., Moreno, R., Guillemi, S., and Cruz, E. (1986). Inspiratory muscle function in unilateral diaphragmatic paralysis. *Am. Rev. Respir. Dis.*, 134:488–492.
72. Zocchi, L., Garzaniti, N., Newman, S., and Macklem, P. T. (1987). Effect of hyperinflation and equalization of abdominal pressure on diaphragmatic action. *J. Appl. Physiol.*, 62:1655–1664.
73. Yan, S., Gauthier, A. P., Similowski, T., Macklem, P. T., and Bellemare, F. (1992). Evaluation of human diaphragm contractility using mouth pressure twitches. *Am. Rev. Respir. Dis.*, 145:1064–1069.
74. Loh, L., Goldman, M., and Newsom, Davis, J. (1977). The assessment of diaphragmatic function. *Medicine*, 56:165–169.
75. Roussos, C., and Macklem, P. T. (1977). Diaphragmatic fatigue in man. *J. Appl. Physiol.*, 43:189–197.
76. Bellemare, F., and Grassino, A. (1983). Force reserve of the diaphragm in patients with chronic obstructive pulmonary disease. *J. Appl. Physiol.*, 55:8–15.
77. Pourriat, J. L., Lamberto, Ch., Hoang, P. H., Fournier, J. L., and Vasseur, B. (1986). Diaphragmatic fatigue and breathing pattern during weaning from mechanical ventilation in COPD patients. *Chest*, 90:703–707.
78. Macklem, P. T., Gross, D., Grassino, A., and Roussos, C. (1978). Partitioning of inspiratory pressure swings between diaphragm and intercostal/accessory muscles. *J. Appl. Physiol.*, 44:200–208.
79. Macklem, P. T. (1985). Inferring the actions of the respiratory muscles. In *The Thorax*. Edited by C. Roussos and P. T. Macklem. New York, Marcel Dekker, pp. 531–538.
80. Macklem, P. T. (1979). A mathematical and graphical analysis of inspiratory muscle action. *Respir. Physiol.*, 38:153–171.
81. Loring, S. H., and Mead, J. (1982). Action of the diaphragm on the rib cage inferred from a force-balance analysis. *J. Appl. Physiol.*, 53:756–760.

82. Mead, J., and Loring, S. H. (1982). Analysis of volume displacement and length changes of the diaphragm during breathing. *J. Appl. Physiol.*, 53:750–755.
83. Konno, K., and Mead, J. (1967). Measurement of the separate volume changes of rib cage and abdomen during breathing. *J. Appl. Physiol.*, 22:407–422.
84. Bye, P. T., Esau, S. A., Walley, K. R., Macklem, P. T., and Pardy, R. L. (1984). Ventilatory muscles during exercise in air and oxygen in normal men. *J. Appl. Physiol.*, 56:464–471.
85. Whitelaw, W. A., Derenne, J. P., and Milic-Emili, J. (1975). Occlusion pressure as a measure of respiratory center output in conscious man. *Respir. Physiol.*, 23:181–199.
86. Aubier, M., Murciano, D., Fournier, J. L., and Milic-Emili, J. (1980). Central respiratory drive in acute respiratory failure of patients with COPD. *Am. Rev. Respir. Dis.*, 122:191–200.
87. Marazzini, L., Cavestri, R., Gori, D., Gatti, L., and Longhini, E. (1978). Difference between mouth and esophageal occlusion pressure during CO_2 rebreathing in chronic obstructive pulmonary disease. *Am. Rev. Respir. Dis.*, 118:1027–1033.
88. Aubier, M., Murciano, D., Viires, N., Lecocguic, Y., Palacios, S., and Pariente, R. (1983). Increased ventilation caused by improved diaphragmatic efficiency during aminophylline infusion. *Am. Rev. Respir. Dis.*, 127:148–154.
89. Herrera, M., Blasco, J., Venegas, J., Barba, R., Doblas, A., and Marquez, E. (1985). Mouth occlusion pressure ($P_{0.1}$) in acute respiratory failure. *Intensive Care Med.*, 11:134–139.
90. Sassoon, C. S. H., Te, T. T., Mahutte, C. K., and Light, R. W. (1987). Airway occlusion pressure. An important indicator for successful weaning in patients with chronic obstructive pulmonary disease. *Am. Rev. Respir. Dis.*, 135:107–113.
91. Murciano, D., Boczkowski, J., Lecocguic, Y., Milic-Emili, J., Pariente, R., and Aubier, M. (1988). Tracheal occlusion pressure: a simple index to monitor respiratory muscle fatigue during acute respiratory failure in patients with chronic obstructive pulmonary disease. *Ann. Intern. Med.*, 108:800–805.
92. McElvaney, G., Blackie, G., Morrison, N. J., Wilcox, P. G., Fairbarn, M. S., and Pardy, R. L. (1989). Maximal static respiratory pressures in the normal elderly. *Am. Rev. Respir. Dis.* 139:277–281.
93. Smyth, R. J., Chapman, K. R., and Rebuck, A. S. (1984). Maximal inspiratory and expiratory pressures in adolescents. *Chest*, 86:568–572.
94. Decramer, M. (1989). Effects of hyperinflation on the respiratory muscles. *Eur. Respir. J.*, 1989;2:299–302.
95. Rochester, D. F., and Braun, N. M. T. (1985). Determinants of maximal inspiratory pressure in chronic obstructive pulmonary disease. *Am. Rev. Respir. Dis.*, 132:42–47.
96. Gilbert, R., Auchincloss, J. H. Jr., and Bleb, S. (1978). Measurement of maximum inspiratory pressure during routine spirometry. *Lung*, 155:23–32.
97. De Troyer, A., and Yernault, J. C. (1980). Inspiratory muscle force in normal subjects and in patients with interstitial lung disease. *Thorax*, 35:92–100.
98. Black, L. F., and Hyatt, R. E. (1971). Maximal static respiratory pressures in generalized neuromuscular disease. *Am. Rev. Respir. Dis.*, 103:641–650.
99. Braun, N. M. T., Arora, N. S., and Rochester, D. F. (1983). Respiratory muscle and pulmonary function in polymyositis and other proximal myopatheis. *Thorax*, 38:616–623.
100. O'Donohue, W. J. Jr., Baker, J. P., Bell, G. M., Muren, O., Parker, C. L., and Patterson, J. L. Jr. (1976). Respiratory failure in neuromuscular disease: management in a respiratory care unit. *JAMA*, 235:733–735.
101. Sahn, S. A., and Lakshminarayan, S. (1973). Bedside criteria for discontinuation of mechanical ventilation. *Chest*, 63:1002–1005.
102. Cohen, C., Zagelbaum, G., Gross, D., Roussos, C., and Macklem, P. T. (1982). Clinical manifestations of inspiratory muscle fatigue. *Am. J. Med.*, 73:308–316.
103. Marini, J. J., Smith, T. C., and Lamb, V. (1986). Estimation of inspiratory muscle strength in mechanically ventilated patients: the measurement of maximal inspiratory pressure. *J. Crit. Care*, 1:32–38.
104. Multz, A. S., Aldrich, T. K., Prezant, D. J., Karpel, J. P., and Hendler, J. M. (1990).

Maximal inspiratory pressure is not a reliable test of inspiratory muscle strength in mechanically ventilated patients. *Am. Rev. Respir. Dis.*, 142:529–532.

105. De Troyer, A., Borenstein, S., and Cordier, R. (1980). Analysis of lung volume restriction in patients with respiratory muscle weakness. *Thorax*, 35:603–610.

106. Laroche, C. M., Mier, A. K., Moxham, J., and Green, M. (1988). The value of sniff esophageal pressures in the assessment of global inspiratory muscle strength. *Am. Rev. Respir. Dis.*, 138:598–603.

107. Arora, N. S., and Gal, T. J. (1981). Cough dynamics during progressive expiratory muscle weakness in healthy curarized subjects. *J. Appl. Physiol.*, 51:494–498.

108. Byrd, R. B., and Burns, J. R. (1975). Cough dynamics in the post-thoracotomy state. *Chest*, 67:654–657.

109. De Troyer, A., and Estenne M. (1981). Limitations of measurement of transdiaphragmatic pressure in detecting diaphragmatic weakness. *Thorax*, 36:169–174.

110. Hershenson, M. B., Kikuchi, Y., and Loring, S. H. (1988). Relative strengths of the chest wall muscles. *J. Appl. Physiol.*, 65:852–862.

111. Sahn, S. A., Lakshminarayan, S., and Petty, T. L. (1976). Weaning from mechanical ventilation. *JAMA*, 235:2208–2212.

112. Laporta, D., and Grassino, A. (1985). Assessment of transdiaphragmatic pressure in humans. *J. Appl. Physiol.*, 58:1469–1476.

113. Hillman, D. R., Markos, J., and Finucane, K. E. (1990). Effect of abdominal compression on maximum transdiaphragmatic pressure. *J. Appl. Physiol.*, 68:2296–2304.

114. Miller, J. M., Moxham, J., and Green, M. (1985). The maximal sniff in the assessment of diaphragm function in man. *Clin. Sci.*, 69:91–96.

115. Esau, S. A., Bellemare, F., Grassino, A., Permutt, S., Roussos, C., and Pardy, R. L. (1983). Changes in relaxation rate with diaphragmatic fatigue in humans. *J. Appl. Physiol.*, 54:1353–1360.

116. Esau, S. A., Bye, P. T., and Pardy, R. L. (1983). Changes in rate of relaxation of sniffs and with diaphragmatic fatigue in humans. *J. Appl. Physiol.*, 55:731–735.

117. Aubier, M., Murciano, D., Lecocguic, Y., Viires, N., and Pariente, R. (1985). Bilateral phrenic stimulation: a simple technique to assess diaphragmatic fatigue in humans. *J. Appl. Physiol.*, 58:58–64.

118. Koulouris, N. G., Vianna, L. G., Mulvey, D. A., Green, M., and Moxham, J. (1989). Maximal relaxation rates of esophageal, nose, and mouth pressures during a sniff reflect inspiratory muscle fatigue. *Am. Rev. Respir. Dis.*, 139:1213–1217.

119. Goldstone, J. C., Koulouris, N. G., Mulvey, D. A., Green, M., and Moxham, J. (1989). Measurement of intrathoracic and upper airway relaxation rate (MRR) using a Starling resistor. *Am. Rev. Respir. Dis.*, 139:A351.

120. Davies, S. W., Pertuze, J., Winter, R., Watson, A. Lipkin, D., and Pride, N. B. (1989). Non-invasive assessment of respiratory muscle fatigue-mouth pressure gasps through Starling resistor. *Am. Rev. Respir. Dis.*, 139:A344.

121. Goldstone, J. C., Allen, K., Mulvey, D. A., et al. (1990). Respiratory muscle fatigue in patients weaning from mechanical ventilation. *Am. Rev. Respir. Dis.*, 141:A370.

122. Mulvey, D. A., Koulouris, N. G., Elliott, M. W., Moxham, J., and Green, M. (1991). Maximal relaxation rate of inspiratory muscle can be effort-dependent and reflect the activation of fast-twitch fibers. *Am. Rev. Respir. Dis.*, 144:803–806.

123. Mak, V. H. F., and Spiro, S. G. (1989). Sternomastoid relaxation rate: a simple technique to assess fatigue. *Am. Rev. Respir. Dis.*, 139:A346.

124. Bellemare, F., and Bigland-Ritchie, B. (1984). Assessment of human diaphragm in vivo. *Respir. Physiol.*, 58:263–277.

125. Bellemare, F., Bigland-Ritchie, B., and Woods, J. J. (1986). Contractile properties of the human diaphragm in vivo. *J. Appl. Physiol.*, 61:1153–1161.

126. Hubmayr, R. D., Litchy, W. J., Gay, P. C., and Nelson, S. B. (1989). Transdiaphragmatic twitch pressure. Effects of lung volume and chest wall shape. *Am. Rev. Respir. Dis.*, 139:647–652.

127. Mier, A., Brophy, C., Moxham, J., and Green, M. (1987). Phrenic nerve stimulation in normal subjects and in patients with diaphragmatic weakness. *Thorax*, 42:885–888.
128. Gandevia, S. C., and McKenzie, D. K. (1985). Activation of the human diaphragm during maximal static efforts. *J. Physiol.*, 367:45–56.
129. Aubier, M., Farkas, G., De Troyer, A., Mozes, R., and Roussos, C. (1981). Detection of diaphragmatic fatigue in man by phrenic stimulation. *J. Appl. Physiol.*, 50:538–544.
130. McKenzie, D. K., and Gandevia, S. C. (1985). Phrenic nerve conduction times and twitch pressures of the human diaphragm. *J. Appl. Physiol.*, 58:1496–1504.
131. Mier, A., Brophy, C., Moxham, J., and Green, M. (1989). Twitch pressures in the assessment of diaphragm weakness. *Thorax*, 44:990–996.
132. Smith, J., and Bellemare, F. (1987). Effect of lung volume on in vivo contraction characteristics of human diaphragm. *J. Appl. Physiol.*, 62:1893–1900.
133. Mier, A., Brophy, C., Moxham, J., and Green, M. (1990). Influence of lung volume and rib cage configuration on transdiaphragmatic pressure during phrenic nerve stimulation in man. *Respir. Physiol.*, 80:193–202.
134. Similowski, T., Yan, S., Gauthier, A. P., Macklem, P. T., and Bellemare, F. (1991). Contractile properties of the human diaphragm during chronic hyperinflation. *N. Engl. J. Med.*, 325:917–923.
135. Similowski, T., Fleury, B., Launois, S., Cathala, H. P., Bouche, P., and Derenne, J. P. (1989). Cervical magnetic stimulation: a new painless method for bilateral phrenic nerve stimulation in conscious humans. *J. Appl. Physiol.*, 67:1311–1318.
136. Wragg, S., Aguilina, R., Goldstone, J., Green, M., and Moxham, J. (1991). Cervical magnetic stimulation of the phrenic nerves. *Eur. Respir. J.* (suppl 4):309S.
137. Murphy, K., Mier, A., Adams, L., and Guz, A. (1990). Putative cerebral cortical involvement in the ventilatory response to inhaled CO_2 in conscious man. *J. Physiol. (London)*, 420:1–18.

39

Performance of Respiratory Muscles In Situ

DUDLEY F. ROCHESTER

University of Virginia Health Sciences
  Center
Charlottesville, Virginia

GASPAR A. FARKAS

State University of New York at Buffalo
Buffalo, New York

I. Introduction

A. Wallace Fenn's Insights

Wallace Fenn compared the performance of respiratory and limb skeletal muscles in situ, with regard to pattern of contraction, operating lengths, the extent of maximum shortening, and the force-velocity relationship (Fenn, 1963). He pointed out that the resting length of the respiratory muscles is set by the balance between the inward recoil of the lung and the outward recoil of the chest wall. Based on its dimensions, Fenn suggested that the diaphragm could shorten by 50%, in agreement with the Weber-Fick law. He developed equations for respiratory muscle contractile force as functions of both the velocity and the extent of muscle shortening. Fenn calculated diaphragmatic wall tension per unit of thoracic circumference, based on trans-diaphragmatic pressure (P_{di}) and thoracic cross-sectional area (TCSA). He calculated the volume swept by the diaphragm as the product of TCSA and diaphragmatic excursion. This chapter about the performance of the respiratory muscles in situ in intact animals and humans owes much to Fenn's landmark review and insightful ideas.

B. Basic Determinants of Contractile Force

Respiratory muscle performance in situ is governed by the same basic relationships that hold for isolated, perfused muscle strips. These are the modulation of force output according to the precontractile or resting length of the muscle (force-length or length-tension relationship), the hyperbolic relationship between the force output of a muscle and its shortening rate (force-velocity relationship), and the force response to the frequency of external stimulation or neural drive (force-frequency relationship). In addition, respiratory muscle performance in situ is modified by other factors such as neural recruitment strategies, mechanical linkages between the muscles, and linkages between the muscles and the thorax. Under some circumstances, the function of the diaphragm and perhaps the abdominal muscles may also be influenced by the Laplace relationship between pressure and wall tension.

II. The Effects of Length on Force-Generating Capacity

A. Force-Length Relationship in Vitro

Many properties of muscle are length dependent and therefore can be expressed as functions of length. The length-tension or force-length relationship of the excised, perfused diaphragm muscle strip in vitro is a leading example. The force generated in response to supramaximal stimulation of the muscle is more or less symmetrical around a peak force that is developed at the optimal resting length (L_o). Force falls to zero at lengths of approximately 50% and 160% of L_o (McCully and Faulkner, 1983).

This property of muscle derives mainly from the sliding filament model. The smallest functional unit of striated skeletal muscle is the sarcomere, bounded at either end by a Z-band. Contractile force is developed in the zones of overlap between thick and thin filaments, and this overlap is optimal over a relatively small range of sarcomere length (Gordon et al., 1966). In the passively shortened muscle, much of the loss of force in a shortened muscle results from mechanical folding of thin filaments that collide with the Z-bands. However, some force loss may also result from impaired muscle activation and calcium release from the terminal cisternae of the sarcoplasmic reticulum (Ridgway and Gordon, 1975; Lopez et al., 1981). In any case, as muscle length deviates from optimal, the active force produced by a given stimulation frequency decreases.

McCully and Faulkner showed that the in vitro length-tension relationship of mammalian diaphragm is fairly uniform across species. However, the shape of the length-tension relationship varies among the respiratory muscles. For example, the length-tension relationship of canine intercostal muscles is markedly compressed along the length axis (Farkas et al., 1985; Farkas and De Troyer, 1987). Therefore, at lengths shorter than L_o, the intercostal muscles generate considerably less force than the diaphragm (Farkas et al., 1985). Among canine respiratory muscles, the costal diaphragm has the broadest length-tension curve, while the parasternal intercostal muscles have the narrowest. Thus, costal diaphragm maintains force generation over a relatively wide range of operating lengths, whereas the parasternals are the most vulnerable to loss of force-generating capacity when they are shortened below L_o.

B. In Situ Pressure-Volume Relationships

It has long been recognized that maximal respiratory pressures measured at the mouth vary with lung volume (Agostoni and Mead, 1964), and it is generally accepted that these relationships reflect the force-length properties of the inspiratory and expiratory muscles (Rahn et al., 1946). Maximal static inspiratory pressure (P_{Imax}) is greatest at residual volume (RV), falls off slightly at functional residual capacity (FRC), and declines to zero at total lung capacity (TLC). By way of contrast, maximal static expiratory pressure (P_{Emax}) is greatest at TLC and declines progressively as lung volume is decreased through FRC to RV. Maximal respiratory pressures in patients with asthma and chronic obstructive pulmonary disease (COPD) follow much the same relationships as found in age-matched normal subjects (Decramer et al., 1980; Rochester and Braun, 1985), that is, they tend to lie on the same curve as the normal subjects, but at higher lung volume.

To obtain the pressures developed by the respiratory muscles (P_{mus}), one must correct maximal static pressures measured at the mouth for respiratory system recoil (P_{rs}). P_{rs} is approximately -40 cm H_2O at TLC, zero at FRC, and $+40$ cm H_2O at RV. Thus, the curve relating expiratory P_{mus} to lung volume retains the shape of the P_{Emax}-volume curve, but its pressure amplitude is reduced, up to approximately 40 cm H_2O at RV. The curve relating inspiratory P_{mus} to lung volume has a different shape than the P_{Imax}-volume curve. Peak inspiratory P_{mus} is developed at or just below FRC, with less negative pressures at higher and lower lung volumes. Moreover, at TLC, the inspiratory P_{mus} curve does not fall to zero, but rather is approximately -40 cm H_2O, or about 35% of the FRC value.

Transdiaphragmatic pressure (P_{di}) varies with lung volume in humans in much the same way as P_{Imax}. In normal humans, twitch P_{di} falls by 60% between RV and TLC (Smith and Bellemare, 1987). The P_{ga} component of P_{di} is virtually unaffected, but the P_{es} component decreases from 58% of P_{di} at RV to 42% at FRC and is less than 5% at TLC. With maximal voluntary effort against a closed airway (Müller's maneuver), peak P_{di} is attained near supine FRC (approximately 40% TLC), and P_{di} is lower at lung volumes above and below supine FRC (Milic-Emili et al., 1964). This relationship is consistent with the expected force-length behavior of the diaphragm. However, with maximal voluntary efforts the diaphragm may not be fully activated at RV (Hershenson et al., 1988). Twitch P_{di} responses to stimulation of the phrenic nerves progressively increased as lung volume is decreased from FRC to RV (Mier et al., 1990). Thus the optimal resting length of the human diaphragm in situ may be at RV rather than between RV and FRC.

C. In Situ Resting Length

The relationship between in situ resting length and optimal force-generating length (L_o) has been evaluated systematically for most of the inspiratory and expiratory muscles of the dog. Length was measured using sonomicrometry (Newman et al.,

1984; Road et al., 1986). To this end, a pair of piezoelectric crystal transducers, 1–2 mm in diameter, were surgically implanted 10–20 mm apart in the muscle of interest. One transducer emits a burst of ultrasound that propagates through muscle at 1.58 m/ms. The other transducer detects the sound wave and the time of its arrival. Distance is measured as the product of the velocity of sound in muscle and the signal transit time.

In these experiments, the operating length of a given respiratory muscle was assessed in situ, then the segment of the muscle bearing the sonomicrometry crystals muscle was excised with the crystals remaining in place (Fig. 1). This muscle bundle was then mounted in a muscle bath for determination of in vitro contractile properties (Fig. 1). Muscle length in the bath was set to L_0, and the distance between the crystals was again recorded sonomicrometrically. Thus it was possible to evaluate precisely the relationship between the in situ length at FRC (L_{FRC}) and L_0. When the ratio L_{FRC}/L_0 is less than 1.0, the muscle is operating on the ascending limb of its length-tension curve, and its L_0 lies at a lung volume lower than FRC. Conversely, when L_0/L_{FRC} is less than 1.0, the muscle is operating on the descending limb of its length-tension curve, and its L_0 lies at a lung volume that is higher than FRC.

Values of L_{FRC}/L_0 for canine inspiratory and expiratory muscles are summarized in Tables 1 and 2, respectively. It should be noted that L_{FRC} was almost always measured in the supine, anesthetized dog, so operating lengths in awake animals in normal canine postures are likely to be somewhat different (Margulies et al., 1990). It is of interest that studies of muscles of mastication reveal that the length of a muscle in situ is adjusted so that the L_0 lies not at the resting length, but at the

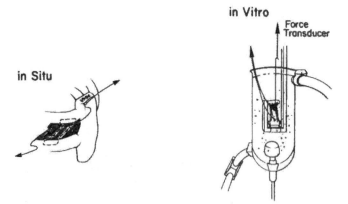

Figure 1 Parasternal intercostal muscle preparation (Farkas et al., 1985). To determine the in situ length (L_r) of the respiratory muscles with respect to their optimal force-producing length (L_0), length transducers (piezoelectric crystals) are inserted in individual muscles in the intact animal and L_r is measured. The muscle bundle containing the length transducers was excised with the transducers in place, and L_0 of the muscle segment was measured in an in vitro chamber.

Table 1 Length of Canine Inspiratory Muscles In Situ at FRC (L_{FRC}) Expressed as Percent of Optimal Resting Length (L_o)

Muscle	L_{FRC}/L_o (%)	Ref.
Costal diaphragm	95 ± 4	Farkas and Rochester, 1988a
	97 ± 2	Farkas and Rochester, 1988b
	≈94	Kim et al., 1976
	105	Road et al., 1986
	100 ± 3	Margulies et al., 1990
	88 ± 4[a]	Margulies et al., 1990
Crural diaphragm	84 ± 3	Farkas and Rochester, 1988a
	89 ± 3	Farkas and Rochester, 1988b
	92	Road et al., 1986
	91 ± 4	Margulies et al., 1990
	78 ± 4[a]	Margulies et al., 1990
Parasternal intercostal	117 ± 4	Farkas and De Troyer, 1987
	115 ± 3	Farkas et al., 1985
External intercostals	96 ± 3	Farkas et al., 1985
Scalenes	86 ± 1	Farkas and Rochester, 1986
Sternomastoids	75 ± 2	Farkas and Rochester, 1986

[a]Prone posture; all other animals supine.

length where the muscle is most active (Herring et al., 1984). If this applies to respiratory muscles, then L_{FRC}/L_o will be 1.0 at the lung volume where the particular muscle is most likely to be actively recruited. Consistent with this hypothesis, the L_{FRC}/L_o of costal diaphragm of the supine, anesthetized dog is 0.95–0.97. Thus, the costal diaphragm is ideally sized for its role as the primary muscle of breathing.

Table 2 Length of Canine Expiratory Muscles In Situ at FRC (L_{FRC}) Expressed as Percent of Optimal Resting Length (L_o)

Muscle	$LFRC/L_o$ (%)	Ref.
Triangularis sterni	75 ± 6	Farkas and De Troyer, 1987
Internal intercostals	97 ± 3	Farkas et al., 1985
External oblique	83 ± 2	Farkas and Rochester, 1988a
	88 ± 2	Farkas, 1992
	77 ± 2[a]	Farkas, 1992
Rectus abdominis	105 ± 3	Farkas and Rochester, 1988a
Transversus abdominis	74 ± 3	Farkas, 1992
	77 ± 2[a]	Farkas, 1992

[a]Prone posture; all other animals supine.

D.   Adaptation of Acute Hyperinflation of the Lungs

The range of resting lengths shown in Tables 1 and 2 has implications concerning interactions among respiratory muscles. The muscles must be able to function effectively in situ over a wide range of conditions, in health and in acute and chronic pulmonary disease. Acute increases in lung volume, such as would accompany asthma attack, produce unequal degrees of shortening in the inspiratory muscles. For example, passively increasing the lung volume of supine, anesthetized dogs from FRC to TLC shortens the diaphragm by 25–35% (Newman et al., 1984; Farkas et al., 1985; Road et al., 1986; Farkas and Rochester, 1988b), whereas the parasternal intercostal muscles shorten by only 10% (Farkas et al., 1985: Decramer et al., 1986a) and the neck inspiratory muscles shorten by only 5% (Farkas and Rochester, 1986). At TLC, the ratio L_{FRC}/L_o is approximately 0.7 for the diaphragm, 0.8 for scalene and sternomastoid muscles, and 1.0 for the parasternal intercostal muscles. Thus, the neck inspiratory and parasternal intercostal muscles function much better than the diaphragm at high lung volumes (Jiang et al., 1989). Because the parasternal muscles shorten to nearer their L_o while other respiratory muscles shorten away from their L_o (Farkas et al., 1985; Farkas and De Troyer, 1987), the integrated inspiratory muscle apparatus has a broader effective force-length range than any single inspiratory muscle.

E.   Force-Length Relationship in Situ

Diaphragmatic force-length behavior must account for the effect of lung volume on P_{Imax} and P_{DImax}, but to verify that this is the case, it is necessary to relate P_{di} to diaphragm length. The length of the diaphragm and other respiratory muscle lengths can be measured directly in intact animals using several techniques. These include the diaphragm slip preparation (Kim et al., 1976), sonomicrometry (Newman et al., 1984; Farkas et al., 1985; Road et al., 1986; Newman et al., 1986), and fluoroscopy to measure the distance between markers sewn to the muscle (Knight et al., 1990). In humans, the lengths of the diaphragm silhouette have been measured on chest x-rays taken under static conditions at different lung volumes (Braun et al., 1982; Loring et al., 1985). In like fashion, one can measure interrib distances that reflect the length of intercostal muscles (Sharp et al., 1986). Three-dimensional information about the human diaphragm has been obtained using computerized tomography (Whitelaw, 1987; Krayer et al., 1989) or magnetic resonance imaging (Paiva et al., 1992).

In humans and dogs, the in situ diaphragm muscle can shorten by approximately 40% over the entire vital capacity (VC) (Braun et al., 1982; Farkas et al., 1985; Road et al., 1986). In contrast, the lateral and parasternal intercostal muscles and the neck inspiratory muscles shorten by only 10% between RV and TLC (Farkas et al., 1985; Sharp et al., 1986: Farkas and Rochester, 1986). The relationship between P_{di} and diaphragm length in situ resembles the in vitro force-length relationship (Kim et al., 1976; Braun et al., 1982; Road et al., 1986), and the relationship between inspiratory P_{mus} and diaphragm length closely resembles that between P_{di} and diaphragm length (Braun et al., 1982). Given the prominent shortening capacity of the diaphragm and the lesser shortening of the other inspiratory muscles, it is likely that the relationship between P_{Imax} and lung volume results primarily from the force-length properties of the diaphragm.

Much less is known about the force-length properties of the expiratory muscles. Excised canine abdominal muscles have force-length properties similar to those of other canine respiratory muscles (Farkas and Rochester, 1988a; Farkas, 1992). The rectus abdominis undergoes minimal length change from FRC to TLC, but the external oblique lengthens by about 10%. The triangularis sterni length-tension curve in vitro is nearly identical to that of the parasternal intercostals, and it lengthens approximately 12% from FRC to TLC (Farkas and De Troyer, 1987). In humans, the ratio of abdominal muscle EMG to abdominal pressure (EMG_{ab}/P_{ab}) was constant between FRC and FRC + 2 L, and linear dimensions of the abdomen changed by less than 5% (Hill et al., 1984). Below FRC, the abdomen was indrawn, and the abdominal muscles may have been shorter or flatter. In any case, the ratio EMG_{ab}/P_{ab} increased below FRC. Thus, the length behavior of the abdominal oblique and rectus muscles are unlikely to explain the marked dependence of expiratory P_{mus} on lung volume. It is also unlikely that the relatively small degree of shortening in internal intercostal muscles (Sharp et al., 1986) is responsible. It may be that deeper muscles such as the transversus abdominis and triangularis sterni are more affected by changes in lung volume. Alternatively, the relationship between expiratory P_{mus} and lung volume might depend on the degree of neural activation (see Sec. IV.C).

F. Shape of the Diaphragmatic Pressure-Length Curve

The force-length behavior of the human diaphragm in situ was not entirely the same as the relationship in vitro, in that the P_{di}-L_{di} curve had a flat top, with no identifiable peak (Braun et al., 1982). However, P_{di} and diaphragm length were not measured at 40–50% TLC where diaphragm muscle might be at its optimal resting length (L_o). It was subsequently found that P_{di} amplitude was greatest at 40% TLC, suggesting that diaphragmatic L_o lies at this volume (Lu et al., 1984). However, the decrement of P_{di} at RV can be also be explained by submaximal activation at RV (Hershenson et al., 1988).

Another estimate of the location of L_o for the in situ human diaphragm is provided by twitch P_{di} responses to bilateral stimulation of both phrenic nerves (Smith and Bellemare, 1987). The twitch P_{di} is greatest at RV, and it is only 5% less at 40% TLC, which corresponds to supine FRC. The twitch P_{di} is even lower at 50% TLC, which corresponds to upright FRC. Thus, the L_o for the in situ human diaphragm probably lies at a lung volume that is well below upright FRC, between RV and supine FRC. The L_o of the canine also lies below FRC (Kim et al., 1976; Road et al., 1986; Farkas and Rochester, 1988b; Margulies et al., 1990).

G. Rib Cage vs. Abdominal Displacement

Grassino et al. (1978) introduced the concept that shortening of the diaphragm was reflected more accurately by the outward displacement of the abdomen than by increases in lung volume. Subsequently, Loring et al. (1985) showed that diaphragmatic length depends on both lung volume and thoracoabdominal configuration. Contrary to expectation, diaphragmatic shortening during breaths made without abdominal displacement was approximately 70% of the shortening in breaths with outward inspiratory abdominal excursion. This indicates that the diaphragm has a significant effect on the excursion of the rib cage as well as the abdomen and that abdominal displacements alone do not accurately reflect shortening of the diaphragm.

H. Laplace Law

The Laplace law describes the relationship between pressure in a deformable medium and tension in the wall of the container. Wall tension (T) is proportional to the product of pressure (P) and the radius of curvature (R) of the container wall, and in a sphere $T = PR/2$. Kim et al. (1976) used both a diaphragm slip preparation and Walton strain gauges attached to the in situ canine diaphragm to show that the ratio T_{di}/P_{di} was virtually constant between RV and TLC. They concluded that the radius of curvature of the diaphragm must have been constant over VC. Subsequently, Loring et al. (1985) showed that the shape of the dome of the human diaphragm was also quite constant between RV and TLC. Thus it seems highly unlikely that the Laplace law has a significant impact on the function of the diaphragm in normal subjects.

I. Passive Tension

When isolated, perfused strips of respiratory muscle are stretched in the absence of stimulation, passive tension is not usually apparent until the muscle is longer than its L_o (McCully and Faulkner, 1983; Farkas et al., 1985; Farkas and Rochester, 1986; Farkas and Rochester, 1988a,b). Occasionally one sees minimal passive tension down to 90% L_o (Gauthier et al., 1993). The passive tension behavior of the isolated muscle strips does not account for the observation that freshly excised whole respiratory muscles shorten by 30% to approximately 60% of their L_o (Margulies et al., 1990; Tao and Farkas, 1992a). This phenomenon is not blocked by curarization, and it is probably not due to muscle contraction. However, it is not clear whether the recoil force is a function of the muscle per se or its fascial investment.

By way of contrast, there is substantial passive tension in the in situ diaphragm at lengths as short as 80% L_o (Fig. 2). The data points for the diaphragm in situ were obtained by using the relationship between L_{FRC} and L_o (Farkas and Rochester, 1988b) to reanalyze the data of Kim et al. (1976) and Road et al. (1986). The length at which either active tension or P_{di} was maximal was taken as L_o. These results are consistent with observations of other investigators. Most parts of the diaphragm

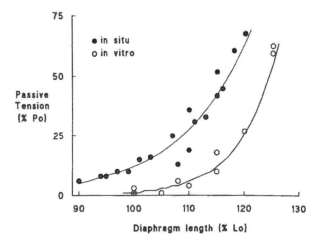

Figure 2 Relationship between passive tension and diaphragm muscle length in the canine diaphragm (Rochester, 1992). The in situ diaphragm exhibits significant passive tension below L_o. Isolated, perfused diaphragm strip data (open circles) are from McCully and Faulkner (1983) and Farkas et al. (1985). The in situ data (closed circles) were recalculated from Kim et al. (1976) and Road et al. (1986). Dashed and solid lines represent logarithmic regressions.

of supine and prone dogs are stretched during passive lung deflation from TLC (Sprung et al., 1990). On inflation above FRC, regional diaphragmatic area decreased in all but the costal region near the rib cage insertion (Pean et al., 1991). The diaphragm of supine humans is under passive tension up to approximately 70% TLC (Agostoni and Mead, 1964). Whitelaw et al. (1983) calculated that the diaphragm of upright humans supports a low level of passive tension at FRC, and the diaphragm is also passively tensed at zero gravity (Edyvean et al., 1991).

The physiological significance of passive tension lies in several areas. First, it enables the diaphragm to shorten passively, without external deformation such as wrinkling. Second, it contributes to the elastance of the rib cage (Kikuchi et al., 1991), and the recoil of the diaphragm is the major component of respiratory system recoil near RV (Agostoni and Mead, 1964). The passive elastance of the canine rectus abdominis is about three times greater than that of the external oblique (Farkas and Rochester, 1988a), so the rectus appears to be ideally suited to its role as a strap to retain the abdominal contents.

III. Effect of Shortening Velocity on Force Production

A. Force-Velocity Relationship In Vitro

Isolated, perfused strips of diaphragm muscle contract without shortening when they have a large afterload but shorten during contraction against afterloads that are less than maximal specific force (Ritchie, 1954). The velocity of shortening varies inversely and hyperbolically with the magnitude of the afterload. In the rat, the maximal velocity of shortening is approximately 10 L_o per second, whereas in the human it is 2.5 L_o per second (Edwards, 1979). The power output of the diaphragm at high velocity of shortening stems mainly from its fast fibers. Faulkner (1986) estimated that a diaphragm with 50% slow and 50% fast fibers would have 55% of the power of a muscle composed entirely of fast fibers and that fast fibers in such a diaphragm would contribute 95% of the power.

B. Force-Velocity Relationship In Situ

Studies of respiratory muscle shortening velocity in situ have utilized graded resistances to attain variable flow rates during maximal voluntary inspiratory or expiratory efforts. Agostoni and Fenn (1960) found that alveolar pressure was higher when flow was retarded by the resistance. The work done by the inspiratory muscles was inversely related to the reciprocal of inspiratory time, and inspiratory alveolar pressure was inversely related to inspiratory flow rate. These results are consistent with the hypothesis that peak inspiratory and expiratory pressures in humans are limited by the velocity of inspiratory and expiratory muscle shortening, rather than by the mechanics of the lungs or airways. Pengelly et al. (1971) found that P_{di} elicited by stimulation of phrenic nerves was linearly and inversely related to mean inspiratory flow rate in cats and in humans. Moreover, the slope of the P_{di}-flow relationship in humans was the same during maximal voluntary efforts as with external stimulation of the phrenic nerves. Similar results were obtained by other investigators (Hyatt and Flath, 1966; Mognoni et al., 1968).

   The shortening rate of respiratory muscles can also be slowed by blocking the neuromuscular junction with d-tubocurarine. Gal and Arora showed that inspiratory and expiratory flow rates fell by 60% and 25%, respectively, when P_{Imax} and P_{Emax} were reduced to 40% and 20% of control (Gal and Arora, 1982). Part of the fall in inspiratory flow rate could be attributed to an increase in upper airway resistance. The dynamic peak inspiratory alveolar pressure fell by only 30%, as compared to a 60% fall in P_{Imax}. The difference between the modest decrement in alveolar pressure and the large fall in static P_{Imax} can be attributed to slowing of the velocity of inspiratory muscle shortening by the increased upper airway resistance.

   During maximal voluntary dynamic efforts with no added external resistance, the velocity of shortening is high enough to exert significant effects on maximal available inspiratory pressures. This occurs during forced inspiratory and expiratory flow-volume curves, maximal voluntary ventilation, and high-intensity exercise. Leblanc et al. (1988) found that maximal dynamic inspiratory P_{es} fell by 5% for every liter per second of inspiratory flow, so the total reduction due to the velocity of inspiratory shortening was 25% at peak exercise ventilation.

C. Shape of the In Situ Force-Velocity Relationship

Some investigators found that the relationship between alveolar pressure, P_{es} or P_{di}, and inspiratory flow rate was linear (Agostoni and Fenn, 1960; Pengelly et al., 1971; Topulos et al. 1987), whereas others found that respiratory muscle force was hyperbolically related to shortening velocity in situ, as it is in vitro. For example, Goldman et al. (1978) demonstrated that the relationship between P_{di} and inspiratory flow rate was hyperbolic, provided that chest wall configuration is such that diaphragmatic shortening is represented by outward displacement of the abdomen. Kikuchi et al. (1982) estimated expiratory muscle length and wall tension by calculating the dimensions of a spherical model of the thorax. They estimated that the velocity of shortening was 3.3 circumferences per second and that wall tension at TLC and FRC was 11.3 and 7.7 N/cm, respectively, corresponding to P_{Emax} of 221 cm H_2O at TLC and 181 cm H_2O at FRC. After correcting for the effect of the series elastic element, expiratory muscle force was also found to be related hyperbolically to the velocity of shortening.

Otis showed on theoretical grounds how an inverse linear relationship between driving pressure and airflow could result from a hyperbolic inspiratory muscle force-velocity relationship, coupled with an exponential relationship for pressure dissipated in the internal impedance of the respiratory system (Otis, 1977). In the absence of direct measurement of in situ respiratory muscle shortening rates, the issue remains in limbo. We agree with Otis (1977) that respiratory muscle force-velocity relationships are likely to be hyperbolic, as found for diaphragm muscle in vitro (Ritchie, 1954).

IV. Effect of Stimulation Rate on Force Output

A. In Vitro Force-Frequency Relationship

The force output of isolated, perfused muscle strips increases as the frequency of external stimulation increases (Rack and Westbury, 1969). Generally, maximal tetanic force is four to five times higher than twitch force. The curve relating force to frequency rises in sigmoid fashion to plateau at a stimulation frequency that is dependent on the intrinsic contractile speed of the particular muscle being studied. Contraction velocities are faster in small animals than in large ones (Sant'Ambrogio and Saibene, 1970; Edwards and Faulkner, 1985), and intrinsic phrenic nerve-firing frequencies are faster in smaller animals than in large ones (Sant'Ambrogio et al., 1969; Iscoe et al., 1976; Kong and Berger, 1986; Lee et al., 1990).

At low stimulation frequencies, the contractile response of a fast muscle will resemble a series of twitches, with a notched contour. In contrast, a slow muscle stimulated at the same frequency will exhibit a smoothed force contour because the successive impulses produce fused force waves. Fusion occurs when the muscle is restimulated before it has had a chance to relax completely from the preceding contraction. This requires a higher stimulation frequency in the fast muscle than in the slow muscle. A corollary of this is that at low stimulation frequencies, the slow muscle will generate higher force than the fast muscle, even though both may generate the same maximal force response to high stimulation frequencies.

B. In Situ Force-Frequency or Pressure-Frequency Relationships

The force developed by contraction of the sternomastoid muscle can be assessed by measuring the horizontal vector of force developed in the coronal plane by flexion and rotation of the head (Moxham et al., 1980). Tetanic stimulation of the sternomastoid muscle at frequencies ranging from 5 to 100 Hz generate a force-frequency response that is virtually identical to that of the adductor pollicis and the quadriceps muscles. Typically, force more than doubles as stimulation frequency is increased from 10 to 20 Hz, and it is 85–90% maximal at 30 Hz. Beyond 50 Hz, there is no further increase in force.

Transdiaphragmatic pressure (P_{di}) responses to stimulation of the phrenic nerves mimic the responses of isolated, perfused diaphragm muscle strips to external stimulation in animals (Aubier et al., 1981; Moxham et al., 1981; Bellemare et al., 1986) and in humans (Edwards, 1979). Pressure generated by the in situ canine diaphragm approximately doubles when stimulation frequency is increased from 10 to 20 Hz (Road et al., 1987). In humans, bilateral tetanic stimulation of human phrenic nerves begins to fuse the P_{di} contour at 8 impulses per second (Bellemare et al., 1986). The magnitude of P_{di} is about 20% of maximal voluntary P_{di} in a twitch, about 50% of maximal voluntary P_{di} at 16 Hz, and 82% at 35 Hz (Bellemare et al., 1986).

The contractile profile of P_{di} during a single twitch exhibits values for time-to-peak-tension (TPT) and half-relaxation (1/2RT) that are characteristic of the species and muscle fiber type distribution. In humans, the delay from stimulus to the onset of the muscle compound action potential (M wave) is approximately 6 ms, and there is another delay of 18 ms until the onset of the mechanical twitch (Bellemare et al., 1986). TPT is approximately 85 ms and 1/2RT is 66 ms.

The P_{di} twitch response to bilateral supramaximal stimulation of the phrenic nerves is the sum of the responses measured in the esophageal and gastric pressures (P_{es}, P_{ga}) (Bellemare et al., 1986). The TPT and 1/2RT of P_{es} are 92 and 65 ms, respectively, whereas the corresponding values for P_{ga} are 71 and 65 ms, respectively. Thus the P_{ga} responses are faster than the P_{es} responses, and P_{di} timing is intermediate. With the abdomen unbound, twitch P_{di} averaged 33 cm H_2O, and 40% of this was P_{ga}. Tightly binding the abdomen increased twitch P_{di} to 42 cm H_2O, with 55% being P_{ga}. Finally, twitch P_{di} with bilateral stimulation is 32% greater than the sum of twitch P_{di} from right- and left-sided unilateral stimulation.

The magnitude of diaphragmatic twitch responses to bilateral single shock stimulation of the phrenic nerves can be assessed indirectly by measuring mouth pressure (Yan et al., 1992). To this end, the subject inhales to TLC and then relaxes while exhaling through a linear resistance back to FRC. During this slow exhalation, as many as 15 twitches can be recorded. The mouth pressure (P_{mo}) responses are linearly related to both the P_{es} and P_{di} responses and are similar in magnitude to P_{es}. The relationship of P_{mo} to either P_{di} or P_{es} is essentially the same at different lung volumes, and it is also the same before and after induction of diaphragmatic fatigue. The P_{mo} responses are also highly reducible over time.

The contractile state of the diaphragm can be evaluated, even when the number of stimuli in the tetanic train is limited to four or two impulses (Yan et al., 1993). The advantage of using paired stimuli is that this form of stimulation can be tolerated by awake human subjects, whereas tetanic stimulation of the phrenic nerves generally cannot. With paired stimuli, the second twitch of the pair (P_2) decreases in intensity as the stimulation frequency increases. As a result, the force-frequency curve of the diaphragm plateaus at lower force or pressure with two stimuli as compared with four, and the plateau with four stimuli is earlier and lower than with a full tetanic train. The ratio (P_2 response at 10 Hz)/(P_2 response at 100 Hz) provides valuable information about low- and high-frequency fatigue (Yan et al., 1993).

Collectively, these observations illustrate the fact that diaphragmatic contraction in situ is strongly influenced by the synchrony of contraction of both diaphragms, as well as by the relative compliances of the abdomen, rib cage, and thoracic gas. Of interest, mass loading the human rib cage had little effect on twitch P_{di}, whereas increasing lung volume to 1 L above FRC reduced P_{di} by 25% (Hubmayr et al., 1989). In addition to its effect on diaphragmatic length, the volume of thoracic gas may exert an independent effect on P_{di}. In anesthetized dogs, shortening responses to tetanic stimulation are well preserved at high lung volumes, but P_{di} responses to tetanic stimulation fall off at high lung volume more than can be explained by the effect of lung volume on diaphragm length (Rochester and Farkas, 1987).

C. Activation of the Respiratory Muscles

In order to compare performance of in situ respiratory muscles with in vitro studies of isolated, perfused muscle strips, it is necessary to know the extent to which the respiratory muscles are activated during spontaneous or voluntary efforts. For example, the in situ diaphragm must be maximally activated to generate maximal transdiaphragmatic pressure (P_{dimax}). The procedure used to test the level of activation during voluntary contractile efforts is referred to as the twitch-occlusion technique. To perform this test, P_{di} twitches produced by bilateral stimulation of the phrenic nerves are superimposed onto voluntary P_{di} efforts of graded intensity (Bellemare and Bigland-Ritchie, 1984; Gandevia and McKenzie, 1985). The magnitude of the twitch decreases linearly as the magnitude of the voluntary contraction increases.

Typically, P_{dimax} during maximal voluntary inspiratory efforts is approximately 125 cm H_2O (Gandevia and McKenzie, 1985), whereas P_{dimax} in maximal expulsive efforts or combined inspiratory and expulsive efforts exceeds 200 cm H_2O (Bellemare and Bigland-Ritchie, 1984; Gandevia and McKenzie, 1985). In all three types of maneuvers, P_{di} twitch is zero during the maximal voluntary effort. Thus the diaphragm is maximally activated. Moreover, the ratio P_{di} twitch/P_{dimax} is 0.21 (Bellemare and Bigland-Ritchie, 1984), which is similar to that in isolated perfused diaphragm muscle strips. Again, this suggests that there is maximal activation. Extrapolation of the line that relates twitch P_{di} to voluntary P_{di} to its intercept on the x-axis indicates that maximal P_{di} should be approximately 200 cm H_2O. Such extrapolation is a useful technique to assess P_{dimax} when subjects are unable to achieve maximal activation by voluntary effort.

Hershenson et al. (1988) showed that sometimes the respiratory muscles are not maximally activated, despite a maximal voluntary effort. For example, during inspiratory Müller's maneuvers, P_{di} is less than during abdominal expulsive maneuvers. That is because activation of the diaphragm is submaximal in Müller's maneuvers, whereas it is maximal in abdominal expulsive maneuvers. In contrast, McKenzie et al. (1988) found that during maximal inspiratory efforts the diaphragm was maximally activated, but the inspiratory intercostal muscles were not.

Similar considerations apply to the abdominal muscles. At high lung volume, abdominal pressure (P_{ab}) generated against a closed glottis is substantially greater than P_{ab} generated with the glottis open. The latter maneuver requires that the abdominal muscles contract against the diaphragm. Thus it was concluded that activation of the abdominal muscles is submaximal in open-glottis expulsive efforts (Hershenson et al., 1988; Gandevia et al., 1990). Moreover, the EMG signals from abdominal muscles were greater during trunk flexion than in expulsive maneuvers, and the EMG of the rib cage and neck inspiratory muscles was greater in tasks requiring head and neck flexion than in maximal inspiratory Müller efforts (Gandevia et al., 1990). Hershenson et al. (1988) concluded that when one respiratory muscle group contracts against another, the weaker group is maximally activated and the stronger group is submaximally activated to maintain balance. This means that in antagonistic contractions, the maximal pressure generated reflects the strength of the weaker muscle group.

D. Muscle Length and Contractile Speed

Shortening the resting length of a muscle shifts its pattern of contraction towards a faster twitch profile (Rack and Westbury, 1969; Wallinga-de Jonge et al., 1980). The mechanism appears to be related to the effect of muscle length on the calcium-activating system (Ridgway and Gordon, 1975; Lopez et al., 1981). Both slow and fast muscles exhibit similar alterations in twitch profile when resting length is varied (Wallinga-de Jonge et al., 1980). One would expect all of the respiratory muscles to respond in like fashion, and they do. Acute shortening of respiratory muscles reduces their twitch force, TPT, and 1/2RT. This has been demonstrated in mammalian diaphragm muscle in vitro (Farkas and Roussos, 1984; Tao and Farkas, 1992b) as well as in other animal diaphragms in situ (Sant'Ambrogio and Saibene, 1970; Edwards and Faulkner, 1985; Road et al., 1986). Acute shortening also increases the contractile speed of the in situ human diaphragm (Smith and Bellemare, 1987) and sternocleido-mastoid muscle (Moxham et al., 1980; Edwards and Faulkner, 1985).

The interrelationships among resting length, twitch profile, and force production are illustrated in Figure 3, which depicts the force-frequency curve of the isolated canine costal diaphragm at L_0 (Tao and Farkas, 1992b). At a stimulation frequency of 5 Hz, the force produced is approximately 40% of maximum (point A). At a stimulation frequency of 100 Hz, the force output is maximal. The length-tension properties of the isolated, perfused canine diaphragm are such that reducing length to 70% L_0 reduces maximal force at 100 Hz by 40%. If the twitch profile of the muscle were unchanged by shortening, tension at all other frequencies would also be reduced by 40%, as shown by the dashed predicted curve. Thus, to generate the force obtained by a stimulation frequency of 5 Hz at L_0, one would predict that it would be necessary to stimulate the shortened muscle at 20 Hz (point B). However, because of the change in twitch profile, one actually has to stimulate the muscle at 40 Hz (point C) to generate 40% of the maximal force at L_0.

E. Maximal vs. Submaximal Force Generation

The physiological range of neural firing frequency ranges from 5–70 Hz, but most respiratory activity is governed by frequencies of 5–30 Hz. In this range of firing

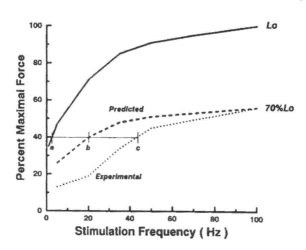

Figure 3   Force-frequency relationship of canine costal diaphragm at optimal length (L_0) and at 70% L_0. The predicted curve at 70% L_0 was calculated by assuming that the loss in force at all frequencies was similar to that observed at 100 Hz. Note that at all submaximal frequencies, actual force loss is greater than that predicted based on the tetanic length-tension properties. (Modified from Tao and Farkas, 1992b.)

frequency, force output is submaximal. In terms of normal breathing, this effect is more important than the effect of changes in length. For example, by doubling firing frequency from 10 to 20 Hz, contractile force is also approximately doubled. It is evident from the example in Figure 3 that submaximal force output is extremely sensitive to shifts in the twitch profile.

The length-tension property of a muscle is an assessment of the maximum force-generating capacity of the muscle. That is, the length-tension curve defines the outer limits of the force-length area in which the muscle can operate. During normal breathing, the force required of the respiratory muscles is far below maximal, and if force is potentially limited by a reduction in resting length, the deficit can be made up at least transiently by increasing neural drive. The diaphragm shortened to 70% L_o can still produce 65% of maximum force at L_o, but it requires inordinately high drive to attain that force. At very high firing frequencies, isolated, perfused muscles are highly susceptible to fatigue because of impaired transmission at the level of the neuromuscular junction (Krnjevic and Miledi, 1958) or impaired excitation-contraction coupling (Edwards, 1979). The susceptibility to fatigue is even greater when the muscle is acutely shortened (Gauthier et al., 1993).

There is yet another disadvantage to making up for shortening by increasing firing frequency. It lies in the force produced relative to maximal force produced at the given length and stimulation frequency. Fatigue of the in situ diaphragm occurs when a given transdiaphragmatic pressure (P_{di}) is too high a fraction of maximal transdiaphragmatic pressure (P_{dimax}) (Bellemare and Grassino, 1982). In the acutely shortened muscle, P_{di}/P_{dimax} is much higher than normal, and it is not surprising that the acutely shortened diaphragm fatigues relatively easily, both in vitro (Farkas and Roussos, 1984) and in situ (Roussos et al., 1979; Tzelepis et al., 1988).

F. Maximal Contractile Pressure and Force

The maximal specific force of mammalian diaphragm muscle strips in vitro is 20–25 newtons (N) per cm^2 of muscle cross-sectional area (McCully and Faulkner, 1983). In normal human volunteers, bilateral tetanic stimulation of the phrenic nerves yields a P_{di} of approximately 200 cm H_2O (Bellemare and Bigland-Ritchie, 1984; McKenzie et al., 1988). This is approximately the same as the P_{di} produced by maximal voluntary effort using a combined inspiratory and expulsive contraction pattern (Bellemare and Bigland-Ritchie, 1984; Laporta and Grassino, 1985). It should be noted that P_{di} can also be increased by abdominal compression, but this increase occurs at the expense of P_{es} (Hillman et al., 1990). From Eq. (3) below, it can be seen that a P_{di} of 200 cm H_2O corresponds to a contractile force of 24 N/cm^2, in excellent agreement with the in vitro data.

The specific contractile force that corresponds to P_{dimax} in humans can be estimated using an analysis based on the dimensions of the thorax and diaphragm (Rochester et al., 1981). The relevant thoracic dimensions are thoracic cross-sectional area (TCSA), the circumference of the zone of apposition (C_{za}) and the transverse and anteroposterior diameters of the thorax (D_1 and D_2, respectively). The transverse diameter of the thorax (D_1) runs from the right to left lateral interior aspect of the rib cage, approximately halfway between anteror and posterior portions of the ribs. The anteroposterior diameter (D_2) runs from the posterior to the anterior aspects of the ribs in a plane that is approximately midway between the midline and the most lateral aspect of the chest wall. At the level of the 10th–11th thoracic vertebral interspace, TCSA lies within the zone of apposition at RV and near the top of the zone at FRC. The exact level is not critical, because the anteroposterior and lateral walls of the human thorax are essentially parallel in this region (Loring et al., 1985). The human thorax is cylindrical in the zone of apposition, whereas the canine thorax is distinctly conical (Petroll, 1990).

TCSA and C_{za} can be estimated to within 5% by the formulas: TCSA $\approx (\Pi/4)$ $\times (D_1 \times D_2)$, $C_{za} \approx (\Pi \times D_1)$, and TCSA/$C_{za} \approx D_2/4$. These formulas were derived empirically, then tested using computerized tomographic images on which TCSA was measured by planimetry and circumference was measured by a map wheel device (Rochester et al., 1981). The relevant diaphragmatic dimension is the thickness of its muscle. The thickness of the human diaphragm at necropsy (TH_{di}) is 0.43 cm measured ultrasonographically (Wait et al., 1989) and 0.35 cm when calculated as the ratio of diaphragm muscle mass to diaphragm muscle surface area (Arora and Rochester, 1982). These represent values at or near supine FRC; averaging them and multiplying by 0.75 to adjust thickness for the increase in diaphragm length at RV yields a value of 0.3 cm for TH_{di} at RV.

When the diaphragm contracts in a maximal effort at RV, the force of contraction (F) is the product of P_{di} and the thoracic cross-sectional area (TCSA). The force of contraction also equals the product of the wall tension in the diaphragm (T_{di}) and muscle cross-sectional area (MCSA). MCSA, in turn, is the product of the circumference of the zone of apposition (C_{za}, approximately 70 cm) and diaphragm muscle thickness (TH_{di}). Thus:

$$F = P_{di} \times TCSA = T_{di} \times MCSA \tag{1}$$

$$T_{di} = P_{di} \times \frac{TCSA}{MCSA} \tag{2}$$

P_{di} can be measured, and reasonable values for the other terms in the equation are TCSA = 250 cm^2 and MCSA = 21 cm^2. Thus:

$$T_{di}(N/cm^2) \approx 0.12\ P_{di}(cm\ H_2O) \tag{3}$$

Although the maximally activated human diaphragm appears to be able to attain levels of contractile force similar to those measured in vitro, the same is not true for animal preparations. When the abdomen is unbound, tetanic stimulation of the phrenic nerves at FRC seldom evokes pressures higher than 50 cm H_2O (Mognoni et al., 1968; Delpierre et al., 1985). When the abdomen is bound, higher pressures can be achieved (Watchko et al., 1986), but the limit is still approximately 120 cm

H_2O (Bellemare et al., 1983). When animals are stimulated by asphyxia to make vigorous inspiratory efforts against a closed airway, the inspiratory pressure responses are much higher than with phrenic stimulation (Bendixen and Bunker, 1962; Euler and Fritts, 1963; Oliven et al., 1986), approaching 90 cm H_2O. Similar inspiratory pressures are attained by anesthetized cats made to sniff or gasp (Tomori et al., 1993), by normal human infants while crying (Shardonofsky et al., 1991), and by patients who are subjected to transient asphyxia (Truwit and Marini, 1992).

V.   Diaphragmatic Shortening and Volume Displacement

A.   Diaphragmatic Shortening Response to Stimulation

Neutral drive or external stimulation causes the diaphragm to shorten. In experiments in which the diaphragm has been subjected to external stimulation, either directly or via the phrenic nerves, the diaphragm shortens approximately 1.0% L_o per external impulse (Mardini and McCarter, 1987; Rochester and Farkas, 1987). The magnitude of the shortening response is remarkably robust. The shortening of the isolated, perfused rat diaphragm strip, expressed as percent of L_o per impulse, is well preserved at afterloads of up to 0.2 P_o (Mardini and McCarter, 1987). One can calculate from Mardini and McCarter's data that between 0.1 and 0.6 P_o the shortening response decreases by 5% for a 10% increase in P_o. In other words, diaphragmatic shortening would be intact up to an in situ P_{di} of approximately 50 cm H_2O. That is approximately the value of P_{di} generated by tetanic stimulation of both phrenic nerves at FRC (Rochester and Farkas, 1987; Hubmayr et al., 1990). In the anesthetized dog, the shortening response was maintained even when inflating the lung passively shortened the diaphragm to 80% L_o (Rochester and Farkas, 1987).

B.   Relating Tidal Volume to Neural Drive

The tidal volume during spontaneous quiet breathing is essentially constant across species lines, being 7–8 ml per kg of body weight (Stahl, 1967). The same values were found in human infants (American Thoracic Society/European Thoracic Society, 1993) and adults (Gilbert et al., 1972; Hirsch and Bishop, 1982; Tobin et al., 1983). Central ventilatory drive per breath also appears to be relatively constant across species lines. Although the firing frequency of phrenic motoneurons or diaphragmatic motor units varies threefold or more among species, one can ascertain from reports on rats, rabbits, cats, and dogs (Sant'Ambrogio et al., 1969; Sakai et al., 1973; Iscoe et al., 1976; Arita and Bishop, 1983; Citterio et al., 1983; Sieck et al., 1984; Kong and Berger, 1986; Lee et al., 1990) that there are approximately 10–20 neural impulses per breath in all these animals. Mean inspiratory flow rate (V_T/T_i) is proportional to $BW^{0.74}$, and (V_T/T_i)/BW is proportional to $BW^{-0.26}$ (Boggs and Tenney, 1984). That is, relative to body weight, V_T/T_i is higher in smaller animals. Based on the relative constancy of neural drive per breath, it is likely that the relatively higher inspiratory flow rate in smaller animals can be attributed to faster contraction of the inspiratory muscles, as suggested by Boggs and Tenney (1984).

In six species, from mouse to human, the length of costal diaphragm muscle, from its origin at the central tendon to insertion on the chest wall, is proportional to $FRC^{0.33}$, as shown in Figure 4 (Rochester, 1992). Conversely, tidal volume is proportional to $FRC^{2.87}$. During spontaneous quiet breathing, the quadruped diaphragm in situ shortens from 5 to 15% (Road et al., 1987; Easton et al., 1989; Torres et al., 1989; Knight et al., 1990). It can be estimated from dimensions of the diaphragm and thorax (Rochester et al., 1987) that the human diaphragm shortens approximately 10% for a tidal volume of 7 ml/kg. The tidal excursion of the in situ human diaphragm is approximately 1 cm, and the full excursion from RV to TLC is approximately 8 cm (Wade, 1954; Braun et al., 1982).

VI. Diaphragm Swept Volume

A. Definition and Quantification

This section addresses the issue of how much the diaphragm contributes to the inspired volume. Diaphragm swept volume (DSV) is defined as volume displaced by the diaphragm as it descends within the thorax. It is important to emphasize that the DSV need not result from active contraction of the diaphragm. In normal adults, the end-expiratory position of the diaphragm is under mild passive stretch, in the upright position (Whitelaw et al., 1983) as well as in the supine position (Agostoni and Mead, 1964). Contraction of the abdominal muscles during expiration increases

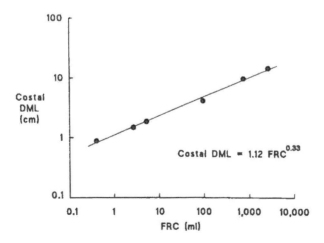

Figure 4 Allometric relationship between length of costal diaphragm muscle (DML) and functional residual capacity (FRC) in six species. DML is proportional to the cube root of FRC. (From Rochester, 1992.)

transdiaphragmatic pressure (Mier et al., 1985; Puddy et al., 1992) and lengthens the diaphragm (Farkas and Rochester, 1988a). Relaxtion of the abdominal muscles permits substantial early inspiratory diaphragmatic descent with volume displacement and inspiratory airflow in the absence of active diaphragmatic contraction (De Troyer, 1983; Easton et al., 1993).

If there were no change in thoracic diameter with inspiration, the volume swept by the diaphragm would lie in a cylinder with a cross-section corresponding to the shape of the interior of the lower rib cage. When there is an increase in lower rib cage diameters with inspiration, DSV includes volume below (caudal to) the initial position of the diaphragm that is attributable to expansion of the lower rib cage, as well as volume swept in the path of the original cylinder.

The DSV for a given volume increment (ΔV) can be calculated as the product of the change in diaphragm length (ΔDL) and the TCSA that corresponds to the volume segment. In upright adults, anteroposterior and transverse diameters of the lower rib cage increase approximately 15% between RV and TLC, so that TCSA increases by approximately 30% (Braun et al., 1982).

B. Measurement of Diaphragm Length

To measure the length of the human diaphragm in situ, chest roentgenograms were made of normal volunteers in anteroposterior and lateral projections at four or five lung volumes from RV to TLC (Braun et al., 1982; Lu et al., 1984). The technique used to achieve the various lung volumes was not controlled, so it is not possible to ascertain whether the x-rays were exposed with breath held actively versus relaxed against a closed airway. In addition, the posture required for exposing the x-rays may have altered chest configuration (Pierce et al., 1979). Thoracic gas volume was measured using a roentgenographic technique (Barnhard et al., 1960; Reger et al., 1972). Spirometry was used to control lung volumes, so that maximal static inspiratory Müller's maneuvers to obtain P_{di} could be performed at the same volume.

The intersections of diaphragm and chest wall shadows seen on the full inspiration (TLC) films probably mark the upper boundary of the insertional ring of the diaphragm. These sites were located for lateral costal, anterior sternal, and posterior crural parts of the right hemidiaphragm on films taken at TLC. Then using skeletal landmarks, the same sites were identified on films exposed at volumes lower than TLC. The width of the zone of apposition was measured as the distance along the anterior, lateral, and posterior aspects of the chest wall from the diaphragm insertions to the beginning of the dome, and the contours of the right hemidiaphragm dome were also measured at each volume. On the PA x-ray films, the dome was measured from chest wall to midline; on lateral views, the dome contour was measured from posterior to anterior chest wall. The length of the entire right hemidiaphragm was taken as the sum of the lengths along the dome and in the zone of apposition.

The diaphragm lengths so obtained were normalized by expressing them as cm diaphragm length per cm height (diaphragm length index, DLI). This eliminated differences between males and females, and the normalization is justified since the y-intercept of the regression equation relating diaphragm length to height was not significantly different from zero. Loring and Mead used chest x-rays to assess the curvature of the diaphragmatic dome by measuring the length of the arc along the visible portion of the diaphragmatic dome and the chord connecting the ends of the arc (Loring et al., 1985). The ratio of arc to chord changed relatively little between RV and TLC, so by this index the shape of the dome is also relatively constant over the VC range.

The coronal and right sagittal diameters of the diaphragm measured at necropsy were comprised of 75% muscle and 25% central tendon (Arora and Rochester, 1982). Unlike excised animal respiratory muscles (Tao and Farkas, 1992a), the transverse diameter of the human diaphragm did not shorten after excision (Arora and Rochester, 1982). The difference may lie in the time of excision, which was immediately postmortem in the animal studies (Tao and Farkas, 1992a), as compared with approximately 12 h postmortem in the human study (Arora and Rochester, 1982).

It was assumed that the necropsy lung volume was equivalent to supine FRC. Thus, the length of the central tendon was calculated at 25% of in situ diaphragm length at 40% TLC (PA and lateral views). This value was subtracted from diaphragm length measured at other volumes to yield values for diaphragm muscle length.

C. Thoracic Cross-Sectional Area

Thoracic cross-sectional area (TCSA) was measured as described in Section IV.F. The cross-sectional area of the thorax at the level of the zone of apposition can be estimated using the transverse and anteroposterior diameters in the formula for an ellipse: $A \approx \Pi/4(D_1 D_2)$. Similarly, the circumference of the inner aspect of the rib cage can be approximated using the transverse diameter in the formula for a circle: $C \approx \Pi D_1$. Thus the ratio $A/C \approx D_2/4$ (Rochester et al., 1981).

D. Diaphragm Swept Volume and Inspired Volume

We constructed a model to estimate diaphragmatic performance in situ, based on previously published thoracic and diaphragmatic dimensions (Braun et al., 1982). Two variables, diaphragm length (DL, cm) and thoracic cross-sectional area (TCSA, cm^2), were related to lung volume (LV, liters) as follows: $DL = 30.4 \, LV^{-0.367}$ and $TCSA = 30.2 \, LV + 190.9$. The relationship between diaphragm swept volume (DSV) and inspired volume is illustrated in Figure 5. Note that DSV is on average approximately 80% of inspired volume between RV and FRC, 60% of inspired tidal volume, and 45% of inspired volume above the tidal volume range. Over the entire vital capacity, the DSV represents approximately 60% of the inspired volume.

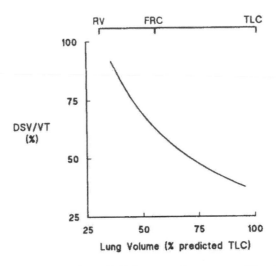

Figure 5   Diaphragm swept volume (DSV) expressed as percent of inspired tidal volume (V_T). On average, DSV is approximately 80% of VT below FRC, 60% of VT just above FRC, and 45% of VT at higher lung volumes.

Other investigators who used roentgenographic techniques to determine diaphragmatic displacement obtained similar results (Table 3). Whitelaw reconstructed diaphragm contours from conventional computerized tomography images and showed that volume displaced by the diaphragm was 68% of the inspired volume, between FRC and FRC + 1 L (Whitelaw, 1987). Krayer used three-dimensional computerized tomography to show that DSV/VT in awake subjects was

Table 3   Diaphragm Swept Volume (DSV) as a Percent of Inspired Volume in Upright Normal Subjects

| | DSV | | | |
RV-FRC	FRC-TLC	VC	V_T	Ref.
81	48	60	—	Agostoni et al., 1965
—	—	—	50	Konno and Mead, 1967
—	—	—	60	Wang and Josenhans, 1971
—	—	—	31	Sharp et al., 1975
78	44	61	51	Rochester et al., 1987
69	58	63	64	Verschakelen et al., 1989
76	50	61	51	Mean values

RV = Residual volume; FRC = functional residual capacity; TLC = total lung capacity; VC = vital capacity; V_T = tidal volume.

higher when they were supine than when they were prone (Krayer et al., 1989). Anesthesia and paralysis reduced the DSV to 52%. During spontaneous breathing, the dorsal excursion of the diaphragm was greater than the ventral excursion in both prone and supine postures. Verschakelen et al. (1989) determined diaphragmatic displacement both fluoroscopically and using respiratory inductance plethysmography. The two estimates of DSV agree well with each other (Verschakelen et al., 1989, 1992). The axial displacement between RV and TLC was greatest posteriorly and approximately 40% less anteriorly. Paiva et al. (1992) studied the diaphragm using magnetic resonance imaging and concluded from its shape that the diaphragm did not function like a piston in a cylinder. Verschakelen et al. (1992) concluded that although the diaphragm did not behave like a piston topographically or anatomically, its functional behavior over the VC is like a piston.

The model results are also consistent with most estimates of diaphragmatic displacement obtained by measuring external dimensions of the rib cage and abdomen. Konno and Mead (1967) and Sharp et al. (1975) found that the contribution of the abdomen (diaphragm) to quiet breathing was larger in the supine posture than upright. Agostoni et al. (1965) showed that the rib cage of upright subjects accounted for much less of the inspired volume between RV and FRC than between FRC and TLC. However, in the supine position, the rib cage accounted for the same proportion of inspired volume across the entire VC. Krayer et al. (1989) showed that DSV accounted for all the tidal volume in anesthetized supine subjects and 80% of tidal volume in prone anesthetized subjects. Hedenstierna et al. (1981) found in awake, supine, spontaneously breathing subjects that the rib cage contributed 40% to the tidal volume, as compared to 60% when the subjects were anesthetized, paralyzed, and mechanically ventilated. On average, the diaphragmatic contribution to the tidal volume in supine normal subjects was 67%.

Wade measured diaphragmatic excursion and change in thoracic circumference during tidal breathing, and also over the expiratory reserve volume, inspiratory capacity, and vital capacity, in 10 upright and supine normal subjects (Wade, 1954). Regression analysis of these data yields the following relationships between inspired volume (V, liter) and diaphragmatic excursion (EXC_{di}, cm) and/or change in chest circumference (ΔC, cm):

$$V = 0.080 + 0.481\ EXC_{di} \qquad (r^2 = 0.904)$$
$$V = 0.502 + 0.524\ \Delta C \qquad (r^2 = 0.837)$$
$$V = 0.111 + 0.342\ EXC_{di} + 0.175\ \Delta C \qquad (r^2 = 0.921)$$

Again, the diaphragmatic excursion in these subjects accounted for most of the lung volume inspired from RV to FRC, especially in the supine position, whereas the change in circumference of the chest had a greater effect at lung volumes above FRC, especially in the upright position (Wade and Gilson, 1951; Wade, 1954).

Josenhans and Wang (1970) used a ballistic technique to measure the axial mass displacement caused by breathing and found that displacement of the abdomen (diaphragm) accounted for 60% of tidal volume in supine normals (Wang and

Josenhans, 1971). In patients with ankylosing spondylitis, which limits rib cage excursion, the diaphragmatic contribution to tidal volume was 85% (Josenhans et al., 1971). Bergofsky (1964) used a specially designed plethysmograph to estimate that the diaphragatic contribution to tidal volume was approximately 33%.

E. Diaphragm Swept Volume in Animals

Decramer et al. (1986b) found that the relationship between changes in canine diaphragm length (ΔDL) and abdominal volume (ΔV_{ab}) determined during passive inflation predicted ΔDL fairly accurately for crural diaphragm but not for costal diaphragm. Petroll et al. (1990) used computerized tomography to show that a conical model to predict DSV in dogs was far superior to a cylindrical model. Knight et al. showed that DSV always exceeded ΔV_{ab}, and that DSV/ΔV_{ab} was proportional to abdominal compliance. Moreover, DSV was better correlated with shortening of the costal than of the crural diaphragm. There was an even stronger correlation with the difference between DSV and ΔV_{ab}, and shortening of the costal diaphragm (Petroll et al., 1990; Knight et al., 1991).

The DSV accounted for 49–67% of the inspired volume in dogs (Krayer et al., 1988; Warner et al., 1989; Petroll et al., 1990; Ward et al., 1992). In rabbits, DSV/VT was 72% prior to vagotomy and 86% after vagotomy. Expiratory muscles contributed half the thoracic volume displacement in spontaneously breathing supine dogs (Warner et al., 1989). Expiratory muscles contributed approximately half the tidal volume in prone or supine anesthetized dogs (Farkas and Schroeder, 1993) and 62% of V_T in upright animals (Farkas et al., 1989).

F. Predicted Maximal Dynamic Performance

Transdiaphragmatic pressures can be added to diaphragmatic and thoracic dimensions in the model described above see (Sec. VI.D) to predict the dynamic performance characteristics of the human diaphragm in situ during a maximal unimpeded inspiratory effort from RV to TLC (Rochester et al., 1987). Outcome variables include the velocity of diaphragmatic shortening, its effect on maximal static transdiaphragmatic pressure, the diaphragmatic contribution to tidal volume and inspiratory airflow, and diaphragmatic power. The model based on previous data (Braun et al., 1982) was extended by observations from a subsequent study (Lu et al., 1984).

In this model, the assumed inspiratory flow profile was based on typical normal values. The volume axis was divided into 0.5-L volume segments. The mean flow for each volume segment was determined graphically, and the time required to inspire across the volume segment (Δt) was calculated as the quotient of segment volume and mean flow. The mean velocity of diaphragmatic shortening across a segment could then be estimated as the quotient of diaphragmatic shortening across the segment (ΔL) and the time (Δt) required to inspire the segment volume of 0.5 L.

The results of the model calculations are summarized in Table 4. The velocity of shortening accelerates quickly to a maximum below FRC and then decelerates approximately linearly from FRC to TLC. The highest in situ rate of shortening is approximately 40% of the V_{max} determined for human diaphragm in vitro (Edwards, 1979). Static P_{di} is highest between RV and FRC, but dynamic P_{di} obtained from the velocity of shortening and the force-velocity curve is almost constant across the whole vital capacity. At peak shortening velocity, dynamic P_{di} is only 25% of maximal static P_{di}. Diaphragmatic power is the product of the maximal dynamic P_{di} and the diaphragmatic contribution to inspiratory flow. The power output of the diaphragm is highest around FRC, and it too declines as lung volume increases from FRC to TLC. The peak power output is almost 13 W.

VII. Summary

A. Limits of Contractility

Respiratory muscles in situ are governed by the same relationships that determine the contractile force of isolated, perfused muscles in vitro. That is, the development of respiratory pressures depends on the resting length of the muscles, the velocity of shortening, and the degree of neural activation. In addition, the performance of respiratory muscles in situ is modified by mechanical linkages among the muscles,

Table 4 Dynamic Performance of Diaphragm Calculated from Model Based on Diaphragmatic and Thoracic Dimensions

LV (%TLC)	$\Delta L / \Delta t$ (L_o/s)	F_v/F_o (%)	P_{didyn} (cm H_2O)	Power (W)
40	1.42	30	38	10.8
49	1.71	25	34	12.8
57	1.56	28	35	12.6
66	1.32	35	37	11.7
74	0.99	43	39	9.9
83	0.60	58	39	6.2
91	0.22	83	37	2.2

LV = Lung volume; L = length of right hemidiaphragm; F_v and F_o = diaphragmatic force in response to maximal stimulation with shortening at velocity (v) and without shortening (o); P_{didyn} = transdiaphragmatic pressure during dynamic contraction of the diaphragm.

and between the muscles and the chest wall, and sometimes by the Laplace relationship.

Among the respiratory muscles, the diaphragm has the greatest capacity for shortening and volume displacement, and it is closest to its optimal resting length at FRC. All inspiratory muscles become shorter when the lung is inflated above FRC. Interactions among inspiratory muscles, which depend in part on their in situ resting lengths, make for a wider range of high force output than could be achieved by any one muscle group alone. Passive tension in respiratory muscles stretched beyond their L_0 contributes to the recoil of the respiratory system and plays a significant role in breathing. The velocity of inspiratory muscle contraction, especially diaphragmatic shortening, causes maximal dynamic inspiratory pressures to be substantially lower than maximal static pressures. This effect is particularly pronounced during maximal voluntary ventilation, maximal exercise, and maximal inspiratory flow volume maneuvers over the full vital capacity.

Analysis of transdiaphragmatic pressure responses to stimulation of the phrenic nerves provides substantial insight into the in situ activation and contractility of the human diaphragm. The twitch-occlusion technique can be used to determine the extent of activation during voluntary efforts and to predict maximal transdiaphragmatic pressure. The technique of paired stimulation to assess the in situ force-frequency relationship is especially promising, because it yields information about both low-frequency and high-frequency fatigue. Even with abdominal binding there may be some shortening of the diaphragm, and the diaphragm shortens markedly in response to tetanic stimulation when the abdomen is not bound. Therefore, although diaphragmatic pressure responses to stimulation of the phrenic nerves mimic in vitro force-length and force-frequency relationships, it is difficult to fit the in situ responses into any single force-length or force-frequency curve.

B. Physiological Range of Function

Neural drive expressed as impulses per breath is constant across species lines. This produces a constant degree of shortening of the diaphragm, expressed as percent of L_0. Since the length of diaphragm muscle is scaled to the cube root of lung volume, a constant relative shortening yields a constant tidal volume when tidal volume is normalized to body weight.

Normal breathing does not require the respiratory muscles to approach the limits of their contractile performance. Only the diaphragmatic excursion approaches its limits near residual volume and total lung capacity. Respiratory pressures are far from maximal during quiet breathing but may near the dynamic maximum at the extremes of physical exercise. Neural activation is also submaximal except at very high levels of voluntary effort. Because the respiratory system operates well within its outer limits, multiple strategies are available to compensate for impediments to breathing and alterations in respiratory muscle function. When the diaphragm is shortened substantially, it can still generate a needed respiratory pressure if it receives more neural drive. Other muscles can be recruited to take over for an impaired diaphragm. Thus, the whole respiratory system is highly versatile.

C. Diaphragmatic Shortening and Volume Displacement

Shortening of the diaphragm accounts for approximately 60% of the vital capacity and the tidal volume during quiet breathing. In standing humans, diaphragmatic volume displacement accounts for a higher fraction of the expiratory reserve volume and a lower fraction of the inspiratory capacity. The maximal dynamic trans-diaphragmatic pressure is approximately 25% of peak static transdiaphragmatic pressure, and unlike the static pressure the dynamic pressure is relatively constant from residual volume to total lung capacity. That is, at high lung volumes, the loss of static pressure consequent to the shorter length is offset by the fact that the diaphragm is shortening much less rapidly. Peak power output and peak static pressure are both developed at or just below FRC.

References

Agostoni, E., Mognoni, P., Torri, G., and Saracino, F. (1965). Relation between changes of rib cage circumference and lung volume. *J. Appl. Physiol.*, 20:1179–1186.

Agostoni, E., and Fenn, W. O. (1960). Velocity of muscle shortening as a limiting factor in respiratory air flow. *J. Appl. Physiol.*, 15:349–353.

Agostoni, E., and Mead, J. (1964). Statics of the respiratory system. In *Handbook of Physiology Section 3: Respiration*. Edited by W. O. Fenn and H. Rahn. Bethesda, MD, American Physiological Society, pp. 387–409.

American Thoracic Society/European Thoracic Society (1993). Respiratory mechanics in infants: physiologic evaluation in health and disease. *Am. Rev. Respir. Dis.*, 147:474–496.

Arita, H., and Bishop, B. (1983). Firing profile of diaphragm single motor unit during hypercapnia and airway occlusion. *J. Appl. Physiol.*, 55:1203–1210.

Arora, N. S., and Rochester, D. F. (1982). Effect of body weight and muscularity on human diaphragm muscle mass, thickness, and area. *J. Appl. Physiol.*, 52:64–70.

Aubier, M., Farkas, G., De Troyer, A., Mozes, R., and Roussos, C. (1981). Detection of diaphragmatic fatigue in man by phrenic stimulation. *J. Appl. Physiol.*, 50:538–544.

Barnhard, H. J., Pierce, J. A., Joyce, J. W., and Bates, J. H. (1960). Roentgenographic determination of total lung capacity. *Am. J. Med.*, 28:51–60.

Bellemare, F., and Bigland-Ritchie, B. (1984). Assessment of human diaphragm strength and activation using phrenic nerve stimulation. *Respir. Physiol.*, 58:263–277.

Bellemare, F., and Grassino, A. (1982). Effect of pressure and timing of contraction on human diaphragm fatigue. *J. Appl. Physiol.*, 53:1190–1195.

Bellemare, F., Rigland-Ritchie, B., and Woods, J. J. (1986). Contractile properties of the human diaphragm in vivo. *J. Appl. Physiol.*, 61:1153–1161.

Bellemare, F., Wight, D., Lavigne, C. M., and Grassino, A. (1983). Effect of tension and timing of contraction on the blood flow of the diaphragm. *J. Appl. Physiol.*, 54:1597–1606.

Bendixen, H. H., and Bunker, J. P. (1962). Measurement of inspiratory force in anesthetized dogs. *Anesthesiology*, 23:315–323.

Bergofsky, E. H. (1964). Relative contributions of the rib cage and diaphragm to ventilation in man. *J. Appl. Physiol.*, 19:698–706.

Boggs, D. F., and Tenney, S. M. (1984). Scaling respiratory pattern and respiratory 'drive'. *Respir. Physiol.*, 58:245–251.

Braun, N. M. T., Arora, N. S., and Rochester, D. F. (1982). Force-length relationship of the normal human diaphragm. *J. Appl. Physiol.*, 53:405–412.

Citterio, G., Sironi, S., Piccoli, S., and Agostoni, E. (1983). Slow to fast shift in inspiratory muscle fibers during heat tachypnea. *Respir. Physiol.*, 52:259–274.

De Troyer, A. (1983). Mechanical action of the abdominal muscles. *Bull. Eur. Physiopathol. Respir.*, 19:575–581.

Decramer, M., Demedts, M., Rochette, F., and Billiet, L. (1980). Maximal respiratory pressures in obstructive lung disease. *Bull. Eur. Physiopathol. Respir.*, 16:479–490.

Decramer, M., Kelly, S., and De Troyer, A. (1986a). Respiratory and postural changes in intercostal muscle length in supine dogs. *J. Appl. Physiol.*, 60:1686–1691.

Decramer, M., Xi, J. T., Reid, M. B., Kelly, S., Macklem, P. T., and Demedts, M. (1986b). Relationship between diaphragm length and abdominal dimensions. *J. Appl. Physiol.*, 61:1815–1820.

Delpierre, S., Fornaris, M., Pelissier, J. F., and Payan, M. J. (1985). Contractile and histochemical characteristics of the rabbit diaphragm in elastase-induced emphysema. *Lung*, 163:221–232.

Easton, P. A., Fitting, J. W., Arnioux, R., Guerraty, A., and Grassino, A. E. (1989). Recovery of diaphragm function after laparotomy and chronic sonomicrometer implantation. *J. Appl. Physiol.*, 66:613–621.

Easton, P. A., Fitting, J-W., Arnoux, R., Guerraty, A., and Grassino, A. E. (1993). Costal and crural diaphragm function during CO_2 rebreathing in awake canines. *J. Appl. Physiol.*, 74:1406–1418.

Edwards, R. H. T. (1979). The diaphragm as muscle. Mechanisms underlying fatigue. *Am. Rev. Respir. Dis.*, 119 (suppl. 2):81–84.

Edwards, R. H. T., and Faulkner, J. A. (1985). Structure and function of the respiratory muscles. In *The Thorax Part A*. Edited by C. Roussos and P. T. Macklem. New York, Marcel Dekker, pp. 297–326.

Edyvean, J., Estenne, M., Paiva, M., and Engel, L. A. (1991). Lung and chest wall mechanics in microgravity. *J. Appl. Physiol.*, 71:1956–1966.

Euler, C. V., and Fritts, H. W., Jr. (1963). Quantitative aspects of respiratory reflexes from the lungs and chest walls of cats. *Acta Physiol. Scand.*, 57:284–300.

Farkas, G. A. (1992). Mechanical characteristics and functional length of canine expiratory muscles. *Respir. Physiol.*, 90:87–98.

Farkas, G. A., Decramer, M., Rochester, D. F., and De Troyer, A. (1985). Contractile properties of intercostal muscles and their functional significance. *J. Appl. Physiol.*, 59:528–535.

Farkas, G. A., and De Troyer, A. (1987). The ventral rib cage muscles in the dog: Contractile properties and operating lengths. *Respir. Physiol.*, 68:301–309.

Farkas, G. A., Estenne, M., and De Troyer, A. (1989). Expiratory muscle contribution to tidal volume in head-up dogs. *J. Appl. Physiol.*, 67:1438–1442.

Farkas, G. A., and Rochester, D. F. (1986). Contractile characteristics and operating lengths of canine neck inspiratory muscles. *J. Appl. Physiol.*, 61:220–226.

Farkas, G. A., and Rochester, D. F. (1988a). Characteristics and functional significance of canine abdominal muscles. *J. Appl. Physiol.*, 65:2427–2433.

Farkas, G. A., and Rochester, D. F. (1988b). Functional characteristics of canine costal and crural diaphragm. *J. Appl. Physiol.*, 65:2253–2260.

Farkas, G. A., and Roussos, C. (1984). Acute diaphragmatic shortening: in vitro mechanics and fatigue. *Am. Rev. Respir. Dis.*, 130:434–438.

Farkas, G. A., and Schroeder, M. A. (1993). Functional significance of expiratory muscles during spontaneous breathing in anesthetized dogs. *J. Appl. Physiol.*, 74:238–244.

Faulkner, J. A. (1992). Power output of the human diaphragm. *Annual Meeting Highlights*: 1081–1083.

Fenn, W. O. (1963). A comparison of respiratory and skeletal muscles. In *Perspectives in Biology. Houssay Memorial Papers*. Edited by C. F. Cori, V. G. Foglia, L. F. Leloir, and S. Ochoa. Amsterdam, Elsevier, pp. 293–300.

Gal, T. J., and Arora, N. S. (1982). Respiratory mechanics in supine subjects during progressive partial curarization. *J. Appl. Physiol.*, 52:57–63.

Gandevia, S. C., and McKenzie, D. K. (1985). Activation of the human diaphragm during maximal static efforts. *J. Physiol.*, 367:45–56.

Gandevia, S. C., McKenzie, D. K., and Plassman, B. L. (1990). Activation of human respiratory muscles during different voluntary manoeuvres. *J. Physiol.*, 428:387–403.

Gauthier, A. P., Faltus, R. E., Macklem, P. T., and Bellemare, F. (1993). Effects of fatigue on the length-tetanic force relationship of the rat diaphragm. *J. Appl. Physiol.*, 74:326–332.

Gilbert, R., Auchincloss, J. H., Jr., Brodsky, J., and Boden, W. (1972). Changes in tidal volume, frequency and ventilation induced by their measurement. *J. Appl. Physiol.*, 33:252–254.

Goldman, M. D., Grassino, A., Mead, J., and Sears, T. A. (1978). Mechanics of the human diaphragm during voluntary contraction: dynamics. *J. Appl. Physiol.*, 44:840–848.

Gordon, A. M., Huxley, A. F., and Julian, F. J. (1966). The variation in isometric tension with sarcomere length in vertebrate muscle fibers. *J. Physiol.*, 184:170–192.

Grassino, A., Goldman, M. D., Mead, J., and Sears, T. A. (1978). Mechanics of the human diaphragm during voluntary contraction: statics. *J. Appl. Physiol.*, 44:829–839.

Hedenstierna, G., Lofstrom, B., and Lundh, R. (1981). Thoracic gas volume and chest-abdomen dimensions during anesthesia and muscle paralysis. *Anesthesiology*, 55:499–506.

Herring, S. W., Grimm, A. F., and Grimm, B. R. (1984). Regulation of sarcomere number in skeletal muscle: a comparison of hypotheses. *Muscle Nerve*, 7:161–173.

Hershenson, M. B., Kikuchi, Y., and Loring, S. H. (1988). Relative strengths of the chest wall muscles. *J. Appl. Physiol.*, 65:852–862.

Hill, A. R., Kaiser, D. L., and Rochester, D. F. (1984). Effects of thoracic volume and shape on electromechanical coupling in abdominal muscles. *J. Appl. Physiol.*, 56:1294–1301.

Hillman, D. R., Markos, J., and Finucane, K. E. (1990). Effect of abdominal compression on maximum transdiaphragmatic pressure. *J. Appl. Physiol.*, 68:2296–2304.

Hirsch, J. A., and Bishop, B. (1982). Human breathing patterns on mouthpiece or face mask during air, CO_2 or low O_2. *J. Appl. Physiol.*, 53:1281–1290.

Hubmayr, R. D., Litchy, W. J., Gay, P. C., and Nelson, S. B. (1989). Transdiaphragmatic twitch pressure: effects of lung volume and chest wall shape. *Am. Rev. Respir. Dis.*, 139:647–652.

Hubmayr, R. D., Sprung, J., and Nelson, S. (1990). Determinants of transdiaphragmatic pressure in dogs. *J. Appl. Physiol.*, 69:2050–2056.

Hyatt, R. E., and Flath, R. E. (1966). Relationship of air flow to pressure during maximal respiratory effort in man. *J. Appl. Physiol.*, 21:477–482.

Iscoe, S., Dankoff, J., Migicovsky, R., and Polosa, C. (1976). Recruitment and discharge frequency of phrenic motoneurons during inspiration. *Respir. Physiol.*, 26:113–128.

Jiang, T. X., Deschepper, K., Demedts, M., and Decramer, M. (1989). Effects of acute hyperinflation on the mechanical effectiveness of the parasternal intercostals. *Am. Rev. Respir. Dis.*, 139:522–528.

Josenhans, W. T., and Wang, C. S. (1970). A modified ballistic method for measuring axial mass displacement caused by breathing. *J. Appl. Physiol.*, 28:679–684.

Josenhans, W. T., Wang, C. S., Josenhans, G., and Woodbury, J. F. L. (1971). Diaphragmatic contribution to ventilation in patients with ankylosing spondylitis. *Respiration*, 28:331–346.

Kikuchi, Y., Sasaki, H., Sekizawa, K., Aihara, K., and Takishina, T. (1982). Force-velocity relationship of expiratory muscles in normal subjects. *J. Appl. Physiol.*, 52:930–938.

Kikuchi, Y., Stamenovic, D., and Loring, S. H. (1991). Dynamic behavior of excised dog rib cage: dependence on muscle. *J. Appl. Physiol.*, 70:1059–1067.

Kim, M. J., Druz, W. S., Danon, J., Machnach, W., and Sharp, J. T. (1976). Mechanics of the canine diaphragm. *J. Appl. Physiol.*, 41:369–382.

Knight, H., Petroll, W. M., Adams, J. M., Shaffer, H. A., and Rochester, D. F. (1990). Videofluoroscopic assessment of muscle fiber shortening in the in situ canine diaphragm. *J. Appl. Physiol.*, 68:2200–2207.

Knight, H., Petroll, W. M., and Rochester, D. F. (1991). Relationships between abdominal and diaphragmatic volume displacements. *J. Appl. Physiol.*, 71:565–572.

Kong, F. J., and Berger, A. J. (1986). Firing properties and hypercapnic responses of single phrenic motor axons in the rat. *J. Appl. Physiol.*, 61:1999–2004.

Konno, K., and Mead, J. (1967). Measurement of the separate volume changes of rib cage and abdomen during breathing. *J. Appl. Physiol.*, 22:407–422.

Krayer, S., Rehder, K., Vettermann, J., Didier, E. P., and Ritman, E. L. (1988). Volume quantification of chest wall motion in dogs. *J. Appl. Physiol.*, 65:2213–2220.

Krayer, S., Rehder, K., Vettermann, J., Didier, E. P., and Ritman, E. L. (1989). Position and motion of the human diaphragm during anesthesia-paralysis. *Anesthesiology*, 70:887–890.

Krnjevic K., and Miledi, R. (1958). Failure of neuromuscular propagation in rats. *J. Physiol.*, 140:440–461.

Laporta, D., and Grassino, A. (1985). Assessment of transdiaphragmatic pressure in humans. *J. Appl. Physiol.*, 58:1469–1476.

LeBlanc, P., Summers, E., Inman, M. D., Jones, N. L., Campbell, E. J. M., and Killian, K. J. (1988). Inspiratory muscles during exercise: a problem of supply and demand. *J. Appl. Physiol.*, 64:2482–2489.

Lee, B. P., Green, J., and Chiang, S. T. (1990). Responses of single phrenic motoneurons to altered ventilatory drives in anesthetized dogs. *J. Appl. Physiol.*, 68:2150–2158.

Lopez, J. R., Wanek, L. A., and Taylor, S. R. (1981). Skeletal muscle: length-dependent effects of potentiating agents. *Science*, 214:79–82.

Loring, S. H., Mead, J., and Griscom, N. T. (1985). Dependence of diaphragmatic length on lung volume and thoracoabdominal configuration. *J. Appl. Physiol.*, 59:1961–1970.

Lu, J.-Y., Farkas, G. A., and Rochester, D. F. (1984). The optimal length of the in situ human diaphragm (abstr). *Clin. Res.*, 32:432A.

Mardini, I. A., and McCarter, R. J. M. (1987). Contractile properties of the shortening rat diaphragm in vitro. *J. Appl. Physiol.*, 62:1111–1116.

Margulies, S. S., Farkas, G. A., and Rodarte, J. R. (1990). Effects of body position and lung volume on in situ operating length of canine diaphragm. *J. Appl. Physiol.*, 69:1702–1708.

McCully, K. K., and Faulkner, J. A. (1983). Length-tension relationship of mammalian diaphragm muscles. *J. Appl. Physiol.*, 54:1681–1686.

McKenzie, D. K., Plassman, B. L., and Gandevia, S. C. (1988). Maximal activation of the human diaphragm but not inspiratory intercostal muscles during static inspiratory efforts. *Neurosci. Lett.*, 89:63–68.

Mier, A., Brophy, C., Estenne, M., Moxham, J., Green, M., and De Troyer, A. (1985). Action of abdominal muscles on rib cage in humans. *J. Appl. Physiol.*, 58:1438–1443.

Mier, A., Brophy, C., Moxham, J., and Green, M. (1990). Influence of lung volume and rib cage configuration on transdiaphragmatic pressure during phrenic nerve stimulation in man. *Respir. Physiol.*, 80:193–202.

Milic-Emili, J., Orzalesi, M. M., Cook, C. D., and Turner, J. M. (1964). Respiratory thoraco-abdominal mechanics in man. *J. Appl. Physiol.*, 19:217–223.

Mognoni, P., Saibene, F., Sant'Ambrogio, G., and Agostoni, E. (1968). Dynamics of the maximal contraction of the respiratory muscles. *Respir. Physiol.*, 4:193–202.

Moxham, J., Wiles, C. M., Newham, D., and Edwards, R. H. T. (1980). Sternomastoid muscle function and fatigue in man. *Clin. Sci.*, 59:463–468.

Moxham, J., Morris, A. J. R., Spiro, S. G., Edwards, R. H. T., and Green, M. (1981). Contractile properties and fatigue of the diaphragm in man. *Thorax*, 36:164–168.

Newman, S., Road, J., Bellemare, F., Clozel, J. P., Lavigne, C. M., and Grassino, A. (1984). Respiratory muscle length measured by sonomicrometry. *J. Appl. Physiol.*, 56:753–764.

Newman, S. L., Road, J. D., and Grassino, A. (1986). In vivo length and shortening of canine diaphragm with body postural change. *J. Appl. Physiol.*, 60:661–669.

Oliven, A., Supinski, G. S., and Kelsen, S. G. (1986). Functional adaptation of diaphragm to chronic hyperinflation in emphysematous hamsters. *J. Appl. Physiol.*, 60:225–231.

Otis, A. B. (1977). Pressure-flow relationships and power output of breathing. *Respir. Physiol.*, 30:7–14.

Paiva, M., Verbanck, S., Estenne, M., Poncelet, B., Segebarth, C., and Macklem, P. T. (1992).

Mechancial implications of in vivo human diaphragm shape. *J. Appl. Physiol.*, 72:1407–1412.

Pean, J. L., Chuong, C. J., Ramanathan, M., and Johnson, R. L., Jr. (1991). Regional deformation of the canine diaphragm. *J. Appl. Physiol.*, 71:1581–1588.

Pengelly, L. D., Alderson, A. M., and Milic-Emili, J. (1971). Mechanics of the diaphragm. *J. Appl. Physiol.*, 30:797–805.

Petroll, W. M., Knight, H., and Rochester, D. F. (1990). A model approach to assess diaphragmatic volume displacement. *J. Appl. Physiol.*, 69:2175–2182.

Pierce, R. J., Brown, D. J., Holmes, M., Cumming, G., and Denison, D. M. (1979). Estimation of lung volumes from chest radiographs using shape information. *Thorax*, 34:726–734.

Puddy, A., Giesbrecht, G., Sanii, R., and Younes, M. (1992). Mechanism of detection of resistive loads in conscious humans. *J. Appl. Physiol.*, 72:2267–2270.

Rack, P. M. H., and Westbury, D. R. (1969). The effects of length and stimulus rate on tension in the isometric cat soleus muscle. *J. Physiol.*, 204:443–460.

Rahn, H., Otis, A. B., Chadwick, L. E., and Fenn, W. O. (1946). The pressure-volume diagram of the thorax and lung. *Am. J. Physiol.*, 146:161–178.

Reger, R. B., Young, A., and Morgan, K. C. (1972). An accurate and rapid radiographic method of determining total lung capacity. *Thorax*, 27:163–168.

Ridgway, E. B., and Gordon, A. M. (1975). Muscle activation: effects of small length changes on calcium release in single fibers. *Science*, 189:881–883.

Ritchie, J. M. (1954). The relation between force and velocity of shortening in rat muscle. *J. Physiol.*, 123:633–639.

Road, J., Newman, S., Derenne, J. P., and Grassino, A. (1986). In vivo length-force relationship of canine diaphragm. *J. Appl. Physiol.*, 60:63–70.

Road, J., Vahi, R., Del Rio, P., and Grassino, A. (1987). In vivo contractile properties of fatigued diaphragm. *J. Appl. Physiol.*, 63:471–478.

Rochester, D. (1992). Respiratory muscles: structure, size, and adaptive capacity. In *Breathlessness: The Campbell Symposium*. Edited by N. L. Jones and K. J. Killian. Hamilton, Ontario, Boehringer Ingelheim, pp. 2–12.

Rochester, D. F., Arora, N. S., and Braun, N. M. T. (1981). Maximum contactile force of human diaphragm muscle, determined in vivo. *Trans. Am. Clin. Climatol. Assoc.*, 93:200–208.

Rochester, D. F., and Braun, N. M. T. (1985). Determinants of maximal inspiratory pressure in chronic obstructive pulmonary disease. *Am. Rev. Respir. Dis.*, 132:42–47.

Rochester, D. F., and Farkas, G. A. (1987). Airway pressure responses to phrenic stimulation: dependence on lung volume as well as diaphragm length. *Am. Rev. Respir. Dis.*, 135:A330.

Rochester, D. F., Farkas, G. A., and Lu, J.-Y. (1987). Contractility of the in situ human diaphragm: assessment based on dimensional analysis. In *Respiratory Muscles and Their Neuromotor Control*. Edited by G. C. Sieck, S. C. Gandevia, and W. E. Cameron. New York, A.R. Liss, pp. 327–336.

Roussos, C., Fixley, M., Gross, D., and Macklem, P. T. (1979). Fatigue of inspiratory muscles and their synergic behavior. *J. Appl. Physiol.*, 46:897–904.

Sakai, Y., Dal Ri, H., and Schmidt, G. (1973). Über die Wirkung von Atropin auf die Entladungs-frequenz in Phrenicus-einzelfasern der Ratte. *Arch. Toxicol.*, 30:161–174.

Sant'Ambrogio, G., Decandia, M., and Gantchev, G. N. (1969). The composite structure of the diaphragm of the rabbit. *Arch. Fisiol.*, 67:27–39.

Sant'Ambrogio, G., and Saibene, F. (1970). Contractile properties of the diaphragm in some mammals. *Respir. Physiol.*, 10:349–357.

Shardonofsky, F. R., Perez-Chada, D., and Milic-Emili, J. (1991). Airway pressures during crying: an index of respiratory muscle strength in infants with neuromuscular disease. *Pediatr. Pulmonology*, 10:172–177.

Sharp, J. T., Goldberg, N. B., Druz, W. S., and Danon, J. (1975). Relative contributions of rib cage and abdomen to breathing in normal subjects. *J. Appl. Physiol.*, 39:608–618,

Sharp, J. T., Beard, G. A. T., Sunga, M., Kim, T. W., Modh, A., Lind, J., and Walsh, J.

(1986). The rib cage in normal and emphysematous subjects: a roentgenographic approach. *J. Appl. Physiol.*, 61:2050–2059.

Sieck, G. C., Trelease, R. B., and Harper, R. M. (1984). Sleep influences on diaphragmatic motor unit discharge. *Exp. Neurol.*, 85:316–335.

Smith, J., and Bellemare, F. (1987). Effect of lung volume on in vivo contraction characteristics of human diaphragm. *J. Appl. Physiol.*, 62:1893–1900.

Sprung, J., Deschamps, C., Margulies, S. S., Hubmayr, R. D., and Rodarte, J. R. (1990). Effect of body position on regional diaphragm function in dogs. *J. Appl. Physiol.*, 69: 2296–2302.

Stahl, W. R. (1967). Scaling of respiratory variables in mammals. *J. Appl. Physiol.*, 22:453–460.

Tao, H.-Y., and Farkas, G. A. (1992a). Predictability of ventilatory muscle optimal length based on excised dimensions. *J. Appl. Physiol.*, 72:2024–2028.

Tao, H.-Y., and Farkas, G. A. (1992b). Mechanics of acutely shortened canine diaphragm in vitro. *J. Formosan Med. Assoc.*, 91:69–74.

Tobin, M. J., Chadha, T. S., Jenouri, J., Birch, S. J., Gazeroglu, H. B., and Sackner, M. A. (1983). Breathing patterns 1. Normal subjects. *Chest*, 84:202–205.

Tomori, Z., Donic, V., and Kurpas, M. (1993). Comparison of inspiratory effort in sniff-like aspiration reflex, gasping and normal breathing in cats. *Eur. Respir. J.*, 6:53–59.

Topulos, G. P., Reid, M. B., and Leith, D. E. (1987). Pliometric activity of inspiratory muscles: maximal pressure-flow curves. *J. Appl. Physiol.*, 62:322–327.

Torres, A., Kimball, W. R., Qvist, J., Stanek, K., Kacmarek, R. M., Whyte, R. I., Montalescot, G., and Zapol, W. M. (1989). Sonomicrometric regional diaphragmatic shortening in awake sheep after thoracic surgery. *J. Appl. Physiol.*, 67:2357–2368.

Truwit, J. D., and Marini, J. J. (1992). Validation of a technique to assess maximal inspiratory pressure in poorly cooperative patients. *Chest*, 102:1216–1219.

Tzelepis, G. E., McCool, F. D., Leith, D. E., and Hoppin, F. G., Jr. (1988). Increased lung volume limits endurance of inspiratory muscles. *J. Appl. Physiol.*, 64:1796–1802.

Verschakelen, J. A., Deschepper, K., Jiang, T. X., and Demedts, M. (1989). Diaphragmatic displacement measured by fluoroscopy and derived by Respitrace. *J. Appl. Physiol.*, 67:694–698.

Verschakelen, J. A., Deschepper, K., and Demedts, M. (1992). Relationship between axial motion and volume displacement of the diaphragm during VC maneuvers. *J. Appl. Physiol.*, 72:1536–1540.

Wade, O. L. (1954). Movements of the thoracic cage and diaphragm in respiration. *J. Physiol.*, 124:193–212.

Wade, O. L., and Gilson, J. C. (1951). The effect of posture on diaphragmatic movement and vital capacity in normal subjects with a note on spirometry as an aid in determining radiological chest volumes. *Thorax*, 6:103–126.

Wait, J. L., Nahormek, P. A., Yost, W. T., and Rochester, D. F. (1989). Diaphragmatic thickness-lung volume relationship in vivo. *J. Appl. Physiol.*, 67:1560–1568.

Wallinga-de Jonge, W., Boom, H. B. K., Boon, K. L., Griep, P. A. M., and Lammeree, G. C. (1980). Force development of fast and slow skeletal muscle at different muscle lengths. *Am. J. Physiol.*, 239:C98–C104.

Wang, C. S., and Josenhans, W. T. (1971). Contribution of diaphragmatic/abdominal displacement to ventilation in supine man. *J. Appl. Physiol.*, 31:576–580.

Ward, M. E., Paiva, M., and Macklem, P. T. (1992). Vector analysis in partitioning of inspiratory muscle action in dogs. *Eur. Respir. J.*, 5:219–227.

Warner, D. O., Krayer, S., Rehder, K., and Ritman, E. L. (1989). Chest wall motion during spontaneous breathing and mechanical ventilation in dogs. *J. Appl. Physiol.*, 66:1179–1189.

Watchko, J. F., LaFramboise, W. A., Standaert, T. A., and Woodrum, D. E. (1986). Diaphragmatic function during hypoxemia: neonatal and developmental aspects. *J. Appl. Physiol.*, 60:1599–1604.

Whitelaw, W. A. (1987). Shape and size of the human diaphragm in vivo. *J. Appl. Physiol.*, 62:180–186.

Whitelaw, W. A., Hajdo, L. E., and Wallace, J. A. (1983). Relationships among pressure, tension and shape of the diaphragm. *J. Appl. Physiol.*, 55:1899–1905.

Yan, S., Gauthier, A. P., Similowski, T., Macklen, P. T., and Bellemare, F. (1992). Evaluation of human diaphragm contractility using mouth pressure twitches. *Am. Rev. Respir. Dis.*, 145:1064–1069.

Yan, S., Gauthier, A. P., Similowski, T., Faltus, R., Macklem, P. T., and Bellemare, F. (1993). Force-frequency relationships of in vivo human and in vitro rat diaphragm using paired stimuli. *Eur. Respir. J.* 6:211–218.

40

Strength of the Respiratory Muscles

FRANÇOIS BELLEMARE

University of Montreal
Hôtel-Dieu Hospital
Montreal, Quebec, Canada

The strength of skeletal muscles in situ is generally measured as the maximum force these muscles can develop against an external load when the position of the relevant structures and articulations is optimally adjusted. With the exception of some of the neck accessory muscles, the force developed by the respiratory muscles cannot be directly measured. As an alternative, the strength of the respiratory muscles can be defined as the transmural pressure these muscles can develop across the respiratory wall structures when maximally activated. However, the force developed by the respiratory muscles can be estimated from the transmural pressure measurements based on known geometrical features of the chest wall (Fenn, 1963; Rochester et al., 1981; Kikuchi et al., 1982; Loring and Mead, 1982) (see also Chap. 39).

The relevant pressures are the airway opening pressure or mouth pressure (P_{ao}; P_{mouth}), which is the pressure across the entire respiratory system; the pleural pressure (P_{pl}), which is the transmural pressure across that part of the rib cage facing the lungs or pulmonary rib cage, the transdiaphragmatic pressure (P_{di}), which is the pressure across the diaphragm, and the transabdominal pressure (P_{ab}), which is the pressure across the abdominal wall. P_{pl} also represents the pressure across the lumped diaphragm-abdomen. Because of the elastic behavior of the respiratory structures, their recoil pressure must be subtracted from the measured pressure to obtain the pressure developed by the respiratory muscles. In this chapter the notation ΔP_{ao}, ΔP_{pl}, ΔP_{di}, and ΔP_{ab} indicates that elastic recoil of the relevant structures has been subtracted. Respiratory muscle strength defined this way should depend on the muscle's mass, contractility, mechanical advantage, operating length, and velocity of shortening.

Several methods have been devised to assess the strength of the respiratory muscles. They fall into three major categories, depending on whether they are based on maximum voluntary effort, artificial motor nerve stimulation, or a combination of both.

I. Maximum Static Voluntary Efforts

A. Transrespiratory System Pressure

The measurement of mouth pressure during maximum inspiratory or expiratory efforts lasting about one second and performed against a closed airway is the method most frequently employed to evaluate the strength of the inspiratory (P_{Imax}) and expiratory muscles (P_{Emax}). When lung volume is constant and the respiratory muscles are relaxed, the mouth pressure (P_{mouth}) reflects the elastic recoil pressure of the respiratory system. If lung volume remains constant, mouth pressure changes should reflect pleural surface pressure changes and both should reflect corresponding changes in the pressure exerted by the respiratory muscles (P_{mus}) (Rahn et al., 1946).

Usually, a small leak is introduced in the mouthpiece to ensure that the glottis is at least partially opened and mouth pressure equals alveolar pressure. When measured this way, the mouth pressure swing reflects the net pressure developed by all respiratory muscles (both inspiratory and expiratory) recruited by the voluntary effort. Therefore it is not possible with this measurement to draw definite conclusions about a specific muscle or muscle group (see below). Furthermore, this measurement is also dependent on the level of voluntary effort expended, and may thus be affected by the degree of alertness, motivation, and practice of the subject and the quality of the instructions given. Additionally, at lung volumes other than that at which the elastic recoil pressure of the respiratory system is zero, it is influenced by the system's elastic properties independently of muscle strength. The elastic recoil pressure of the respiratory system is a difficult parameter to evaluate in untrained subjects (Agostoni and Mead, 1964), and in most conditions in which the strength of the respiratory muscles has been evaluated, no corrections were made for respiratory system recoil. Typically the recoil pressure varies in a sigmoidal fashion as a function of lung volume from –30 cm H_2O at normal RV to +40 cm H_2O at normal total lung capacity. Proper correction of respiratory system recoil requires that lung volume changes due to gas compression or rarefaction during expiratory and inspiratory efforts, respectively, be taken also in consideration. This, in turn, requires knowledge of the absolute lung volume or that the measurements be performed in a body plethysmograph.

The values of P_{mus} obtained by this method have been shown to vary with lung volume, those recorded during inspiratory efforts showing a decrease and those recorded during expiratory efforts an increase with increasing lung volume (Rohrer, 1916; Rahn et al., 1946). These early findings have been largely confirmed in subsequent studies (Cook et al., 1964; Milic-Emili et al., 1964; Ringqvist, 1966) (Fig. 1). In general, the reported maximal expiratory pressures are considerably greater (between 50 and 100% in different studies) than the maximal inspiratory ones.

The dependency of maximum inspiratory and expiratory pressures on lung volume has been interpreted as reflecting the basic length-tension properties of the respiratory muscles, the inspiratory ones increasing their length and number of cross-bridges as lung volume decreases, the opposite occurring for the expiratory muscles. However, the length changes of the different respiratory muscles with lung inflation and deflation are not uniform. The length change of the diaphragm (Sharp et al., 1974) and the abdominal muscles (Leevers and Road, 1989) over the vital capacity is about three times as large as that of the intrinsic muscles of the rib cage and of the accessory muscles of the neck (Sharp et al., 1974) (see also Chap. 39). It is, therefore, tempting to attribute the volume dependency of maximum inspiratory and expiratory pressures to the diaphragm and abdominal muscles, respectively.

Residual volume (RV) and total lung capacity (TLC) have been generally identified as the optimal respiratory positions to assess the strength of the inspiratory and expiratory muscles, respectively. However, when a correction is made for respiratory system recoil, a more intermediate optimal position is found for the inspiratory muscles (Ringqvist, 1966). Maximum inspiratory (P_{Imax}) and expiratory (P_{Emax}) pressures measured at RV and TLC but uncorrected for respiratory system recoil have been found to be about 30% greater in adult males than in adult females (Cook et al., 1964; Ringqvist, 1966; Black and Hyatt, 1969; Leech et al., 1983; Vincken et al., 1989; McElvaney, 1989) (Fig. 2). The differences in P_{Imax} and P_{Emax}

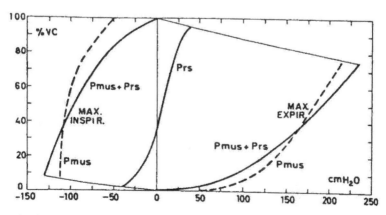

Figure 1 Lung volume against alveolar pressure during maximum inspiratory and expiratory efforts and during relaxation. The broken lines indicate the pressure contributed by the muscles. (From Rohrer, 1916, as modified by Agostoni and Mead, 1964.)

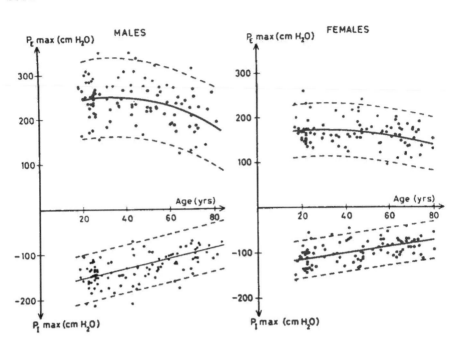

Figure 2   Variations with age of the maximum expiratory (P_{Emax}) and inspiratory (P_{Imax}) pressures in male and females. Regression lines ± 2 SD are shown. (From Ringqvist, 1966.)

between males and females increase rapidly from childhood to early adolescence but are present even before puberty (Cook et al., 1964; Wilson et al., 1984; Gaultier and Zinman, 1983). However, in crying infants between 3 months and 3 years of age, the maximum pressures during inspiratory or expiratory efforts were not different in males and females (Shardonowski et al., 1989).

P_{Imax} and P_{Emax} have been found to decrease with age both in males and females (Cook et al., 1964; Ringvist, 1966; Black and Hyatt, 1969; Vincken et al., 1989) (see Fig. 2). For the inspiratory muscles, this decrease is linear over the entire age range investigated, whereas for the expiratory muscles the effect of age is best described by a parabolic function showing a decrease beyond 40–50 years of age (Ringqvist, 1966; Black and Hyatt, 1969; Vincken et al., 1987).

P_{Imax} and P_{Emax} values have been shown to be increased by specific strength training programs but are not affected by endurance type training programs (Leith and Bradley, 1976). Accordingly, no difference was found in maximum inspiratory pressures between sedentary subjects and athletes engaged in endurance exercise (Cost et al., 1990). It is of interest, however, that Ringqvist (1966) found that a significant portion of the intersubject variability in P_{Imax} and P_{Emax} could be explained by intersubject variations in airway resistance, which was viewed as an adaptation of the respiratory muscles to the prevailing respiratory load. Likewise, the finding that the optimal respiratory positions established for inspiratory and expiratory muscle strength appear to correspond to those at which they are usually requested to perform ventilatory tasks may also be interpreted as a functional adaptation of the respiratory muscles. The above-mentioned effects of age, sex, and level of activity parallel similar findings in limb muscles and have been interpreted as reflecting corresponding changes in muscle mass.

In crying infants from 3 months to 3 years of age (Shardonowsky et al., 1989) as well as in children between 7 and 11 years of age (Cook et al., 1966; Gaultier and Zinman, 1983; Wilson et al., 1984), the values of P_{Imax} and P_{Emax} are not markedly different from adults in spite of obvious differences in inspiratory muscle strength. The relatively well-preserved inspiratory and expiratory pressure generating capacity in infants and children despite markedly smaller respiratory muscle mass has been attributed to better mechanical advantage of the respiratory muscles possibly related to a smaller radius of curvatures of the chest wall structures (Cook et al., 1964; Gaultier and Zinman, 1983) (see also Chap. 16). However, when the maximum respiratory pressures are corrected for intersubject variations in non-respiratory muscle strength, the differences between adult males and females disappear, in spite of obvious differences in the mechanical advantage of the respiratory muscles between the sexes (Ringqvist, 1966). The lower values of P_{Imax} and P_{Emax} frequently reported in patients with thoracic deformities may in part be explained by mechanical disadvantage of the respiratory muscles in addition to muscle weakness (Cooper et al., 1984; Lisboa et al., 1985). Although Hyatt, as reported in Chapter 16, found no difference in the values of P_{Imax} and P_{Emax} between the upright and the supine postures, smaller values have been found in the supine than in the seated posture by Koulouris et al. (1989), a difference that could in part be related to the different geometry of the chest wall structures of the two postures (see Chap. 16).

After the effects of age and sex have been taken into account, there is still substantial variability in the values of maximum inspiratory and expiratory pressures measured at the volume extremes both among different individuals and among different studies. Rochester (1988) has reviewed a number of studies in normal subjects and obtained a coefficient of variation for P_{Imax} and P_{Emax} of about 25% with a range of 8–37% in different studies. The most detailed and comprehensive analysis of intersubject variability has been conducted by Ringqvist (1966). For both sexes together, age, bony dimensions, and lung volumes (TLC; RV/TLC) were found to have significant negative effects, whereas pulmonary resistance and nonrespiratory muscle strength had significant positive influences, the nonrespiratory muscle strength being the most important factor. About 65% of the variance in P_{Imax} and P_{Emax} was explained by these factors, including sex. Considering the error involved in measuring some of these factors, up to 75% of the variance could potentially be explained by these factors alone. Other factors that could explain this variability are variations in respiratory system recoil, in the way the maneuvers are performed by different subjects, in the degree of coordination among various muscle groups, or in the level of effort exerted. Because of this large intersubject variability, a large change in muscle pressure will be needed before a decision can be made as to whether a given measured value is abnormal. However, the coefficients of variation for repeated measurements in the same subject are much smaller (8–9%), and little practice seems to be required such that changes in respiratory muscle strength may be reliably evaluated when a subject serves as his or her own control (Cook et al., 1964; Ringqvist, 1966; Gaultier and Zinman, 1983; McElvaney et al., 1989).

The range of normal values also varies widely among different studies. Several factors could account for this variability, including variations in the characteristics of the population examined, the quality of the instructions given and their degree of enforcement, the number of trials performed, etc. Part of the variability could be related to the different types of mouthpieces employed by different investigators. Indeed, a review of the literature and direct experimental evidence (Cook et al., 1964; Koulouris et al., 1988) suggests that higher values of P_{Imax} and P_{Emax} can be achieved with a rigid rubber tube pressed around the lips than with a regular flanged mouthpiece positioned between the lips and teeth, particularly during expiratory efforts. The tube mouthpiece, by providing a better seal, may allow the subject to exert higher pressures (and level of muscle activation), whereas the seal provided by the flanged mouthpiece may also be determined by the strength of the facial muscles. In view of the large variability among different studies and of the many factors that could affect the measurement of maximum respiratory pressures, it is generally recommended that normal standards be established by each laboratory. The problems associated with the use of a mouthpiece can be overcome by keeping the glottis closed and recording esophageal pressure changes as index of pleural pressure changes during inspiratory and expiratory efforts with a balloon-catheter system positioned in the middle third of the esophagus. In intubated patients the problem is overcome by measuring tracheal pressure (Marini et al., 1986). A recent study pointed out, however, that the measurement of P_{Imax} in intubated patients may not be relied upon to estimate their inspiratory muscle strength, the measurements being poorly reproducible in a given patient and also dependent on the investigator controlling the test (Multz et al., 1990). Nevertheless, the measurements of P_{Imax} and P_{Emax} have been used extensively to investigate the strength of the respiratory muscles in various clinical conditions affecting the lungs, the chest wall, or the neuromuscular system (pertinent reviews can be found in other chapters of this book).

B. Trans–Rib Cage, Transabdominal, and Transdiaphragmatic Pressures

As indicated above, the transrespiratory system pressure can only give the net pressure developed by all the respiratory muscles, both agonists and antagonists, that are recruited simultaneously. A separation between antagonistic respiratory muscle activity can only be made at the abdominal boundary of the respiratory system through the measurement of transdiaphragmatic pressure (P_{di}) and transabdominal pressure (P_{ab}) (Agostoni and Rahn, 1960). These pressures are usually obtained with the aid of air-filled balloon-catheter systems introduced via the upper airways into the esophagus and the stomach. Under most circumstances these pressures approximate pleural (P_{pl}) and abdominal (P_{ab}) pressure changes. At isolung volume, when the glottis is opened:

$$\Delta P_{ao} = \Delta P_{pl} = \Delta P_{di} + \Delta P_{ab} \tag{1}$$

It is clear from Eq. (1) that ΔP_{ao} or ΔP_{pl} during maximum inspiratory or expiratory efforts will be smaller than the maximum pressure the diaphragm or the abdominal muscles can generate if these two sets of muscles are recruited simultaneously. Values of ΔP_{pl} smaller than ΔP_{di} during inspiratory efforts and smaller than ΔP_{ab} during expiratory efforts have now been reported by several investigators (Agostoni and Mead, 1964; Mead et al., 1964, DeTroyer and Estenne, 1981; Gibson et al., 1981), clearly reflecting the limitation of ΔP_{ao} and ΔP_{pl} when assessing the strength of the inspiratory or expiratory muscles.

The difficulty resulting from the simultaneous recruitment of antagonistic muscles cannot be overcome by simply recording ΔP_{di} or ΔP_{ab} since the values obtained will also be determined by the strength and/or level of recuitment of the antagonistic muscle or muscle group. Indeed, in untrained subjects, not only is the ΔP_{di} measured during maximum inspiratory efforts markedly variable among different subjects (DeTroyer and Estenne, 1981; Gibson et al., 1981), but those with low values of ΔP_{di} can rapidly learn to generate higher ΔP_{ab} and ΔP_{di} values by simultaneously recruiting the abdominal muscles (DeTroyer and Estenne, 1981). Their low initial ΔP_{di} likely results, therefore, from a submaximal activation of their diaphragms. By contrast, in highly trained subjects, the pattern of pressure generation is remarkably uniform, P_{ab} remaining close to relaxation values during maximum static inspiratory efforts at any given lung volume (Milic-Emili et al., 1964; Mead et al., 1964; Hershenson et al., 1988). In those subjects, higher ΔP_{di} values can be recorded during expulsive efforts requiring the co-activation of the abdominal muscles, again suggesting that during inspiratory efforts, the diaphragm is submaximally activated. Similarly, higher values of ΔP_{ab} have generally been found in the same subjects during expulsive than during expiratory efforts at the same lung volume (Agostoni and Rahn, 1960; Milic-Emili et al., 1964; Hershenson et al., 1988), again suggesting that the abdominal muscles are not maximally activated during expiratory efforts. That the diaphragm can be maximally activated during expulsive efforts or during combined inspiratory and expulsive efforts has now been demonstrated using the technique of twitch occlusion (see below) (Bellemare and Bigland-Ritchie, 1984; Gandevia et al., 1985, 1992; Hershenson et al., 1988). Whether the diaphragm is submaximally activated during inspiratory efforts performed without increasing abdominal pressure is, however, controversial (Hershenson et al., 1988; McKenzie et al., 1988; Gandevia et al., 1985, 1992). Maximal activation of abdominal muscles does not appear possible with any maneuvers (Gandevia et al., 1990).

Not surprisingly, reported values of maximal P_{di} vary markedly among different individuals as well as among different studies. For maximum inspiratory efforts, reported values of maximal ΔP_{di} are between 36 and 200 cm H_2O in different subjects and mean values are between 108 and 175 cm H_2O in different studies. For expulsive or combined inspiratory-expulsive efforts, corresponding values are between 165 and 265 cm H_2O for individual subjects and between 180 and 218 cm H_2O for study groups (Agostoni and Rahn, 1960; Milic-Emili et al., 1964; Roussos and Macklem, 1977; Gibson et al., 1981; DeTroyer and Estenne, 1981; Braun et al., 1982; Bellemare and Bigland-Ritchie, 1984; Laporta and Grassino, 1985; Hershenson et al., 1988; Koulouris et al., 1989; Levy et al., 1990). Maximal values are usually recorded in the mid–lung volume range (Milic-Emili et al., 1964; Gibson et al., 1977, 1981; Hershenson et al., 1988), and, although only limited data are available, there appears to be little difference between males and females (DeTroyer and Estenne, 1981). Maximal P_{di} during inspiratory efforts is closely related to the length of the diaphragm as measured from x-ray films for lung volumes comprised between FRC and TLC (Braun et al., 1982). The variability among subjects can be markedly reduced by displaying the P_{di} signal or the P_{es} and P_{ga} signals as feedback to the subject (Laporta and Grassino, 1985). Using this biofeedback method, maximal diaphragmatic activation has been consistently demonstrated in normal subjects (Bellemare and Bigland-Ritchie, 1984; Levy et al., 1990) and patients with chronic obstructive lung disease (Similowski et al., 1991) when the diaphragm is fresh and not fatigued. In the presence of diaphragmatic fatigue, maximal activation of the diaphragm may not be achieved whatever the method employed (Bellemare and Bigland-Ritchie, 1987; see also McKenzie et al., 1992).

No matter how trained the subject is and irrespective of the condition under which this has been tested, the maximal P_{di} the diaphragm can generate is considerably greater (between 30 and 100%) than the minimum pleural or mouth pressure that can be developed. The implication of this high pressure-generating capacity that is incompletely transformed into pleural pressure has often been questioned (e.g., Gibson et al., 1981; DeTroyer and Estenne, 1981; Laporta and Grassino, 1985). A large force reserve may serve the purpose of preventing fatigue of the diaphragm by increasing the fatigue threshold (Bellemare and Grassino, 1983), or may serve to compensate for the fall in force due to force-velocity properties of muscles as the level of ventilation increases (McCool et al., 1992). Also, that part of P_{di} that goes into P_{ab} serves to displace the abdomen and the rib cage during breathing, thereby making room for lung expansion (Loring and Mead, 1982) (see also Sec. III.B).

Maximal abdominal pressures during expulsive efforts performed with opened glottis are nearly equal to the maximal P_{di} during expulsive efforts (see above). These values are consistently smaller than the maximal values of ΔP_{ab} that can be recorded during expiratory or expulsive efforts with the glottis closed (Agostoni and Rahn, 1960; Milic-Emili et al., 1964; Agostoni and Mead, 1964; Hershenson et al., 1988; Gandevia et al., 1990). Few maximum values have been reported with the latter maneuver. They range between 250 and 400 cm H_2O in different subjects and are usually recorded at high lung volumes, i.e., near TLC. These are greater than the maximum pressures that can be developed by the diaphragm or the rib cage muscles.

C. Relative Strengths of Chest Wall Muscles

It is clear from the preceding section that the maximum pressures that can be developed by different respiratory muscle groups are not matched. Hershenson et al. (1988) hypothesized that the level of activation of antagonistic muscles when recruited simultaneously is regulated in such a way as to minimize chest wall distortions. This hypothesis led them to suggest that the maximum pressure measured in a given maneuver should reflect the strength of the weaker antagonistic muscle or muscle group. In their analysis, the diaphragm was considered antagonistic to both the abdominal muscles and the inspiratory muscles of the rib cage on the basis that the latter would lengthen when the diaphragm shortens at iso-lung volume. Having found like others that P_{di} is greater during expulsive efforts than during inspiratory efforts performed without increasing abdominal pressure, they concluded that the change in P_{pl} (or P_{ao}) during inspiratory efforts reflect the strength of the weaker inspiratory rib cage muscles. They supported their conclusion by demonstrating more negative values of ΔP_{pl} (and also ΔP_{di}) when the rib cage muscles are assisted by negative pressure applied around the thorax. Similarly, having found higher values of ΔP_{ab} during expulsive maneuvers, with glottis closed than with open glottis, they concluded that with the latter ΔP_{ab} reflects the strength of the weaker diaphragm. They supported their conclusion by showing with twitch occlusion (see below) and electromyogram (EMG) recordings that, at functional residual capacity (FRC), the diaphragm was indeed maximally activated during open glottis expulsive maneuver, but submaximally activated during inspiratory efforts and by showing, also with EMG recordings, a greater activation of abdominal muscles during closed glottis than during open glottis expulsive maneuvers. The strength of the inspiratory rib cage muscles during inspiratory efforts, of the diaphragm during open glottis expulsive effort or combined inspiratory-expulsive efforts, and of the abdominal muscles during closed glottis expulsive efforts at different lung volumes in their normal subjects is shown in Figure 3. This shows that in normal subjects, the diaphragm is stronger than the inspiratory rib cage muscles at all lung volumes, even though it is submaximally activated at lung volumes less than FRC, and that the abdominal muscles are stronger than the diaphragm over most of the vital capacity (i.e., above 20% VC). In addition, their results clearly show that the smaller values of maximum ΔP_{di} at RV than at FRC (Milic-Emili et al., 1964; Gibson et al., 1977) are due to a reduced capacity of the subjects to maximally activate it and strongly argue in favor of a more intermediate position to test the diaphragm with voluntary efforts, even though maximal P_{di} values should be recorded at RV, as was demonstrated by artificial bilateral phrenic nerve stimulation (Smith and Bellemare, 1987; Johnson et al., 1993).

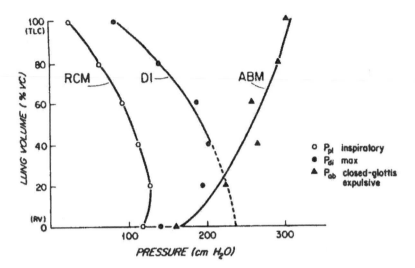

Figure 3   Relative strengths of respiratory muscles at different lung volumes. Estimates are based on measurements of maximal inspiratory pressure (inspiratory muscles of rib cage, RCM), maximal P_{di} (diaphragm, DI), and maximal abdominal pressure during closed-glottis expulsive efforts (abdominal muscles, ABM). Line representing diaphragm strength is dashed below 40% vital capacity (VC), because diaphragmatic activation was probably submaximal during expulsive and combined maneuvers at these lung volumes. (From Hershenson et al., 1988.)

The analysis of Hershenson et al. (1988) offers, as a first approximation, a method to assess the relative strengths of the weaker chest wall muscles. By comparing the ΔP_{di} during inspiratory and expulsive efforts and the ΔP_{ab} during open and closed glottis expulsive maneuver, one could determine which of the diaphragm, the rib cage, or the abdominal muscles is the weaker during inspiratory and expiratory efforts. This method has been employed to investigate the effect of fatigue on the strength of different respiratory muscle groups (McCool et al., 1992). Whether this approach can be useful clinically remains to be established. Patients may have difficulty learning how to perform the different required maneuvers properly. Furthermore, it may not be possible with this method alone to evaluate the strength of the stronger muscle. For instance, Gandevia et al. (1990) found higher levels of abdominal muscle EMG activity during postural tasks than during closed glottis expulsive maneuvers, thus showing the potential for higher transabdominal pressures, which they directly demonstrated by stimulating the motor cortex transcranially (see below). The consideration by Hershenson et al. (1988) of the diaphragm and the inspiratory rib cage muscles as antagonists may be an oversimplification even when P_{ab} does not increase because it neglects the direct insertional action of the diaphragm on the rib cage (Loring and Mead, 1982). Thus the ΔP_{pl} during inspiratory effort may not simply reflect the strength of the weaker rib cage muscles. The measurement of ΔP_{pl} as a measure of trans–rib cage pressure, in addition to being determined in part by the diaphragm, can only reflect the strength of the rib cage muscles facing the lung surface. As the surface of the rib cage exposed to the lungs varies from about 20% to about 90% of the total rib cage surface between TLC and RV, the measurement of ΔP_{pl} will reflect the strength of a progressively smaller fraction of the rib cage musculature as lung volume decreases. Because the rib cage muscles not facing the lung presumably remain active at all lung volumes, their action on that part of the rib cage must be balanced by antagonistic muscle activity. In the absence of abdominal muscle contraction, this activity must be from the rib cage itself, which further complicates the interpretation of ΔP_{pl} during inspiratory efforts.

Clearly, the mechanism governing the level of activation of the respiratory muscles in different maneuvers and particularly in trained individuals remains to be elucidated. A mechanism aimed at minimizing chest wall distortion independently from the voluntary effort, as suggested by Hershenson et al. (1988), may not generally apply, since inspiratory efforts can be performed that markedly distort the chest wall without any discomfort by preferentially recruiting the diaphragm (Hillman et al., 1990). In this instance the diaphragm shortens and its capacity to generate pressure decreases. Gandevia et al. (1992) have now shown using radiography that the diaphragm can shorten by as much as 20% of its initial length during inspiratory efforts in which abdominal pressure increases by up to 25 cm H_2O, whereas the length does not change or increases slightly during expulsive efforts. The change in length in their experiment was in fact sufficient to account for the difference in maximal P_{di} measured in both conditions, a finding consistent with their previous demonstration of maximal diaphragmatic activation under similar conditions (Gandevia et al., 1985, 1990). Because diaphragmatic shortening can only reduce maximal P_{di} while, in most instances, also increasing P_{ab}, P_{pl} may not be increased or may even be reduced at the expense of further increasing diaphragmatic activation. It seems possible, therefore, that in trained subjects, respiratory muscle recruitment be coordinated in such a way as to optimize performance in the required task. Because of the unusual character of those tasks for most subjects, some practice or training may be required before optimal coordination is attained. Of course, optimizing performance in terms of pleural pressure changes may also require that chest wall distortions be minimized. It is of particular interest that highly trained subjects seem to be able to achieve higher lung volumes with lower transdiaphragmatic pressure changes than untrained individuals (Mead et al., 1963).

II. Maximum Dynamic Voluntary Efforts

A. Maximum Pressure-Flow Relationships

Dynamic contractions can also be employed to evaluate the strength of the respiratory muscles. In fact, the maximum inspiratory or expiratory pressures measured under static conditions are not the maximum pressures the respiratory muscles can develop. Topoulos et al. (1987) have now shown that the inspiratory muscles can generate high higher pressures when attempting to prevent lung emptying by an external pressure source than under static conditions at the same lung volume, a characteristic resembling that of the other skeletal muscles when being stretched while active (i.e., during pliometric contractions).

When inspiratory or expiratory efforts are performed against external resistances, the maximum inspiratory or expiratory pressures that can be recorded at a set volume are smaller than under static conditions and inversely related to the prevailing inspiratory or expiratory flow (Agostoni and Fenn, 1960; Hyatt and Flath, 1966; Topoulos et al., 1987). These findings have also been interpreted on the basis of the force-velocity characteristics of skeletal muscles. By contrast with the curvilinear in vitro force-velocity relation of skeletal muscles, the reported pressure-flow relationships for the respiratory muscles in situ are generally linear, a discrepancy that has not yet been resolved (see, however, Goldman et al., 1978, and Kikuchi et al., 1982).

The maximum pressure-flow relationships are rarely employed to evaluate the function of the respiratory muscles. Their determination is time consuming and could be tiring. In addition, because of the dependency of maximum pressure-flow curves on lung volume (Pengelly et al., 1971), normal standards would be difficult to establish. Nevertheless, under some circumstances requiring high respiratory minute volume, such as heavy exercise, the capacity of the respiratory muscles to generate pressure at high flow rates may be more meaningful physiologically than the maximum static pressure these muscles can generate (Leblanc et al., 1986). The recent demonstration of diaphragmatic fatigue in normal subjects during heavy exercise (Johnson et al., 1993) combined with the observation that fatigue induced by high-flow tasks preferentially fatigues the diaphragm and reduces maximum flow (McCool et al., 1992) suggest that the maximum pressure-flow relationships could be of use in evaluating the role of the respiratory muscles in limiting maximum exercise performance.

B. Time Course of Maximum Voluntary Contractions

The dynamics of the maximal voluntary contractions of the respiratory muscles have been studied by Mognoni et al. (1968) in normal subjects by analyzing the time course of esophageal and gastric pressure changes during the quickest maximum inspiratory and expiratory efforts, respectively. After the first 30–50 ms, during which the pressure rises more slowly, the pressure rises as a simple exponential function of time with a half time of about 50 ms for both the inspiratory and the expiratory efforts (Mognoni et al., 1968). Similar values for the half-time have been found in normal subjects and patients with chronic obstructive pulmonary disease (COPD) by Marazzini et al. (1972). These values of half time are about the same as for other skeletal muscles during artificially stimulated tetanic contractions

(Merton, 1954) and for the diaphragm stimulated with twin pulses at 10-ms intervals (McKenzie et al., 1992) and suggest that the respiratory motor units that are recuited by maximum voluntary efforts are also tetanically activated (Mognoni et al., 1968). More recently, a similar conclusion has been reached for the diaphragm using a completely different technique (bilateral phrenic nerve stimulation) both in normals (Bellemare and Bigland-Ritchie, 1984; Gandevia et al., 1990) and in patients with COPD (Similowski et al., 1991) (see below). The time course of the initial pressure change is about the same whether the airways are opened or closed, suggesting that also for dynamic contractions, the maximum pressures are not slowed by neural factors (Mognoni et al., 1968). Because of its simplicity, this method could be of use when evaluating the extent to which the respiratory muscles are exerted during various dynamic respiratory maneuvers.

C. Maximum Sniffs and Coughs

The recording of diaphragmatic movement during a maximum sniff maneuver has been introduced as a diagnostic test to detect diaphragm paralysis (Alexander 1966). The sniff maneuver has subsequently been used in combination with mouth, esophageal, and transdiaphragmatic pressure measurements to evaluate the rate of diaphragmatic relaxation (Esau et al., 1983; Levy et al., 1984) and to evaluate the strength of the diaphragm (Miller et al., 1985; Mier et al., 1989) or of all inspiratory muscles (Laroche et al., 1988; Koulouris et al., 1989). When used for the purpose of measuring inspiratory muscle strength, the nose during a sniff is considered to act as a Starling resistor such that the nasal flow would be largely independent of the applied pressure, an assumption that does not appear to have been tested. The maximal nasal, esophageal, or transdiaphragmatic pressures during maximal sniffs performed at FRC have been found to require less practice, to be more reproducible, to have a smaller range of normal values, and to be the same or even higher than the corresponding pressures measured in the same subjects during maximum static inspiratory efforts performed at RV (Miller et al., 1985; Laroche et al., 1988). Differences between men and women are also smaller for maximum sniffs than for static inspiratory efforts (Miller et al., 1985). Some of these differences could, however, be related to the different lung volume at which the two maneuvers were performed. Furthermore, none of these differences were very large such that the superiority of the sniff over the usual static maneuvers is not clearly established. The nasal resistance could be affected by several other factors, including allergic reactions, that may be difficult to control and could affect the measured pressures. As for any voluntary contractions, the measured pressure will be determined by the level of voluntary effort exerted, a factor that, because of the transient character of the maneuver, would be difficult to evaluate. Measuring the time course of the maximum pressure change as described above could potentially be employed for this purpose (Mognoni et al., 1968).

In much the same way as the maximum sniff maneuver for the inspiratory muscles, maximum cough maneuvers could potentially be employed to evaluate the strength of the expiratory muscles. Arora and Gal (1981) have shown that the maximum esophageal pressures measured during maximum coughs and during maximum static expiratory efforts decline in the same proportion with progressive curarization in normal subjects, suggesting that the pressures measured with either method could reliably reflect the strength of the expiratory muscles. A potential advantage of coughs over maximum static expiratory efforts is that maximum expiratory pressures can easily be recorded as a function of lung volume during a single series of coughs started at TLC. Even though coughs, like sniffs, may be more natural maneuvers than maximum static efforts, their superiority over conventional measurements has not yet been firmly established. Nevertheless, they represent useful alternatives or complements available when the performance of other maneuvers is in doubt.

III. Respiratory Muscle Responses to Artificial Stimulation

Human muscle strength can be most directly measured during maximal tetanic stimulation of the motor nerve. This overcomes the usual problems associated with voluntary contractions. By varying the stimulation frequency, the force-frequency relationship can be constructed, which can yield additional information concerning the contractile properties of the muscle and helps distinguish different types of fatigue (Edwards et al., 1977). In addition, a comparison of the maximal voluntary force with that of an artificially stimulated contraction yields an objective estimate of the degree of muscle activation by voluntary effort (Merton, 1954). This can also be evaluated directly by delivering single supermaximal shocks during ongoing voluntary contractions, since the amplitude of the resulting twitches detects the force reserve left for full muscle activation by the central nervous system (Merton, 1954). These methods have been employed successfully in a number of experimental conditions in various limb muscles (Merton, 1954; Bigland-Ritchie et al., 1978, 1983; Edwards et al., 1977; Grimby et al., 1981; Belanger and McComas, 1981; Bellemare and Bigland-Ritchie, 1984; Bellemare and Garzaniti, 1988). Among the respiratory muscles, the sternomastoid (Moxham et al., 1980; Edwards et al., 1977; Wilson et al., 1984), the diaphragm (Pengelly et al., 1971; Moxham et al., 1981; Aubier et al., 1981; Bellemare et al., 1986), and the abdominal muscles (Mier et al., 1985; Gandevia et al., 1992) are also amenable to this form of testing.

A. The Sternomastoid Muscle

The sternomastoid can be easily stimulated with a surface electrode (cathode) over its midpoint, where it receives its innervation from the spinal accessory nerve, the anode being placed over the manubrium. The strength of the sternomastoid

contraction can be recorded as alternate force vectors. When rotation of the head
to the contralateral side is prevented, a lateral force vector in the coronal plane can
be recorded with a force transducer applied over the mastoid process. Alternatively,
a force transducer can be pressed against the sternal tendon of the sternomastoid
and an anterior force vector recorded in the sagittal plane. The force-frequency
curves obtained by either method were found to be similar (Moxham et al., 1980).
Forces well in excess of 15 N have been recorded by these methods, but normal
standards have not yet been established (Moxham et al., 1980; Wilson et al., 1984b).
So far, no attempts have been made to compare the forces developed by this muscle
during voluntary and stimulated contractions. The intensity of the stimulus can be
controlled by monitoring the output from the stimulator. A force plateau can be
reached with increasing stimulus intensity, indicating a maximum muscle activation,
although this may be too painful for routine clinical use (Wilson et al., 1984b).

Force-frequency curves of the sternomastoid muscles have a shape similar to
those of the diaphragm and other human limb muscles (Moxham et al., 1980) (Fig.
4). These have shown a decreased contractility and revealed the presence of
low-frequency fatigue in normal subjects after respiratory loading (Moxham et al.,
1981). The latter can be estimated by calculating the ratio of the force measured at 20
Hz stimulation with that at 100 Hz. Normal values of this ratio are around 0.75–0.8
and typically decrease to 0.5–0.6 in the presence of low-frequency fatigue (Moxham
et al., 1980). As for phrenic nerve stimulation, tetanic stimulation of the sternomastoid

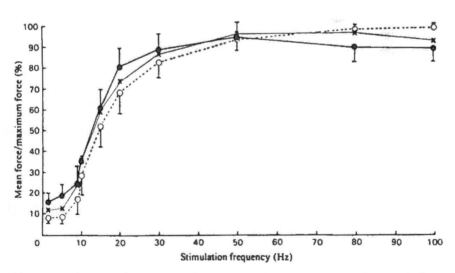

Figure 4   Frequency/force curve of the sternomastoid, quadriceps, and adductor pollicis in
normal subjects. Closed circles, sternomastoid (mean ±SD, n = 10); open circles, adductor
pollicis (mean ±SD, n = 10); crosses, quadriceps (mean only for clarity, n = 40). In different
subjects maximum force was achieved at different frequencies. The mean maximal values
are therefore less than 100%. (From Moxham et al., 1980.)

muscle at maximal intensies can be painful, which may limit the applicability of this test. Reproducible force frequency curves can, however, be obtained with submaximal but constant intensities (pulse duration: 0.5 ms; stimulator output: 50–80 V), which is more acceptable to the patient (Moxham et al., 1980; Wilson et al., 1984b; Eftimiou et al., 1987). By this method, and assuming the stimulus remains the same, changes in sternomastoid strength can be followed over time in a given patient and the presence of high- or low-frequency fatigue documented. The clinical significance of this test is not clear, however, as the sternomastoid muscle is not normally involved in resting breathing. In normal subjects it is only recruited at high levels of ventilation. They are reportedly often active in patients with severe airways obstruction who must rely on extradiaphragmatic muscles for quiet breathing (Campbell, 1970), although this has recently been questioned (Peche et al., 1993). A relatively rare recruitment of these muscles could explain the low incidence of low-frequency fatigue detected in this muscle in patients presenting in a hospital emergency setting with severe dyspnea (Eftimiou et al., 1989). Nevertheless, in patients with severe respiratory muscle weakness who must rely on the sternomastoid muscle for normal breathing, this test should be useful. For instance, patients with high cervical cord lesions can breathe with these muscles alone for only a few hours each day presumably because these muscles become fatigued (Danon et al., 1979; DeTroyer et al., 1986). Moxham et al. (1981b) reported the case of one patient with poliomyelitis with relative sparing of the sternomastoid muscle who developed severe low-frequency fatigue of this muscle after one hour of quiet breathing in the supine posture. They also documented the case of a patient with myasthenia gravis in which a selective loss of force at high stimulation frequencies (high-frequency fatigue) could be demonstrated by this method (Moxham et al., 1981b).

B. The Diaphragm

The diaphragm is innervated by the C3–C5 phrenic nerve roots, and all three branches are accessible to artificial stimulation in the neck, posteriorly to the sternomastoid muscle and at the level of the cricoid cartilage. An accessory branch to the phrenic nerve originating from the brachial plexus has been found in a majority of patients (Gray, 1976), however, its relative contribution to the motor innervation of the diaphragm is not known. The contraction of the diaphragm lowers pleural pressure and increases abdominal and transdiaphragmatic pressures, and all three pressures have been used to record the mechanical output of the diaphragm in response to artificial nerve stimulation.

Several methods have been described to stimulate the phrenic nerves in humans. Electrical stimulation of the phrenic nerves can be achieved transcutaneously with surface electrodes of various sizes (cathode) (Sarnoff et al., 1951; Delhez, 1965; Newsom-Davis, 1967, Bellemare and Bigland-Ritchie, 1984; Gandevia et al., 1985, 1990) or percutaneously with needles (Maclean and Mattioni, 1981; Aubier et al., 1985; Hershenson et al., 1988; Wilcox et al., 1988) or fine wire (Hubmayr et al., 1989) electrodes inserted at this site and positioned close to the phrenic nerve. In all these instances a large plate is usually fixed over the manubrium and serves as anode. No detailed comparison of these methods has yet been made, but the following may serve as a guide.

Selective and reproducible stimulation of the phrenic nerves and activation of the diaphragm has been reported with either method. Graded responses up to maximum can also be obtained with any of these methods by increasing the current or voltage applied. To this end, the electrical responses (M-waves) from the diaphragm to each nerve shock can be recorded with surface electrodes over the lower intercostal spaces (Newsom Davis, 1967) or with esophageal leads (Delhez, 1965). The stimulation is considered maximal when further increasing the stimulus intensity produces no further increase in the M-wave's size. Usually, currents or voltages 20–30% greater than that producing maximal responses are employed to ensure a constant maximal stimulation. Because of the high impedance of the skin, higher currents are generally required with transcutaneous (15–30 mA) than with percutaneous stimulation (8–15 mA) (the pulse duration being the same). However, when single shocks are employed, the higher currents of transcutaneous stimulation are well accepted by most subjects (Bellemare and Bigland-Ritchie, 1984; Similowski et al., 1993). Local anesthesia of the skin may be required before the insertion of needles in the neck (Aubier et al., 1985, 1987, 1989) or when repetitive tetanic stimulation of the phrenic nerves with surface electrodes is employed (Bellemare et al., 1986). With insertion of needles in the neck, there is a risk of damaging the phrenic nerve and of inducing a pneumothorax, although no such side effects have been reported. Because of its proximity, the vagus nerve may also be stimulated, although no side effects have been noted (Sarnoff et al., 1951). The time required for proper placement of the stimulating electrodes is considerably longer when using needle electrodes (up to 1 h according to Hershenson et al., 1988) than with transcutaneous stimulation (<15 min). Thus, for routine use and when only single shocks are employed, a trancutaneous approach seems preferable.

Other methods have been described that activate the phrenic nerves indirectly. Transcranial stimulation of the motor cortex with electric currents or with pulsed magnetic fields can activate the phrenic nerves via corticofugal pathways (Gandevia et al., 1987, 1988). Pulsed magnetic fields can also be applied dorsally at the cervical level that activate the phrenic nerves bilaterally (Similowski et al., 1989). By these methods, the intensity of stimulation is not directly controlled. With transcranial stimulation, other conducting pathways are involved and the threshold for excitation is determined by the level of underlying cortical activity, i.e., the threshold is smaller during voluntary contractions of the muscle being tested. Pulsed magnetic fields do not depolarize motor nerves directly. Instead, motor nerve activation is determined by local currents being created in the vicinity of the nerve by the magnetic field (Barker et al., 1987). Both transcranial stimulation and cervical magnetic stimulation techniques stimulate many other truncal muscles in addition to the diaphragm. This nonselectivity complicates the interpretation of mechanical responses. Tetanic stimulation is not possible with these two methods, but uncontrolled repetitive activations of some phrenic motor neurons can be produced by transcranial stimulation (Gandevia et al., 1987).

Tetanic Responses

The transdiaphragmatic pressure response to tetanic stimulation was first reported by Pengelly et al. (1971), who stimulated one phrenic nerve at several constant but submaximal intensities. The ΔP_{di} thus obtained was found to decrease linearly with increasing lung volume and at a lung volume close to FRC to decrease linearly with increasing inspiratory flow, thereby reflecting the intrinsic force-length and force-velocity properties of the diaphragm (Pengelly et al., 1971).

Transdiaphragmatic pressure-frequency relationships have been constructed using maximal unilateral (Moxham et al., 1981; Aubier et al., 1981) and bilateral phrenic nerve stimulation (Bellemare et al., 1986; Johnson et al., 1993) at a lung volume close to FRC. In all these studies the abdomen and lower rib cage were rigidly bound to limit chest wall distortions and shortening of the diaphragm. The shape of the pressure-frequency relationships thus obtained was found to be comparable to the force-frequency relationship reported for other human muscles with a mixed fiber type composition and intermediate contractile properties such as the quadriceps femoris (Fig. 5). However, owing to the unavoidable distortion of

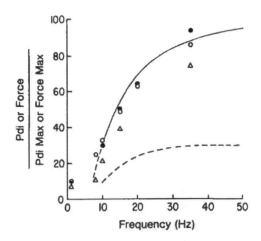

Figuer 5   Relationship between transdiaphragmatic pressure (P_{di}) and stimulation frequency during bilateral stimulation in three subjects (different symbols). Solid line shows force/frequency relationship adapted from Edwards et al. (1977) for quadriceps and adductor pollicis in vivo. Dotted lines shows P_{di}/frequency relationship for unilateral left side stimulation calculated from results of Aubier et al. (1981). P_{di} is expressed as percentage of maximum voluntary P_{di}. Force is expressed as percentage of maximum tetanic force (100 Hz). (From Bellemare et al., 1986.)

the diaphragm during unilateral stimulation, the transdiaphragmatic pressure response to any stimulation frequency is approximately three times greater during bilateral than during unilateral stimulation (Bellemare et al., 1986). Only two studies attempted to compare the ΔP_{di} developed by maximum voluntary effort with that which can be produced by artificial bilateral tetanic stimulation (Bellemare et al., 1986; Gandevia et al., 1990). In one normal subject studied by Gandevia et al., ΔP_{di} during a maximum voluntary inspiratory effort (130 cm H_2O) was almost the same as in response to tetanic stimulation at 100 Hz (128 cm H_2O), both values being, however, less than during maximum expulsive effort (175 cm H_2O). In the study of Bellemare et al. (1986) maximal stimulation of both phrenic nerves simultaneously could not be achieved at stimulation frequencies greater than 35 Hz because of unavoidable contraction of the neck muscles displacing the stimulating electrodes. Therefore, no direct comparison could be made. Nevertheless, in three subjects, the P_{di} at 35 Hz was 82% of the maximal voluntary P_{di} measured during expulsive efforts (200 ± 38 cm H_2O), a fraction equal to that predicted by the force-frequency relationship for this and other human muscles (Fig. 5). In that study the abdomen and lower rib cage were rigidly bound at FRC, which could explain the substantially greater P_{di} values. These limited comparisons do support the notion that volitional efforts can generate P_{di} values comparable to those of the tetanically activated muscle. The pressure-frequency relationship of the diaphragm also showed characteristic changes with fatigue and during recovery that are indicative of impaired contractility and of preferential pressure losses at low stimulation frequencies (low-frequency fatigue), respectively (Aubier et al., 1981; Moxham et al., 1981). Comparable changes in the diaphragmatic response to low-stimulation frequencies have also been documented with bilateral stimulation in normal subjects after exhausting high-intensity exercise (Johnson et al., 1993).

As already mentioned, maximal tetanic phrenic nerve stimulation is difficult to achieve at rates greater than 35 Hz. Tetanic stimulation in the neck can also be painful, particularly when measurements are repeatedly performed. Although this sensory problem can be overcome by local anesthesia of the skin under the cathode, these difficulties are compounded by the necessity of stimulating the phrenic nerves bilaterally if the artificial response is to be compared with that of a voluntary contraction and if the normal geometry of the diaphragm is to be retained. Thus, although tetanic stimulation of the phrenic nerves may be an ideal test to evaluate the function of the diaphragm, it is clearly too difficult and painful to be recommended for routine use in patients or naive subjects. Recently, reproducible pressure-frequency relationships of the diaphragm have been contructed using paired shocks instead of trains of shocks and by varying the interval between the two stimuli (Yan et al., 1993). The amplitude of the P_{di} response to the second impulse of each pair can be measured after subtraction of the first response (which is equal to a single twitch) from the total response. The amplitude of the second response thus measured declines as the interval between the stimuli decreases, reflecting the progressive fusion of successive twitches as the instantaneous stimulation frequency increases. This method proved to be much easier to perform than tetanic stimulation and was well tolerated by normal subjects. It provided similar information as the tetanic responses concerning the evaluation of high- vs. low-frequency diaphragmatic fatigue. It could potentially be applicable clinically. For this and other forms of tetanic phrenic nerve stimulation it has been found necessary to restrict the motion of the lower rib cage and abdomen by rigid binding. For clinical application this procedure will need to be further standardized.

Single Responses

As an alternative to tetanic or paired phrenic nerve stimulation, recording of the muscle twitch in response to a single maximal nerve shock can be employed to evaluate the strength of the diaphragm. This approach is virtually painless and well accepted by patients and naive subjects. It is particularly suited for repeated determinations. It does not require any effort on the part of the patient. So far its application has been restricted to the diaphragm, but it could be applied to other respiratory muscles as well.

When recorded from the relaxed muscle at normal functional residual capacity, the amplitude of the diaphragmatic twitches is approximately 20–25% of the maximal tetanic P_{di} (Bellemare and Bigland-Ritchie, 1984; Aubier et al., 1985; Similowski et al., 1989; Levy et al., 1990). This value lies well within the range of the twitch-to-tetanus ratio reported for other mamalian muscles at normal body temperature (Close, 1972) and suggests that most if not all diaphragmatic motor units can be recruited by each nerve shock. From these twitches, several other indexes of diaphragmatic contractile properties can also be measured such as the twitch contraction and relaxation rates (Bellemare et al., 1986; Similowski et al., 1991; Wilcox et al., 1989; Levine et al., 1988; Johnson et al., 1993) and the ratio of pleural pressure to transdiaphragmatic pressure changes, which is a measure of the inspiratory function of the diaphragm (see below). Reported values of twitch P_{di} during relaxation at FRC in the seated posture in normal subjects of both sexes range from 18 to 52 cm H_2O with mean values ranging from 25 to 35 cm H_2O in different studies (Bellemare and Bigland-Ritchie, 1984; Gandevia et al., 1990; Hubmayr et al., 1989; Johnson et al., 1993; Similowski et al., 1989).

Several factors that could affect the amplitude of single twitches must be controlled. Whereas it is essential that both phrenic nerves be stimulated simultaneously, it is not necessary that both be maximally activated, for twitch P_{di} remains maximal provided that 70% of the diaphragmatic fibers on one side and 100% of the fibers on the contralateral side (as judged from the size of the corresponding M-waves) are recruited simultaneously (Nava et al., 1987).

Isolated contractions of the diaphragm in vivo are not isometric but involve a variable degree of movement, and hence shortening of the diaphragm, the magnitude of which will be determined by the balance between the strength of diaphragmatic contractions and the mechanical impedance of chest wall structures that the diaphragm displaces. Rigid binding of the abdomen and lower rib cage, which increases diaphragm length and reduces the extent of diaphragm shortening, has been shown to increase twitch P_{di} by 20–40% (Bellemare et al., 1986; Koulouris et al., 1989; Wilcox et al., 1988). Comparable changes in twitch P_{di} would be expected if the major antagonists of the diaphragm, the abdominal muscles and the rib cage muscles, are simultaneously recruited. It is therefore important to ensure that these other muscles are also relaxed when recording single twitches from the relaxed diaphragm.

Changes in posture affect diaphragm length and chest wall impedance in opposite directions (see Chap. 16) and may be expected to have variable effects on twitch P_{di}. Koulouris et al. (1989) found no difference in twitch P_{di} between sitting and supine postures. By contrast, unpublished results from our laboratory in five normal subjects showed twitch P_{di} to be significantly smaller in four and significantly greater in one subject when supine than when seated (group results are shown in Table 1). Thus the gain in P_{di} due to diaphragm lengthening in the supine posture may be offset to a variable extent by a greater shortening of the diaphragm during the twitch caused by the smaller abdominal impedance in this posture. The upright or seated postures are thus preferred when evaluating diaphragm function by this method.

Recent reports have indicated that P_{di} twitches can be potentiated when preceded by a maximal voluntary contraction of the diaphragm. McKenzie et al. (1992) reported a 20% increase in twitch P_{di} following a series of brief maximum voluntary contractions. A comparable increase can be calculated from the records shown in Figure 6. Much larger increases have recently been reported by Moxham et al. (1993) (mean increase 40%) and by Mador et al. (1993) (mean increase 66%). According to these two reports, amplitude returns to control levels within 3–15 min after the end of voluntary contractions. It is not always clear, however, whether these increases in twitch P_{di} solely reflect the phenomenon of twitch potentiation as observed in other skeletal muscles contracting isometrically or whether this is also caused by incomplete relaxation of other chest wall muscles that are co-activated with the diaphragm. Nevertheless, these results suggest that it may be necessary to control the contraction history of the diaphragm when evaluating the strength of this muscle with single twitches, particularly when the level of underlying diaphragmatic activity is high.

Table 1 Inspiratory Function of the Diaphragm

	Sitting	Sitting bound	Supine
ΔP_{di} (cm H_2O)	27.3 ± 1.6	35.3 ± 1.6[a]	24.8 ± 1.6
$-\Delta P_{pl}$ (cm H_2O)	15.5 ± 2.6	18.2 ± 2.7	17.3 ± 3.1
$-\Delta P_{pl}/\Delta P_{di}$	0.56 ± 0.03	0.49 ± 0.04	0.70 ± 0.05[a]

[a]Significantly different from sitting posture, $p < 0.05$.
Unpublished observations from the author.

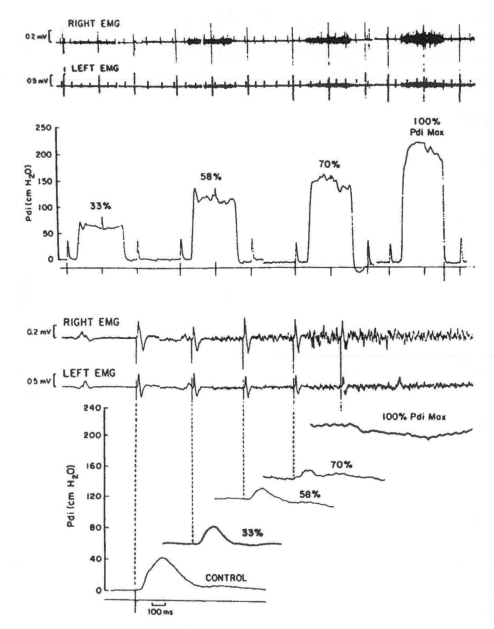

Figure 6 Top: Typical EMG (upper) and P_{di} (lower) records when maximal shocks were delivered between and during combined Müller-expulsive maneuvers of different $\%P_{dimax}$ in the sitting position. Bottom: Portions of the same records displayed on a faster time base. The lower trace in top records and the vertical dotted lines in bottom records mark the time at which the stimulus was applied. (From Bellemare and Bigland-Ritchie, 1984.)

When the above conditions are carefully controlled, P_{di} twitches are highly reproducible in a given subject over extended periods of time (Bellemare and Bigland-Ritchie, 1984; Aubier et al., 1985; Similowski et al., 1989; Yan et al., 1992). Their amplitude can therefore be used to assess changes in diaphragm strength when a subject serves as his or her own control (Aubier et al., 1985a,b, 1987, 1989; Bellemare and Bigland-Ritchie, 1987; Yan et al., 1990; Levine et al., 1988; Levy et al., 1990; McKenzie et al., 1990; Johnson et al., 1993), as well as when comparing groups of subjects or patients (Mier et al., 1988, 1989; Similowski et al., 1991).

Because diaphragm length is dependent on lung volume and chest wall shape, diaphragmatic twitches may also be affected by these factors. Indeed, studies in normal subjects (Smith and Bellemare, 1987; Hubmayr et al., 1989; Yan et al., 1990; Mier et al., 1990; Johnson et al., 1993) and in patients with chronic obstructive lung disease (Similowski et al., 1991) have shown that twitch P_{di} decreases with increasing lung volume. By contrast, the effects of changes in chest wall configuration on twitch P_{di} at any given lung volume appear to be small or negligible in relation to those produced by lung volume changes (Hubmayr et al., 1989; Mier et al., 1990). Similarly, marked changes in chest wall configuration were found to have relatively little effect on the maximal P_{di} that can be generated voluntarily during various maneuvers (Hershenson et al., 1988). As shown by Loring and Mead (1985), it may be that the length of the diaphragm is less dependent on chest wall configuration than was previously thought. Nevertheless, it is clear that, when evaluating diaphragm contractility, it is necessary to take lung volume into account. For this purpose the linear relationship between twitch P_{di} and lung volume can be advantageously employed. For example, using this approach, Yan et al. (1990) and Johnson et al. (1993) have shown that fatigue causes a greater decrease in diaphragm contractility when measured at high than at low lung volumes. Similarly, an improved diaphragm contractility could be demonstrated in stable patients with COPD, by comparison with a group of sex- and age-matched normal subjects, despite a 200% increase in FRC in the patient group, thus showing an adaptation of the diaphragm to the chronic hyperinflation of the lungs (Similowski et al., 1991).

Estimation of Diaphragm Activation and Maximal Strength

The ratio of twitch P_{di} to maximal tetanic P_{di} varies in different subjects between 0.16 and 0.35. Because of this high intersubject variability, P_{dimax} cannot be reliably estimated by recording single twitches from the relaxed muscle. For a more precise determination of P_{dimax} or to evaluate the level of diaphragmatic activation by the central nervous system, the twitch occlusion method can be employed (Bellemare and Bigland-Ritchie, 1984, 1987; Levy et al., 1990; Gandevia et al., 1990; Hershenson et al., 1988; Similowski et al., 1991).

As was shown by Merton (1954), for the adductor pollicis muscle contracting isometrically, when single supermaximal nerve shocks are superimposed to ongoing voluntary contractions, the amplitude of the resulting superimposed twitches declines almost linearly as a function of the voluntary force developed (twitch occlusion; Fig. 6). If all motor units are already recruited and fully activated by the natural activity, then an extra nerve shock will superimpose no additional force on the voluntary tension record. The amplitude of the superimposed twitches thus detects the force reserve left for full muscle activation by the central nervous system. Extrapolation of the relationship between the amplitude of the superimposed twitches and the voluntary force developed to the abcissa yields an objective estimate of the maximal muscle strength that is independent of the voluntary effort developed (Fig. 7). Merton (1954) showed that the maximum strength estimated this way corresponds to that which can be measured by maximum tetanic stimulation of the motor nerve, thus showing that both methods are equally valid in estimating muscle strength.

This method has been employed successfully in a number of experimental conditions in various limb muscles (Merton, 1954; Belanger and McComas, 1981; Bellemare et al., 1983; Bigland-Ritchie et al., 1986). In the respiratory system, Bellemare and Bigland-Ritchie (1984) showed that it can also be used to evaluate the strength and level of activation of the human diaphragm. They showed that the relationship between the amplitude of P_{di} twitches and the voluntary P_{di} developed is linear in the P_{di} range of 0–70% P_{dimax} (Fig. 7). Because of a slight nonlinearity at P_{di} greater than 70% P_{dimax}, extrapolation of this relationship from submaximal P_{di} levels to the abcissa underestimated the true P_{dimax} by about 10%. The extent of diaphragm activation for any breathing effort can also be calculated from the ratio of the superimposed to the relaxed twitches (Bellemare and Bigland-Ritchie, 1984, 1987; Gandevia et al., 1990).

The technique of twitch occlusion has since been used in a number of human

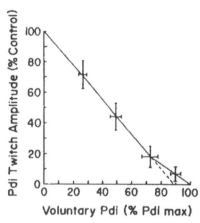

Figure 7 Twitch occlusion diagram. Pooled data from nine subjects, the twitch amplitude and the voluntary P_{di} each expressed as % of the corresponding relaxed twitch amplitude and the observed P_{dimax}, respectively. (From Bellemare and Bigland-Ritchie, 1984.)

studies to investigate the effect of fatigue (Bellemare and Bigland-Ritchie, 1987; McKenzie and Gandevia, 1991), of pharmacological agents (Levy et al., 1990), of different respiratory maneuvers (Bellemare and Bigland-Ritchie, 1984; Hershenson et al., 1988; Gandevia et al., 1990), and of chronic hyperinflation (Similowski et al., 1991) or asthma (Gandevia et al., 1993) on the maximum strength of the diaphragm and the extent of diaphragm activation by voluntary effort. This method has also been tested in an in vivo preparation of cat diaphragm (Dick and Kelsen, 1989). Although no direct comparison has been made, the twitch occlusion diagrams for the diaphragm appear to be similar whether the phrenic nerves are stimulated transcutaneously with surface electrodes (Bellemare and Bigland-Ritchie, 1984, 1987; Levy et al., 1990; Gandevia et al., 1990), percutaneously with needle electrodes (Hershenson et al., 1988), or with cervical magnetic stimulation (Similowski et al., 1993).

A suggestion has been made that the technique of twitch occlusion may not be relied on to estimate diaphragm strength and the level of diaphragm activation when inspiratory efforts are performed without co-activation of the abdominal muscles because of the low impedence to motion of the abdominal wall under this condition (Hershenson et al., 1988). Indeed, because of the greater extent and speed of shortening of the diaphragm during the twitch, twitch P_{di} would be smaller than expected in relation to the available maximal muscle strength leading to an underestimation of P_{dimax} and overestimation of the level of diaphragm activation. This hypothesis was put to test by Loring and Hershenson (1993) using Merton's model of adductor pollicis muscle. They compared the twitch occlusion test during isometric contractions and when contracting with the same initial length against an elastic or compliant load. As in Merton's study (1954), the twitch occlusion relationship was linear during isometric contractions. By contrast, when contracting against the compliant load, not only was the twitch amplitude smaller at any given level of voluntary force, but the twitch occlusion relationship became markedly curvilinear with an upward concavity, a finding that was well explained by the marked increases in the speed and extent of muscle shortening during the twitch. Extrapolation of these relationships from submaximal force levels markedly underestimated the maximal muscle force (Loring and Hershenson, 1993).

It is not clear whether the same conclusion can be extended to the respiratory system and in particular to the diaphragm. Although, as stated above, the contraction of the diaphragm in vivo is not isometric and hence dependent on the mechanical properties of the chest wall, the extent of diaphragmatic shortening during a twitch is probably substantially smaller than in the experiments of Loring and Hershenson on the thumb (1993). Considering the effect of rigid binding of the lower rib cage and abdomen on twitch P_{di} (Bellemare et al., 1986), the normal chest wall elastance causes the diaphragmatic twitch to be about 21% less than the isometric twitch. By comparison, the elastic load used by Loring and Hershenson (1993) to test the adductor pollicis caused the twitch to be 50% or less of the isometric twitch. Furthermore, in the case of the diaphragm, the effect of chest wall elastance is likely to be substantially less than calculated above because diaphragm length was also increased by abdominal and lower rib cage binding. Finally, and in contrast to the thumb contracting against a constant compliant load, the elastance of the chest wall is not constant but increases in proportion to the effort exerted by the subject or patient (Barnas et al., 1986), thereby further reducing the extent of diaphragm shortening during the twitch. Hence the degree of curvilinearity in the twitch occlusion diagram and hence the error in estimating the strength of the diaphragm from submaximal force levels is in all probability small and certainly substantially less than predicted by Hershenson et al. (1988). The slight curvilinearity shown in Figure 7 is unlikely explained by diaphragmatic shortening during a twitch, for in that experiment the abdomen and lower rib cage were also rigidly bound. Furthermore, as shown by Gandevia et al. (1990), there appears to be little difference, if any, in the degree of curvilinearity of the twitch occlusion diagram between inspiratory and expulsive efforts, whereas this would be expected if the difference in P_{dimax} between the two maneuvers estimated by extrapolation of the twitch occlusion diagram was to be accounted for by this mechanism alone (Gandevia et al., 1990). It is also worth mentioning that a similar or even greater curvilinearity in the twitch occlusion diagram has been reported for isometric contractions of the plantar flexors and extensors (Belanger and McComas, 1981) and for the quadriceps muscle (Bigland-Ritchie et al., 1986). The twitch occlusion technique thus seems to be valid also in the case of the diaphragm contracting in situ, even though the size of the twitch is reduced due to shortening and particularly at low levels of effort.

Inspiratory Function of the Diaphragm and Noninvasive Evaluation of Diaphragm Strength

Although transdiaphragmatic pressure measurements can give reliable and specific information regarding the strength of diaphragmatic contractions, it gives no indication as to how effectively this can be transformed into inspiratory pressure on the lungs. The implication of the large maximal P_{di} values in relation to the maximal pleural pressure changes has also been questioned (Gibson et al., 1981). The capacity of the diaphragm to transform its force of contraction into effective inspiratory pressure (i.e., its inspiratory function) cannot be evaluated during voluntary contractions because other muscles are contributing to the measured pressures. The technique of phrenic nerve stimulation offers a unique opportunity to evaluate the inspiratory function of the diaphragm in addition to the strength and contractile properties of its muscle fibers. The inspiratory function of the diaphragm can be defined as the ratio between the pleural pressure change and the transdiaphragmatic pressure change ($\Delta P_{pl}/\Delta P_{di}$) during isolated diaphragmatic contractions (Smith and Bellemare, 1987; Similowski et al., 1991; Yan et al., 1992). Furthermore, if the ratio of $\Delta P_{pl}/\Delta P_{di}$ remains relatively constant, mouth pressure changes (which should equal pleural pressure changes) may be substituted to P_{di} for the noninvasive evaluation of diaphragm function (Yan et al., 1992; Similowski et al., 1993).

To obtain some insight into the inspiratory function of the diaphragm during phrenic nerve stimulation, it is necessary to consider the two major pathways for lung volume changes (ΔV_l), i.e., the rib cage pathway (ΔV_{rc}) and the abdominal pathway (ΔV_{ab}). ΔV_{rc} can be further subdivided into a pulmonary rib cage (ΔV_{rc_p}) and an abdominal rib cage (ΔV_{rc-ab}) pathway (see Chap. 16). However, because of the low mechanical coupling between the two parts of the rib cage (D'Angelo and Sant'Ambrogio, 1974; Xiang et al., 1986; Urmey et al., 1986), it is only necessary for the present purposes to consider the net rib cage displacement (ΔV_{rc} = ΔV_{rc_p} + ΔV_{rc_ab}). The pressure inflating the lung is transpulmonary pressure ($\Delta P_l = \Delta P_{ao} - \Delta P_{pl}$), and when the airways are opened it is equal to $-\Delta P_{pl}$. The diaphragm can lower P_{pl} by lowering its dome relative to the spine with a consequent increase in abdominal pressure and outward displacement of the abdomen or by inflating the rib cage either directly by way of its insertions on the rib cage or indirectly by way of abdominal pressure transmission through the diaphragm in the area of apposition (Mead, 1977; Loring and Mead, 1982). Loring and Mead (1982) expressed the insertional and appositional actions of the diaphragm on the rib cage as a single pressure equivalent $B\Delta P_{di}$ in which the factor B can vary between 0 and 1. When the other respiratory muscles are relaxed, the pressure displacing the passive rib cage (ΔP_{rc}) is given by $\Delta P_{rc} = \Delta P_{pl} + B\Delta P_{di}$ (see also Chap. 16). Under sufficiently slowly changing conditions, the motions of the chest wall and lungs can be described only with pressures and compliances (C_l, lung compliance; C_{rc}, rib cage compliance; C_{ab}, abdominal wall compliance):

$$\Delta V_l = \Delta V_{rc} + \Delta V_{ab} = -\Delta P_{pl} * C_l \qquad (2)$$
$$\Delta V_{rc} = \Delta P_{rc} * C_{rc} = (\Delta P_{pl} + B\Delta P_{di}) * C_{rc} \qquad (3)$$
$$\Delta V_{ab} = \Delta P_{ab} * C_{ab} \qquad (4)$$
$$-\Delta P_{pl} * C_l = [(\Delta P_{pl} + B\Delta P_{di}) * C_{rc}] + (\Delta P_{ab} * C_{ab}) \qquad (5)$$

Dividing Eq. (5) by ΔP_{di}, replacing $\Delta P_{ab}/\Delta P_{di}$ by $(1 + \Delta P_{pl}/\Delta P_{di})$ and the expression ($C_{rc} + C_{ab}$) by C_w, the total chest wall compliance, and solving for the ratio $\Delta P_{pl}/\Delta P_{di}$ yields the following expression:

$$- \Delta P_{pl}/\Delta P_{di} = \frac{B*C_{rc} + C_{ab}}{C_l + C_w} \qquad (6)$$

According to Eq. (6), the inspiratory function of the diaphragm as defined increases as the lung compliance decreases. An increase in airway resistance would have a similar effect. This is a useful feature, which by allowing the diaphragm to transform a greater fraction of its transdiaphragmatic pressure into pleural pressure can overcome larger lung impedances. At the limit where $C_l = 0$, such as occurs when the airways are closed, the inspiratory function of the diaphragm would increase as the ratio C_{ab}/C_w increases and, for values of B less than 1, as the ratio C_{rc}/C_w decreases. Recruitment of the rib cage muscles by decreasing C_{rc} (Barnas et al., 1989) would be expected to increase the inspiratory function of the diaphragm when recruited simultaneously. By contrast, simultaneous recruitment of the abdominal muscles would reduce the inspiratory function of the diaphragm because this reduces C_{ab}. Although this approach is clearly an oversimplification of the action of the diaphragm on the rib cage and abdomen and of how this can be assessed, a number of observations support this analysis.

The ratio $-\Delta P_{pl}/\Delta P_{di}$ is about the same during single twitches and during tetanic stimulation, at least when the abdomen and lower rib cage motions are restricted (Bellemare et al., 1986). Thus is spite of their transient character, single twitches can provide an accurate estimate of the inspiratory function of the diaphragm.

In line with the predictions of Eq. (6), we found in five normal subjects that strapping the abdomen reduced the ratio $-\Delta P_{pl}/\Delta P_{di}$ during diaphragmatic twitches at FRC, whereas the opposite was found when C_{ab} was increased by placing the subjects in the supine posture (Table 1). If the diaphragm had no action on the rib cage other than through the fall in pleural pressure, the value of B would be O and the ratio $-\Delta P_{pl}/\Delta P_{di}$ during twitches simply given by the ratio C_{ab}/C_w. For normal values of C_{ab} and C_w (Estenne et al., 1985) the ratio $-\Delta P_{pl}/\Delta P_{di}$ in the neighborhood of FRC during phrenic nerve stimulation would only be about 0.15 in the seated posture and about 0.4 in the supine posture. Measured values in normal subjects for both postures are about 0.56 and 0.7, respectively, suggesting that the diaphragm action on the rib cage is substantial in both postures as was suggested previously (Loring and Mead, 1982). According to these figures, the value of B would be about 0.5 in both the seated and the supine postures at FRC. This value of B corresponds to that estimated by Loring and Mead (1982) during attempted voluntary isolated diaphragmatic contractions in normal subjects at FRC.

The $-\Delta P_{pl}/\Delta P_{di}$ ratio decreases systematically with increasing lung volume from about 0.4–0.6 at FRC to 0.15–0.3 at lung volumes close to TLC (Smith and Bellemare, 1987; Yan et al., 1992; Similowski et al., 1991). This finding is consistent with a reduction in the value of B secondary to a progressively smaller zone of apposition of the diaphragm with the rib cage as lung volume increases (Loring and Mead, 1982). However, a decrease in C_{ab} with lung inflation may also contribute to this finding (Kono and Mead, 1967). All of the above clearly suggest that meaningful information on the transformation of diaphragmatic strength into effective inspiratory pressure can be obtained by recording the ratio $-\Delta P_{pl}/\Delta P_{di}$ during twitches at FRC or as a function of lung volume (Smith and Bellemare, 1989; Similowski et al., 1991; Yan et al., 1992). For instance, an improvement of the inspiratory function of the diaphragm, as was found in patients with COPD (Similowski et al., 1991), can compensate at least in part for the reduction in diaphragmatic strength caused by diaphragmatic shortening with hyperinflation of the lungs. For this analysis it is essential that the diaphragm be stimulated in isolation. The techniques of transcranial or cervical magnetic stimulation which activate other muscles in addition to the diaphragm could not be employed for this purpose.

A high ratio $-\Delta P_{pl}/\Delta P_{di}$ during single twitches also suggests that mouth pressure twitches should also be substantial and could potentially be employed to evaluate diaphragm contractility noninvasively. This possibility was investigated in normal subjects by Yan et al. (1992) and in patients with COPD by Similowski et al. (1993).

In normal subjects, highly significant correlations between mouth and esophageal pressure twitches have been found during passive slow exhalation against a resistance from TLC to FRC (Fig. 8). In that study, mouth pressure twitches were only about 12% smaller than esophageal pressures twitches, a difference that could be accounted for by nonuniform pleural pressure changes (Yan et al., 1992). Mouth and transdiaphragmatic pressure twitches were also highly correlated, and both were also correlated to lung volume changes and showed comparable changes as a result of diaphragmatic fatigue. All of these relationships were highly reproducible in a given subject over extended periods of time. The noninvasive recording of mouth pressure twitches can thus provide objective information about changes in diaphragm contractility as a result of changes in lung volume or as a result of fatigue. It requires little equipment and is easily performed. It is likely to be useful clinically.

Comparable relationships between mouth, esophageal, and transdiaphragmatic pressure twitches were also reported in patients with COPD when recorded during graded inspiratory efforts (Similowski et al., 1993). Their amplitude declined as the

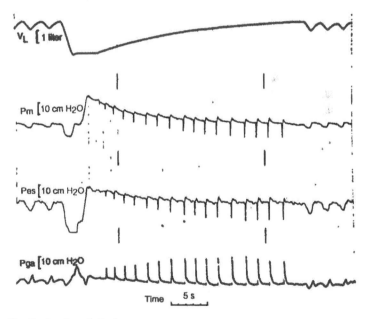

Figure 8 Evaluation of diaphragm contractility using mouth pressure twitches. Representative experimental recordings of the changes in lung volume (V_L), mouth pressure (P_m), esophageal pressure (P_{es}), and gastric pressure (P_{ga}) for one normal subject during relaxed exhalation against a high resistance. The diaphragmatic twitches are clearly detected as a sharp negativity in the P_m and P_{es} records and a sharp positivity in the P_{ga} record. V_L increases downward. (From Yan et al., 1992.)

level of inspiratory effort and of diaphragm recuitment increased. As the ratio between mouth and transdiaphragmatic pressure twitches remained constant at different levels of inspiratory effort, the recording of mouth pressure twitches as a function of the mouth pressure generated by the inspiratory effort could also be employed to evaluate the level of diaphragm activation by twitch occlusion. However, whereas the mouth pressure twitches reflect the action of the diaphragm alone (when using electrical stimulation techniques), the mouth pressure generated by the inspiratory effort reflects the net pressure developed by all respiratory muscles being recuited. Thus the relationship between mouth pressure during a twitch and during an inspiratory effort could vary depending on the level of recruitment of the different respiratory muscles. In the study of Similowski et al. (1993) the relationship between the amplitude of mouth pressure twitches and the level of inspiratory effort was negatively sloped and linear in five subjects, indicating a proportionate recruitment of the diaphragm and the other respiratory muscles (see also Gandevia et al., 1985). In another subject, however, no relationship was found, indicating a variable recuitment of the diaphragm during inspiratory effort. When using transcranial or cervical magnetic stimulation techniques, mouth pressure twitches will also be affected by the other respiratory muscles that are being stimulated (both inspiratory and expiratory) such that it may not be possible to draw conclusions about the diaphragm with this measurement alone.

In patients with COPD, no relationship was found between mouth and esophageal pressure twitches during relaxation at FRC (Similowski et al., 1993). Mouth pressure twitches were smaller and time lagged with respect to esophageal pressure twitches. Because of the high airway resistance of these patients, there may have been insufficient time for alveolar and mouth pressures to equilibrate during a twitch (Marazzini et al., 1978). A similar phenomenon could also occur in normal subjects or patients with normal lungs if the glottis is partially opened and the resistance is high. Because the compliance of the upper airways plays an important role in delaying pressure equilibration between the alveoli and the mouth when airway resistance is increased (Murciano et al., 1982), it is important that it be reduced as much as possible when recording mouth pressure twitches. Either positive or negative pressures applied at the mouth would be expected to reduce upper airway compliance (Jaeger, 1982). In the study of Yan et al. (1992) positive pressure was provided by the respiratory system recoil at lung volumes greater than FRC. In the study of Similowski et al. (1993), negative pressure was provided by the inspiratory effort. In both circumstances rapid equilibration of airway pressure occurred during a twitch. In intubated or tracheostomized patients, the problem of pressure equilibration would be overcome by recording tracheal pressure instead of mouth pressure twitches, thereby bypassing the upper airways (Murciano et al., 1982).

The Phonomyogram as a Noninvasive Measure of Diaphragm Strength and Contractility

Contracting skeletal muscles when put under tension vibrate at their resonant frequencies and emit sounds that are related to the force of contraction (Barry and

Cole, 1990). Muscle sounds, or phonomyogram, have been recorded from muscles in vivo to monitor force production and fatigue (Oster and Jaffee, 1980; Barry et al., 1989). The acoustic signal of the diaphragm in response to single phrenic nerve shocks was first recorded by Newsom Davis (1967) to determine the onset of the mechanical response of the diaphragm. More recently, the phonomyogram of the diaphragm was recorded with electret micophones fixed bilaterally to the skin over the lower intercostal spaces laterally during unilateral and bilateral phrenic nerve stimulation (Petitjean et al., 1993). Good linear correlations were found between the size of the acoustic signal and the size of the P_{di} twitches during bilateral stimulation and of the M-waves recorded ipsilaterally, suggesting that this method could be useful in evaluating diaphragm contractility noninvasively. This is a simple test that is applicable clinically and that can be extended to other respiratory muscles whose force or pressure output cannot be easily measured.

C. The Abdominal Muscles

The rectus abdominis and external oblique muscles can be stimulated transcutaneously with large pad electrodes applied on the skin overlying the muscles (Mier et al., 1986; Gandevia et al., 1990). By this method intramuscular nerve terminals are being stimulated and graded responses can be obtained by increasing the current or voltage applied. The abdominal muscles can also be stimulated with electric currents applied paraspinally over the appropriate thoracic segments (T8–T11) or transcranially at the vertex (Gandevia et al., 1990). As mentioned above for the diaphragm, these later forms of stimulation do not selectively activate the abdominal muscles. Whether maximal activation of the abdominal muscles can be achieved by any of these methods is not known. Abdominal muscle contraction increases abdominal and pleural pressures and, to the extent that the diaphragm is tensed, increases transdiaphragmatic pressure. Abdominal pressure changes should therefore be recorded when evaluating the strength of abdominal muscle contractions. None of the above-mentioned techniques have been employed to evaluate the strength of the abdominal muscles. In the study of Gandevia et al. (1993), abdominal muscle stimulation was employed to evaluate whether these muscles were maximally activated by various expulsive efforts as well as by postural tasks. They were able to demonstrate with these techniques the persistence of superimposed abdominal pressure twitches during the various tasks indicating a submaximal activation of the abdominal muscles in those circumstances. In the study of Mier et al. (1985) the abdominal muscles were stimulated tetanically at submaximal intensities to evaluate the effect of abdominal muscle contraction on chest wall motion.

References

Agostoni, E., and Rahn, H. (1960). Abdominal and thoracic pressures at different lung volumes. *J. Appl. Physiol.*, 15:1087–1092.
Agostoni, E., and Fenn, W. O. (1960). Velocity of muscle shortening as a limiting factor in respiratory air flow. *J. Appl. Physiol.*, 15:349–353.

Agostoni, E., and Mead, J. (1964). Statics of the respiratory system. In *Handbook of Physiology. Section 3, Respiration.* Vol. 1. Edited by W. O. Fenn and H. Rahn. Washington, D.C., American Physiological Society, pp. 387–409.

Alexander, C. (1966). Diaphragm movement and the diagnosis of diaphragm paralysis. *Clin. Radiol.*, 17:79–83.

Arora, N. S., and Gal, T. J. (1981). Cough dynamics during progressive expiratory muscle weakness in healthy curarizes subjects. *J. Appl. Physiol.*, 51:494–498.

Aubier, M., Farkas, G., De Troyer, A., Mozes, R., and Roussos, C. (1981). Detection of diaphragmatic fatigue in man by phrenic stimulation. *J. Appl. Physiol.*, 50:538–544.

Aubier, M., Murcianno, D., Lecocguic, Y., Viires, N., and Pariente, R. (1985a). Bilateral phrenic stimulation: a simple technique to assess diaphragmatic fatigue in humans. *J. Appl. Physiol.*, 58:58–64.

Aubier, M., Murciano, D., Lecocguic, Y., Viires, N., Jacquens, Y., Squara, P., and Pariente, R. (1985b). Effect of hypophosphatemia on diaphragmatic contractility in patients with acute respiratory failure. *N. Engl. J. Med.*, 313:420–424.

Aubier, M., Murciano, D., Viires, N., Lebargy, F., Curran, Y., Seta, J. P., and Pariente, R. (1987). Effects of digoxin on diaphragmatic strength generation in patients with chronic obstructive pulmonary disease during acute respiratory failure. *Am. Rev. Respir. Dis.*, 135:544–548.

Aubier, M., Murciano, D., Mewnu, Y., Boczkowski, J., Mal, H., and Pariente, R. (1989). Dopamine effects on diaphragmatic strength during acute respiratory failure in chronic obstructive pulmonary disease. *Ann. Intern. Med.*, 110:17–23.

Barker, A. T., Freeston, I. L., Jalinous, R., and Jaratt, J. A. (1987). Magnetic stimulation of the human brain and peripheral nervous system: an introduction and the results of an initial clinical evaluation. *Neurosurgery*, 20:100–109.

Barnas, G. M., Heglund, N. C., Yager, D., Yoshino, K., Loring, S. H., and Mead, J. (1989). Impedance of the chest wall during sustained respiratory muscle contraction. *J. Appl. Physiol.*, 66:360–369.

Barry, T. D., and Cole, N. M. (1990). Muscle sounds are emitted at the resonant frequencies of skeletal muscle. *IEEE Trans. Biomed. Eng.*, 37:525–531.

Belanger, A. Y., and McComas, A. J. (1981). Extent of motor unit activation during effort. *J. Appl. Physiol.*, 51:1131–1135.

Bellemare, F., and Grassino, A. E. (1983). Force reserve of the diaphragm in patients with chronic obstructive pulmonary disease. *J. Appl. Physiol.*, 55:8–15.

Bellemare, F., Woods, J. J., Johansson, J. J., and Bigland-Ritchie, B. (1983). Motor-unit discharge rates in maximal voluntary contractions of three human muscles. *J. Neurophysiol.*, 50:1380–1392.

Bellemare, F., and Bigland-Ritchie, B. (1984). Assessment of human diaphragm strength and activation using phrenic nerve stimulation. *Respir. Physiol.*, 58:263–277.

Bellemare, F., Bigland-Ritchie, B., and Woods, J. J. (1986). Contractile properties of the human diaphragm in vivo. *J. Appl. Physiol.*, 61:1153–1161.

Bellemare, F., and Bigland-Ritchie, B. (1987). Central components of diaphragmatic fatigue assessed by phrenic nerve stimulation. *J. Appl. Physiol.*, 62:1307–1316.

Bellemare, F., and Garzaniti, N. (1988). Failure of neuromuscular propagation during human maximal voluntary contractions. *J. Appl. Physiol.*, 74:1084–1093.

Bigland-Ritchie, B., Jones, D. A., Hosking, G. P., and Edwards, R. H. T. (1978). Central and peripheral fatigue in sustained maximal voluntary contractions of human quadriceps muscles. *Clin. Sci. Mol. Med.*, 54:609–614.

Bigland-Ritchie, B., Johansson, R., Lippold, O. C. J., and Woods, J. J. (1983). Contractile speed and EMG changes during fatigue of sustained maximal voluntary contractions. *J. Neurophysiol.*, 50:313–324.

Bigland-Ritchie, B., Furbush, F., and Woods, J. J. (1986). Fatigue of intermittent, submaximal voluntary contractions: central and peripheral factors. *J. Appl. Physiol.*, 61:421–429.

Black, L. F., and Hyatt, R. E. (1969). Maximal respiratory pressures: normal values and relationship to age and sex. *Am. Rev. Respir. Dis.*, 99:696–702.

Braun, N. M. T., Arora, N. S., and Rochester, D. F. (1982). Force-length relationship of the normal human diaphragm. *J. Appl. Physiol.*, 53:405–412.

Campbell, E. J. M. (1970). Accessory muscles. In *The Respiratory Muscles*. Edited by E. J. M. Campbell, E. Agostoni, and J. Newsom Davis. Philadelphia, W. B. Saunders, pp. 181–193.

Close, R. I. (1972). The dynamic properties of mammalian skeletal muscles. *Physiol. Rev.*, 52:129–197.

Coast, J. R., Clifford, P. S., Henrich, T. W., Stray-Gundersen, J., and Johnson, R. L. (1990). Maximal inspiratory pressure following exercise in trained and untrained subjects. *Med. Sci. Sports Exerc.*, 22:811–815.

Cook, C. D., Mead, J., and Orzalesi, M. M. (1964). Static volume-pressure characteristics of the respiratory system during maximal efforts. *J. Appl. Physiol.*, 19:1016–1022.

Cooper, D. M., Velasquez Rojas, J. Mellins, R. B., Keim, H. A., and Mansell, A. L. (1984). Respiratory mechanics in adolescents with idiopathic scoliosis. *Am. Rev. Respir. Dis.*, 130:16–22.

D'Angelo, E., and Sant'Ambrogio, G. (1974). Direct action of contracting diaphragm on the rib cage in rabbits and dogs. *J. Appl. Physiol.*, 36:715–719.

Danon, J., Druz, W. S., Goldberg, N. B., and Sharp, J. T. (1979). Function of the isolated paced diaphragm and the cervical accessory muscles in C1 quadriplegics. *Am. Rev. Respir. Dis.*, 119:909–919.

Decramer, M., Demedts, M., Rochette, F., and Billet, L. (1980). Maximal transrespiratory pressures in obstructive lung disease. *Bull. Eur. Physiopathol. Respir.*, 16:479–490.

Delhez, L. (1965) Modalités chez l'homme normal, de la réponse électrique des piliers du diaphragme à la stimulation électrique des nerfs phréniques par des chocs uniques. *Arch. Int. Physiol. Biochim.*, 73:832–839.

De Troyer, A., and Estenne, M. (1981). Limitations of measurement of transdiaphragmatic pressure in detecting diaphragmatic weakness. *Thorax*, 36:169–174.

De Troyer, A., Estenne, M., and Vincken, W. (1986). Rib cage motion and muscle use in high tetraplegics. *Am. Rev. Respir. Dis.*, 133:1115–1119.

Dick, T. E., and Kelsen, S. G. (1989). Relationship between diaphragmatic activation and twitch tension to superimposed electrical stimulation in the cat. *Respir. Physiol.*, 76:337–346.

Edwards, R. H. T., Young, A., Hosking, G. P., and Jones, D. A. (1977). Human skeletal muscle function: description of tests and normal values. *Clin. Sci. Mol. Med.*, 52:283–290.

Edwards, R. H. T., Moxham, J., Newham, D., Wiles, C. M. (1980). Alternative techniques for recording the frequency-force curve of the sternomastoid muscle in man. *J. Physiol.* (London), 305:4P–5P.

Eftimiou, J., Flemming, J., and Spiro, S. G. (1987). Sternomastoid muscle function and fatigue in breathless patients with severe respiratory disease. *Am. Rev. Respir. Dis.*, 136:1099–1105.

Esau, S. A., Bye, P. T. P., and Paedy, R. L. (1983). Changes in rate of relaxation of sniffs with diaphragmatic fatigue in humans. *J. Appl. Physiol.*, 55:731–735.

Estenne, M., Yernault J., and De Troyer, A. (1985). Rib cage and diaphragm-abdomen compliance in humans: effects of age and posture. *J. Appl. Physiol.*, 59:1842–1848.

Fenn, W. O. (1963). A comparison of respiratory and skeletal muscles. In *Perspectives in Biology*. *Houssay Memorial Papers*. Edited by C. F. Cori, V. G. Foglia, L. F. Leloir, and S. Ochoa. Amsterdam, Elsevier Publishing Co., pp. 293–300.

Fiz, J. A., Texido, A., Izquierdo, J., Ruiz, J., Roig, J. and Morera, J. (1990). Postural variation of the maximum inspiratory and expiratory pressures in normal subjects. *Chest*, 97:313–314.

Gandevia, S. C., and McKenzie, D. K. (1985). Activation of the human diaphragm during maximal static efforts. *J. Physiol.* (London), 367:45–56.

Gandevia, S. C., and Rothwell, J. C. (1987). Activation of the human diaphragm from the motor cortex. *J. Physiol.* (London), 384:109–118.

Gandevia, S. C., and Plassman, B. L. (1988). Responses of human intercostal and truncal muscles to motor cortical and spinal stimulation. *Respir. Physiol.*, 73:325–338.

Gandevia, S. C., McKenzie, D. K., and Plassman, B. L. (1990). Activation of human respiratory muscles during different voluntary maneuvres. *J. Physiol.* (London), 428:387–403.

Gandevia, S. C., Gorman, R. B., McKenzie, D. K., and Southon, F. C. G. (1992). Dynamic changes in human diaphragm length: maximal inspiratory and expulsive efforts studied with sequential radiography. *J. Physiol.* (London), 457:167–176.

Gaultier, C., and Zinman, R. (1983). Maximal respiratory pressures in healthy children. *Respir. Physiol.*, 51:46–61.

Gibson, G. J., Edmonds, J. P., and Hughes, G. R. V. (1977). Diaphragm function and lung involvement in systemic lupus erythematosus. *Am. J. Med.*, 63:926–932.

Gibson, G. J., Clark, E., and Pride, N. B. (1981). Static transdiaphragmatic pressures in normal subjects and in patients with chronic hyperinflation. *Am. Rev. Respir. Dis.*, 124:685–689.

Goldman, M. D., Grassino, A., Mead, J. and Sears, T. A. (1978). Mechanics of the human diaphragm during voluntary contraction: dynamics. *J. Appl. Physiol.*, 44:840–848.

Gray, H. (1976). *Anatomy of the Human Body*. Edited by C. M. Goss. Philadelphia, Lea and Febiger.

Grimby, L., Hannerz, J., and Hedman, B. (1981). The fatigue and voluntary discharge properties of single motor units in man. *J. Physiol.* (London), 316:545–554.

Hershenson, M. B., Kikuchi, Y., and Loring, S. H. (1988). Relative strengths of the chest wall muscles. *J. Appl. Physiol.*, 65:852–862.

Hillman, D. R., Markos, J., and Finucane, K. E. (1990). Effect of abdominal compression on maximum transdiaphragmatic pressure. *J. Appl. Physiol.*, 68:2296–2304.

Hubmayr, R. D., Litchy, W. J., Gay, P. C., and Nelson, S. B. (1989). Transdiaphragmatic twitch pressure. Effects of lung volume and chest wall shape. *Am. Rev. Respir. Dis.*, 139:647–652.

Hyatt, R. E., and Flath, R. E. (1966). Relationship of air flow to pressure during maximal respiratory effort in man. *J. Appl. Physiol.*, 21:477–482.

Jaeger, M. J. (1982). Effect of the cheeks and the compliance of alveolar gas on the measurement of respiratory variables. *Respir. Physiol.*, 47:325–340.

Jiang, T., Demedts, M., and Decramer, M. (1988). Mechanical coupling of upper and lower canine rib cages and its functional significance. *J. Appl. Physiol.*, 64:620–626.

Johnson, B. D., Babcock, M. A., Suman, O. E., and Dempsey, J. A. (1993). Exercise-induced diaphragmatic fatigue in healthy humans. *J. Physiol.* (London), 460:385–405.

Kikuchi, Y., Sasaki, H., Sekizawa, K., Aihara, K., and Takishima, T. (1982). Force-velocity relationship of expiratory muscles in normal subjects. *J. Appl. Physiol.*, 52:930–938.

Konno, K., and Mead, J. (1968). Static volume-pressure characteristics of the rib cage and abdomen. *J. Appl. Physiol.*, 24:544–548.

Koulouris, N., Mulvey, D. A., Laroche, C. M., Green, M., and Moxham, J. (1988). Comparison of two different mouthpieces for the measurement of Pimax and Pemax in normal and weak subjects. *Eur. Respir. J.*, 1:863–867.

Koulouris, N., Mulvey, D. A., Laroche, C. M., Sawicka, E. H., Green, M., and Moxham, J. (1989a). The measurement of inspiratory muscle strength by sniff esophageal, nasopharyngeal, and mouth pressure. *Am. Rev. Respir. Dis.*, 139:641–646.

Koulouris, N., Mulvey, D. A., Laroche, C. M., Goldstone, J., Moxham, J., and Green, M. (1989b). The effect of posture and abdominal binding on respiratory pressures. *Eur. Respir. J.*, 2:961–965.

Laporta, D., and Grassino, A. (1985). Assessment of transdiaphragmatic pressure in humans. *J. Appl. Physiol.*, 58:1469–1476.

Laroche, C. M., Mier, A. K., Moxham, J., and Green, M. (1988). The value of sniff esophageal pressures in the assessment of global inspiratory muscle strength. *Am. Rev. Respir. Dis.*, 138:598–603.

Leblanc, P., Summers, E., Inman, M. D., Jones, N. L., Campbell, E. J. M., and Killian, K. J. (1988). Inspiratory muscles during exercise: a problem of supply and demand. *J. Appl. Physiol.*, 64:2482–2489.

Leech, J. A., Ghezzo, H., Stevens, D., and Becklake, M. R. (1983). Respiratory pressures and function in young adults. *Am. Rev. Respir. Dis.*, 128:12–23.

Leevers, A. M., and Road, J. D. (1989). Mechanical response to hyperinflation of the two abdominal muscle layers. *J. Appl. Physiol.*, 66:2189–2195.

Leith, D. E., and Bradley, M. (1976). Ventilatory muscle strength and endurance training. *J. Appl. Physiol.*, 41:508–516.

Levine, S., and Henson, D. (1988). Low-frequency diaphragmatic fatigue in spontaneously breathing humans. *J. Appl. Physiol.*, 64:672–680.

Levy, R. D., Esau, S. A., Bye, P. T. P., and Pardy, R. L. (1984). Relaxation rate of mouth pressure with sniffs at rest and with inspiratory muscle fatigue. *Am. Rev. Respir. Dis.*, 130:38–41.

Levy, R. D., Nava, S., Gibbons, L., and Bellemare, F. (1990). Aminophylline and human diaphragm strength in vivo. *J. Appl. Physiol.*, 68:2591–2596.

Loring, S. H., and Mead, J. (1982). Action of the diaphragm on the rib cage inferred from a force-balance equation. *J. Appl. Physiol.*, 53:756–760.

Loring, S. H., Mead, J., and Griscom, N. T. (1985). Dependence of diaphragmatic length on lung volume and thoracoabdominal configuration. *J. Appl. Physiol.*, 59:1961–1970.

Loring, S. H., and Hershenson, M. B. (1992). Effects of series compliance on twitches superimposed on voluntary contractions. *J. Appl. Physiol.*, 73:516–521.

MacLean, I. C., and Mattioni, T. A. (1981). Phrenic nerve conduction studies: a new technique and its application in quadriplegic patients. *Arch. Phys. Med Rehabil.*, 62:70–73.

Mador, M. J., Magalang, U. J., and Kufel, T. J. (1993). Twitch potentiation following voluntary diaphragmatic contraction. *Am. Rev. Respir. Dis.*, 147:A699.

Marazzini, L., Rizzato, G., and Vezzoli, F. (1972). Dynamics of the maximal contraction of the respiratory muscles in chronic obstructive lung disease. *Respiration*, 29:488–496.

Marini, J. J., Smith, T. C., and Lamb, V. (1986). Estimation of inspiratory muscle strength in mechanically ventilated patients: the measurement of maximal inspiratory pressure. *J. Crit. Care*, 1:32–38.

McCool, F. D., Hershenson, M. B., Tzelepis, G. E., Kikuchi, Y., and Leith, D. E. (1992). Effect of fatigue on maximal inspiratory pressure-flow capacity. *J. Appl. Physiol.*, 73:36–43.

McElvaney, G., Blackie, S., Morrison, N. J., Wilcox, P. G., Fairbarn, M. S., and Pardy, R. L. (1989). Maximal static respiratory pressures in the normal elderly. *Am. Rev. Respir. Dis.*, 139:277–281.

McKenzie, D. K., Plassman, B. L., and Gandevia, S. C. (1988). Maximal activation of the human diaphragm but not inspiratory intercostal muscles during static inspiratory efforts. *Neurosci. Lett.*, 89:63–68.

McKenzie, D. K., Bigland-Ritchie, B., Gorman, R. B., and Gandevia, S. C. (1992). Central and peripheral fatigue of human diaphragm and limb muscles assessed by twitch interpolation. *J. Physiol.* (London), 454:643–656.

McKenzie, D. K., Allen, G. M., Gandevia, S. C., and Hickie, I. (1993). Impaired voluntary drive to breathe: a possible risk factor for death from asthma. *Am. Rev. Respir. Dis.*, 147:A701.

Mead, J. (1979). Functional significance of the area of apposition of the diaphragm to rib cage. *Am. Rev. Respir. Dis.*, 119(part 2, suppl):31–32.

Mead, J., Milic-Emili, J., and Turner, J. M. (1963). Factors limiting depth of a maximum inspiration in human subjects. *J. Appl. Physiol.*, 18:295–296.

Merton, P. A. (1954) Voluntary strength and fatigue. *J. Physiol.* (London), 123:553–564.

Mier, A., Brophy, C., Estenne, M., Moxham, J., Green, M., and De Troyer, A. (1985). Action of abdominal muscles on rib cage in humans. *J. Appl. Physiol.*, 58:1438–1443.

Mier, A., Brophy, C., Moxham, J., and Green, M. (1989). Twitch pressures in the assessment of diaphragm weakness. *Thorax*, 44:990–996.

Mier, A., Brophy, C., Moxham, J., and Green, M. (1990). Influence of lung volume and rib cage configuration on transdiaphragmatic pressure during phrenic nerve stimulation. *Respir. Physiol.*, 80:193–202.

Mier-Jedrzejowicz, A., and Green, M. (1988). Respiratory muscle weakness associated with cerebellar atrophy. *Am. Rev. Respir. Dis.*, 137:673–677.

Mier-Jedrzejowicz, A., Brophy, C., Moxham, J., and Green, M. (1988). Assessment of diaphragm weakness. *Am. Rev. Respir. Dis.*, 137:877–883.

Milic-Emili, J., Orzalesi, M. M., Cook, C. D., Turner, J. M. (1964). Respiratory thoracoabdominal mechanics in man. *J. Appl. Physiol.*, 19:217–223.

Miller, J. M., Moxham, J., and Green, M. (1985). The maximal sniff in the assessment of diaphragm function in man. *Clin. Sci.*, 69:91–96.

Mognoni, P., Saibene, F., Sant'Ambrogio, G., and Agostoni, E. (1968). Dynamics of the maximal contraction of the respiratory muscles. *Respir. Physiol.*, 4:193–202.

Moxham, J., Wiles, C. M., Newham, D., and Edwards, R. H. T. (1980). Sternomastoid muscle function and fatigue in man. *Clin. Sci.*, 59:463–468.

Moxham, J., Morris, A. J. R., Spiro, S. G., Edwards, R. H. T., and Green, M. (1981). Contractile properties and fatigue of the diaphragm in man. *Thorax*, 36:164–168.

Moxham, J., Wiles, C. M., Newham, D., and Edwards, R. H. T. (1981b). Contractile function and fatigue of the respiratory muscles in man. In *Human Muscle Fatigue: Physiological Mechanisms*. London, Pitman Medical (Ciba Foundation Symposium 82) pp. 197–212.

Multz, A. S., Aldrich, T. K., Prezan, D. J., Karpel, J. P., and Hendler, J. M. (1990). Maximal inspiratory pressure is not a reliable test of inspiratory muscle strength in mechanically ventilated patients. *Am. Rev. Respir. Dis.*, 142:529–532.

Mulvey, D. A., Koulouris, N., Elliott, M. W., Moxham, J., and Green, M. (1991). Maximal relaxation rate of inspiratory muscle can be effort dependent and reflect the activation of fast-twitch fibers. *Am. Rev. Respir. Dis.*, 144:803–806.

Murciano, D., Aubier, M., Bussi, S., Derenne, J. P., Pariente, R., and Milic-Emili, J. (1982). Comparison of esophageal, tracheal, and mouth occlusion pressure in patients with chronic obstructive pulmonary disease during acute respiratory failure. *Am. Rev. Respir. Dis.*, 126:837–841.

Nava, S., Levy, R. D., Gibbons, L., and Bellemare, F. (1987). Determinants of diaphragmatic response to bilateral phrenic nerve stimulation in man. *Am. Rev. Respir. Dis.*, 135:A332.

Newsom Davis, J. (1967). Phrenic nerve conduction in man. *J. Neurol. Neurosurg. Psychiatry*, 30:420–426.

Oster, G., and Jaffee, J. S. (1980). Low frequency sounds from sustained contraction of human skeletal muscle. *Biophys. J.*, 30:119–127.

Peche, R., Estenne, M., Yernault, J. C., and De Troyer, A. (1993). Scalene and sternocleidomastoid muscle activity in patients with severe chronic obstructive pulmonary disease. *Am. Rev. Respir. Dis.*, 147 (part 2):A700.

Pengelly, L. D., Alderson, A. M., and Milic-Emili, J. (1971). Mechanics of the diaphragm. *J. Appl. Physiol.*, 30:797–805.

Petitjean, M., Yan, S., Macklem, P. T., and Bellemare, F. (1993). Phonomyogram of the diaphragm during unilateral and bilateral phrenic nerve stimulation. *Am. Rev. Respir. Dis.*, 147(part 2):A693.

Rahn, H., Otis, A. B., Chadwick, L. E., and Fenn, W. O. (1946). The pressure-volume diagram of the thorax and lung. *Am. J. Physiol.*, 146:161–178.

Ringqvist, T. (1966). The ventilatory capacity in healthy subjects. *Scand. J. Clin. Lab. Invest.*, 18 (suppl 88):1–113.

Rochester, D. (1988). Tests of respiratory muscle function. *Clin. Chest Med.*, 9:249–261.

Rochester, D. F., Arora, N. S., and Braun, N. M. T. (1981). Maximum contractile force of human diaphragm muscle, determined in vivo. *Trans. Am. Clin. Climatol. Assoc.*, 93:200–208.

Rochester, D. F., and Braun, N. M. T. (1985). Determinants of maximal inspiratory pressure in chronic obstructive pulmonary disease. *Am. Rev. Respir. Dis.*, 132:42–47.

Rohrer, F. (1916). Der Zusammenhang der Atermkräfte und ihre Abhängigkeit vom Dehungszustand der Atmungsorgane. *Pflugers Arch. Ges. Physiol.*, 165:419–444.

Roussos, C. S., and Macklem, P. T. (1977). Diaphragmatic fatigue in man. *J. Appl. Physiol.*, 43:189–197.

Sarnoff, S. J., Sarnoff, L. C., and Wittenberger, J. L. (1951). Electrophrenic respiration. VII. The motor point of the phrenic nerve in relation to external stimulation. *Surg. Gynecol. Obstet.*, 93:190–196.

Sharp, J. T., Danon, J., Druz, W. S., Goldberg, N. B., Fishman, H., and Machnach, W. (1974).

Respiratory muscle function in patients with chronic obstructive pulmonary disease: its relationship to disability and to respiratory therapy. *Am. Rev. Respir. Dis.*, 110 (suppl):154–167.

Smith, J., and Bellemare, F. (1987). Effect of lung volume on in vivo contraction characteristics of human diaphragm. *J. Appl. Physiol.*, 62:1893–1900.

Shardonofsky, F. R., Perez-Chada, D., Carmuega, E., and Milic-Emili, J. (1989). Airway pressures during crying in healthy infants. *Pediatr. Pulmon.*, 6:14–18.

Similowski, T., Fleury, B., Launois, S., Cathala, H. P., Bouche, P., and Derenne, J. P. (1989). Cervical magnetic stimulation: a new painless method for bilateral phrenic nerve stimulation in conscious humans. *J. Appl. Physiol.*, 67:1311–1318.

Similowski, T., Yan, S., Gauthier, A. P., Macklem, P. T., and Bellemare, F. (1991). Contractile properties of the human diaphragm during chronic hyperinflation. *N. Engl. J. Med.*, 325:917–923.

Similowski, T., Gauthier, A. P., Yan, S., Macklem, P. T., and Bellemare, F. (1993). Assessment of diaphragm function using mouth pressure twitches in chronic obstructive pulmonary disease patients. *Am. Rev. Respir. Dis.*, 147:850–856.

Topoulos, G. P., Reid, M. B., and Leith, D. E. (1987). Pliometric activity of inspiratory muscles: maximal pressure-flow curves. *J. Appl. Physiol.*, 62:322–327.

Urmey, W., Loring, S., Mead, J., Slutsky, A. S., Sarkarati, M., Rossier, A., and Brown, R. (1986). Upper and lower rib cage deformation during breathing in quadriplegics. *J. Appl. Physiol.*, 60:618–622.

Vincken, W., Ghezzo, H., and Cosio, M. G. (1987). Maximal static respiratory pressures in adults: normal values and their relationship to determinants of respiratory function. *Bull. Eur. Physiopathol. Respir.*, 23:435–439.

Wilcox, P. G., Eisen, A., Wiggs, B. J., and Pardy, R. L. (1988). Diaphragmatic relaxation rate after voluntary contractions and uni- and bilateral phrenic nerve stimulation. *J. Appl. Physiol.*, 65:675–682.

Wilson, S. H., Cook, N. T., Edwards, R. H. T., and Spiro, S. G. (1984a). Predicted normal values for maximal respiratory pressures in Caucasian adults and children. *Thorax*, 39:535–538.

Wilson, S. H., Cooke, N. T., Moxham, J., and Spiro, S. G. (1984b). Sternomastoid muscle function and fatigue in normal subjects and in patients with chronic obstructive pulmonary disease. *Am. Rev. Respir. Dis.*, 129:460–464.

Wragg, S., Hamnegard, C., Road, J., Goldstone, J., Green, M., and Moxham, J. (1993). Twitch Pdi depends on contractile history. *Am. Rev. Respir. Dis.*, 147:A699.

Yan, S., Similowski, T., Gauthier, A. P., Macklem, P. T., and Bellemare, F. (1992a). Effect of fatigue on diaphragmatic function at different lung volumes. *J. Appl. Physiol.*, 72:1064–1067.

Yan, S., Gauthier, A. P., Similowski, T., Macklem, P. T., and Bellemare F. (1992b). Evaluation of human diaphragm contractility using mouth pressure twitches. *Am. Rev. Respir. Dis.*, 145:1064–1069.

Yan, S., Gauthier, A. P., Similowski, T., Faltus, R., Macklem, P. T., and Bellemare, F. (1993). Force-frequency relationships of in vivo human and in vitro rat diaphragm using paired stimuli. *Eur. Respir. J.*, 6:211–218.

41

Respiratory Muscle Endurance in Humans

THOMAS L. CLANTON

Ohio State University
Columbus, Ohio

I. Introduction

Endurance is a term that, when applied to skeletal muscle, is synonymous with "resistance to fatigue." It is a basic property of muscle that is a function of certain complex variables such as fiber type, blood flow, substrate availability, mitochondrial density, and the concentration of particular metabolic enzymes (Saltin and Gollnick, 1983; Faulkner, 1985). It can be functionally distinguished from strength and augmented by endurancelike conditioning stimuli (Leith and Bradley, 1976; Saltin and Gollnick, 1983; Faulkner, 1985). Finally, it can be uniquely compromised by certain pathophysiological conditions that are not uncommon in clinical settings (Cohen et al., 1982; Grassino and Macklem, 1984; Tobin, 1988).

Endurance would seem to be an important feature of the respiratory muscles, since the lack of it could potentially result in inadequate ventilation in the face of increased mechanical loads, low blood flow, and/or high ventilatory requirements. Though in normal humans there are only a few occasions when the reserve of respiratory muscle function is utilized sufficiently to cause fatigue (e.g., Loke et al., 1982), there are certain patient groups where the endurance properties of the respiratory muscles may be critical to survival or necessary for adequate exercise tolerance (Cohen et al., 1982; Grassino and Macklem, 1984; Tobin, 1988). Therefore, it has become important to develop techniques for quantifying the endurance properties of the respiratory muscles and to identify factors that influence its measurement.

II. Basic Methodologies

A. Endurance Time Measurements

One of the most basic approaches to studying the endurance properties of any synergic muscle group is the measurement of the duration a specific submaximal load or task can be maintained, sometimes referred to as Tlim (i.e., the "time limit"). The differences between techniques for measuring Tlim primarily involve the nature of the load on the respiratory pump and are summarized below.

Endurance Time to High Ventilatory Loads: Ventilatory Endurance

A number of investigations have measured the Tlim at various levels of elevated minute ventilation ($\dot{V}_E$) in normals (Zocche et al., 1960; Tenny and Reese, 1968; Leith and Bradley, 1976; Bai et al., 1984; Jones et al., 1985) and in patients (Keens et al., 1977; Belman and Mittman, 1980; Aldrich et al., 1982; Levine et al., 1986; reviewed in Rochester, 1988). Using various methods, subjects attempt to maintain a high target $\dot{V}_E$ for as long as possible and are usually kept isocapnic throughout the test. A typical relationship between $\dot{V}_E$ and Tlim is illustrated in Figure 1. Mathematically, the axes of this relationship should be reversed; however, it is still most commonly described in this way. As can be seen, Tlim increases with gradually decreasing levels of $\dot{V}_E$ and can be described by a simple exponential curve (Leith and Bradley, 1976) of the following form:

$$\dot{V}_E(t) = ae^{-kt} + b \tag{1}$$

The asymptote appears at a $\dot{V}_E$ (described by parameter "b") between 50 and 80% of maximum voluntary ventilation (MVV), a value that varies somewhat between investigators and between patient groups (Rochester, 1988). It is called the maximum "sustainable" ventilation (MSV), approximating the maximum level of $\dot{V}_E$ that the respiratory pump can maintain for prolonged periods. Any levels of $\dot{V}_E$ above this threshold would result is fatigue.

This approach to studying respiratory muscle endurance might be considered a "high-output" experimental model of respiratory failure, where the mechanical load is directly proportional to the level of $\dot{V}_E$ and the intrinsic impedance of the thorax to inflation and deflation. Its advantage is that it is applicable to conditions of high ventilatory requirement such as exercise. Furthermore, the recruitment patterns of the respiratory muscles are probably physiologically relevant. However, there are also some disadvantages. Patients with airflow obstruction may have a limited MVV because of expiratory airflow obstruction (Aldrich et al., 1982). Therefore, comparison of MSV with MVV may provide a distorted view of the endurance qualities of their respiratory muscles when compared to normals.

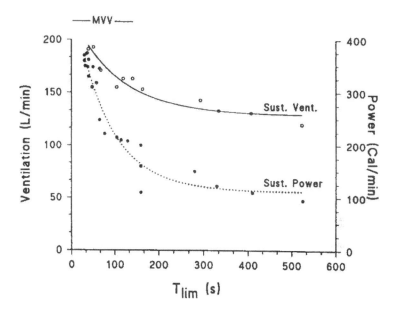

Figure 1 Ventilatory and respiratory power output endurance curves. Curves were fit to equation 1, in text. Open circles: ventilation measurements. Closed circles: power output for same data plus additional runs with He breathing. (Data from Tenney and Reese, 1968).

Furthermore, MVV maneuvers are somewhat dependent on breathing strategy and optimization. As will be reviewed later, respiratory muscle performance can be greatly affected by flow, lung volume, breathing rhythm, intrinsic thoracic impedance, and end-expiratory lung volume.

In order to account for some of these factors on measurements of endurance, Tenny and Reese (1968) proposed that the rate of mechanical work of breathing (power output) was the relevant variable determining T_{lim}. They found that when T_{lim} is plotted against the power output, a strong relationship can be obtained (Fig. 1, right axes, dotted line). Power–endurance time relationships are often fit to simple hyperbolic functions when applied to the limb musculature (Hill, 1927; Carnevale and Gaesser, 1991), but this has rarely been used for the respiratory muscles. It is interesting that sustainable power output is a smaller fraction of maximum power than MSV is for MVV (Fig. 1). This is probably because the relationship between power output and ventilation is nonlinear at elevated levels of ventilation (reviewed in Roussos and Campbell, 1986).

Endurance Time to External Mechanical Loading

A second approach to measuring the endurance characteristics of the respiratory pump is to determine the time an external resistive, elastic, or threshold load can be maintained. This approach might be considered a "low-output" model of respiratory failure, being more relevant to conditions of acute respiratory failure (Cohen et al., 1982) than exercise limitation. Roussos et al. (1977, 1979) were among the first to use this methodology to measure endurance times for the diaphragm and the respiratory muscles working in synergy (Fig. 2). In these early experiments, breathing pattern was not tightly controlled, and there was more variability in the Tlim measurement at specific loads than is generally seen when breathing pattern is controlled (e.g., Bellemare and Grassino, 1982; Clanton et al., 1985b). Certain innovations such as the use of the threshold loading device (Nickerson and Keens, 1982), discussed later, have made the application of the resistive load easier and more quantitative.

Considerations to the Interpretation of Endurance Time

What does endurance time actually measure? The event that occurs at T_{lim} is sometimes referred to as the "point of fatigue" or the "point of task failure." Unfortunately, these phrases imply that there is some underlying event occurring at T_{lim} which could be viewed as a sudden mechanical failure. That this is not what is happening is illustrated Figure 3, where a subject was asked to target an inspiratory flow-resistive load at a constant breathing pattern and flow using a constant flow

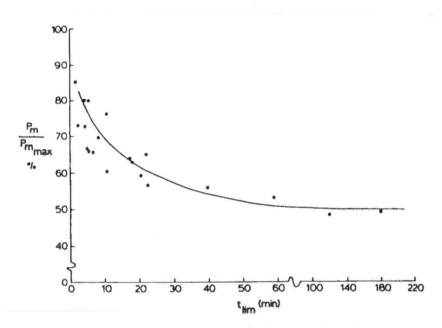

Figure 2 Endurance curve for pressures generated at the mouth (P_m) by the synergic pump against resistive loads. (From Roussos et al., 1979.)

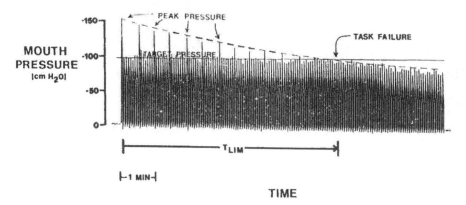

Figure 3 Changes in the capacity to generate pressure (peak values) during a submaximal endurance run. See text for details. (From Grassino et al., 1991.)

generator (Clanton and Ameredes, 1988b). Intermittently, the subject made a maximum inspiratory effort resulting in a peak dynamic pressure. As can be seen, the peak declined over time until the maximum pressure intersected with the targeted submaximal pressure load. This intersection defines T_{lim}. The fatigue process was actually measurable early in the endurance run but is hidden from view under normal endurance testing conditions. The higher the load on the muscles, the faster the loss of muscle function and the earlier task failure occurs. Sustainable loads represent those loads in which no intersection occurs.

Is the measurement of endurance time to one submaximal load strictly a function of endurance properties of the muscles involved? As shown in Figure 4, theoretical changes in strength (B) and endurance (C) can have large effects on the shape of the endurance curve, compared to a baseline curve (A). Although strength and endurance are often closely associated in a given individual, each can be altered independently depending on the conditioning stimuli, as shown by Leith and Bradley (1976). Both adaptations could theoretically result in an increase in T_{lim} in the midrange of submaximal, fatiguing loads. Therefore, the measurement of endurance time to one submaximal load, which is a common approach to the study of the effects of human inspiratory muscle training (e.g., Clanton et al., 1985a, 1987; Larson et al., 1988), has some limitations with respect to interpretation.

B. Sustainable Pressure and Ventilation Measurements

The measurement of sustainable pressure development (the asymptote of the endurance curve) or sustainable ventilation would theoretically be a better assessment of the endurance properties of the muscles involved since it is less likely to be influenced by strength. However, using the techniques described above, several days of measurements are usually required to accurately find the highest sustainable

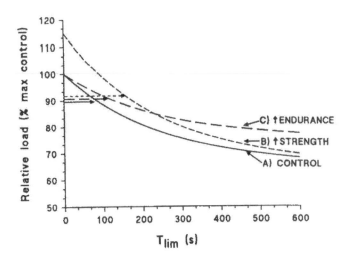

Figure 4 Theoretical effects of isolated changes in strength (curve B) and endurance (curve C) compared to control (curve A) endurance curves. The arrows indicate the endurance time to a submaximal load of approximately 90% of maximum. Isolated changes in strength or endurance can increase endurance time to one submaximal load.

levels of ventilation or pressure load a given subject can maintain. To overcome this problem, several investigative techniques have been employed.

Sustainable Ventilation

Belman et al. (1988) described a procedure (similar to that of Keens et al., 1977) whereby subjects target a minute ventilation of approximately 70% of their MVV. During the first 2 min of the test, when ventilation falls most rapidly as the muscles fatigue (Zocche et al., 1960), the target is adjusted to a level slightly above the subject's best effort. The average ventilation achieved over the last 8 min of the 10-min test is considered MSV. Using this method, normal elderly subjects were found to sustain approximately 60–65% of their MVV (Belman and Gaesser, 1988). Since in younger subjects MSV is closer to 75–80% of the MVV and in obstructed patients it may be similarly elevated (Rochester, 1988), the initial target ventilation needs to be adjusted appropriately or alternatively increased as the test proceeds (Keens et al., 1977).

Sustainable Pressure Development

Nickerson and Keens (1982) took advantage of a threshold loading device for measurements of respiratory muscle endurance. The threshold loading system has proven useful both for testing and training of the respiratory muscles (e.g., Clanton et al., 1985b; Clanton et al., 1987; Larson et al., 1988). The advantage of threshold loads compared to the more common resistive loading systems (usually simple orifice type resistances) is that the external pressure the inspiratory muscles must work against can be easily controlled without a great deal of visual feedback on the part of the subject. If the device is used correctly, pressure is nearly independent of inspiratory flow, therefore approaching conditions of isotonic contraction. To establish sustainable pressures using Nickerson and Keens' technique (1982), the inspiratory pressure load is gradually reduced in 5% increments for succeeding endurance runs, starting from maximum inspiratory pressure (MIP). The sustainable inspiratory pressure (SIP) is established as the pressure the subject can maintain for 10 min. On the average, untrained subjects can sustain 68 ± 3% of MIP. In general, no attempt is made to control breathing pattern or flow rate with this method. This fact is no doubt important for repeated testing as Martyn et al. (1987) have shown that the Nickerson and Keens method (1982) substantially underestimates true SIP, because subjects can adjust their pattern of breathing and attain higher sustainable loads with practice. Approximately 2 h is required to establish SIP using the Nickerson and Keens method.

Interestingly, there is a paucity of information concerning SIP in patients using any of the resistive loading techniques. However, patients with asthma and cystic fibrosis have been shown to have elevated sustainable pressures (Nickerson et al., 1981) as fractions of their MIP.

Repeated Maximum Contractions (Isoflow Technique and Repeated MIP Maneuvers)

Clanton and Ameredes (1988b) have described an isoflow method for establishing sustainable pressures, which was designed to be analogous to isokinetic testing of limb musculature in humans, i.e., Cybex systems (Thorstensson et al., 1977; Barnes, 1981). Subjects inspire from a constant flow generator that triggers "on" when small negative pressures are generated at the mouth and "off" with positive pressures. Using visual feedback, they are instructed to inspire with maximal effort over a controlled inspiratory period as their lungs are inflating at a constant rate. Breathing rhythm, tidal volume, and $ETCO_2$ are controlled. The pressure measurements at the mouth have a characteristic shape (Fig. 5) where peak pressure is reached early in the inspiration and gradually declines as lung volume increases and the inspiratory muscles shorten. This shape of the pressure wave form makes it necessary to express pressure as peak (P_{pk}), average (P_{av}), or integrated pressures (pressure-time integral). With each succeeding maximum inspiration, the pressure generated gradually declines over time, in a predictable, exponential fashion (Fig. 5). The data are fit to Eq. (1). Sustainable levels of pressure development are usually approached at approximately 5 min (depending on breathing rhythm). Subjects can sustain approximately 60–80% of their maximum "dynamic" pressure (maximum pressures with flow) at rest, which represents about 40–50% of static MIP (i.e., without flow, against an occlusion). However, this value is highly dependent on the breathing

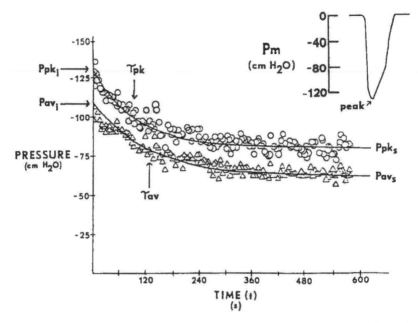

Figure 5 Isoflow endurance curves for a single subject. P_{pk_i} and P_{av_i} are initial maximum peak and average pressure/inspiration. τ = the time constants of the two exponential decay curves [1/k in Eq. (1)]. P_{pk_s} and P_{av_s} are the calculated sustainable pressures. (Adapted from Clanton and Ameredes, 1988b.)

pattern (Clanton et al., 1990), as will be discussed later. The isoflow method has proven useful for physiological testing in normals because most of the important variables that can affect the endurance measurement are controlled and the test is completed in a short time period. In addition, recent data have demonstrated that the sustainable pressures obtained with the isoflow method are nearly identical to those obtained with submaximal loading (Julian et al., 1991). However, its applicability to the study of endurance properties in patient populations has yet to be evaluated.

A second test that may be useful for its simplicity has been described by Gandevia et al. (1983) and McKenzie et al. (1986). It involves 12 repeated MIP maneuvers lasting 15 s, with 7.5 s of rest (duty cycle = 0.67; lower duty cycles do not result in fatigue of the inspiratory muscles over 12 contractions). In normal subjects the MIP pressures drop approximately 23%. Asthma patients show a significantly higher MIP at the end of the 12 contractions compared to normals, suggesting additional respiratory muscle endurance in this population (McKenzie and Gandevia, 1986). One of the advantages of this test is that the load is static and therefore independent of alterations in chest wall or lung mechanics. In addition, the test is relatively short and has been shown to be reproducible (Gandevia et al.,

1983). A potential disadvantage is that the endurance characteristics of the muscles may reflect the anaerobic capacity of the muscles to sustain force, since it is likely that blood flow is occluded during prolonged contraction (Bellemare et al., 1986).

Considerations Concerning the Interpretation of Sustainable Pressures

On a theoretical basis, sustainable ventilation or pressure development must represent an equilibrium between the processes contributing to the loss of contractile function, due to fatigue, and processes that sustain contractile function. Since an individual can remain at this equilibrium for a prolonged period (e.g., Fig. 5), it has been possible to test the influence of various factors that may affect the fatigue process (Ameredes and Clanton, 1988; Clanton et al., 1988a; Ameredes and Clanton, 1989; Ameredes et al., 1991). However, some factors may have unique influences on endurance to loads higher than sustainable (e.g., hypoxemia in Roussos and Macklem, 1977). One has to consider that different fatigue mechanisms may predominate or the activity of certain fiber types may be prevalent in response to various levels of fatiguing stimuli (Faulkner, 1985; Grassino and Clanton, 1991).

It is of considerable interest that the concept of sustainable maximum activities of the respiratory muscles appears be a phenomenon more easily identified in the in vivo situation. Sustainable activities of isolated diaphragm strips or in situ diaphragm strips are extremely low when these muscles are stimulated maximally for prolonged periods (Ameredes et al., 1991). It is possible that protective mechanisms within the central nervous system inhibit complete activation of the respiratory muscles by voluntary stimulation, thus preventing potential injury to the muscles or substantial neuromuscular fatigue and allowing a certain level of sustainable activity to be maintained. Such protective mechanisms would presumably be overridden in the artificially stimulated muscle.

C. Incremental Resistive Loading Procedures

Martyn et al. (1987) have described an incremental threshold loading technique, similar in concept to incremental exercise testing but applied to the inspiratory muscles. Subjects begin inspiring at a pressure load of approximately 30% of MIP, and the load is increased every 2 min by approximately 5–10% of MIP until the subject cannot inspire against the load. The maximum pressure thus achieved is referred to as P_{mPeak} and represents approximately 88% of MIP. Despite the fact that breathing pattern is not controlled, subsequent studies of McElvaney et al. (1989) have demonstrated a high degree of reproducibility of this measurement in a given subject compared to the more common Tlim measurements. There are numerous advantages to this test, not the least of which is the fact that it is tolerated well by normals, elderly, and moderate to severe COPD patients (Morrison et al., 1989a; Pruesser et al., 1992), and similar testing procedures have been shown to be very sensitive to the effects of respiratory muscle training in COPD (Pruesser et al., 1992).

However, the exact relationship between the P_{mPeak}, measured in this way, and the endurance versus strength of the inspiratory muscles is not clear because P_{mPeak} appears to lie somewhere between MIP and SIP (Julian et al., 1991). Furthermore, the potential influence of breathing pattern could lead to inaccuracies in some patients, although Martyn et al. (1987) found that this was not a significant problem when individuals are evaluated on subsequent days.

Interestingly, Morrison et al. (1989a) have found that in patients with obstructive lung disease the P_{mPeak} obtained during incremental loading is reduced compared to normals when expressed as a fraction of MIP. This suggests that the "functional capacity" of the muscles of these patients may be compromised to a greater extent than is generally appreciated.

D. Endurance of the Diaphragm

Roussos and Macklem (1977) made the first attempt to study the endurance of the diaphragm in humans by having subjects try to sustain various target trans-diaphragmatic pressures (P_{di}) during inspiration against an external resistance. The target P_{di} was obtained by a combination of positive abdominal pressure (P_{ab}) and a negative pleural pressure (P_{pl}) generation. Endurance curves, similar to Figure 2, were generated but with P_{di} on the y-axis. It was found that subjects could only sustain approximately 40% of maximum transdiaphragmatic pressure. The approach was greatly refined in the studies of Bellemare and Grassino (1982), who systematically matched $+P_{ab}$ and $-P_{es}$ to obtain target P_{di} values during the endurance runs. They found results similar to those of Roussos and Macklem (1977) but they carefully controlled breathing rhythm and their analyses included the important application of the tension-time index, described in detail in a later section. It is interesting that based on the above results, the diaphragm appears to be more sensitive to fatigue than the inspiratory muscles working in synergy. The inspiratory muscles can generally sustain 50–80% of maximum inspiratory pressure under most contraction conditions, whereas the diaphragm can apparently only sustain about 40%. This phenomenon cannot be explained by differences in fiber type or blood flow, since the diaphragm is believed to contain at least as many fatigue-resistant fibers as the accessory muscles (reviewed in Sharp and Hyatt, 1986), and the capacity for blood flow of the diaphragm is believed to be extremely high (reviewed in Supinski, 1988). One explanation may be the method by which the maximum pressures for the diaphragm are estimated (P_{dimax}) versus the way in which maximum pressures are estimated for the inspiratory muscles working in synergy (MIP). Hillman et al. (1990), using fluoroscopic analyses and other methods, have recently suggested that the usual way of determining maximum P_{di}, which includes a significant abdominal muscle contraction, results in a net lengthening of the diaphragm, allowing it to generate higher pressures due to the force-length relationship of skeletal muscle. In contrast, for the determination of MIP, no attempt is made to limit thoracic configuration, and generally the highest values are obtained under conditions of considerable distortion of the lower thorax (Saunders et al., 1979), probable diaphragm shortening (Newman et al., 1984), and accessory muscle shortening due to gas decompression. Therefore, comparing the fractions, SIP/MIP and sustainable P_{di}/P_{dimax} may give a skewed idea of the relative fatigabilities of these two muscle groups.

Determining the endurance of the diaphragm in naive subjects is more difficult to perform than determining the endurance of the inspiratory muscles working in synergy because considerable coordination is involved in maintaining appropriate pressures on either side of the diaphragm. Loading the diaphragm correctly (Bellemare and Grassino, 1982) results in a chest wall configuration that somewhat opposes normal thoracic expansion during loaded breathing. Therefore, it has only rarely been applied to patient populations. One can study the changes in P_{di} that occur concurrently with fatigue of the whole inspiratory pump (Clanton et al., 1990), but it is difficult to infer to what extent the diaphragm is contributing to the overall loss of pressure development and to what extent it is simply following changes that are occurring in the chest wall musculature (Hershenson et al., 1988). Our understanding of the intrinsic behavior and fatigability of the diaphragm during large inspiratory efforts, resulting in fatigue, is inadequate.

E. Expiratory Muscle Endurance

Less attention has been paid to measuring the endurance of the expiratory muscles. On a theoretical basis, expiratory muscle fatigue would appear to be much less important since even in the presence of severe expiratory flow limitation, the largest mechanical burden is taken up by the inspiratory muscles. This is presumably due to the fact that large positive pleural pressures are not particularly useful in increasing expiratory flow over a large portion of the flow-volume relationship because of maximum expiratory flow limitation (Hyatt, 1986). In patients with obstructive lung disease, the ability to increase ventilation by expiratory muscle recruitment is greatly limited, and they must encroach on their inspiratory capacity and hyperinflate in order to use their reserve of lung elastic recoil to keep the airways open (Pride and Macklem, 1986). This, of course, puts a much larger burden on the inspiratory muscles compared to normal subjects. Nevertheless, it has been estimated that 25% of the work of breathing is performed by the expiratory muscles in COPD patients at rest (McIlory and Christie, 1954), and they are recruited during highly aerobic activity and may be subject to fatigue. For example, maximum expiratory pressures can drop 30% or more after a marathon run (Loke et al., 1982). Therefore, there is some interest in understanding the endurance properties of the expiratory muscles.

McKenzie and Gandevia (1986), using the repeated maximum static contraction technique, discussed above, showed that the expiratory muscles in normals and asthma patients demonstrate greater decreases in pressure compared to similar tests on the inspiratory muscles, suggesting their endurance characteristics are reduced. More recently, Suzuki et al. (1991) induced expiratory muscle fatigue by having normal subjects expire against varying resistances. Interestingly, loads amounting to approximately 16% of maximum expiratory pressure (MEP) resulted in task failure in 75% of the subjects (the tension-time index for the expiratory muscles with this load was approximately 11%). This suggests that the expiratory muscles are more susceptible than the inspiratory muscles to fatigue, and it is possible that under some conditions, fatigue may occur even when the relative forces or pressures they are generating are modest. More surprising, Suzuki et al. (1991) demonstrated that immediately following an expiratory loading protocol, MEP was reduced by 16%, and MIP by 13%, suggesting some "crossover" influence of fatigue between these antagonist muscle groups.

III. Factors That Influence Respiratory Muscle Endurance

Using the above approaches to study respiratory muscle endurance, a number of investigations have been made into various factors that can influence endurance measurements. There are countless other physiological or pharmacological variables that affect the fatigue process. However, the following paragraphs are restricted to a discussion of influences that are directly relevant to the measurement of respiratory muscle endurance in humans and have been studied using the above approaches to endurance testing.

A. Hypoxemia and Altered O_2 Delivery

The question as to the extent to which hypoxemia can influence endurance measurements has been an important one because of the potential coupling between respiratory failure and hypoxemia in patients. Although it is clear that if O_2 delivery to the respiratory muscles is reduced sufficiently their contractile function will be diminished, it is still reasonably unclear how relevant the availability of O_2 is to respiratory muscle function and endurance under conditions in which the circulation or blood oxygenation are not greatly compromised. For example, it has been proposed that endurance time in normals is a function of the imbalance between energy supply and demand in the muscle (Monod and Scherrer, 1965), sometimes called the "energy imbalance hypothesis." Since early experiments demonstrated that decreases in inspired O_2 reduce endurance time (Roussos and Macklem, 1977), it appeared likely that the critical substrate for energy supply was O_2. Taking it one step further, sustainable muscle activity in this model would reflect the balance between the muscle's ability to absorb O_2 for energy production and its capacity to utilize energy for contractile force or shortening. This idea, however, under most normal physiological conditions, has been difficult to prove or disprove. The problem is complicated by (1) the fact that other mechanisms of muscle dysfunction or fatigue may predominate under normal physiological conditions (Grassino and Clanton, 1991) and substrate availability may only play an important role in muscles that are already compromised by inadequate perfusion pressures or excessive contraction times, etc., (2) the fact that O_2 (or the lack thereof) may have direct or indirect influences on cellular respiration or blood flow that are independent of energy balance or substrate availability (Barclay, 1986; Hogan and Welch, 1986; Adams et al., 1986), and (3) the fact that the lack of O_2 can cause elevations in hydrogen ion concentration, which can have independent influences on muscle contractile function (Mainwood et al., 1987).

The experimental results of the effects of changes in oxygenation on human respiratory muscle fatigue are mixed. For example, Tenny and Reese (1968) were unable to demonstrate an influence of 9% inspired oxygen on endurance time at any particular fatiguing ventilation and concluded that O_2 availability had little impact on fatigue during these maneuvers. In contrast, Roussos and Macklem (1977), studying diaphragm fatigue during resistive breathing, demonstrated marked reductions in endurance time in response to inspiring 13% FIO_2. Similar results were demonstrated by Jardim et al. (1981). Furthermore, Pardy and Bye (1985) found that diaphragm fatigue was attenuated at elevated levels of inspired O_2. All of this information would suggest that the fatiguing diaphragm is particularly sensitive to relatively modest decreases or increases in blood O_2 content.

Differing results were found by Ameredes and Clanton (1989), who, using the isoflow model, could find no influence of similar levels of hypoxia (13% FIO_2) or hyperoxia (100% FIO_2) on the rate of decay of inspiratory pressure development during fatigue or sustainable pressure development. Further experiments were performed by Ameredes et al. (1991) on the in situ dog diaphragm strip preparation. Essentially no effect of hypoxia or hyperoxia on sustainable tension generation of the diaphragm could be identified until O_2 content fell some 9 vol% to a PaO_2 of 34 mm Hg. Even at approximately 50–60% Sa_{O_2}, the effects were small and occurred only in the shortening diaphragm, not in the diaphragm contracting isometrically. These studies suggest that the extent of diaphragm fatigue in the normally contracting or artificially stimulated conditions is relatively insensitive to moderate changes in blood oxygen. Compensatory mechanisms such as increased perfusion pressure, decreased vascular resistance, or increases O_2 extraction must protect the muscles from hypoxemia in the normally fatiguing diaphragm.

The question remains: Why have all investigators who have looked at endurance time of the diaphragm in humans demonstrated a strong sensitivity of the diaphragm to O_2 availability (Roussos and Macklem, 1977; Jardim et al., 1981; Pardy and Bye, 1985), but other investigators looking at the inspiratory muscles working in synergy have not (Tenny and Reese, 1968; Ameredes and Clanton, 1989)? Some of the differences in results could possibly be explained on the basis of technical factors (Ameredes and Clanton, 1989). However, it is also possible that when the diaphragm contracts with prolonged duty cycles (T_I/T_{TOT}) and when transdiaphragmatic pressures are obtained by generating high positive abdominal pressures, O_2 availability may be more critical compared to conditions of contraction in which pleural pressure is negative but abdominal pressure is reasonably low (typical of experiments studying the fatigue of the synergic respiratory pump). In support of this, Buchler et al. (1985) have shown that positive abdominal pressures tend to diminish diaphragm blood flow.

In summary, the relationship between O_2 availability and endurance under various kinds of muscle contractions is complex and highly integrative. Though it is probable that the energy imbalance hypothesis cannot entirely account for endurance time under all conditions, it is no doubt important under some conditions.

B. Hypercapnia and Respiratory Acidosis

As with the effects of hypoxemia on measurements of endurance, there has been considerable interest in understanding whether hypercapnia contributes to a kind of positive feedback loop driving patients toward muscle pump failure. From a technical viewpoint, understanding whether hypercapnia affects measurements of endurance is also important because many of the resistive loading protocols for measuring endurance result in moderate CO_2 retention at task failure, and these could influence the measurements.

One of the first experiments in humans was performed by Juan et al. (1984), who demonstrated that the "contractility" of the diaphragm was reduced in response to 7.5% $ETCO_2$. It was unaffected by hypocapnia ($FECO_2 = 3\%$). Furthermore, hypercapnic resistive loading caused the H/L ratio of the diaphragm EMG signal to decrease precipitously, suggesting an accelerated rate of the fatigue process compared to control conditions. Similar results on the fatigue process were found by Ameredes and Clanton (1988) using the isoflow model. Although sustainable pressures were essentially unaffected by 7.0% $ETCO_2$, the rare of decay of pressure development was greatly increased and there was no measurable effects of hypocapnia on any endurance measurement. These data are in basic agreement with results in animal preparations (Schnader et al., 1985) and suggest that CO_2 retention and the resultant acidosis may contribute to ventilatory failure. In addition, when possible, $ETCO_2$ should be controlled during measurements of endurance and respiratory muscle function.

C. End-Expiratory Lung Volume and Initial Muscle Length

Many patients with chronic obstructive disease have chronic hyperinflation, which results in certain long-term morphological adaptations to the respiratory muscles (Farkas and Roussos, 1983; Oliven et al., 1986) and chest wall (Thomas et al., 1986). These changes no doubt affect the mechanics and endurance characteristics of the inspiratory pump. However, more relevant to this discussion are the effects of acute hyperinflation that accompany conditions of elevated ventilatory requirement (e.g., exercise) or increased bronchoconstriction in patients with obstructive lung disease (Pride and Macklem, 1986). Increases in lung volume shorten the inspiratory muscles, but do shortened muscles fatigue more? It does not appear that they do. For a given level of neural activation, all studies of isolated muscle or in vivo skeletal muscle demonstrate that muscles fatigue proportional to their activation or, under constant length conditions, their tension development (Aljure and Borrero, 1968; Farkas and Roussos, 1984; Fitch and McComas, 1985). This has led to the hypothesis that what is important in the fatigue process is the number of cross-bridges interacting over time, which is decreased by reductions in muscle length (Aljure and Borrero, 1968). For a given electrical activation, a shortened muscle has less cross-bridge interaction and therefore demonstrates a smaller degree of fatigue (Aljure and Borrero, 1968; Farkas and Roussos, 1984; Fitch and McComas, 1985).

However, hyperinflation is somewhat more complicated than simple shortening of the inspiratory muscles. First, at higher lung volumes the inspiratory muscles see greater intrinsic elastic loads, so that for a given level of external mechanical work, they may fatigue to a greater extent. Second, the efficiency of the inspiratory muscles is reduced at elevated lung volumes (Collett and Engel, 1986), probably due, in part, to the flattening of the diaphragm and the altered configuration or recruitment of the chest wall musculature. Third, if the lung volume is high enough, the capacity of the chest wall musculature to generate pressure may be reduced because of the limitations of the maximum pressure-volume relationship of the thorax (Agostoni and Hyatt, 1986). Under these latter conditions, comparing endurance characteristics between low and high lung volumes is somewhat complicated.

Most experiments on the endurance of the inspiratory muscles at elevated lung volumes have demonstrated a reduction in endurance time when end-expiratory volume was increased (Roussos et al., 1979; McKenzie and Gandevia, 1987; Tzelepsis et al., 1988). Most notably, Tzelepsis et al. (1988) observed a marked decrement in sustainable pressure during endurance runs at elevated lung volumes. In contrast to these results, Clanton et al. (1993) have recently shown (using the isoflow technique) that when end-expiratory lung volume is increased by approximately 1.1 L in normal volunteers, the rate of decline of pressure generation during fatigue is decreased and the sustainable pressures generated are nearly identical to those that could be obtained at normal end-expiratory lung volume. Nevertheless, sustainable transdiaphragmatic pressures were reduced at elevated lung volumes, suggesting that hyperinflation had a unique effect on the diaphragm. The rib cage muscles must have been able to compensate to maintain the pressure development at the airway opening. Careful attention was paid to thoracic impedance at the elevated lung volumes, and therefore the pressures recorded were as close as possible to representing the actual inspiratory muscle pressures (P_{mus}). This latter study suggests that as long as hyperinflation is occurring within a moderate range, the inspiratory muscles (particularly the rib cage muscles) behave much like other skeletal muscles with respect to their endurance characteristics at shortened lengths.

D. Elements of Breathing Pattern

As mentioned, early investigations of respiratory muscle endurance paid little attention to breathing pattern in determining endurance time, and it is still a common practice. The influence of various components of the breathing pattern on inspiratory muscle endurance time is complex, as illustrated in Figure 6. The top three panels describe relative changes in Tlim (compared to control conditions) that occur when the pressure load is kept constant but inspiratory time (T_I), total period (T_{TOT}), or inspiratory flow ($\dot{V}_{TI}$) are altered. In the bottom three panels, the external mechanical work was kept constant but T_I and T_{TOT} or breathing frequency were altered by adjustments in $\dot{V}_{TI}$. Sorting out these factors has been the work of numerous laboratories over the past decade, and the results of these experiments are discussed below.

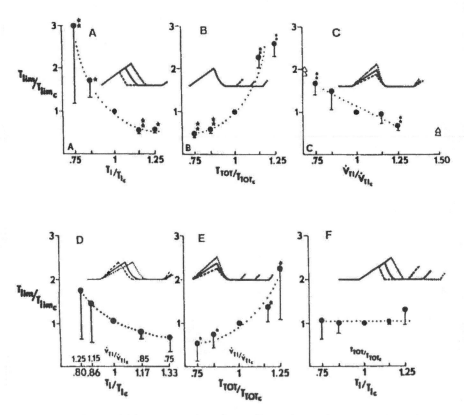

Figure 6 Changes in T_{lim} as a fraction of control T_{lim} (T_{lim_c}) induced by isolated changes in T_I (panel A), T_{TOT} (panel B), and inspiratory flow ($\dot{V}_{TI}$, panel C). Stars indicate significant changes from control. In panels D, E, and F, external power output was kept constant with simultaneous changes in flow or timing. In F, power and pressure-time integral were kept constant while breathing frequency was changed. (From Clanton et al., 1985.)

The Influence of Breath Timing (Duty Cycle and the Pressure-Time Index)

Seminal experiments on the influence of breath timing on respiratory muscle fatigue and endurance in humans were performed by Bellemare and Grassino (1982), who applied the tension-time index to diaphragm fatigue. The concept of the tension-time index has its roots in early investigations of the mechanisms determining oxygen consumption of the right ventricle (Sarnoff et al., 1958) as well as fatigue of limb muscles (Scherrer and Monod, 1960). Rochester and Bettini (1976) also applied the concept to the contracting dog diaphragm to understand relationships between tension development, blood flow, and O_2 consumption. The tension-time index can be defined simply as the average tension generated by a muscle over time (i.e., averaged over the contraction and relaxation phases) and expressed as a fraction of the maximum tension available to the muscle at rest (i.e., MIP or max P_{di}). More recently, the term "pressure-time index" (PTI) has been used. Bellemare and Grassino (1982) found that endurance time for the diaphragm, over a wide variety of breathing rhythms, could be predicted accurately by the pressure-time index. This is illustrated in Figure 7. Values of PTI below 0.15–0.18 were found to be sustainable. The sustainable PTI was subsequently viewed as the "critical PTI" or "threshold" for diaphragm fatigue and has been applied to a number of clinical

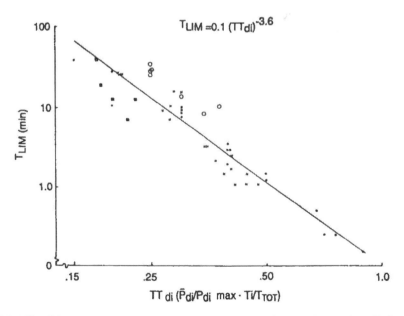

Figure 7 Tlim expressed as an exponential function of tension time index of the diaphragm over a wide range of duty cycles. (From Bellemare and Grassino, 1982.)

situations (e.g., Bellemare and Grassino, 1983). Recent experiments by Fitting et al. (1988) and Zocchi et al. (1992) have obtained a separate PTI for the rib cage muscles of approximately 0.30. This was accomplished by having subjects actively paradox, that is, generate negative abdominal pressures during inspiration, which effectively unloads the diaphragm. One of the characteristics of these estimates of PTI for the diaphragm and rib cage muscles is that tidal volume, inspiratory flow, and thoracoabdominal configuration were limited to reasonably narrow ranges, and therefore their applicability to conditions of higher ventilations may be limited (as will be discussed later). However, the contributions of these investigations clearly defined the influence of breath timing on endurance time and really combined three important variables—T_I, T_{TOT}, and pressure load—into one determining factor on the fatigue process.

Inspiratory Flow Rate, Tidal Volume, and Mechanical Work

The influence of inspiratory flow on endurance time under conditions of constant pressure-time integral were described nearly simultaneously by two laboratories using two different approaches. Clanton et al. (1985b) demonstrated the effects of flow by measuring endurance time to high inspiratory threshold loads (Fig. 6, panel C), and McCool et al. (1986) demonstrated it using inspirations against external orifice resistors. As seen in Figure 8 from McCool et al. (1986), as inspiratory flow increased, the pressure-time index for esophageal pressure (similar to P_{mus}) that

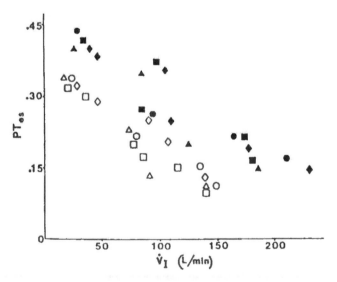

Figure 8 Changes in esophageal pressure-time index that can be sustained for 8 min (open symbols) and 1 min (closed symbols) with changes in inspiratory flow. (From McCool et al., 1986.)

could be maintained for 8 min (open symbols) and 1 min (closed symbols) gradually decreased. Clanton et al. (1988b, 1990) later showed that sustainable inspiratory pressures (using the isoflow technique) are reduced by elevations in inspiratory flow when duty cycle is maintained constant. This effect is quite large; the sustainable pressure-time integral can decrease by about 20% when inspiratory flow is doubled from 0.5 to 1.0 L/s, or from 1.0 to 2.0 L/s (Clanton et al., 1990). From these data, it is quite clear that the pressure-time index, as originally described, cannot entirely account for the endurance properties of the respiratory muscles. Therefore, some aspect related to changes in inspiratory flow, namely, the rate of muscle shortening (flow), muscle length (lung volume), the amount of muscle shortening (tidal volume), or the mechanical work of breathing, must have important consequences with respect to endurance measurements. These are considered below.

Effects of Velocity of Shortening

As muscles contract at increasing velocities of shortening, their capacity to generate force declines as defined by the maximum force-velocity relationship. Although the relationship between flow and velocity of shortening is poorly understood for any of the inspiratory muscles; certainly, as flow increases, so must velocity. However, the effect of flow on pressure development is small over the range of inspiratory flows that are available to the inspiratory pump. For example, at a given lung volume, maximum inspiratory pressures only decrease about 5 cm $H_2O \cdot L^{-1} \cdot s^{-1}$, or about 3–4% per L/s (Topulos et al., 1987; unpublished observations in our laboratory). As pointed out by Rochester (1982) and later discussed by Dodd et al. (1988a), with maximum voluntary efforts, only about 20% of maximum velocity of shortening for the diaphragm can be attained due to the intrinsic impedance of the thoracic pump. Therefore, the influence of velocity of shortening, by itself, cannot fully explain the effects of flow.

Effects of Muscle Length

As inspiratory flow goes up at a constant duty cycle, so must lung volume and the amount of shortening of the muscle. With increasing lung volume the capacity to generate pressure decreases, as defined by the classic maximum pressure-volume relationship for the thorax (Agostoni and Hyatt, 1986). Unlike the influence of flow, this reduction in capacity to generate airway opening pressure against an external load is quite large, decreasing to zero at TLC. It is clear that this reduction in the capacity to generate pressure will cause task failure to a given submaximal load to occur earlier in time and thus cause a reduction in measured endurance time. However, this suggests that at increased flows the muscles are not fatiguing more; they simply have lost capacity to generate pressure. From isoflow experiments (Clanton and Ameredes, 1988b; Clanton et al., 1990), as will be described later, this may not be the whole story for the effect of increases in flow, because the actual sustainable pressure development at a given lung volume is reduced with increasing tidal volumes, independent of the capacity to generate pressure due to the maximum volume-pressure curve. Therefore, there still must be additional influences of shortening on the fatigue process.

Effects of Mechanical Work

What may be of most importance is the fact that as the flow rate increases, the inspiratory muscles shorten further for a given inspiratory period and perform more mechanical work. This results in an increased energy cost to the muscles (Fenn, 1924; Mommaerts, 1970; Homsher and Kean, 1978; Rall, 1982; Kushmerick, 1982). As summarized by Mommaerts (1970), "a muscle doing work mobilizes, over and above that needed for activation and maintenance of tension, energy accounting for the work and for the dissipation of energy accompanying the work process." The additional energy costs of shortening and mechanical work would be expected to contribute to the fatigue process. That shortening muscles fatigue more than nonshortening muscles at a given level of electrical stimulation is therefore not surprising and has been shown conclusively by a number of investigators, most recently by Ameredes et al. (1990) in the in situ diaphragm strip preparation, contracting with an isokinetic ergometer (Fig. 9).

Breathing Frequency

Increases in breathing frequency have the potential to influence measurements of endurance. This is because from an energetics standpoint, there is an independent "activation energy" that is expended in the mobilization and sequestration of Ca^{+2} following initial activation (Homsher and Kean, 1978). Though for twitch contractions this amounts to a reasonably large amount of energy, for tetanic contractions it becomes proportionally less important because of reductions in Ca^{+2} cycling with tetani. From measurements of endurance time to submaximal loads (Clanton et al., 1985b) (Fig. 6F), using the isoflow technique (Julian and Clanton, 1990) or sustained hyperventilation (Tenney and Reese, 1968), no independent effects of breathing frequency on endurance measurements have been identified. Furthermore, when work rate and pressure-time integral are kept constant during resistive breathing,

ISOMETRIC   ISOVELOCITY

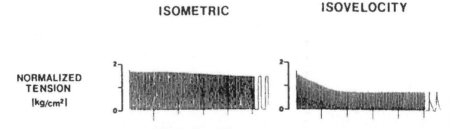

NORMALIZED
TENSION
[kg/cm²]

Figure 9   An example of changes in diaphragm force development in response to maximum intermittent stimulations in the in situ dog diaphragm strip during isometric and isovelocity contractions. (From Ameredes et al., 1990.)

there are no measurable changes in oxygen consumption (Dodd et al., 1988b). Therefore, it appears that at least within a moderate range of frequencies, all of the elements of breathing rhythm can be accounted for through the quantification of duty cycle and/or pressure-time index. Previous studies that have addressed the breathing frequency problem have necessarily increased mechanical work and or pressure-time integral during contraction and have attributed these to breathing frequency (e.g., Morrison et al., 1989b).

Inspiratory Muscle Configuration

Probably the least understood variable with respect to respiratory muscle endurance is the influence of different chest wall configurations on the measurements. Striking differences are seen in configuration when different maneuvers are utilized to attain an external mechanical load. For example, it requires the activation of antagonistic muscles to maintain a targeted submaximal pressure or flow using visual feedback, just as it requires the co-activation of agonists and antagonists to sustain any controlled motor activity. During targeted inspiratory maneuvers there is considerable abdominal muscle contraction, which increases transdiaphragmatic pressure to larger absolute values than esophageal pressure (Clanton et al., 1985b). However, during maximal inspirations against constant flow generators (Clanton and Ameredes, 1988b; Clanton et al., 1990) or against an occluded airway, there is little or no positive abdominal pressure generated; in fact, abdominal pressures often become negative and the load on the diaphragm (with respect to P_{di}) is less than that on the chest wall muscles (Clanton et al., 1990). Therefore, configuration and contraction of antagonist muscles must influence measurements of endurance but the effect is poorly studied or documented. Such influences may be responsible for the loss of coordination that often accompanies the point of task failure during endurance measurements.

Summary of the Effects of Breathing Pattern

In the minimally shortening muscles, the pressure-time index (Bellemare and Grassino, 1982; Zocchi et al., 1992) appears to remain a very good predictor of endurance time and sustainable activity for a given configuration and level of activation of the pump. However, as the muscles begin to shorten substantially (as would occur with increasing flow rates and tidal volumes), the pressure-time index becomes less predictive in terms of endurance characteristics of the inspiratory muscles (Clanton et al., 1985b; McCool et al., 1986; Clanton et al., 1990). This is illustrated in Figure 10, which was obtained from a breath-by-breath recalculation of pressure-time index for the synergic muscle pump during isoflow endurance runs (Clanton et al., 1990). This suggests that there is no single threshold pressure-time index. It may be more appropriate in breathing patterns that employ significant tidal volume excursion to include a factor accounting for mechanical work in addition to the pressure-time factor

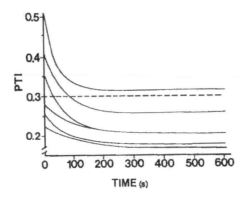

Figure 10 Mean exponential regression lines from six subjects for breath-by-breath pressure-time-index (PTI) for the synergic inspiratory muscles during isoflow experiments. The dashed line represents a threshold PTI of 0.3. The figure illustrates that over a wide range of flows and tidal volumes there is no single critical pressure-time index that determines sustainable pump activity. (From Clanton et al., 1990.)

to take into consideration the influence of shortening on the fatigue process. In support of this idea, Dodd et al. (1988a) have shown that when pressure-time product is kept constant, endurance time can be shown to be a relatively tight function of mechanical work being performed. Nevertheless, the integration of elements of mechanical work with pressure-time index as determinants of endurance time and sustainable activity of the pump have not yet been comprehensively evaluated.

IV. A Model for Understanding the Influence of Varying Contraction Patterns on Inspiratory Muscle Endurance

Using data from a number of investigations largely employing the isoflow technique (Clanton et al., 1985b, 1990, 1992; Clanton and Ameredes, 1988b; Julian and Clanton, 1990), we have developed the following working hypothesis to describe the endurance properties of the synergic inspiratory pump in response to varying types of contractions. It does not relate directly to a discussion of energetics, which is the usual approach to the problem (Monod and Scherrer, 1965; Roussos and Macklem, 1977: Roussos and Campbell, 1986). However, it takes advantage of the close association between energetics and mechanics of contraction (Kushmeric, 1982). The working hypothesis is the following:

> For a given breathing pattern against a fatiguing load, the decay of the dynamic pressure-generating capacity of the inspiratory muscle pump is directly proportional to its pressure-time product, expressed as a fraction of its "capacity" to generate dynamic pressure on the max pressure-flow-volume relationship.

This hypothesis has many aspects in common with the original pressure-time index concept, as described by Bellemare and Grassino (1982), but there are also some important differences. For example, pressure development is referenced to the capacity of the inspiratory muscles to generate "dynamic" pressure at finite flows and lung volumes, and not "static" pressure (MIP) at rest. Furthermore, there is no single threshold pressure-time product that accurately predicts when fatigue will occur; rather, the absolute pressure threshold varies with breathing pattern and the trajectory of the breath within the maximum pressure-flow-volume relationship of the muscles involved.

To understand this, it is helpful to visualize the maximum pressure-flow-volume relationship of the inspiratory muscles (P-F-V$_{insp}$), as seen in Figure 11. This relationship defines the "dynamic" capacity of the pump to generate pressure (z-axis) as a function of thoracic volume and flow (x- and y-axes). It is the composite three-dimensional representation of the classic maximum pressure-volume relationship and the maximum pressure-flow relationship. The figure was obtained from one subject using more than 30 maximum inspirations from RV to TLC against varying types of resistances (Clanton et al., 1991). Surfaces are generated with three-dimensional nonlinear regression analysis of the raw data. Though the relationships between muscle force and pressure development as well as muscle shortening and lung volume are extremely complex and incompletely understood in humans, the maximum P-F-V$_{insp}$ surface is the "functional equivalent" of the maximum force-veloicity-length curve of skeletal muscles (Bahler et al., 1968; Sharp and Hyatt, 1986).

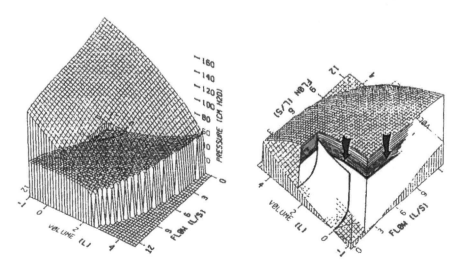

Figure 11   Two viewpoints of the maximum pressure-flow-volume relationship in humans. See text for details.

The lower surfaces in the background of the two graphs in Figure 11 represent the inherent impedance of the thoracic pump, i.e., the pressure required to overcome the elastic and resistive forces opposing thoracic expansion, as a function of inspiratory flow and volume. During normal breathing, without external mechanical loads imposed on the system, the inspiratory muscles produce a pressure (P_{mus}) that is confined to this impedance surface, regardless of breathing pattern or inspiratory effort.

The upper surface comprises the maximum dynamic pressure of the inspiratory muscles (max P_{mus}). It is calculated from the mathematical summation of the maximum pressures that the inspiratory pump can generate at the airway opening against external loads plus the pressures inherent to overcoming thoracic impedance. The difference between upper and lower surfaces is the "reserve" for pressure generation available at any particular flow and volume. At the outer edges, where the two surfaces intersect, TLC or maximum flow are defined where there is no additional P_{mus} reserve.

The graph on the right of Figure 11 is the same relationship as on the left but seen from an alternate viewpoint in space. For purposes of illustration, within the cutout portion, a P_{mus} trajectory is depicted that would occur by inspiring from a submaximal threshold load at a constant inspiratory flow rate (e.g., Clanton et al., 1985b). The large arrows depict the predictable movement of the maximum $P-F-V_{insp}$ surface as the muscles fatigue during an endurance run (see Fig. 4). The figure illustrates that task failure (at T_{lim}) would occur at the point in time in which the curve intersects the targeted load. This inevitably happens at high lung volumes first because of the shape of the maximum $P-F-V_{insp}$ surface. The shift of the maximum $P-F-V_{insp}$ curve with fatigue is parallel across the surface in this depiction, which is consistent with data from our laboratory (Clanton et al., 1988a).

The hypothesis predicts the following findings:

1. *Effects of flow rate*: At a constant duty cycle but with contrasting inspiratory flow rates (and thus tidal volumes), the inspiratory muscles will fatigue approximately the same amount relative to their dynamic capacity to generate pressure at rest. Their sustainable pressures will not, however, be a constant fraction of "static" MIP at rest. This is illustrated in Figure 12, which was generated from the composite breaths of six subjects during fatiguing isoflow runs at two contrasting flow rates (Clanton et al., 1990). The upper tracings are the average maximum dynamic pressures the subjects could generate at rest as they inspired from a constant flow generator; the lower curves are the sustainable maximum dynamic pressures. Note that the sustainable pressures at any specific time point are lower at the higher flow rate, but the ratio of sustainable to initial average dynamic pressure during inspiration (i.e., "sustainable fraction") is constant at the two inspiratory flow rates (approximately 63% in this example). The ratio of average sustainable pressures to maximum "static" pressures is not constant, being 56% at the lower flow and 46% at the higher flow.

2. *Effects of duty cycle*: As duty cycle is increased, there is a greater decay in the capacity to generate dynamic inspiratory pressure as the muscles fatigue (Fig. 13). In addition, the decay rate in maximum dynamic pressure development over time is significantly faster, with increasing duty cycle (Julian and Clanton

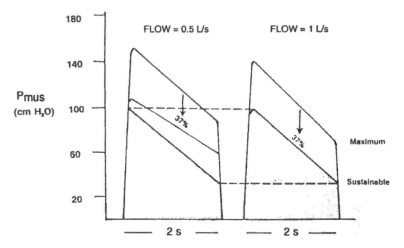

Figure 12 Effects of isolated changes in flow on sustainable pressure development in the time domain. The data are signal averages of six subjects. At both flows, pressure development drops due to fatigue, approximately the same percentage of dynamic maximum (37%) in this example. (From Clanton et al., 1990.)

unpublished observations). As mentioned, there is no effect of isolated changes in breathing frequency on the relationship. Therefore, duty cycle is the predominant variable in breathing rhythm. The overall effect of duty cycle on sustainable fraction of initial pressure-time product is illustrated in Figure 14. In six subjects this relationship has been shown to be linear with a mean slope of -0.38 ± 0.11, independent of tidal volume, breathing rate, or inspiratory flow rate. With respect to the P-F-V_{insp} relationship, increased duty cycle causes a more pronounced inward shift of the maximum P-F-V_{insp} surface as the muscles fatigue. The amount of this shift is determined by the slope of the relationship seen in Figure 14.

3. *Effects of lung volume*: As initial lung volume (end-expiratory volume) increases and the inspiratory muscles shorten, they are less capable of generating pressure and performing external mechanical work (as dictated by the sloping maximum P-F-V_{insp} surface). For a given submaximal load, a subject will reach task failure more quickly because there is less reserve for pressure generation. However, the sustainable dynamic P_{mus} development remains similar to that at lower lung volumes and is actually increased, relative to the dynamic capacity of the inspiratory muscles to generate pressure at rest (Clanton et al., 1992). It is possible that this relationship may not hold at very high lung volumes because efficiency would be greatly reduced (Collett and Engel, 1986).

Despite the influence of initial volume on sustainable pump function, we have been unable to identify a similar effect of tidal volume (independent of flow, mechanical work or pressure-time product) on sustainable fractions of initial

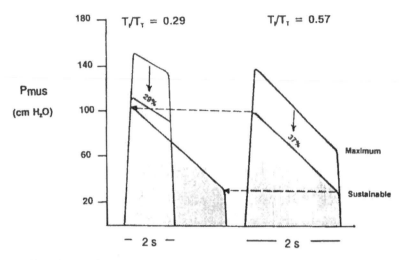

Figure 13 Effects of isolated changes in duty cycle on sustainable pressure development in the time domain. At elevated duty cycles (right), the pressure drops more than at the lower duty cycle (left). (Data signal averaged from Clanton et al., 1990.)

dynamic pressures (Clanton et al., 1990; Julian and Clanton, 1990). Increasing tidal volume increases "average" muscle length during contraction and would presumably have an influence that mirrors initial lung volume effects. The fact that we have not been able to identify such an effect may simply reflect the limited resolution of these types of measurements or the balance between several opposing influences, namely: (1) the additional mechanical work being performed because of shortening (promoting the fatigue process), (2) the diminished ability to activate the shortened muscles (limiting the fatigue process, similar to initial volume effects), and (3) potential decreases in efficiency at elevated lung volumes (Collett and Engel, 1986), also promoting the fatigue process.

4. *A predictive equation*: The above observations lend themselves to the following relationship for predicting the sustainable pressure for a given pattern of contraction:

$$PT_{mus_s} = PT_{mus_i}(1 + S \cdot T_I/T_{TOT}) \tag{2}$$

where PT_{mus_s} and PT_{mus_i} are the sustainable and initial pressure-time products (i.e., integration of pressure over inspiration) of the inspiratory muscles at a given flow rate and inspiratory duration. The PT_{mus_i} might be thought of as a given trajectory on the maximum P-F-V_{insp} surface at rest, prior to fatigue, and the PT_{mus_s} as the trajectory on the sustainable P-F-V_{insp} surface. The slope, S, is the slope of the relationship between sustainable fraction and duty cycle (Fig. 14), dropping at a

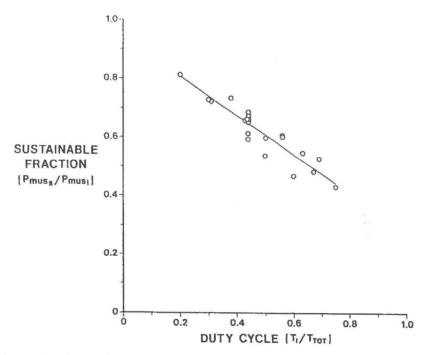

Figure 14 Changes in the sustainable fraction of maximum initial pressure with increasing duty cycle over a wide range of flows, breathing frequencies and tidal volumes. Data from one subject. (From Clanton et al., 1990.)

rate of about 3% for every 0.1 change in duty cycle. Knowing the maximum P-F-V_{insp} relationship, or at least a part of it, appears to make it possible to predict the sustainable pressure development or the sustainable P-F-V_{insp} surface for any given subject at any particular breathing pattern.

Equation (2) suggests that there is no single pressure-time index that adequately predicts the threshold for fatigue or the sustainable pressure development as long as significant tidal volumes are generated. Furthermore, to understand the fatigue characteristics of the inspiratory muscle pump, it is clear that it is useful to be able to evaluate the maximum capacity of the pump to generate dynamic pressure as exhibited by maximum P-F-V_{insp}. MIP does not provide sufficient information for a reference point until its relationship to P-F-V_{insp} is better understood.

V. New Directions

Clearly, one of the most important remaining areas of investigation involves measurements of the extent to which endurance properties of the respiratory muscles are important in various patient groups. Despite the intense level of investigation in this area, the importance of respiratory muscle endurance in the failing patient or the obstructed patient during endurance exercise or other activities is still relatively inadequate. Just as important are the development of better techniques for evaluating respiratory muscle endurance and work capacity in patients. Methods such as those of Martyn et al. (1987) are promising but need further evaluation and development, and the relevance of this and other methods to sustainable ventilatory capacity, sustainable pressure development, and maximum inspiratory pressures needs to be analyzed. Better techniques for indirect assessment of muscle function during fatiguing work (EMG spectral shifts, etc.) will also be important for eventual application to patients.

From a basic science standpoint, understanding the interaction of the variables that are important in determining endurance and fatigue characteristics in the in vivo situation in humans will hopefully lead to a better understanding of the functioning of the respiratory pump under conditions of ventilatory stress. Eventual synthesis of such diverse influences as abdomino-thoracic configuration, energetics, blood flow, changes in neural activation, chest wall mechanics, relationships between force and shortening of agonist and antagonist muscles, and how the interaction between these variables changes with various disease states presents a remarkable challenge to integrative human biology.

References

Adams, R. P., Cashman, P. A. and Young, J. C. (1986). Effect of hyperoxia on substrate utilization during intense submaximal exercise. *J. Appl. Physiol.*, 61(2):523–529.

Agostoni, E., and R. E. Hyatt, (1986) Static behavior of the respiratory system. In *Handbook of Physiology*. Section 3: The Respiratory System. Vol. II. Mechanics of Breathing, Part 1. Edited by A. P. Fishman, P. T. Macklem, and J. Mead. Bethesda, Md., American Physiological Society, p. 113.

Aldrich, T. K., Arora, N. S. and Rochester, D. F. (1982). The influence of obstruction and respiratory muscle strength on maximal voluntary ventilation in lung disease. *Am. Rev. Respir. Dis.*, 126:195.

Aljure, E. F., and Borrero, L. M. (1968). The influence of muscle length on the development of fatigue in toad sartorius. *J. Physiol.*, 199:241–252.

Ameredes, B. T., and Clanton, T. L. (1988). Accelerated decay of inspiratory pressure during hypercapnic endurance trials in humans. *J. Appl. Physiol.*, 65(2):728–735.

Ameredes, B. T., and Clanton, T. L. (1989). Hyperoxia and moderate hypoxia fail to affect inspiratory muscle fatigue in humans. *J. Appl. Physiol.*, 66(2):894–900.

Ameredes, B. T., and Clanton, T. L. (1990). Increased fatigue of isovelocity vs isometric contractions of canine diaphragm. *J. Appl. Physiol.*, 69(2):740–746.

Ameredes, B. T., Julian, M. W. and Clanton, T. L. (1991). Muscle shortening increases sensitivity of fatigue to severe hypoxia in canine diaphragm. *J. Appl. Physiol.*, 71(6):2309–2316.

Bahler, A. S., Fales, J. T., and Zierler, K. L. (1968). The dynamic properties of mammalian skeletal muscle. *J. Gen. Physiol.*, 51:369–384.

Bai, T. R., Rabinovitch, B. J., and Pardy, R. L. (1984). Near-maximal voluntary hyperpnea and ventilatory muscle function. *J. Appl. Physiol.*, 57(6):1742–1748.

Barclay, J. K. (1986). A delivery-independent blood flow effect on skeletal muscle fatigue. *J. Appl. Physiol.*, 61(3):1084–1090.

Barnes, W. S. (1981). Isokinetic fatigue curves at different contractile velocities. *Arch. Phys. Med. Rehabil.*, 62:66–69.

Bellemare, F., and Grassino, A. (1982). Effect of pressure and timing of contraction on human diaphragm fatigue. *J. Appl. Physiol.*, 53(5):1190–1195.

Bellemare, F., and Grassino, A. (1983). Force reserve of the diaphragm in patients with chronic obstructive pulmonary disease. *J. Appl. Physiol.*, 55(1):8–15.

Bellemare, F., Wight, D., Lavigne, C. M., and Grassino, A. (1986). Effect of tension and timing of contraction on blood flow of the diaphragm. *J. Appl. Physiol.*, 54:1597–1606.

Belman, M. J., and Mittman, C. (1980). Ventilatory muscle training improves exercise capacity in chronic obstructive pulmonary disease patients. *Am. Rev. Respir. Dis.*, 121:273–280.

Belman, M. J., and Gaesser, G. A. (1988). Ventilatory muscle training in the elderly. *J. Appl. Physiol.*, 64(3):899–905.

Buchler, B., Magder, S., Katsardis, H., Jammes, Y. and Roussos, C. (1985). Effects of pleural pressure and abdominal pressure on diaphragmatic blood flow. *J. Appl. Physiol.*, 58(3):691–697.

Carnevale, T. J., and Gaesser, G. A. (1991). Effects of pedaling speed on the power-duration relationship for high-intensity exercise. *Med. Sci. Sports Exerc.*, 23(2):242–246.

Clanton, T. L., Dixon, G., Drake, J., and Gadek, J. E. (1985a). Inspiratory muscle conditioning using a threshold loading device. *Chest*, 87:62–66.

Clanton, T. L., Dixon, G. F., Drake, J., and Gadek, J. E. (1985b). Effects of breathing pattern on inspiratory muscle endurance in humans. *J. Appl. Physiol.*, 59(6):1834–1841.

Clanton, T. L., Dixon, G. F., Drake, J., and Gadek, J. E. (1987). Effects of swim training on lung volumes and inspiratory muscle conditioning. *J. Appl. Physiol.*, 62(1):39–46.

Clanton, T. L., Ameredes, B. T., and Kelsen, S. G. (1988a). Shifts in the maximum pressure-flow relationship after inspiratory muscle fatigue. *Physiologist*, 31:A65

Clanton, T. L., and Ameredes, B. T. (1988b). Fatigue of the inspiratory muscle pump in humans: an isoflow approach. *J. Appl. Physiol.*, 64(4):1693–1699.

Clanton, T. L., Ameredes, B. T., Thomson, D. B., and Julian, M. W. (1990). Sustainable inspiratory pressures over varying flows, volumes, and duty cycles. *J. Appl. Physiol.*, 69(5):1875–1882.

Clanton, T. L., Julian, M. W., Borzone, G., and Diaz, P. (1991). Three-dimensional analysis of inspiratory muscle function. *FASEB J.*, 5(4):A746.

Clanton, T. L., Hartman, E., and Julian, M. W. (1993). Preservation of sustainable inspiratory muscle pressure at increased end-expiratory lung volume. *Am. Rev. Respir. Dis.* 147:385–91.

Cohen, C., Zagelbaum, G., Gross, D., Roussos, C. and Macklem, P. T. (1982). Clinical manifestations of inspiratory muscle fatigue. *Am. J. Med.*, 73:308–316.

Collett, P. W., and Engel, L. A. (1986). Influence of lung volume on oxygen cost of resistive breathing. *J. Appl. Physiol.*, 61(1):16–24.

Dodd, D. S., Kelly, S., Collett, P. W., and Engel, L. A. (1988a). Pressure-time product, work rate, and endurance during resistive breathing in humans. *J. Appl. Physiol.*, 64(4):1397–1404.

Dodd, D. S., Collett, P. W., and Engel, L. A. (1988b). Influence of inspiratory flow rate and frequency on O2 cost of resistive breathing in humans. *J. Appl. Physiol.*, 65(2):760–766.

Farkas, G. A., and Roussos, C. (1983). Diaphragm in emphysematous hamsters: sarcomere adaptability. *J. Appl. Physiol.*, 54:1635–1640.

Farkas, G. A., and Roussos, C. (1984). Acute diaphragmatic shortening: in vitro mechanics and fatigue. *J. Appl. Physiol.*, 130:434–438.

Faulkner, J. A. (1985). Structural and functional adaptations of skeletal muscle. In *The Thorax*. Part B. Edited by C. Roussos and P. T. Macklem. New York, Marcel Dekker, p. 1329.

Fenn, W. O. (1924). The relation between the work performed and the energy liberated in muscular contraction. *J. Physiol.*, 58:373–395.

Fitch, S., and McComas, A. (1985). Influence of human muscle length on fatigue. *J. Physiol.*, 362:205–213.

Fitting, J. W., Bradley, T. D., Easton, P. A., Lincoln, M. J., Goldman, M. D., and Grassino,

A. (1988). Dissociation between diaphragmatic and rib cage muscle fatigue. *J. Appl. Physiol.*, 64:659–965.

Gandevia, S. C., McKenzie, D. K., and Neering, I. R. (1983). Endurance properties of respiratory and limb muscles. *Respir. Physiol.*, 53:47–61.

Grassino, A., and Macklem, P. T. (1984). Respiratory muscle fatigue and ventilatory failure. *Ann. Rev. Med.*, 35:625–647.

Grassino, A., and Clanton, T. L. (1991). Respiratory muscle fatigue. *Sem. Respir. Med.*, 12(4):305–321.

Hershenson, M. B., Kikuchi, Y., and Loring, S. H. (1988). Relative strengths of the chest wall muscles. *J. Appl. Physiol.*, 65(2):852–862.

Hill, A. V. (1927). *Muscular Movement in Man: The Factors Governing Speed and Recovery from Fatigue.* New York, McGraw-Hill, p. 41.

Hillman, D. R., Markos, J., and Finucane, K. E. (1990). Effect of abdominal compression on maximum transdiaphragmatic pressure. *J. Appl. Physiol.*, 68(6):2296–2304.

Hogan, M. C., and Welch, H. G. (1986). Effect of altered arterial O_2 tensions on muscle metabolism in dog skeletal muscle during fatiguing work. *Am. J. Physiol.*, 251:C216–C222.

Homsher, E., and Kean, C. J. (1978). Skeletal muscle energetics and metabolism. *Annu. Rev. Physiol.*, 40:93–131.

Hyatt, R. E. (1986). Forced expiration. In *Handbook of Physiology.* Section 3: The Respiratory System. Vol. III. Mechanics of Breathing, Part 1. Edited by A. P. Fishman, P. T. Macklem, and J. Mead. Bethesda, MD, American Physiological Society, p. 295.

Jardim, J., Farkas, G., Prefaut, C., Thomas, D., Macklem, P. T., and Roussos, C. (1981). The failing inspiratory muscles under normoxic and hypoxic conditions. *Am. Rev. Respir. Dis.*, 124:274–279.

Jones, N. L., McCartney, N., Graham, T., Spriet, L. L., Kowalchuk, J. M., Heigenhauser, G. J. F., and Sutton, J. R. (1985). Muscle performance and metabolism in maximal isokinetic cycling at slow and fast speeds. *J. Appl. Physiol.*, 59(1):132–136.

Juan, G., Claverley, P., Talamo, C., Schnader, J., and Roussos, C. (1984). Effect of carbon dioxide on diaphragmatic function in humans. *N. Engl. J. Med.*, 310:874–879.

Julian, M., Kinker, R., Preusser, B., and Clanton, T. L. (1991). Sustainable pressures and venous lactates in two models of human inspiratory muscle fatigue. *FASEB J.*, 5(4):A746.

Julian, M. W., and Clanton, T. L. (1990). Predicting sustainable inspiratory pressures over varying duty cycles, breathing frequencies and tidal volumes. *FASEB J.*, 4(4):865.

Keens, T. G., Krastins, I. R. B., Wannamaker, E. M., et al. (1977). Ventilatory muscle endurance training in normal subjects and patients with cystic fibrosis. *Am. Rev. Respir. Dis.*, 116:853–860.

Kushmerick, M. J. (1982). Energetics of muscle contraction. In *Handbook of Physiology, Skeletal Muscle.* Bethesda, MD, American Physiological Society, p. 189.

Larson, J. L., Kim, M. J., Sharp, J. T. and Larson, D. A. (1988). Inspiratory muscle training with a pressure threshold breathing device in patients with chronic obstructive pulmonary disease. *Am. Rev. Respir. Dis.*, 138:689–696.

Leith, D. E., and Bradley, M. (1976). Ventilatory muscle strength and endurance training. *J. Appl. Physiol.*, 41(4):508–516.

Levine, S., Weiser, P., and Gillen, J. (1986). Evaluation of a ventilatory muscle endurance training program in the rehabilitation of patients with chronic obstructive pulmonary disease. *Am. Rev. Respir. Dis.*, 133:400–406.

Loke, J., Mahler, D. A., and Virgulto, J. A. (1982). Respiratory muscle fatigue after marathon running. *J. Appl. Physiol.*, 52(4):821–824.

Mainwood, G. W., Renaud, J. M., and Mason, M. J. (1987). The pH dependence of the contractile response of fatigued skeletal muscle. *Can. J. Physiol. Pharmacol.*, 65:648–658.

Martyn, J. B., Moreno, R. H., Pare, P. D., and Pardy, R. L. (1987). Measurement of inspiratory muscle performance with incremental threshold loading. *Am. Rev. Respir. Dis.* 135:919–923.

McCool, F. D., McCann, D. R., Leith, D. E., and Hoppin, F. G. (1986). Pressure-flow effects on endurance of inspiratory muscles. *J. Appl. Physiol.*, 60(1):299–303.

McElvaney, G., Fairbarn, M. S., Wilcox, P. G., and Pardy, R. L. (1989). Comparison of two-minute incremental threshold loading and maximal loading as measures of respiratory muscle endurance. *Am. Rev. Respir. Dis.*, 96:557–563.

McIlory, M. B., and Christie, R. V. (1954). The work of breathing in emphysema. *Clin. Sci. Lond.*, 13:147–154.

McKenzie, D. K., and Gandevia, S. C. (1986). Strength and endurance of inspiratory, expiratory and limb muscles in asthma. *Am. Rev. Respir. Dis.*, 134:999–1004.

McKenzie, D. K., and Gandevia, S. C. (1987). Influence of muscle length on human inspiratory and limb muscle endurance. *Respir. Physiol.*, 67:171–182.

Mommaerts, W. F. H. M. (1970). What is the Fenn-effect? *Naturwissenschaft*, 57:326–330.

Monod, H., and Scherrer, J. (1965). The work capacity of a synergic muscular group. *Ergonomics*, 8:329–337.

Morrison, N. J., Richardson, D. P. T., Dunn, L., and Pardy, R. L. (1989a). Respiratory muscle performance in normal elderly subjects and patients with COPD. *Chest*, 95(1):90–94.

Morrison, N. J., Fairbarn, M. S., and Pardy, R. L. (1989b). The effect of breathing frequency on inspiratory muscle endurance during incremental threshold loading. *Chest*, 96:85–88.

Newman, S., Road, J., Bellemare, F., Clozel, J. P., Lavigne, C. M., and Grassino, A. (1984). Respiratory muscle length measured by sonomicrometry. *J. Appl. Physiol.*, 56(3):753–764.

Nickerson, B. G., Richards, W., Wang, C., and Keens, T. G. (1981). Increased ventilatory muscle strength and endurance in children with asthma and cystic fibrosis. *Fed. Proc.*, 40:540A.

Nickerson, B. G., and Keens, T. G. (1982). Measuring ventilatory muscle endurance in humans as sustainable inspiratory pressure. *J. Appl. Physiol.*, 52(3):768–772.

Oliven, A., Supinski, G. S., and Kelsen, S. G. (1986). Functional adaptation of diaphragm to chronic hyperinflation in emphysematous hamsters. *J. Appl. Physiol.*, 60(1):225–231.

Pardy, R. L., and Bye, P. T. P. (1985). Diaphragmatic fatigue in normoxia and hyperoxia. *J. Appl. Physiol.*, 58(3):738–742.

Pride, N. B., and Macklem, P. T. (1986). Lung mechanics in disease. In *Handbook of Physiology, The Respiratory System*. Vol. III, Mechanics of Breathing, Part 2. Edited by A. P. Fishman, P. T. Macklem, and J. Mead. Bethesda, MD, American Physiological Society, P. 659.

Pruesser, B., Clanton, T. and Winningham, M. (1992). Inspiratory muscle interval training in patients with COPD. *Am. Rev. Respir. Dis.*, 145(4):151A.

Rall, J. A. (1982). Sense and nonsense about the Fenn effect. *Am. J. Physiol.*, 242:H1–H6.

Rochester, D. E., and Bettini, G. (1976). Diaphragmatic blood flow and energy expenditure in the dog. Effects of inspiratory airflow and resistance and hypercapnia. *J. Clin. Invest.*, 57:661–672.

Rochester, D. F. (1982). Fatigue of the diaphragm. In *Update: Pulmonary Disease and Disorders*. Edited by A. P. Fishman. New York, McGraw-Hill.

Rochester, D. F. (1988). Tests of respiratory muscle function. In *Respiratory Muscles: Function in Health and Disease*. Edited by M. J. Belman. Philadelphia, W. B. Saunders, p. 249.

Roussos, C., Gross, D. amd Macklem, P. T. (1979). Fatigue of inspiratory muscles and their synergic behavior. *J. Appl. Physiol.*, 46(5):897–904.

Roussos, C., and Campbell, E. J. M. (1986). Respiratory muscle energetics. In *Handbook of Physiology*. Section 3: The Respiratory System. Vol. III. Mechanics of Breathing, Part 2. Edited by A. P. Fishman, P. T. Macklem, and J. Mead. American Physiological Society, p. 481.

Roussos, C. S., and Macklem, P. T. (1977). Diaphragmatic fatigue in man. *J. Appl. Physiol.*, 43(2):189–197.

Saltin, B., and Gollnick, P. D. (1983). Skeletal muscle adaptability: significance for metabolism and performance. In *Handbook of Physiology*. Section 10: Skeletal Muscle. Edited by L. D. Peachey et al. Bethesda, MD, American Physiological Society, p. 556.

Sarnoff, S. J., Braunwald, E., Welch, Jr., G. H., Case, R. B., Stainsby, W. N., and Macruz, R. (1958). Hemodynamic determinants of oxygen consumption of the heart with special reference to the tension-time index. *Am. J. Physiol.*, 192(1):148–156.

Saunders, N. A., Kreitzer, S. M., and Ingram, R. H. (1979). Rib cage deformation during static inspiratory efforts. *J. Appl. Physiol.*, 46(6):1071–1075.

Scherrer, J., and Monod, H. (1960). Le travail musculaire local et la fatigue chez l'homme. *J. Physiol.* (Paris), 52:419–510.

Schnader, J. Y., Juan, G., Howell, S., Fitzgerald, R., and Roussos, C. (1985). Arterial CO_2 partial pressure affects diaphragmatic function. *J. Appl. Physiol.*, 58(3):823–829.

Sharp, J. T., and Hyatt, R. E. (1986). Mechanical and electrical properties of respiratory muscles. In *Handbook of Physiology*. Section 3: The Respiratory System. Edited by A. P. Fishman, P. T. Macklem, and J. Mead. Bethesda, MD, American Physiological Society, p. 389.

Supinski, G. S. (1988) Respiratory muscle blood flow. In *Respiratory Muscles: Function in Health and Disease*. Edited by M. J. Belman. Philadelphia, W.B. Saunders, p. 211.

Suzuki, S., Suzuki, J., and Okubo, T. (1991). Expiratory muscle fatigue in normal subjects. *J. Appl. Physiol.*, 70(6):2632–2639.

Tenny, S. M., and Reese, R. E. (1968). The ability to sustain great breathing efforts. *Respir. Physiol.*, 5:187–201.

Thomas, A. J., Supinski, S., and Kelsen, S. G. (1986). Changes in chest wall structure and elasticity in elastase-induced emphysema. *J. Appl. Physiol.*, 61(5):1821–1829.

Thorstensson, A., Larsson, L., Tesch, P., and Karlsson, J. (1977). Muscle strength and fiber composition in athletes and sedentary men. *Med. Sci. Sports*, 9:26–30.

Tobin, M. J. (1988). Respiratory muscles in disease. In *Respiratory Muscles: Function in Health and Disease*. Edited by M. J. Belman. Philadelphia, W. B. Saunders, p. 263.

Topulos, G. P., Reid, M. B., and Leith, D. E. (1987). Pliometric activity of inspiratory muscles maximal pressure-flow curves. *J. Appl. Physiol.*, 62(1):322–327.

Tzelepis, G., McCool, F. D., Leith, D. E., and Hoppin, Jr., F. G. (1988). Increased lung volume limits endurance of inspiratory muscles. *J. Appl. Physiol.*, 64(5):1796–1802.

Zocche, G. P., Fritts, Jr., H. W., and Cournand, A. (1960). Fraction of maximum breathing capacity available for prolonged hyperventilation. *J. Appl. Physiol.*, 15(6):1073–1074.

Zocchi, L., Fitting, J. W., Majani, U., Fracchia, C., Rampulla, C., and Grassino, A. (1993). Effect of pressure and timing of contraction on human rib cage muscle fatigue. *Am. Rev. Respir. Dis.* 147(4):857–64.

42

Measurement of the Work of Breathing in the Critically Ill Patient

APOSTOLOS ARMAGANIDIS

Evangelismos Hospital
Athens, Greece

CHARIS ROUSSOS

National and Kapodistrian University
   of Athens Medical School
Athens, Greece
McGill University
Montreal, Quebec, Canada

I. Introduction

The work of breathing occupied a quiet spot in the field of physiology until the 1950s (Milic Emili, 1991) although the scientific foundations for much of the subsequent research were provided by Liljestrand (1918) and Rohner (1925) more than 70 years ago. In the last 25 years there has been growing interest in respiratory muscle energetics in the normal subject, and the major issues in this area have been discussed in several excellent reviews and original works (Hill, 1964; Mommaerts, 1969 Wilkie, 1974; Gibbs, 1978; Homsher and Kean, 1978; Curtin and Woldge, 1978; Gibbs and Chapman, 1979; Roussos, 1985).

The development of new modes of partial ventilatory support for difficult to wean patients has also renewed the interest in quantifying the breathing workload in the intensive care unit (ICU) setting. Such an assessment may have important diagnostic and therapeutic implications in critically ill patients with acute respiratory failure, hypoxia, and/or decreased oxygen delivery. In mechanically ventilated patients, for instance, quantification of the work of breathing could be used as a more reliable weaning index as well as to tailor ventilatory support and other therapeutic measures to the specific needs of the individual patient, either during mechanical ventilation or during weaning trials (Marini, 1991).

Although important technical advances have allowed a bedside assessment of external mechanical work and of the energy expenditure of breathing in critically ill patients, their measurement continues to be used more in a research setting than in clinical practice (Marini, 1991; Armaganidis and Roussos, 1991; Civetta, 1993). The limited use of such measurements in the ICU could be related to many factors: (1) the great variability in the estimates of oxygen cost and mechanical efficiency of breathing, (2) the difficulty in performing bedside measurements with a simple and easily calibrated and accurate monitor, and (3) the lack of a precise definition and understanding of the physiological significance and methodological assumptions and limitations of each of the methods used for the assessment of breathing workload (Armaganidis and Roussos, 1991; Civetta, 1993).

The purpose of this chapter is to present the methodology and to discuss the technical problems and the methodological limitations of studies dealing with the work and the energy cost of breathing in the critically ill patient. Such an understanding is necessary in order to assess the accuracy of and mainly the usefulness of the assessment of breathing workload in the management of ICU patients requiring or undergoing mechanical ventilation or performing a weaning trial.

II. General Aspects and Definitions

Although the term "work of breathing" is generally understood to relate to patient effort during breathing activity, the different approaches taken in an attempt to quantify breathing effort assess a specific component of breathing workload in which the physiological meaning must be carefully defined (Marini, 1991). Since each method of measurement is based on a number of theoretical and methodological assumptions, there are a substantial number of physiological and clinical factors that should be taken into consideration to assess the validity of these assumptions and to evaluate the accuracy and usefulness of the measurements of the breathing workload in the individual ICU patient.

In his classic publication on the subject, Otis pointed out that there are two different but complementary approaches of quantifying the work of breathing: (1) estimation of the mechanical work from measurements of the pressures developed and the volumes displaced by the respiratory muscles and (2) estimation of the energy cost of breathing by measuring the oxygen consumption of the muscles of breathing (Otis et al., 1950; Otis, 1954). Otis also pointed out that "the ratio of values obtained by the first method to those obtained by the second provides a measure of the mechanical efficiency of the breathing apparatus" (Otis, 1954). Therefore, an ideal approach for the measurement of the breathing workload should quantify the work performed and the energy expended by the specific respiratory muscles of interest (i.e., diaphragm, intercostal, and accessory respiratory muscles). In fact, during mechanical ventilation or spontaneous breathing investigators are often interested in quantifying not only the total work required to inflate a patient's lungs, but also the subcomponent of the total work performed by a group of respiratory muscles during different ventilatory modes, or the additional workload imposed on the patient by his endotracheal tube and/or external devices, or by the respirator's valves and circuitry. On the other hand, clinicians are interested in knowing how the stress of a weaning trial adds to the total-body oxygen consumption, regardless of the muscle groups involved.

Work is usually measured in calories, joules, or kilograms per meter (1 calorie = 4.186 J; 1 kg/m = 9.8 J). As explained later, the external mechanical work required for the inflation of a given volume (Vt) can be measured by the integration of the product of inflation pressure and the rate of volume change. Therefore, in practical terms 1 J represents the work needed to move a volume equal to 1 L of gas through pressure gradient of 10 cm H_2O.

Since the work per breath varies with the inspired volume (Vt), it is useful to express the inspiratory work per unit of volume. On the other hand, to quantify the total work of breathing required to achieve ventilatory needs of a given patient, we must consider not only his work per breath but also his respiratory frequency or his minute ventilation.

Therefore, the external mechanical work can be expressed as:

1. External mechanical work per breath (W_b), which is the external work needed to inflate the lungs and the chest wall and is measured in joules.
2. External mechanical work per liter of ventilation (W_{vol}), which is the W_b divided by tidal volume (VT). It reflects better the inspiratory load imposed by alterations of mechanical characteristics of the lungs and chest wall and is measured in joules per liter of ventilation.
3. Total mechanical work performed per unit of time (W_{tot}), which is calculated by multiplying the W_b by the breathing frequency of the W_{vol} by the minute ventilation. The W_{tot} reflects the "power output" of the ventilatory pump or the total mechanical work needed to match ventilatory and metabolic requirements of a given patient and is measured in watts (1 watt = 1 J/s).

From a physiological standpoint, measurement of the total mechanical work required for passive inflation is only an approximation of the total work performed by the respiratory muscles (Roussos, 1985). In fact, when a muscle contracts it either shortens, lengthens, or does not change its length. Although muscular activity is always associated with increased energy expenditure, positive external work is performed only in the first case (myometric contraction). In the second case (pliometric contraction), displacement is opposite to the direction of the force exerted by the muscle (negative work). Finally, if no displacement takes place (isometric contraction), no external work is performed (Roussos, 1985).

The integration of the product of pressure developed and the rate of volume change (external mechanical work per breath or per liter of ventilation) measures the work performed by myometric contraction of inspiratory muscles. Although Sharp et al. (1964) did not find any electrical activity in the intercostal and abdominal muscles during the artificial ventilation of relaxed subjects, complete relaxation is often impossible without sedation and neuromuscular paralysis (Marini, 1991).

Since expiration normally is passive, most studies on the work of breathing concern inspiratory work. However, a number of ICU patients may have expiratory muscle activity during inspiration, and this activity must be taken into consideration when the total work and the energy expenditure of the respiratory muscles are measured (Roussos, 1985; Smith et al., 1986; Marini, 1990).

Since measurements of external mechanical work do not take into account isometric and/or pliometric activity of inspiratory muscles during discoordinate contraction and expiratory muscle activity, such an assessment of breathing workload may bear little relationship to the "common sense" of breathing effort. In more practical terms, when a patient is "fighting" his ventilator, the load imposed to his inspiratory and sometimes expiratory muscles and the energy cost due to pliometric and isometric contraction may be substantial (Marini, 1988, 1991). In such patients, the workload imposed on the respiratory muscles could be better assessed by indexes of their metabolic activity, such as the intensity of their electrical stimulation (electromyography) or the rate of their oxygen consumption (Vo_2r).

In the clinical setting, the usual approach is to quantify the Vo_2r by measuring the difference of total body oxygen consumption (ΔVo_2) before and after the application of a breathing stress or a ventilatory mode. Although this ΔVo_2 is attributed to changes of metabolic activity of respiratory muscles due to changes of the breathing workload, variations of Vo_2 may also be a general effect of the "stress of breathing" to the total body metabolism (Marini, 1990). In addition, variations of the efficiency of the respiratory muscles may result in changes of Vo_2 due to an increase of the "energy cost of breathing" without any change in the external mechanical work performed by the patient. Therefore, assessment of oxygen consumption of respiratory muscles (Vo_2r) from variations of total-body oxygen consumption (i.e., the oxygen cost of breathing) does not always allow estimation of the workload imposed on the respiratory muscles.

III. Measurement of External Mechanical Work of Breathing

Two different approaches can be taken in an attempt to quantify the external mechanical work of breathing: (1) direct measurement of external mechanical work by graphic analysis of pressure-volume curves and (2) assessment of the net outcome of respiratory muscle activity from the pressure time product or the pressure time index.

A. Theory of Measurement

Defined in a physical sense, work (W) is a force-length product. When a pressure gradient (P_{ts}) is applied in an area (A) to inflate a distensible structure, the applied force equals pressure multiplied by area. Since the product of area and distance equals volume, the mechanical work performed can be estimated by the integral of the product of volume of gas displaced (V) and the pressure gradient required for this displacement (P_{ts}). Thus, the external work of breathing during the inspiratory time (ti) is equal to:

$$W = \Sigma_0^{ti} P_{ts} V = \int_0^{ti} P_{ts} dV \text{ or } = \int_0^{ti} P_{ts} V_{dt} \tag{1}$$

Similar principles are applied in the computation of mechanical work during expiration, although expiratory work of breathing is usually not taken into consideration since exhalation is normally passive (Marini, 1991).

The pressure time product (PT) is another useful approach in assessing breathing effort. Decomposing the work integral into its components:

$$W = \int_0^{ti} P_{ts} dV = \int_0^{ti} P_{ts} dt \frac{dV}{dt} = \int_0^{ti} \text{"PT product"} \times \text{flow } dt \tag{2}$$

B. Equipment Required and Methodology

To compute and integrate pressure volume loops or pressure flow product, it is necessary to simultaneously measure the airflow and the pressure gradient on either side of the inflated structure. The variations of the airflow can be monitored with a heated pneumotachograph positioned at the proximal end of the endotracheal tube. A flow integrator is used to calculate volume from the electrically time-integrated flow signal.

Measurements of the pressure gradient on either side of the inflated structure (chest wall and/or lungs) requires a continuous monitoring of airway pressure (P_{aw}), intrapleural pressure (P_{pl}), and extrathoracic (atmospheric) pressure with differential pressure transducers.

In the ICU the P_{aw} is usually measured at the proximal end of the endotracheal tube (Marini, 1991). Although the intrapleural pressure (P_{pl}) cannot be measured directly, its changes can be assessed with acceptable accuracy for most clinical purposes from changes of esophageal pressure (P_{es}) (Baydur et al., 1982, 1987). Variations in esophageal pressure are best measured by a balloon (10 cm long and containing approximately 1 ml of air) tied over the end of a narrow, multiperforated polyethylene catheter (Marini, 1991).

A monitoring of transdiaphragmatic pressure (P_{di}) (accessed by the difference of esophageal and gastric pressure) is also used in clinical studies dealing with the mechanical work performed by the diaphragm (Roussos and Macklem, 1977; Field et al., 1984). Special nasogastric-esophageal balloon catheters are commercially available and allow monitoring of esophageal and gastric pressure changes with acceptable accuracy at least for clinical purposes (Gillespie, 1982).

Finally, a recording system and a plotter are needed for drawing pressure-volume curves (Fig. 1). The area beneath the plot of pressure against volume can be

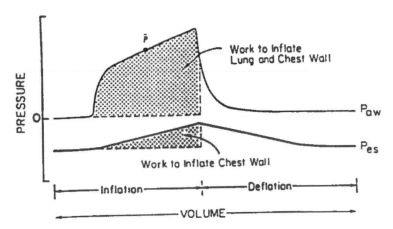

Figure 1 Graphic analaysis of the work of breathing from pressure volume curves of the respiratory system. The external inspiratory work performed by the ventilator during passive inflation of the entire respiratory system and of the chest wall can be estimated by plotting airway pressure (P_{aw}) and esophageal pressure (P_{es}) against inflated volume and measuring the areas included (stippled areas). (From Marini, 1988.)

measured by planimetry or electronic integration (Truwit and Marini, 1988; Marini, 1990; Mancebo, 1990).

C. Measurement of the External Mechanical Work per Breath by Graphic Analysis During Mechanical Ventilation

Theoretically, during controlled mechanical ventilation of a relaxed patient, passive inflation occurs and the increase of P_{aw} produces a volume change of both the lungs and the chest wall. The total work per breath is the sum of the work performed across the lungs (W_l) and the chest wall (W_{cw}) in moving tidal volume against pressure graidents (Truwit and Marini, 1988; Marini, 1988). Therefore, measurement of both W_l and W_{cw} requires the use of an esophageal balloon for estimating changes in pleural pressure (P_{pl}) from changes in esophageal pressure (P_{es}). The work performed by the ventilator on different structures during passive inflation can be calculated as follows:

$$W_{tot} = (P_{aw} - P_{atm}) \times Vt \tag{3}$$
$$W_l = (P_{aw} - P_{es}) \times Vt \tag{4}$$
$$W_{cw} = (P_{es} - P_{atm}) \times Vt \tag{5}$$

where P_{atm} = atmospheric pressure and Vt = tidal volume.

The W_{tot} and W_{cw} can be measured from the area enclosed in the plot of P_{aw} and P_{es} against inspired volume, respectively (Fig. 1).

The W_1 can be divided between work performed across the airways (resistive work) and work performed across the lung parenchyma (elastic work):

$$\text{Resistive work} = (P_{aw} - P_A) \times \text{inflated volume} \tag{6}$$
$$\text{Elastic work} = (P_A - P_{pl}) \times \text{inflated volume} \tag{7}$$

where P_A = alveolar pressure.

Although it is impossible to monitor the P_A, plots of P_{aw} against volume (Fig. 2) allow estimation of these two components of work (Truwit and Marini, 1988), assuming a linear relation for elastic recoil.

During controlled mechanical ventilation of a relaxed or a paralyzed patient, positive pressure is delivered at a constant flow rate and the pressure-volume curve closely resembles a trapezoid (Figs. 1 and 2). Under these specific conditions, time is proportional to volume, so plotting P_{aw} against time will provide a similar loop: the pressure-time product (Fig. 3).

The pressure measured at midcycle (P_{avg}) of a passive inflation (Fig. 3) is the mean pressure inflating the system (P_{ts} or the mean difference between the pressures on either side of the inflated structure, i.e., chest wall or lungs). Since the product of P_{avg} and V_T yields the W_b, $P_{avg} = W_b/V_T$. Thus, P_{avg} may be used to estimate the work per liter of ventilation (Truwit and Marini, 1988). The P_{avg} of tidal inflation (see Fig. 3) can be calculated by the equation of motion of the respiratory system (Otis et al., 1950):

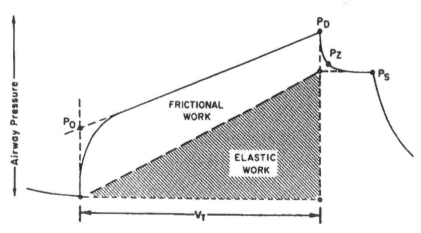

Figure 2 Resistive and elastic inspiratory work. During passive inflation, plots of airway pressure (P_{aw}) against inflated volume allow estimation of resistive and elastic inspiratory work of the thorax. P_D = peak dynamic pressure; P_S = static (plateau) pressure; P_Z = airway pressure at zero flow. (From Truwit and Marini, 1988.)

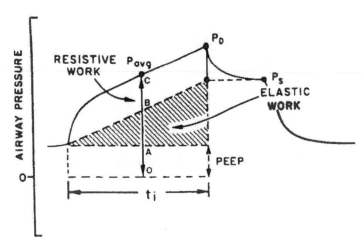

Figure 3 Airway pressure (P_{aw}) tracing over time. During constant-flow mechanical ventilation under passive conditions, time is a linear analogue of volume. Plotting the airway pressure against time permits estimation of the inspiratory work of breathing performed by the ventilator by determining either the area under the curve or the mean distending pressure (P_{avg}), which equals the work per liter of ventilation. From this plotting it is obvious that P_{avg} = OA + AB + BC, where OA = end expiratory pressure (PEEP), AB = (Ps – PEEP)/2 = (V_T/C_2), and BC = F_D – FsR × Flow = R × (V_T/Ti). Po = peak dynamic pressure; Ps = peak static (plateau) pressure; Pz = airway pressure at zero flow; C = compliance. (From Truwit and Marini, 1988.)

$$P_{avg} = \frac{R}{V_T/Ti} + \frac{V_T/C}{2} + P_{ex} \tag{8}$$

where R = resistance, C = compliance, Ti = inspiratory time, Pex = end expiratory pressure, V_T = tidal volume, and V_T/Ti = mean inspiratory flow.

The P_{avg} can be measured directly by recording P_{aw} at the bedside using the standard equipment and methods used for measuring pulmonary arterial pressure. However, as pointed out by Marini (1991), to avoid infection or gas embolism, the transducer utilized for this purpose must not be used for measuring intravascular pressures. Finally, P_{avg} also can be estimated roughly from peak dynamic pressure (P_D) and static pressure (P_s) developed during a passive mechanical inflation using a constant flow (Fig. 2) (Marini et al., 1986a; Truwit and Marini, 1988; Marini, 1988, 1990), according to the formulas:

$$P_{avg} = P_D - \frac{P_s}{2} \tag{9}$$

$$P_{avg} \simeq 0.80 \times P_D \tag{10}$$

D. Measurement of the External Mechanical Work per Breath by Graphic Analysis During Spontaneous Breathing

During spontaneous breathing, the intrapleural pressure becomes more negative during inspiration and opposes chest expansion; therefore, changes of P_{Pl} will no longer displace the chest wall outward, as in patients under mechanical ventilation. Since P_{Pl} no longer reflects the forces distending the thorax (Otis, 1964), the pressure expanding the chest wall is inaccessible to direct measurement. The work done across the entire respiratory system is obtained by adding the W_l, measured from a plot of P_{es} against inspired volume (Fig. 4) to W_{cw} estimated from published values or extrapolated from measurements of W_{cw} or P_{avg} under conditions of passive inflation. Obviously, such an assessment is based on the assumption that W_{cw} is the same during passive inflation and active inflation after contraction of the respiratory muscles (Otis, 1954). The total W_{cw} can also be quantified by using the equation of motion (Marini et al., 1986b; Marini, 1988, 1990), since the average distending pressure against the elastic forces opposed to chest wall expansion may be calculated by the formula:

$$P_{avgcw} = V_T /(2 \times C_{cw}) \tag{11}$$

where C_{cw} = chest wall compliance.

Therefore, the elastic work accomplished during inflation of the chest wall (W_{cwel}) can be assessed by the product of P_{avgcw} and V_T or:

$$W_{(cwel)} = V_T^2/(2 \times C_{cw}) \tag{12}$$

Such an estimation is not very useful in clinical practice since it requires measurement of the compliance of the thorax and it does not include flow-resistive work required

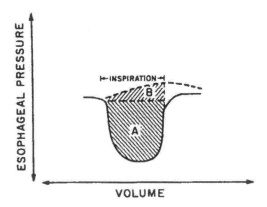

Figure 4 Graphic analysis of the work of breathing during spontaneous ventilation. During spontaneous breathing the work done inflating the lungs and moving volume against resistance can be estimated from a plot of esophageal pressure against volume (area A). The work to expand the chest wall cannot be directly measured, but is approximated by the work to expand the chest wall under passive conditions (area B). (From Truwit and Marini, 1988.)

for chest wall inflation, which may account for as much as 25–36% of the total mechanical work (Bergofsky et al., 1959; Opie et al., 1959; Goldman et al., 1976).

E. Estimation of the Mechanical Work of Breathing from Pressure Time Product (PT) and Tension Time Index (TTI)

The importance of developed tension in respiratory muscle energetics was pointed out initially by McGregor and Becklake, who found a different relationship between work and oxygen cost of breathing during unloaded hyperventilation and during breathing through a resistance. However, the relationship between the force developed by the respiratory muscles and their oxygen consumption was the same under the two conditions (McGregor and Becklake, 1961).

It has been suggested that the product of the pressure developed by the respiratory muscles (e.g., the diaphragm) and the time of muscle contraction reflects muscular effort better than the external work of breathing (Field et al., 1984; Aubier, 1987).

From a mathematical point of view, the *pressure-time product* (PT) is calculated by multiplying the mean pressure generated by the muscle (P_{avg}) with the inspiratory time (T_i). If the P_{avg} is expressed as a fraction of the maximal inspiration of the isometric pressure that can be generated at functional residual capacity (P_{max}) and the inspiratory time (T_i) is expressed as a fraction of the total cycle length (T_{tot}), another index of muscular effort, the *pressure-time index* (TTI) is calculated by the following equation (Bellemare and Grassino, 1982):

$$TTI = \frac{P_{avg}}{P_{max}} \times \frac{T_i}{T_{tot}} \tag{13}$$

Under conditions of varying afterload, the pressure time product parallels the oxygen consumption of respiratory muscles more closely than does the external work (Otis, 1954). In addition, values of the pressure-time index exceeding 0.15 identify highly stressful breathing workload that may induce muscle fatigue (Bellemare and Grassino, 1982).

In spontaneously breathing subjects, the pressure usually measured to calculate PT or TTI is the transdiaphragmatic pressure (gastric minus esophageal pressure), since Field et al. (1982) have demonstrated that the transdiaphragmatic pressure-time index better reflects the oxygen cost of breathing than the measurement of the mean pleural pressure (P_{Pl}) or the pleural pressure-time index.

F. Methodological Limitations, Technical Problems, and Errors

Theoretical Problems

Indirect assessment of external mechanical work of spontaneous or partially supported breaths from passive inflation plots of P_{aw} against V$_T$ is based on two assumptions: (1) average values of resistance, compliance, inspiratory time, VT, and flow rate are similar during spontaneous breathing and mechanical ventilation, and (2) the respiratory system behaves in a similar fashion whether moved by active contraction of the ventilatory muscles or by an external source of positive pressure.

In reality, the validity of these assumptions has never been tested. On the contrary, it is well known that during active inspiration, the respiratory muscles work against five types of forces (Roussos, 1985):

1. Elastic forces developed in the tissues of the lung and chest when a volume change occurs
2. Flow-resistive forces due to airway resistance to gas flow and nonelastic deformation of tissue
3. Inertial forces
4. Gravitational forces
5. Distorting forces of the chest wall

The values of the work of breathing usually reported in the literature include only elastic and resistive work. Inertial forces are considered negligible (Dubois et al., 1956; Mead, 1956) and gravitational forces are included in the measurement of elastic forces, although they can be considered part of the inertial forces (Roussos, 1985). Although there is little or no chest wall distortion during quiet spontaneous breathing, the distorting forces increase in patients with chest wall diseases or deformation, as well as when minute ventilation is high or large external resistive or elastic loads are imposed on the patient (Milic Emili, 1991). Since critically ill patients have altered lung and/or chest wall mechanics (most often with a nonhomogeneous gas distribution) and an external resistive load imposed by the respirators' circuitry and/or the endotracheal tube, distorting forces may contribute to an increase of the work of breathing. However, the importance of the distorting forces during different ventilatory modes has not been measured.

From a physiological point of view, the effect of the endotracheal tube should be quantified, or at least taken into consideration, when comparisons are made between patients or between ventilatory modes in the same patient but with different inspiratory and expiratory flows. Previous correction for the "effect" of the endotracheal tube is also required when measurements of breathing workload are compared with known normal values in spontaneously breathing subjects. On the other hand, for clinical practice, measurements of P_{aw} and external mechanical work should not be corrected for the "effect" of the endotracheal tube in the individual patient since the additional resistance of the tube represents a real increase of the workload of spontaneous or partially supported breathing (Marini et al., 1985a, 1988; Marini, 1986a; Shapiro et al., 1986; Sassoon et al., 1989a,b).

Problems Related to Flow Measurements

The importance of a correct balance of pneumotachograph before volume measurement is well known. The pneumotachograph must sample laminar flow and it must be selected appropriately for the flows under consideration and linearized over that range (Marini, 1991). Since the flow is integrated to yield volume, any imbalance in the electrical baseline will cause a linear drift and an incorrect volume measurement. As mentioned before, when attempting to quantify breathing effort during various ventilatory modes, it is important to check that the flow magnitude and the flow profile, as well as the tidal volume, do not differ substantially (Marini, 1991).

Problems Related to Pressure Measurements

The airway pressure signal (P_{aw}) should be tapped perpendicularly to the airstream axis at a point near the airway opening, i.e., at the proximal end of the endotracheal tube in the intubated patient (Marini, 1991).

Accurate P_{es} measurement requires a strict methodology with special emphasis on a number of technical details. The balloon must be kept filled with the appropriate amount of air since its deflation may lead to the underestimation of intrapleural pressure swings. In spontaneously breathing patients the optimal of air in the balloon is 0.5–1 ml of air; however, during mechanical ventilation (positive pressure conditions), the balloon should first be inflated at 6 ml to fully expand the chamber and then deflate to 1 ml of gas, which is considered the appropriate volume needed to ensure good sensitivity in ventilated patients (Marini, 1991).

The balloon is positioned in the lower third of the esophagus, using the technique of Baydur et al. (1982). After topical anesthesia of the nasal channel, the balloon is advanced into the stomach with pressure guidance, while the patient is given water to swallow and is asked to perform vigorous sniffing efforts. A positive deflection of pressure during sniffing indicates the passage of the distal part of the balloon into the stomach. The patient is then placed in the position required, and only at this moment is the balloon withdrawn slowly, as the patient sniffs intermittently, until the appearance of a negative pressure deflection during sniffing. This deflection indicates the entry of the proximal portion of the balloon into the thorax. The balloon is then withdrawn another 8–10 cm and the subject is then asked to perform a series of inspiratory efforts with the airway occluded. A final adjustment of the balloon is made during these procedures in order to have the best matching of inspiratory deflections of airway and esophageal pressure. Such a good agreement of P_{aw} and P_{es} can be obtained, whatever the posture of the patient may be (Baydur et al., 1987). In paralyzed and/or sedated ICU patients, the airway occlusion positioning technique cannot be undertaken. In such cases, a rough approximation of the appropriate balloon position is used by placing the distal tip of the balloon catheter 40 cm from the nasal opening (Marini, 1991).

Problems Related to Pti Measurements

Although the transdiaphragmatic pressure-time index parallels more closely the oxygen cost of breathing than does the external mechanical work (Field et al., 1982), this may not apply for the entire range of pressure, duty cycle, or frequency of contraction (Bellemare and Grassino, 1983; Buchler et al., 1985). As pointed ouit by Roussos and Macklem (1977), for the pressure-time index to be proportional to Vo_2, and therefore a good approximation of energy demands, the ratio of the average airflow (considered as an expression of the average velocity of shortening) to the muscle efficiency must remain constant, which is not always the case in critically ill patients.

The above methodological limitations, as well as the difficulty in using esophageal and gastric balloons in critically ill patients without, in most cases, the minimum collaboration required, have limited the use of pressure-time product and TTI as a method for the estimation of the work of breathing in the ICU.

G. Results of Clinical Studies and Their Implications

Although it was commonly believed that mechanically ventilated patients are spared the majority of the energy cost of breathing, clinical studies did not confirm this hypothesis. On the contrary, it was shown that many patients under controlled mechanical ventilation but without sedation and neuromuscular paralysis either perform expiratory work or negative inspiratory work (pliometric muscular contraction due to asynchrony between patient and ventilator) or share inspiratory work with their ventilator. This is also true when a mode of providing partial support of ventilation is used, such as synchronized intermittent mandatory ventilation (SIMV), continuous positive airway pressure (CPAP), or pressure support (PS) (Marini et al., 1985b, 1986b; Sassoon et al., 1986, 1988; Ward et al., 1988).

Work of Breathing During Controlled and Assisted Controlled Mechanical Ventilation (CMV and ACMV)

During assisted controlled mechanical ventilation (ACMV) the patient triggers mechanical inflation by lowering airway pressure a small amount. The patient's work component is related only to the effort involved in triggering and should therefore be negligible. However, mechanically assisted breaths usually differ markedly from spontaneous breaths since ventilators deliver fixed-flow waveforms and volumes that differ from spontaneous values and cannot adapt to variations in the patient's inspiratory effort (Marini, 1988, 1990). Since many patients continue their respiratory effort with the onset of the machine-delivered breath, they may perform inspiratory work when: (1) there is a substantial delay between the onset of the patient's inspiratory effort and the moment that full machine support is achieved (Table 1) (Hillman et al., 1986) and (2) the flow provided by the ventilator does not match the patient's needs precisely (Marini et al., 1985b, 1986b; Sassoon

Table 1 Sensitivity, Response Time, and Inspiratory Resistance of Demand Valves of Different Ventilators

Ventilator	Sensitivity (cm H_2O)	Response time (ms)	Inspiratory resistance (cm H_2O/L/min)
Bear I	−1.4 ± 0.1	92 ± 2	0.080 ± 0.002
Bennett MA2B	−0.2 ± 0.1	78 ± 4	0.003 ± 0.003
CPU 1	−0.5 ± 0.1	71 ± 6	0.040 ± 0.005
UVI Draëger	−0.3 ± 0.1	21 ± 5	0.007 ± 0.004
Engstrom Erica	−1.0 ± 0.3	35 ± 2	0.030 ± 0.006
Pulmosystem Z-800	−0.4 ± 0.1	19 ± 2	0.030 ± 0.003
Servo 900B	−0.2 ± 0.1	33 ± 2	0.050 ± 0.003
Servo 900C	−0.7 ± 0.1	26 ± 3	0.100 ± 0.021

From Hillman, 1986.

et al., 1988; Ward et al., 1988). Under such circumstances, although no measurable external work is accomplished, the isometric and pliometric work performed by the patient's respiratory muscles may be substantial.

Provided that inspiratory flow rate and V_T are held constant, the patient's contribution to the work of breathing during assisted mechanical ventilation may be estimated by plotting the P_{aw} against volume (Fig. 5) during assisted and controlled cycles and measuring the difference in the areas included in the plots. Marini et al. used this technique to quantify the work performed by the respiratory muscles during triggered machine cycles in normal subjects (Marini et al., 1985b) and ICU patients with acute respiratory failure of various etiologies (Marini et al., 1986b). They were able to demonstrate an increase in the subject's active inspiratory work with decreasing inspiratory flow rate, trigger sensitivity, and increasing minute ventilation. The inspiratory work performed by a patient under ACMV may represent 30–116% of the work performed during spontaneous breathing (Marini et al., 1986b). Sassoon et al., (1988) confirmed these results and demonstrated that inspiratory work performance by healthy subjects during ACMV is a function of the tidal volume (V_T) and mainly of the inspiratory flow delivered by the ventilator. In contrast to the results of Marini et al. (1986b), these authors reported that changes in the inspiratory work performed by the patient do not affect the mouth occlusion pressure (PO.1), which was similar during ACMV and spontaneous breathing. These results suggest that ventilation did not unload inspiratory work in healthy subjects since, in that case, the response of neuromuscular output (assessed by PO.1) would decrease. Further studies are needed to define the importance of ventilatory drive as a determinant of patient effort in different pathological situations in the ICU.

Ward et al. (1988) compared the pressure-time product and the plots of inflation pressure against volume during controlled and assisted machine cycles, as well as during passive inflation (Fig. 6). They not only confirmed and extended the observations of Marini et al. (1985b, 1986b) in patients with failure of neuromuscular

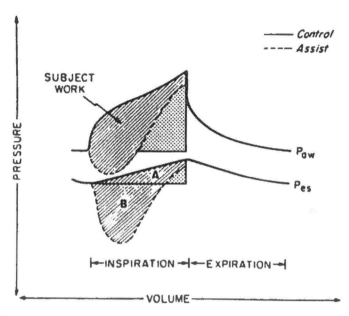

Figure 5 Graphic analysis of the patient's work during assisted mechanical ventilation (AMV). The patient's contribution to the work of breathing during AMV (subject work) can be estimated by plotting airway (P_{aw}) or esophageal pressure (P_{es}) against tidal volume during AMV and during controlled mechanical ventilation and measuring the difference of the areas included in such plots (hatched areas). Area A is subject work performed in moving the chest wall (estimated from the passive analogue; see Fig. 1), and area B is subject work done in moving the lung. (From Marini, 1988.)

apparatus undergoing assisted mechanical ventilation with low inspiratory flows, but also demonstrated that when an inappropriate pattern of breathing is imposed on such patients, they may perform as much as 25% of the total work of breathing during controlled mechanical ventilation. These authors suggested that the stimulus for muscle activation arises within an individual breath in response to the imposition of an inappropriate ventilator setting rather than to a general stimulation of the respiratory drive performed by the patients studied (Ward et al., 1988).

Work of Breathing During Ventilatory Modes with Spontaneous Breaths Partially Supported or Not

Synchronized intermittent mandatory ventilation (SIMV) is a mode of ventilatory support introduced to achieve graded withdrawal of mechanical ventilation and progressive increase in the work of breathing during weaning. (Downs et al., 1973; Kirby et al., 1984). However, as for assisted mechanical ventilation, the assumption that patient effort is spared in proportion to the ventilation provided by the respirator

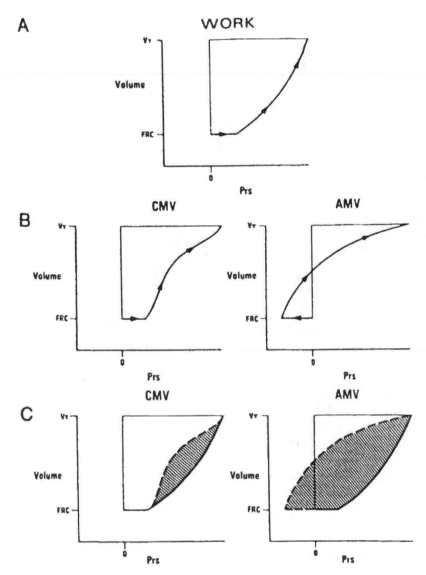

Figure 6 Graphic analysis of the patient's work component during controlled and assisted mechanical ventilation (CMV and AMV, respectively). The patient's contribution to the work of breathing during CMV and AMV can be estimated by plotting inflation pressure (P_{rs}) against volume during completely passive inflation (A) and during CMV cycles and AMV cycles (B). The difference of the area included in such plots (shaded area, C) yields the inspiratory work performed by the patient during each mode of ventilatory support. FRC = functional residual capacity; V_T = tidal volume. (From Ward et al., 1988.)

has not been tested. Since SIMV intermixes machine and spontaneous breaths, the work of breathing accomplished by the patient will be the sum of the work of spontaneous breathing through the ventilator's circuitry and the work performed by the patient during assisted machine cycles. Marini et al. (1988) have shown that, as the rate of synchronized intermittent mandatory ventilation is reduced in patients with acute respiratory failure, the patient's component of the work per assisted machine cycle increases and parallels an increase in respiratory drive. This increased work during assisted breaths was greater than the work performed during spontaneous breaths.

During weaning trials, the patient breathes through an endotracheal tube for a minimum of 30–60 min and often for several hours before extubation. It has been demonstrated that the presence of the endotracheal tube may double the inspiratory resistance (Sahn et al., 1976; Sullivan et al., 1976). Shapiro et al. (1986) evaluated the external work of breathing and the tension-time index of normal volunteers breathing through endotracheal tubes of different internal diameters (6–9 mm). At a constant volume of 500 ml, minute ventilation was increased from 5 to 50 L/min by increasing respiratory frequency. External work and tension-time index increased as tube diameter decreased; the changes were substantially magnified at higher minute ventilation (Fig. 7).

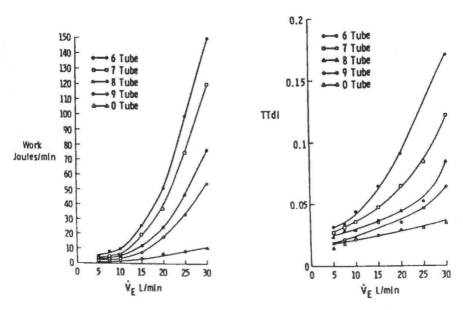

Figure 7   Relationship between the work of breathing or the pressure time index (TTi) and minute ventilation of subjects breathing through endotracheal tubes. The number indicates internal diameter of tube in millimeters. O Tube = no endotracheal tube. (From Shapiro et al., 1986.)

Considerable concern has been expressed recently over the additional work of breathing imposed on the patient, not only by endotracheal tubes, but also by ventilator demand valves and breathing circuits (Gherini et al., 1979; Gibney, 1982; Katz et al., 1985; Viale et al., 1985; Ward, 1985; Marini et al., 1985a; Marini, 1986a; Shapiro et al., 1986; Sassoon et al., 1989b; Mecklenburg et al., 1986; Banner et al., 1986; Easton and Antonishen, 1986; Yang et al., 1988; Petrof et al., 1988; Specht et al., 1988; Swinamer et al., 1989; Bersten et al., 1989). Continuous positive airway pressure (CPAP), for instance, has been proposed as a modality of respiratory support that could decrease mechanical load and facilitate weaning (Martin et al., 1982; Katz and Marks, 1985; Petrof et al., 1988), but several authors reported no change or an increase of the work of breathing with a number of such CPAP systems (Gibney et al., 1982; Cox and Niblett, 1984; Katz et al., 1985). In fact, a number of demand-valve systems for delivering CPAP are slow to respond and impose considerable resistance to ventilation. Therefore, many (Easton and Andonishen, 1986; Lemaire et al., 1986; Petrof et al., 1988; Sassoon et al., 1989b), but again not all (Op't Holt et al., 1982; Henry et al., 1983; Katz et al., 1985; Bersten et al., 1989), studies indicate that continuous-flow systems offer less resistance than demand-flow systems. Finally, expiratory positive pressure valve systems may increase the expiratory work of spontaneous breathing (Martin et al., 1980; Marini et al., 1985a; Banner et al., 1986).

The disagreement of the results of the previously reported studies is not a paradox for several reasons:

1. There are important differences in the mechanical characteristics of different CPAP systems. The effects of such differences in the work of breathing are illustrated from the marked variations of their pressure volume loops (Fig. 8).

2. The work required for spontaneous breaths (partially supported or not) increases every time the patient's inspiratory flow rate exceeds the set rate of flow delivery (Gherini et al., 1979; Cox and Niblett, 1984), as was the case for controlled mechanical ventilation (Marini et al., 1985b, 1986b). Therefore, the workload of breathing depends on the mechanical characteristics of the respiratory device used and on the patient's respiratory mechanics and drive (Gibney et al., 1982; Cox and Niblett, 1984; Katz et al., 1985).

The complexity of estimating the workload in clinical settings has been demonstrated indirectly by Bersten et al. (1989) in an experimental study using a lung simulator. According to this study, inspiratory work increased more than 100% at flow rates usually delivered by ventilators (40–60 L/min) when an 8.0- or 9.0-mm endotracheal tube was utilized (Fig. 9). This effect is much greater as diameter decreases and/or inspiratory flow increases, and it may reach critical levels of work of breathing above which patients become ventilator-dependent (see Fig. 9).

The same authors demonstrated that endotracheal tube and apparatus resist-

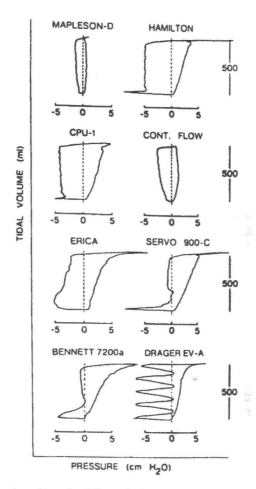

Figure 8 Pressure volume loops for different devices tested at zero end-expiratory pressure at an inspiratory flow rate of 60 L/min. The differing mechanical characteristics of the device are responsible for the marked variation in the appearance of the loops. (From Bersten et al., 1989.)

ances measured separately relate poorly to total respiratory resistance (see Figs. 9, 10, and 11) since the interaction between the tube and the ventilator's components alter flow patterns greatly (Bersten et al., 1989).

Therefore, the combined effect of an endotracheal tube, demand valves, and circuitry cannot be estimated by simple addition of their resistances (measured at a constant flow). From Figures 10 and 11 it is apparent that the diameter of the endotracheal tube has a great influence, not only on the W_b, but also on the magnitude of its change with increasing inspiratory flow (Bersten et al., 1989).

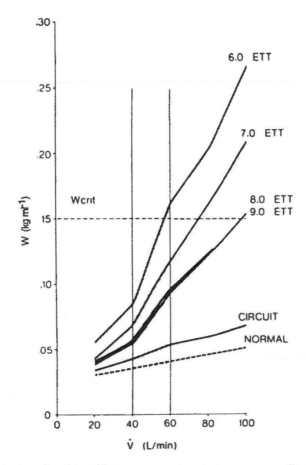

Figure 9 Total work of breathing at zero end-expiratory pressure. Various sizes of endotracheal tubes (ETT) and their connectors are plotted against flow rate. The same device (Mapleson D) was used for all measurements and the normal work of breathing was added to all values plotted. The zone between 40 and 60 L/min indicates clinically relevant inspiratory flow rates and the dotted line represents an inspiratory work value (W_{crit}) above which patients may be ventilator-dependent. V = gas volume per unit time; W = work of breathing. (From Bersten et al., 1989.)

Implications for Clinical Practice

Endotracheal tube resistance increases in proportion to the length of the tube and in inverse proportion to the fourth power of its radius (when flow is laminar). Nasotracheal tubes present greater resistance than do orotracheal or tracheostomy tubes (Marini, 1990).

    During weaning trials, clinicians must pay attention to a number of several points:

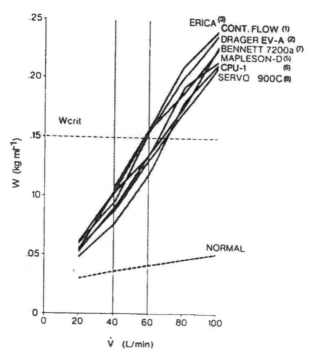

Figure 10 Total work of breathing through a size 7 endotracheal tube, its connector, and one of the seven ventilators tested at 10 cm H_2O continuous positive airway pressure (CPAP) plotted against flow rate. The zone between 40 and 60 L/min indicates clinically relevant inspiratory flow rates, and the dotted line represents an inspiratory work value (W_{crit}) above which patients may be ventilator-dependent. There were no statistically significant differences between work required by the bottom four ventilators, although servo 900 c and CPU = 1 devices required significantly less work than the top three devices. The Erica device required significantly more work than any of the others ($P < 0.005$). V = gas volume per unit; W = work of breathing. (From Bersten et al., 1989.)

1. Narrowing of the endotracheal tube (intraliminal kinks, constrictions, and adherent secretions) should be avoided since it dramatically increases the airway resistance and the work of breathing (especially if the lumen of the tube is small). Such a narrowing of endotracheal tubes could explain why resistance measured in vivo is often higher than in vitro (Marini et al., 1985a).

2. According to Bernsten et al., endotracheal tubes with internal diameter less than 8 mm should be avoided, since the patient's work component imposed by a small tube may contribute to or even be responsible for ventilator dependence (Fig. 9, 10, and 11).

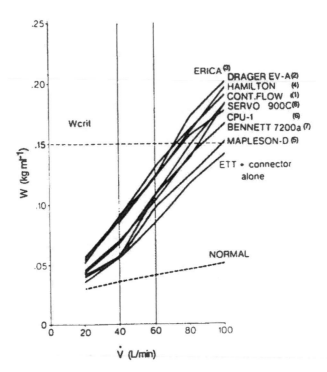

Figure 11 Total work of breathing through size 8 endotracheal tube, its connector, and one of the eight devices tested at 10 cm H_2O CPAP plotted against flow rate. The zone between 40 and 60 L/min indicates clinically relevant inspiratory flow rates. The dotted line represents an inspiratory work value (W_{crit}) above which patients may be ventilator-dependent. At 40 L/min inspiratory flow there was a significant ($P < 0.05$) difference between the Mapleson D and continuous flow circuit, which required the lowest work and the Engstrom, Erica, Ohmeda CPU-1, Drager EV-A, and Hamilton Veolar, which required the highest. V = gas volume per unit time; W = work of breathing. (From Bersten et al., 1989.)

The difficulty with which spontaneous breaths can be drawn through the ventilator's circuitry depends on the resistance of the demand-valve system and its time response. Although many experimental and clinical studies recently have assessed the additional burden imposed by the ventilator's demand valves and breathing circuits during spontaneous breathing, their effect during weaning trials is often not taken into consideration (Marini, 1990). This could be explained in part by the great variability between patients or between devices of different manufacturers used on the same patient (Katz et al., 1985; Lemaire et al., 1986; Sassoon et al., 1989b; Bersten et al., 1989).

Although the patient's work components due to increased apparatus resistance depend mainly on the endotracheal tube and less on the demand valve and circuitry of the device (Bersten et al., 1989), biomedical engineers should take this additional work into account and try to improve the efficiency of spontaneous breathing through ventilators.

Automatic positive end-expiratory pressure (auto-PEEP) or intrinsic positive end-expiratory pressure (PEEPi) can also increase the variability of the work of breathing during weaning trials. As shown in Figure 12, $PEEP_i$ has the same effect as a decrease of trigger sensitivity since the positive P_A must be counterbalanced before an inspiratory flow appears (Smith and Marini, 1988). Figure 13 illustrates that in patients with PEEPi, the difference between Patm and PA results in a higher static equilibrium volume (hyperinflation) and the elastic work necessary for inflation is increased proportionally to the PEEPi (darker shaded area in Fig. 13) (Smith and Marini, 1988; Hubmayr et al., 1990).

Since patients most prone to develop PEEPi are those with increased airway resistance, any additional workload imposed by PEEPi may contribute to ventilator dependence, failure to prevent respiratory muscle fatigue, and unsuccessful weaning (Peters et al., 1972; Proctor and Woolson, 1973; Civetta, 1993).

CPAP can offset the inspiratory effort performed to overcome the increased load due to PEEPi (Fig. 13) and may decrease the work of inspiratory muscles since expiratory muscle contractions may displace the system below its normal equilibrium position and give an inspiratory boost (Fig. 14) (Hubmayr et al., 1990).

A second mode of ventilatory support proposed to offset the effect of the endotracheal tube, demand-valve, and ventilator circuitry during spontaneous breathing is pressure support ventilation (PS) (MacIntyre, 1986a). During PS the flow profile varies but the patient's contribution to the inspiratory work of breathing can be measured in a fashion similar to that for controlled and assisted mechanical ventilation using plot of P_{es} against inspired volume (Marini, 1988). Recent studies have confirmed not only that PS decreases the inspiratory work of breathing, but also that patients' subjective acceptance of this mode is better compared to other

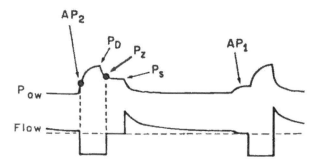

Figure 12 Simultaneous tracings of airway pressure (P_{aw}) and airflow during controlled volume-cycled ventilation in a patient with airflow obstruction and autoPEEP (AP). With flow stopped at the end of inflation, P_{aw} reflects the positive alveolar pressure (AP_1). AutoPEEP can also be estimated from the P_{aw} needed to counterbalance elastic recoil and stop pressure. P_z = airway pressure at zero flow. (From Truwit et al., 1988.)

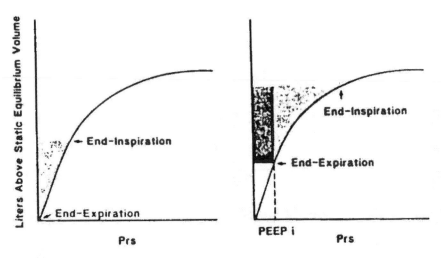

Figure 13   Effect of dynamic hyperinflation (due to autoPEEP) on elastic inspiratory work. The solid curve shows the relationship between volume above static equilibrium volume (SEV) and the recoil of the inspiratory system (P_{rs}). (A) An inspiration is initiated from the SEV and the elastic inspiratory work is shown by the shaded area. In the presence of dynamic hyperinflation (B), inspiration is initiated from volume above SEV. The work of breathing increases, since in addition to the elastic inspiratory work (lighter shaded area), the patient performs work to halt expiratory flow (darker shaded area). The use of continuous positive airway pressure equal to the autoPEEP could spare the patient this additional work. (From Hubmayr et al., 1990.)

modes of mechanical and spontaneous ventilation (MacIntyre, 1986b; Brochard et al., 1987, 1988, 1989; Fiastro et al., 1988). According to Brochard et al. (1988), excess work due to breathing through an endotracheal tube and the ventilator's circuit can be offset by using pressure support on the order of 5–12 cm H_2O.

The interaction of parameters and pathophysiological mechanisms discussed before could explain why a number of ICU patients tolerate much better spontaneous breathing after immediate extubation than partially supported breathing with sophisticated ventilatory modes and respiratory devices. For clinical practice, only careful assessment of each patient in real clinical conditions can suggest the best respiratory support modality for the particular situation.

IV.   Indirect Assessment of Breathing Workload from the Electromyographic Activity of Respiratory Muscles

A.   Theory of Measurement, Equipment Required, and Methodology

The contractile force developed by a muscle and its oxygen uptake are proportional to its electrical activity and therefore to the magnitude of the integrated

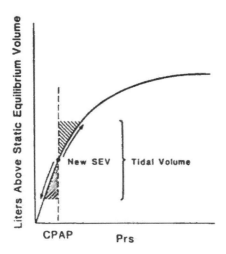

Figure 14 Effect of CPAP on the work performed by respiratory muscles. The solid curve shows the relationship between volume above static equilibrium volume (SEV) and the recoil of the respiratory system (P_{rs}). During CPAP the patient may recruit expiratory muscles and exhale below the SEV. The elastic work performed by the expiratory muscles is represented by the darker shaded area below New SEV. Relaxation of the expiratory muscles inflates the lungs back to the SEV without inspiratory effort. Therefore, CPAP reduces inspiratory muscle work (light shaded area) by letting the expiratory muscles do part of the inspiratory work. (From Hubmayr et al., 1990.)

electromyographic signal (Bigland and Lippold, 1954). Almost 40 years later, the electromyogram (EMG) of the diaphragm remains a valuable research tool, not only for quantifying respiratory muscle effort, but also for detecting muscular fatigue since a decrease of the ratio of high- to low-frequency components of the electromyographic signal indicates that the patient faces a breathing stress that cannot be indefinitely sustained (Gross et al., 1979; Bellemare and Grassino, 1982; Aubier, 1987). Furthermore, when used in conduction with a pneumotachograph and/or a measure of developed pressure, the EMG allows precise separation of muscular activity during the inspiratory and expiratory phases of airflow.

Another promising application of electromyography is the EMG of the sternocleidomastoid muscle, which has been shown to parallel overall breathing stress (Wilson et al., 1984).

Although the technical and methodological details of electromyography are beyond the scope of this chapter, we must discuss a number of methodological and technical problems, which could explain why the EMG remains a research tool and is rarely used as an indirect continuous indicator of respiratory muscle activity in clinical practice.

B. Methodological Limitations and Technical Problems

The major problem with electromyographic activity of respiratory muscles is the difficulty to obtain with a noninvasive methodology a "clean" signal whose quality remains stable over a long period.

Surface electromyography is used to monitor costal diaphragm activity. Although it is not difficult to place surface electrodes in the sixth to seventh interspaces along the anterolateral intercostal spaces (Newsom, 1967; Grassino et al., 1976), the signal transmission from the costal fibers of the diaphragm and its intensity are hampered by suboptimal skin contact, obesity, and/or improper lead placement. In addition, the EMG is usually contaminated by electromyographic signals of other respiratory and nonrespiratory muscles; electrocardiographic contaminating signals are occasionally a problem and must also be filtered out (Bruce and Goldman, 1983). The more invasive monitoring with needle electrodes may be used to obtain a good signal from costal fibers of the diaphragm (Marini, 1991).

From a clinical standpoint, the EMG cannot be used to make comparisons between different patients since amplitude varies widely due to differences in electrical conduction among individuals and may also vary for reasons unrelated to the intensity of muscle activation (Loring and Bruce, 1986). In addition, tracking the activity of any single muscle group (most often crural and/or costal fibers of the diaphragm) may not faithfully reflect total respiratory muscle activity. For all these reasons, clinical applications of the EMG to respiratory problems of critically ill patients remains very limited.

V. Measurement of the Oxygen Cost of Breathing

A. Theory of Measurement

The diaphragm, like the heart and quite likely the other respiratory muscles, obtains its energy almost entirely from oxidative metabolism over a large range of work output. Regardless of the substrate being oxidized, the energy required for the metabolic reactions responsible for adenosine triphosphate production can be estimated quite well from direct or indirect measurements of oxygen consumption (Roussos, 1985).

Direct Measurements

The oxygen consumption of an organ or a tissue is determined by the Fick equation:

$$V_{O_2} = Q \times \Delta(a\text{-}v)O_2 \tag{14}$$

where V_{O_2} = oxygen consumption, Q = blood flow, and $\Delta(a\text{-}v)O_2$ = arteriovenous oxygen content difference.

The oxygen uptake of the inactive diaphragm in dogs during mechanical ventilation is 0.2–0.8 ml of O_2 per minute per 100 g, similar to values for other resting skeletal muscles (Rochester, 1974; Robertson et al., 1977). During quiet breathing, the diaphragm oxygen consumption varies between 0.5 and 2.0 ml of O_2 per minute per 100 g, while during unobstructed hyperventilation it increases to 1.7–3.0 ml/min/100 g (Rochester, 1974; Robertson et al., 1977). The highest levels of oxygen consumption occur during breathing against high inspiratory resistances. At the highest resistance used by Robertson et al. (1977) the diaphragm consumed 24 ml of O_2 per minute per 100 g. Similar information is not available for other respiratory muscles.

Although the results of experimental studies on animals using this technique are interesting, their findings should be extrapolated to humans with caution, since direct measurement of O_2 consumption of the respiratory muscles in humans is not possible.

Indirect Measurements

Liliestrand (1918) has used an indirect method of measuring the oxygen consumption of respiratory muscles. In spontaneously breathing subjects, total-body oxygen consumption (VO_2) and ventilation are measured at rest; ventilation then is increased either voluntarily, by breathing CO_2, or by the addition of dead space, and total-body VO_2 is measured again. Assuming that the increase in oxygen consumption during hyperventilation is due to the increase in aerobic metabolism of the respiratory muscles, their oxygen consumption (VO_2r) can be calculated from the difference of the two values (ΔVO_2). In mechanically ventilated patients, the VO_2r can be estimated as the difference between VO_2 during controlled ventilation (when respiratory muscles are supposed to be at rest) and VO_2 during the application of a ventilatory mode and/or a breathing stress such as a weaning trial.

B.   Equipment Required and Methodology

Computing VO_2 from the product of cardiac output and the oxygen content difference between arterial and mixed venous blood (CaO_2–CVO_2) is a conceptually attractive and easily accomplished method in the ICU setting. However, this technique is subject to multiplicative arithmetic errors of inherently imprecise measurements of cardiac output, CaO_2 and CVO_2 (Marini, 1990).

The reference method for VO_2 measurements remains the Douglas bag technique (Bartlett et al., 1958; Field et al., 1982) but its application in the critically ill patient is cumbersome and its reproducibility is difficult to evaluate. These technical problems become more important in the ICU setting where we need a continuous monitoring of VO_2 rather than an instantaneous measurement. The monitoring of pulmonary gas exchange requires a continuous measurement of minute ventilation and of fractional concentrations of O_2 and CO_2 in the inspired and expired gas. Several measurement systems have been developed in the last 15 years that allow a monitoring of CO_2 production and oxygen consumption in mechanically ventilated patients, without interfering with routine nursing care or ventilatory management.

Measurement Systems Using a Mass Spectrometer

The use of a mass spectrometer is considered the most accurate method for the measurement of the energy expenditure of breathing in the critically ill. The system has four major parts: (1) a mixing chamber connected to the expiratory part of the ventilatory circuit, for the collection of expired gases, (2) a pneumontachograph connected to the output of the mixing chamber for the measurement of the expired volume, (3) a mass spectrometer for the simultaneous and precise measurement of fractional concentrations of oxygen and carbon dioxide in inspired and expired gases, and (4) a computer for data processing.

Bertrand et al. (1986) validated such a system in patients undergoing mechanical ventilation with Fio$_2$ up to 60% and reported an excellent correlation with the reference method, i.e., the Douglas bag technique.

Commercial Measurement Systems

A number of commercial instruments for the monitoring of pulmonary gas exchange have been developed recently. Since most of these systems are compact and easy to use in clinical practice and dispose microcomputer-based autocalibration, data trends, and self-diagnostics, one may expect that their use will contribute to a better understanding of the physiological principles of the workload of breathing in the ICU patient and will result in a more successful application of this knowledge in clinical practice.

The *Engstrom Metabolic Computer* is a commercial instrument developed for the Engstrom ventilators ERICA and ELVIRA. An automatically calibrated electrochemical fuel cell is used for the measurement of inspired and expired oxygen concentrations, while mixed expired CO_2 concentration is measured by an infrared analyzer and minute volume is obtained from the ventilator's flow sensor. The system must be tested before use for possible leaks and calibrated if necessary by a technician. It continuously displays the mean values of Vo$_2$, Vco$_2$, and RQ from the preceding 1-min, 15-min, and 60-min measurement periods. Bredbacka et al. (1984) and Carlsson et al. (1985) have evaluated the system in the laboratory and in critically ill patients and reported a reasonable accuracy for routine clinical use.

With the *Beckman Metabolic Measurement Chart* (MMC), the carbon dioxide is also measured by an infrared analyzer, but a polarographic sensor is used for measuring oxygen concentrations and a turbine with electrooptical detectors measures the expired minute volume. Special transducers are also used for measuring the pressures and temperatures of the gas samples. The inspired and expired gases are dried and analyzed, and a special software program performs the necessary corrections and provides accurate measurements of V_{O_2} and V_{CO_2} in spontaneously breathing as well as in mechanically ventilated patients (Damask et al., 1984).

Finally, the *Deltatrack Metabolic Monitor* utilizes a fast differential paramagnetic oxygen sensor for V_{O_2} measurement and a carbon dioxide infrared sensor for V_{CO_2} measurement. The expired minute volume is measured by a gas dilution technique. The concentration of CO_2 in the expired gas is measured before and after dilution with a constant airflow. Since the ratio of the two different concentrations is equal to the ratio of expired minute volume to the total flow, which is constant, the system allows a continuous monitoring of expired minute volume without a pneumotachograph. The system is a compact unit that can be connected to the expiratory port of any ventilator or used with a canopy for spontaneously breathing patients.

Measurement of the Oxygen Cost of Breathing

In ICU patients, pulmonary gas exchange may be calculated by using a number of well-known formulas of respiratory physiology. For a given inspired and expired minute volume (V_I and V_E, respectively), the amount of carbon dioxide produced (V_{CO_2}) and the oxygen consumption (V_{O_2}) per minute are given by Formulas (1) and (2):

$$V_{CO_2} = V_E \times F_{E_{CO_2}} \tag{15}$$

and

$$V_{O_2} = (V_I \times F_{I_{O_2}}) - (V_E \times F_{E_{O_2}}) \tag{16}$$

where $F_{E_{CO_2}}$ and $F_{E_{O_2}}$ are mixed expired concentrations of CO_2 and $F_{I_{O_2}}$ is the percentage of oxygen in the inspired air.

According to the Haldane hypothesis, the amount of nitrogen going into the body equals the amount of nitrogen going out, so that:

$$V_I \times F_{I_{N_2}} = V_E \times F_{E_{N_2}} \text{ or } V_I = V_E \times \frac{F_{E_{N_2}}}{F_{I_{N_2}}} \tag{17}$$

where $F_{I_{N_2}}$ and $F_{E_{N_2}}$ are the inspired and expired concentrations of nitrogen.

From Eqs. (16) and (17), the V_{O_2} can be calculated without measurement of V_I, as follows:

$$V_{O_2} = V_E \left(F_{I_{O_2}} \times \frac{F_{E_{N_2}}}{F_{I_{N_2}}} - F_{E_{O_2}} \right) \tag{18}$$

Since this equation is valid even in the presence of anesthetic gases, it can be applied during general anesthesia in humans (Auckburg et al., 1985; Viale et al., 1988). In the ICU patient the absence of gases other than O_2, CO_2, and N_2 in the inspired and expired gas allows the calculation of N_2 concentrations by using the formulas $F_{I_{N_2}} = 1 - F_{I_{O_2}}$ and $F_{E_{N_2}} = 1 - F_{E_{O_2}} - F_{E_{CO_2}}$, so that:

$$V_{O_2} = V_E \frac{(1 - F_{E_{CO_2}}) F_{I_{O_2}} - F_{E_{O_2}}}{(1 - F_{I_{O_2}})} \tag{19}$$

From Eq. (19) it is clear that only four variables must be measured to calculate V_{O_2}: three fractional concentrations of gases (F_{IO_2}, F_{EO_2}, and F_{ECO_2}) and minute expired volume. When inspired minute volume (V_I) is used instead of V_E, the equation for V_{O_2} is:

$$V_{O_2} = V_I \frac{(1 - F_{ECO_2})\, F_{IO_2} - F_{EO_2}}{1 - F_{EO_2} - F_{ECO_2}} \tag{20}$$

In clinical studies, the calculation of respiratory quotient (RQ) as a ratio between V_{CO_2} and V_{O_2} provides an indirect estimation of the accuracy of the method used for pulmonary gas analysis.

C. Methodological Limitations, Technical Problems, and Errors

In critically ill patients, especially those under mechanical ventilation, the indirect estimation of the oxygen consumption of respiratory muscles from differences in total V_{O_2} measurements presents many methodological problems. The importance of analytical and computational errors discussed below is amplified by the fact that the energy cost of breathing is usually only a small fraction of the total body oxygen requirement (only 1–2% of total-body V_{O_2}), and an even smaller fraction of the large amounts of oxygen washes into and out of the lungs of a patient ventilated with large minute volumes and a high level of F_{IO_2}. In a normal subject, for instance, the fractional concentrations of oxygen in the inspired of expired gases are 21% and 16%, respectively, at rest (when the classic open-circuit method is used). In an ICU patient with the same V_{O_2} but ventilated with a minute volume increased from 7 to 15 L/min and breathing 60% of oxygen, the fractional concentration of oxygen in the expired gas will be about 57.6%. An analytical error of 0.1% in the measured fractional concentrations of oxygen in the inspired or expired gases will cause 4% of V_{O_2} error in the estimate of total body V_{O_2}, i.e., two or three times the likely increase of oxygen consumption of the respiratory muscles.

Theoretical Problems

One of the major theoretical problems in the assessment of the work of breathing from V_{O_2} measurements is the difficulty in estimating the efficiency of respiratory muscles (Roussos, 1985). For practical purposes, the mechanical efficiency of muscle contraction (E) has been defined as:

$$E = \frac{W}{Q + W} \tag{21}$$

where W = external mechanical work and Q = energy transformed into heat.

Measurement of the energy expenditure of respiratory muscles does not allow an accurate assessment of the mechanical work of breathing since there are important fluctuations of the efficiency of inspiratory and expiratory muscles. Efficiencies between 10% to 25% have been reported (Cain and Otis, 1949; Milic Emili, 1960) with large variations between subjects and between different ventilatory modes in the individual patient. From the overall standpoint of physiological economics, the efficiency of breathing is probably nearer 10% and in disease it may fall to 1–2% (Roussos, 1985).

When the Vo_2r is indirectly estimated from variations of total-body Vo_2, it is difficult to achieve a sufficiently stable nonrespiratory Vo_2 at rest since it is well known that Vo_2 variations may be the result of metabolic activity of other muscles and/or tissues apart from the group of respiratory muscles of interest. During artificial ventilation, for instance, complete muscular relaxation is impossible in most ICU patients without sedation and eventually neuromuscular paralysis. As mentioned before, some ICU patients may have expiratory muscle activity during inspiration and increase the energy expenditure of breathing (Roussos, 1985; Smith et al., 1986; Marini, 1990) while in patients "fighting" their ventilators, the energy cost of pliometric and isometric contraction may be substantial. On the other hand, during hyperventilation a number of nonrespiratory muscles may become active and other organs, most notably the heart, may be responsible for the increase in total-body Vo_2. Under these circumstances, the measured variations of Vo_2 during weaning assess the "real oxygen cost of breathing," which is usually higher than the real oxygen consumption of respiratory muscles since the increased oxygen consumption includes components related to the expiratory work of breathing and the energy expended by nonrespiratory tissues. Therefore, even the ratio of simultaneously measured external mechanical work and oxygen cost of breathing does not always provide the efficiency of the respiratory muscles of interest.

Problems Related to the Accuracy of Measurements in Patients Ventilated with High Levels of FiO₂ and Large Minute Volumes

It is well known that any increase of the absolute value of the FiO_2 will amplify the random measurement error in the determination of the Vo_2 (Ultman and Bursztein, 1981). Although it is generally admitted that the measurement of Vo_2 should be limited to patients ventilated with an FiO_2 lower than 60%, it is obvious that the high FiO_2 level used in the majority of critically ill patients (40–60%) will increase the possibility of computational errors. Obviously, at high FiO_2 there is no error amplification in the computation of VcO_2.

Another problem related to the FiO_2 in ICU patients is that with usual ventilator air mixers, FiO_2 is unstable during inspiration (Annat et al., 1991) and may also vary with time (personal observations; Fig. 15). The addition of an inspiratory mixing chamber is essential for an accurate measurement of Vo_2, since it attenuates eventual fluctuations of FiO_2 (Fig. 16) (Kinney et al., 1970; Annat, 1991).

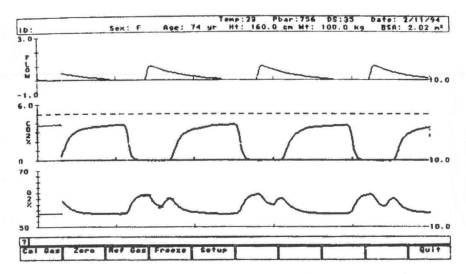

Figure 15 Recordings of flow, CO_2, and O_2 concentration in the airways of a patient under controlled ventilation. The use of a system allowing a breath-by-breath analysis of the concentration of oxygen in the inspired gas indicates an important variation of O_2 concentration during inspiratory time (personal observation).

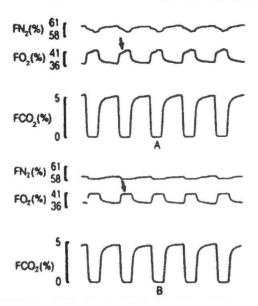

Figure 16 Simultaneous recordings of airway F_{N_2}, F_{O_2}, and F_{CO_2} in a patient under controlled ventilation. Note that the F_{IO_2} is unstable in A. The use of an external air mixer is necessary in order to have a constant value of F_{O_2} throughout inspiration (B). (From Annat et al., 1991.)

Problems Related to Changes in Oxygen and Carbon Dioxide Body Stores

Assessment of metabolic gas exchange of the total body from measurements on pulmonary gas exchange is based on the assumption that no gas is deposited in or withdrawn from the body stores. This situation is defined as a "steady state" (Fahri and Rahn, 1955) and must be reached in all patients before Vo_2 is measured. Since body stores are much smaller and more rapidly exchangeable for oxygen than for carbon dioxide, the time required to reach a new steady state is much more rapid for oxygen than for carbon dioxide.

Obviously, in the ICU setting, not only is it difficult to be sure that the patient is under steady-state conditions throughout the study, but also a great number of events (such as shivering, variations of minute volume, functional residual capacity, and changes in body temperature or metabolic requirements) may lead to variations of body stores of O_2 and CO_2. Continuous measurement of the respiratory quotient (RQ) may provide indirect evidences of a non-steady-state situation and/or computational errors (especially when variations are very important or absolute values are not in the physiological range). Long-term continuous measurements of Vo_2, Vco_2, and RQ are therefore needed to attenuate the effects of eventual external events and/or changes in the patient's minute volume and metabolic rate.

From a practical point of view, a stable end-tidal CO_2 value ($Petco_2$) for 15–20 min may be considered an indirect but useful index to verify the stability of CO_2 body stores. For an accurate assessment of metabolic gas exchanges from Vo_2 and Vco_2 measurements at the mouth, a period of 20–30 min should be respected after any therapeutic or accidental modification of parameters susceptible to produce a change in body stores of O_2 and/or CO_2 (Annat, 1991).

Problems Related to Artificial Respiratory Cycles

During continuous pulmonary gas exchange monitoring, routine nursing care, tracheal aspirations, or even cough efforts may lead to erroneous computation. Since data provided during such events must be disregarded, the commercially available measurement systems must allow identification of artificial respiratory cycles and automatically correct for their effects (Annat, 1991).

D. Results of Clinical Studies and Their Implications

The Oxygen Cost of Breathing During Spontaneous or Mechanical Ventilation

Experimental studies have shown that the oxygen consumption of the respiratory muscles (Vo_2r) is about 0.2–0.8 ml O_2/min 100 g at rest, and 0.5–2.0 ml O_2/min/ 100 g during quiet breathing (Rochester, 1974; Roberts et al., 1977). During resistive breathing, the Vo_2 may increase from a control value of about 150 ml of O_2 per minute to 200 ml of O_2 per minute due to an increased oxygen extraction by the respiratory muscles. About 50% of this increase of extraction (i.e., 25 ml of oxygen) may be taken up by the diaphragm alone (Roussos, 1985).

We must reemphasize that, as explained in Chapter 25, the Vo_2 of the respiratory muscles increases hyperbolically with the increase of minute ventilation (see also Fig. 11 of that chapter) and that the slope of the hyperbola varies greatly between subjects (Roussos, 1985). In patients with altered chest mechanics the resting Vo_2 of the respiratory muscles is nearly double the normal amount and the hyperbolic increase with increased ventilation is early and steep (Cambell et al., 1957; Cherniak, 1959).

When Vo_2r is assessed from variations of total-body Vo_2 in humans, the range of normal values is between 0.25 and 2.5 ml of O_2/min/L of ventilation (1–4% of total Vo_2) (Bartlett et al., 1958; Campbell et al., 1958; Fritts et al., 1959; Milic Emili, 1960; Harden et al., 1962; Hilman et al., 1986). However, substantially higher percentages of total-body Vo_2 have been reported after transition from machine-assisted ventilation to spontaneous breathing in ICU patients. In 1963 Thung et al. reported a 13% increase in the oxygen cost of breathing of 12 patients after cardiac surgery. It is interesting that the mean oxygen cost of breathing was 6% of the total Vo_2 in the absence of postoperative complications (six patients), but increased to 21% in patients with cardiopulmonary problems (four patients with congestive heart failure, one with severe left arterial hypertension, and one with pulmonary hypertension and poor pulmonary compliance). Similar values of oxygen cost of breathing were reported by Wilson et al. (1973) in patients with cardiopulmonary disease (oxygen cost of breathing = 8.7 ± 9.9 ml of O_2 per liter of ventilation, representing about 24% of total Vo_2), while Savino et al. (1985) observed a Vo_2 increase of 11% in a group of surgical patients. In the postoperative period after cardiac surgery an increase in Vo_2 of 15–20% was found when patients were switched from controlled ventilation to spontaneous breathing or an intermittent mandatory ventilation rate of 4–5 (Prakash et al., 1985). More recently, Kemper et al. (1987) and Viale et al. (1988b) found oxygen cost of breathing on the order of 10% in postoperative patients; the increase in Vo_2 was similar during intermittent mandatory ventilation and CPAP trials (Kemper et al., 1987). Finally, in patients with multiple injuries, extensive burns, or sepsis, the oxygen cost of breathing varies from normal to values greater than 30% of total Vo_2 (Bursztein et al., 1978), and values up to 59% have been reported in COPD patients who failed extubation (Brochard et al., 1989).

During controlled mechanical ventilation, all modern ICU ventilators are powerfully sufficient to perform the entire work of chest expansion during passive inflation despite the impedance of inflation due to thoracopulmonary compliance and airway resistance. However, many ICU patients without sedation and neuromuscular paralysis perform inspiratory efforts and accomplish part of the total external work whenever the inspiratory flow demand exceeds the flow delivered by the ventilator. According to Ward et al. (1988), patients undergoing controlled mechanical ventilation performed about 25% of the total work of breathing at the lowest flow studied (20 ml/min). The patient's work, representing an attempt to reach a more comfortable inspiratory flow rate, decreased with increasing ventilator inspiratory flow rate until the patient's contribution was insignificant at 65 L/min.

During assisted mechanical ventilation, the energy cost of breathing may be about 25–50% of the energy expenditure during spontaneous breathing in a variety of clinical settings (Sassoon et al., 1989; Marini, 1990, 1991). This percentage can also increase greatly during vigorous breathing or mechanical ventilation with suboptimal ventilator settings. The main determinant of how much work the patient performs in such a clinical setting is the ventilatory drive, which is related to the minute ventilation requirement and to the presence of dyspnea (Marini, 1990).

Manipulations of ventilator settings during assisted mechanical ventilation may influence the patient's work profoundly. The less sensitive the ventilator's threshold (trigger sensitivity) and the greater the response time of the demand valve, the more work that will be performed by the patient. If assisted mechanical ventilation is used to minimize the respiratory work load while allowing the patient to retain control of minute ventilation, trigger sensitivity should be minimized and the inspiratory flow should be set at a level higher than the peak inspiratory flow of the patient, i.e., about four times the minute ventilation required, or in the range of 60–80 L/min (Marini, 1990).

Clinicians also must be concerned about the expiratory work of breathing, since Smith et al. (1986) reported that expiratory work represented as much as 44% of the total work of breathing in 17 of 21 patients during assisted controlled ventilation.

In conclusion, if mechanical ventilation is used to spare patients the energy expenditure of breathing and/or to allow recovery from muscular fatigue, special attention should be paid to inappropriate ventilator settings, which may increase the patient's work substantially even during controlled mechanical ventilation or assisted mechanical ventilation (Marini, 1986b). In fact in a number of clinical situations, the work performed by the patient (Ward et al., 1988) or the oxygen cost of breathing (Berry and Pontoppidan, 1968; Field et al., 1982) was found to be greater during mechanical ventilation than during spontaneous breathing.

In such patients, assisted mechanical ventilation may induce a iatrogenic ventilator dependency (Banner et al., 1986; Civetta, 1993). On the other hand, it seems likely that the muscle activity associated with active breathing efforts during mechanical ventilation is sufficient to prevent atrophy of the respiratory muscles (Marini et al., 1985b). Therefore, it is unclear whether the respiratory muscles should be rested completely by the use of mechanical ventilation and what the appropriate balance is between rest and "respiratory muscle training" (Rochester et al., 1977).

The Oxygen Cost of Breathing in Patients During Weaning Trials

As already discussed, the total inspiratory work required for spontaneous breathing is influenced by the breathing pattern (depth or V_T, rate and mean inspiratory flow rate) and the impedance characteristics of the respiratory system (compliance and resistance). When a high minute ventilation is required, inspiratory flow rate and VT increase. The resulting effect on the total work of breathing is doubly important, since both work per liter of ventilation and minute ventilation are increased.

Pathological conditions that decrease compliance (lung edema, pleural effusion, pneumothorax, acute respiratory distress syndrome, lung or chest restrictive disease) or increase resistance (bronchospasm, retained secretions, external loads) will increase the ventilatory workload. Several authors have reported a tenfold increase in the work of breathing over normal resting values in spontaneously breathing ICU patients with acute respiratory failure and such an increase may lead to respiratory muscle fatigue and a need for mechanical ventilation (Roussos and Macklem, 1982; Cohen et al., 1982).

During weaning trials, therefore, patients should be positioned to minimize chest wall distance, i.e., sitting upright rather than supine, so that the hydrostatic forces of abdominal weight do not press on the diaphragm, thereby loading inspiration. Diuretics can be used to minimize lung water and improve lung compliance, especially during cardiogenic pulmonary edema (Lemaire and Teboul, 1989), and large fluid collections should be drained (Marini, 1990).

In critically ill patients, clinicians must keep in mind that although the energy expenditure of breathing increases with external work performed, the extent of the increase depends mainly on the mechanical efficiency of breathing. The analysis of the interplay between the work performed, the energy available for breathing, and the efficiency of respiratory muscles is a difficult but necessary analysis for the intensivist who tries to define optimal ventilator settings.

Take, as an example, Figure 17, used also in Chapter 25. The lower right quadrant of this figure shows the relationship between power output and ventilation when the resistance imposed on the patient is increased. The right upper quadrant illustrates the relationship betwen energy expenditure and power output at different levels of respiratory muscle efficiency (1–20%). Energy is expressed in kg/m/min or in the equivalent milliliters of oxygen per minute. According to the lower right quadrant, the work of breathing required for a given minute ventilation may increase greatly in patients with airway obstruction and/or breathing through endotracheal tubes and respirator valves and circuitry. As indicated in the upper right quadrant, for a given rate of work of breathing or power (10 kg/m/min, for instance, which is a common value in disease), oxygen consumption will increase as the efficiency decreases from 20% to 1%. Theoretically, critically ill patients with a low efficiency of the respiratory muscles may require up to 400 ml of O_2/min for the metabolic requirements of respiratory muscles. However, according to the left upper quadrant, the relationship between respiratory muscle blood flow and oxygen cost of breathing varies greatly with the arteriovenous oxygen content differences across the muscle. Clearly, for any given oxygen cost of breathing, the smaller the arteriovenous difference (as in septic shock, anemia, and hypoxemia), the greater the required

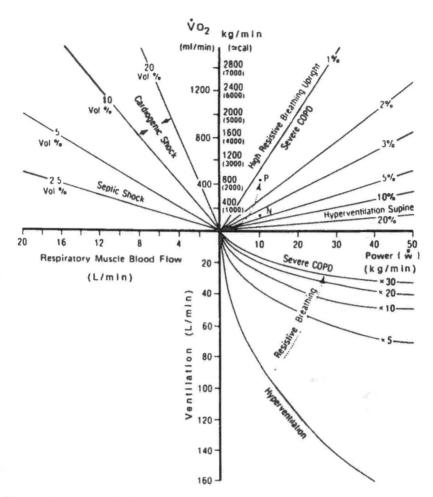

Figure 17 Relationship between respiratory muscle energetics and overall body economy in health and disease. For details, see text. Vo_2 = oxygen uptake; COPD = chronic obstructive pulmonary disease. (From Roussos, 1985.)

blood flow. In other words, in the critically ill patient, the percentage of cardiac output used by the respiratory muscles may vary enormously even for the same level of minute ventilation, power output efficiency, and oxygen consumption.

Under normal conditions, high blood flow and oxygen requirements of the respiratory muscle pose no threat to the body as a whole. However, high requirements of blood flow by respiratory muscles may have important consequences in patients with decreased oxygen delivery (i.e., decreased cardiac output, hypoxemia, anemia, altered oxygen extraction) and/or high total-body Vo_2 (fever, agitation, release of catecholamines, sepsis). In fact, experimental studies on animals in circulatory shock caused by pericardial tamponade showed that during spontaneous ventilation the respiratory muscles received 20% of the cardiac output, compared to 3% in paralyzed and mechanically ventilated animals (Viires et al., 1983). This large fraction of cardiac output to the respiratory muscles inevitably reduces flow to the brain, liver, and other skeletal muscles if mechanical ventilation is not used (Fig. 18) and could be responsible for the higher mortality of spontaneously breathing animals than of ventilated ones (Aubier et al., 1981). For the same reason, the cardiac stress accompanying the breathing workload during weaning could lead to unsuccessful weaning in patients with chronic obstructive pulmonary disease and congestive heart failure (Lemaire et al., 1988; Permutt, 1988).

The logical implication of the above analysis and experimental evidence is clear: when the cardiac output is depressed and/or the patient is anemic or hypoxemic, the high oxygen cost of breathing may deprive the rest of the body of

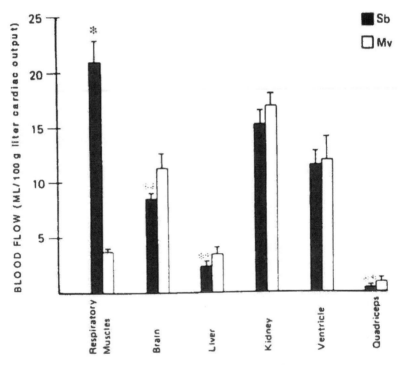

Figure 18 Comparison of the fractional distribution of cardiac output during tamponade in spontaneous breathing dogs (Sb, solid columns) and in mechanically ventilated dogs (MV, open columns). The significantly decreased perfusion of the brain, liver, and quadriceps in Sb animals is due to the fact that their respiratory muscles received a significantly greater portion of cardiac output. (From Viires et al., 1983.)

desperately needed energy supplies. Conversely, blood and oxygen uptake by other body tissues may deprive the respiratory muscles of blood, thereby inducing anaerobic metabolism and eventually fatigue and alveolar hypoventilation. Placing the respiratory muscles at rest by appropriately adjusted mechanical ventilation appears to be the best solution for such critically ill patients.

References

Annat G, Viale JP, Bertrand O, et al. Measurement of oxygen consumption and carbon dioxide production in artificially ventilated patients. In Pulmonary Function in Mechanically Ventilated Patients. Edited by J. L. Vincent. Berlin, Springer Verlag, 1991, pp 62–80.

Armaganidis A, Roussos CH. Work of breathing in the critically ill patient. In Current Pneumology, edited by D. H. Simmons. St. Louis, Mosby-Year Book, 1987, pp 51–86.

Aubier M, Trippenbach T, Roussos CH. Respiratory muscle fatigue during cardiogenic shock. J Appl Physiol 1981; 51:499–508.

Aubier M. Role of respiratory muscles in weaning. In Update on Intensive and Emergency Medicine. Edited by J. L. Vincent. Brussels, Springer Verlag, 1987, pp 240–249.

Aukburg SJ, Geer RT, Wollman H, Neufeld GR. Errors in measurement of oxygen uptake due to anesthetic gases. Anesthesiology 1985; 62:54–59.

Banner MJ, Lampotang S, Boysen PG, et al. Flow resistance of expiratory positive pressure valve systems. Chest 1986; 90:212–219.

Bartlett RG, Brubach MF, Specht H. The oxygen cost of breathing. J Appl Physiol 1958; 12:413–434.

Baydur A, Behrakis K, Zin A. A simple method for assessing the validity of esophageal balloon technique. Am Rev Respir Dis 1982; 126:788–791.

Baydur A, Cha E, Sassoon CSH. Validation of esophageal balloon technique at different lung volumes and postures. J Appl Physiol 1987; 62:315–321.

Bellemare F, Grassino A. Effect of pressure and timing of contraction on human diaphragm fatigue. J Appl Physiol 1982; 53:1190–1195.

Bellemare F, Grassino A. Force reserve of the diaphragm in patients with chronic obstructive pulmonary disease. J Appl Physiol 1983; 55:8–15.

Bergofsky EH, Turino GM, Fishman AP. Cardiorespiratory failure in kyphoskoliosis. Medicine 1959; 38:263–317.

Berry PR, Pontoppidan H. Oxygen consumption and blood gas exchange during controlled and spontaneous ventilation in patients with respiratory failure. Anesthesiology 1968; 29:177–178.

Bersten AD, Rutten AJ, Vedig EA, et al. Additional work of breathing imposed by endotracheal tubes, breathing circuits and intensive care ventilators. Crit Care Med 1989; 17:671–677.

Bertrand O, Viale JP, Annat G, et al. Mass spectrometer system for long-term continuous measurements of V_{O_2} and V_{CO_2} during artificial ventilation. Med Biol Eng Comput 1986; 24:174–181.

Bigland B, Lippold OCJ. The relationship between force, velocity and integrated electrical activity in human muscles. J Physiol (Lond) 1954; 123:214–224.

Bredbacka S, Kawachi S, Norlander O, Kirk B. Gas exchange during ventilator treatment: a validation of a computerised technique and its comparison with the Douglas bag method. Acta Anaesthesiol Scand 1984; 28:462–468.

Brochard L, Pluskwa F, Lemaire F. Improved efficiency of spontaneous breathing with inspirator pressure support. Am Rev Respir Dis 1987; 136:411–415.

Brochard L, Rua F, Lorino, et al. The extra work of breathing due to the endotracheal tube is abolished during inspiratory pressure support breathing. Am Rev Respir Dis 1988; 137:A646.

Brochard L, Harf A, Lorino H, Lemaire F. Inspiratory pressure support prevents diaphragmatic fatigue during weaning from mechanical ventilation. Am Rev Respir Dis 1989; 139:513–521.

Browning JA, Linberg SE, Turney SZ, et al. The effects of a fluctuating FIO_2 on metabolic measurements in mechanically ventilated patients. Crit Care Med 1982; 10:82–85.

Bruce EN, Goldman MB. High frequency oscillations in human respiratory electromyograms during voluntary breathing. Brain Res 1983; 269:259–265.

Buchler B, Magder S, Roussos CH. Effects of pleural pressure and abdominal pressure on the diaphragmatic blood flow. J Appl Physiol 1985; 58:691–697.

Bursztein S, Taitelman U, DeMyrrenaere S, et al. Reduced oxygen consumption in catabolic states with mechanical ventilation. Crit Care Med 1978; 6:162–164.

Cain CC, Otis AB. Some physiological effects resulting from added resistance to respiration. J Aviat Med 1949; 20:149–160.

Campbell EJM, Westlake EK, Cherniack RM. Simple methods of estimating oxygen consumption and efficiency of the muscles of breathing. J Appl Physiol 1958; 11:303–308.

Carlsson M, Forsberg E, Thorne A, Nordenstrom J, Hedenstierna G. Evaluation of an apparatus for continuous monitoring of gas exchange in mechanically ventilated patients. Int J Clin Mon Comput 1985; 1:211–220.

Cherniak RM. The oxygen consumption and efficiency of respiratory muscles in health and emphysema. J Clin Invest 1959; 38:494–499.

Civetta JM. Nosocomial respiratory failure or iatrogenic ventilator dependency. Crit Care Med 1993; 21:171–173.

Cohen Ca, Zagelbaum G, Gross D, et al. Clinical manifestations of inspiratory muscle fatigue. Am J Med 1982; 73:308–316.

Collett PW, Perry C, Engel LA. Pressure time product, flow and oxygen cost of resistive breathing in humans. J Appl Physiol 1985; 58:1263–1272.

Cox D, Niblett DJ. Studies on continuous positive airway pressure breathing systems. Br J Anaesth 1984; 56:905–908.

Curtin NA, Woldge RC. Energy changes and muscular contraction. Physiol Rev 1978; 58:670–761.

Damask MC, Weissman C, Askanasi J, et al. A systematic method for validation of gas exchange measurements. Anesthesiology 1982; 57:213–218.

Downs JB, Klein EF, Desautels D et al. Intermittent mandatory ventilation: A new approach to weaning patients from mechanical ventilators. Chest 1973; 64:331–335.

Dubois AB, Brody AW, Lewis DH, et al. Oscillation mechanics of lungs and chest in man. J Appl Physiol 1956; 8:587–594.

Easton PA, Antonishen NR. Spontaneous ventilation through a mechanical ventilator. The ventilatory effects of a demand valve. Am Res Pespir Dis 1986; 133:A121.

Fahri LE, Rahn H. Gas stores of the body and the unsteady state. J Appl Physiol 1955; 7:472–484.

Fiastro FJ, Habib MP, Quan SF. Pressure support compensation for inspiratory work due to endtracheal tubes and demand continuous positive airway pressure. Chest 1988; 93:499–505.

Field S, Kelly SM, Macklem PT. The oxygen cost of breathing in patients with cardiorespiratory disease. Am Rev Respir Dis 1982; 126:9–13.

Field S, Sanci S, Grassino A. Respiratory muscle oxygen consumption estimated by the diaphragm pressure time index. J Appl Physiol 1984; 57:44–51.

Fritts HW Jr, Filler J, Fishman AP, et al. The efficiency of ventilation during voluntary hyperpnea: Studies in normal subjects and in dyspneic patients with early chronic pulmonary emphysema or obesity. J Clin Invest 1959; 38:1339–1348.

Gherini S, Peters RM, Virgilio RW. Mechanical work on the lungs and work of breathing with positive end expiratory pressure and continuous positive airway pressure. Chest 1979; 76:251–256.

Gibbs CL. Cardiac energetics. Physiol Rev 1978; 58:174–254.

Gibbs CL, Chapman JB. Cardiac energetics. In Handbook of Physiology, Section 2: The Cardiovascular System, vol 1: The heart. Edited by RM Berne, Sperelakis S, Geiger S, Washington DC., American Physiologic Society, 1979, pp 775–804.

Gibney RTN, Wilson RS, Pontoppidan H. Comparison of work of breathing on high gas flow and demand valve continuous positive airway pressure systems. Chest 1982; 82:692–695.

Gillespie DJ. Comparison of intraesophageal balloon pressure with nasogastric-esophageal balloon system in volunteers. Am Rev Respir Dis 1982; 126:583–585.

Goldman MD, Grimby G, Mead J. Mechanical work of breathing derived from rib cage and abdominal P-V partitioning. J Appl Physiol 1976; 41:752–763.

Grassino A, Whitelaw WA, Milic Emili J. Influence of lung volume and electrode position on electromyography of the diaphragm. J Appl Physiol 1976; 40:971–975.

Gross D, Grassino A, Roos WRD, et al. Electromyographic pattern of diaphragmatic fatigue. J Appl Physiol 1979; 46:1–7.

Harden KA, Bartlett RG, Barnes H, et al. The cost of breathing. Part I. Am Rev Respir Dis 1962; 85:387–391.

Henry WC, West GA, Wilson RS. A comparison of the oxygen cost of breathing between a continuous flow CPAP system and a demand flow CPAP system. Respir Care 1983; 28:1273–1281.

Hill AV. The variation of total heat production in a twitch with velocity of shortening. Proc R Soc Lond (Biol) 1964; 159:596–605.

Hillman K, Friedlos J, Davey A. A comparison of intermittent mandatory systems. Crit Care Med 1986; 14:499–502.

Homsher E, Kean CJ. Skeletal muscle energetics and metabolism. Annu Rev Physiol 1978; 40:93–131.

Hubmayr RD, Abel MD, Rehder K. Physiologic approach to mechanical ventilation. Crit Care Med 1990; 18:103–113.

Katz JA, Marks JD. Inspiratory work with and without continuous positive airway pressure in patients with acute respiratory failure. Anesthesiology 1985; 63:598–603.

Katz JA, Kraemer RW, Gjerde GE. Inspiratory work and airway pressure with continuous positive airway pressure delivery systems. Chest 1985; 88:519–526.

Kemper M, Weissman C, Askanazi J, et al. Metabolic and respiratory changes during weaning from mechanical ventilation. Chest 1987; 92:979–983.

Kinney JM, Duke JH, Long CL, Gump FE. Tissue fuel and weight loss after injury. J Clin Pathol 1970; 23:64–72.

Kirby R, Smith RA, Desautels DA. Mechanical ventilation. In Respiratory Care: A Guide to Clinical Practice, 2nd ed. Edited by Burton GG, Hodgkin JE. Philadelphia, JB Lippincott, 1984, pp 571–573.

Lemaire F, Rieuf P, Rauss A, et al. A clinical comparison of the work of breathing through demand valve systems. Am Rev Respir Dis 1986; 133:A121.

Lemaire F, Teboul JL, Cinotti L, et al. Acute left ventricular dysfunction during unsuccessful weaning from mechanical ventilation. Anesthesiology 1988; 69:171–179.

Lemaire F, Teboul JL. Acute left ventricular dysfunction during unsuccessful weaning from mechanical ventilation. Anesthesiology 1989; 69:157–160.

Liljestrand G. Untersechungen uber die atmungsarbeit. Scand Arch Physiol 1918; 35:199–293.

Loring SH, Bruce EN. Methods for study of the chest wall. In Handbook of Physiology. Edited by Fishman AP, Mead J. Bethesda, American Physiological Society, 1986, pp 415–428.

Lourenco RV, Cherniack NS, Malm JR, et al. Nervous output from the respiratory center during obstructed breathing. J Appl Physiol 1966; 21:527–533.

MacIntyre NR. Respiratory function during pressure support ventilation. Probl Pulmon Dis 1986a; 2:1–8.

MacIntyre NR. Respiratory function during pressure support ventilation. Chest 1986b; 89:677–683.

Mancebo J, Brochard L, Amaro P, et al. Effect of bronchodilators on the work of breathing in intubated patients weaning from mechanical ventilation. Am Rev Respir Dis 1989; 139:A97.

Mancebo J. Measurement of the work of breathing in the mechanically ventilated patient. In Update on Intensive Care and Emergency Medicine. Edited by JL Vincent. Brussels, Springer Verlag, 1990, pp 252–259.

Marini JJ, Culver GH, Kirk BW. Flow resistance of exhalation valves and positive end expiratory pressure devices used in mechanical ventilation. Am Rev Respir Dis 1985a; 131:850–854.

Marini JJ, Capps JS, Culver BH. The inspiratory work of breathing during assisted mechanical ventilation. Chest 1985b; 87:612–618.

Marini JJ. The role of the inspiratory circuit in the work of breathing during mechanical tubes. Crit Care Med 1986a; 14:1028–1031.

Marini JJ. The physiologic determinants of ventilator dependence. Respir Care 1986b; 31:271–282.

Marini JJ, Smith TC, Lamb VJ. Rapid estimation of the inspiratory work of spontaneous breathing. Am Rev Respir Dis 1986a; 133:A120.

Marini JJ, Rodriguez M, Lamb V. The inspiratory workload of patient-initiated mechanical ventilation. Am Rev Respir Dis 1986b; 134:902–909.

Marini JJ. Monitoring during mechanical ventilation. Clin Chest Med 1988; 9:73–100.

Marini JJ, Smith TC, Lamb VJ. External work output and force generation during synchronised intermittent mechanical ventilation. Am Rev Respir Dis 1988; 138:1169–1179.

Marini JJ. Work of breathing during mechanical ventilation. In Update on Intensive Care and Emergency Medicine. Edited by J. L. Vincent. Berlin, Springer Verlag, 1990, pp 239–251.

Marini JJ. Assessment of the breathing workload during mechanical ventilation. In Pulmonary Function in Mechanically Ventilated Patients. Edited by J. L. Vincent. Berlin, Springer Verlag, 1991, pp 62–80.

Martin JG, Shore S, Engel LA. Effect of continuous positive airway pressure on respiratory mechanics and pattern of breathing in induced asthma. Am Rev Respir Dis 1982; 126:812–816.

Martin JG, Habib M, Engel LA. Inspiratory muscle activity during hyperinflation. Respir Physiol 1980; 39:303–311.

McGregor M, Becklake M. The relationship of oxygen cost of breathing to respiratory mechanical work and respiratory force. J Clin Invest 1961; 40:971–980.

Mead J. Measurement of intertia of the lungs at increased ambient pressure. J Appl Physiol 1956; 9:208–212.

Mecklenburgh JS, Latto IP, Al-Obaidi TAA, et al. Excessive work of breathing during intermittent mandatory ventilation. Br J Anesth 1986; 58:1048–1053.

Milic Emili J, Petit JM. Mechanical efficiency of breathing. J Appl Physiol 1960; 15:359–362.

Milic Emili J, Mead J, Turner JM, Glauser EM. Improved technique for estimating pleural pressure from esophageal balloons. J Appl Physiol 1964; 19:207–211.

Milic Emili J. Work of breathing. In The Lung, Chapter 5.1.2.8. Edited by RG Crystal, JB West, et al. New York, Raven Press, 1991, pp 1065–1075.

Mommaerts WFHM. Energetics of muscular contraction. Physiol Rev 1969; 49:427–508.

Newsom DJ. Phrenic nerve conduction in man. J Neurol Nurosurg Psychiatry 1967; 30:420–426.

Opie LH, Spalding JMK, Scott FD. Mechanical properties of the chest during intermit tent positive pressure respiration. Lancet 1959; 1:545–550.

Op't Holt TB, Hall MW, Bass JB, et al. Comparison of changes of airway pressure during continuous positive airway pressure (CPAP) between demand valve and continuous flow devices. Respir Care 1982; 27:1200–1209.

Otis AB. The work of breathing. Physiol Rev 1954; 34:449–458.

Otis AB, Fenn WO, Rahn H. Mechanics of breathing in man. J Appl Physiol 1950; 2:592–607.

Otis AB. The work of breathing. In Handbook of Physiology, section 3, Vol I. Edited by Fenn WO, Rahn H. Washington DC, American Physiological Society, 1964, pp 463–476.

Pepe PE, Marini JJ. Occult positive end expiratory pressure in mechanically ventilated patients with airflow obstruction. Am Rev Respir Dis 1982; 126:166–170.

Permutt S. Circulatory effects of weaning from mechanical ventilation: The importance of transdiaphragmatic pressure (editorial). Anesthesiology 1988; 69:157–160.

Peters RM, Hilberman M, Hogan JS, et al. Objective indications for respiratory therapy in post trauma and postoperative patients. Am J Surg 1972; 124:262–268.

Petrof B, Legare M, Goldberg P, et al. Effects of continuous positive airway pressure (CPAP) on respiratory muscle function during weaning from mechanical ventilation in COPD. Am Rev Respir Dis 1988; 137:A65.

Prakash O, Meij SH. Oxygen consumption and blood gas exchange during controlled and intermittent mandatory ventilation after cardiac surgery. Crit Care Med 1985; 13:556–559.

Proctor HJ, Woolson R. Prediction of respiratory muscle fatigue by measurements of the work of breathing. Surg Gynecol Obstet 1973; 136:367–370.

Robertson CH, Pagel MA, Johnson RL. The distribution of blood flow, oxygen consumption, and work output among the respiratory muscles during obstructed hyperventilation. J Clin Invest 1977; 59:43–50.

Rochester DF. Measurement of diaphragmatic blood flow and oxygen consumption in the dog by Kety-Schmidt technique. J Clin Invest 1974; 53:1126–1221.

Rochester DF, Braun NMT, Laine S. Diaphragmatic energy expenditure in chrinic respiratory failure: The effects of assisted ventilation with body repirators. Am J Med 1977; 63:223–229.

Rohrer F. Physiologie der Atembewegung. In Handbuch der normalen und pathologischen Physiologie, vol 2. Edited by Bethe ATJ, von Bergmann G, Embden G, Ellinger A. Berlin, Springer Verlag, 1925, pp 70–127.

Roussos CH, Macklem PT. Diaphragmatic fatigue in man. J Appl Physiol 1977; 43:189–197.

Roussos CH, Macklem, PT. The respiratory muscles. N Engl J Med 1982; 307:786–795.

Roussos CH. Structure and function of the thorax: Energetics. In The Thorax. Edited by Ch Roussos and PT Macklem. New York, Marcel Dekker, 1985; pp 437–492.

Sahn SA, Lakshminarayan, Petty TL. Weaning from mechanical ventilation. JAMA 1976; 235:2208–2212.

Sassoon CSH, Te T, Mahutte CK, et al. Inspiratory work of breathing: A function of the ventilatory inspiratory flow rates and tidal volume during assisted ventilation. Am Rev Respir Dis 1986; 133:A120.

Sassoon CSH, Mahutte CK, Te T, et al. Work of breathing and airway occlusion pressure during assistmode mechanical ventilation. Chest 1988; 93:571–576.

Sassoon CSH, Lodia R, Zari ZE, et al. Effects of T-piece, continuous positive airway pressure mechanical ventilation. Am Rev Respir Dis 1989a; 139:A97.

Sassoon CH, Giron AE, Ely EA, et al. Inspiratory work of breathing on flow-by and demand-flow continuous positive airway pressure. Crit Care Med 1989b; 17:1108–1114.

Savino JA, Dawson JA, Agarwal N, et al. The metabolic cost of breathing in critical surgical patients. J Trauma 1985; 25:1126–1133.

Shapiro M, Wilson RK, Casar G, et al. Work of breathing through different sized endotracheal tubes. Crit Care Med 1986; 14:1028–1031.

Sharp J, Henry JP, Sweany SK, et al. The total work of breathing in normal and obese men. J Clin Invest 1964; 43:728–739.

Smith TC, Marini JJ, Lamb VJ. Active expiratory work of breathing during mechanical ventilation. Am Rev Respir Dis 1986; 133:A121.

Smith TC, Marini JJ. Impact of PEEP on lung mechanics and work of breathing in severe airflow obstruction. J Appl Physiol 1988; 65:1488–1499.

Specht NL. Killeen T, Roos PJ, et al. Comparison of intermittent mandatory ventilation and T-piece as a method of mechanical ventilation. Am Res Respir Dis 1988; 137:66.

Sullivan MJ, Paliotta J, Saklad M. Endotracheal tube as a factor in measurement of respiratory mechanics. J Appl Physiol 1976; 41:590–595.

Swinamer DL, Fedoruk LM, Jones RL, et al. Energy expenditure associated with CPAP and T-piece spontaneous ventilatory trails: Changes following prolonged mechanical ventilation. Chest 1989; 96:867–872.

Thung N, Herzog P, Christlieb I, et al. The cost of respiratory effort in postoperative cardiac patients. Circulation 1963; 28:552–559.

Truwit JD, Marini JJ. Evaluation of thoracic mechanics in the ventilated patient. Part II: Applied mechanics. J Crit Care 1988; 3:199–213.

Ultman JS, Bursztein S. Analysis of error in the determination of respiratory gas exchange at varying FiO2. J Appl Physiol 1981; 50:210–216.

Viale JP, Annat G, Betrand O, et al. Additional inspiratory work in intubated patients breathing with continuous positive airway pressure systems. Anesthesiology 1985; 63:536–540.

Viale JP, Annat G, Betrand O, et al. Continuous measurement of pulmonary gas exchange during general anaesthesia in man. Acta Anaesthesiol Scand 1988a; 32:691–697.

Viale JP, Annat GJ, Bouffard YM, et al. Oxygen cost of breathing in postoperative patients: pressure support ventilation versus positive airway pressure. Chest 1988b; 93:506–509.

Viires N, Sillye N, Aubier M, et al. Regional blood flow distribution in dog during induced hypotention and low cardiac output. J Clin Invest 1983; 72:935–947.

Ward ME, Corbeil C, Gibbons W, et al. Work of breathing during mechanical ventilation as a function of peak inspiratory flow rate. Am Rev Respir Dis 1985; 31:A131.

Ward ME, Corbeil C, Gibbons W, et al. Optimization of respiratory relaxation during mechanical ventilation. Anesthesiology 1988; 69:29–35.

Wilkie DR. The efficiency of muscular contraction. J Mechanochem Cell Motil 1974; 2:257–267.

Wilson SH, Looke NT, Maxham J, Spiro SJ. Sternomastoid muscle function and fatigue in normal subjects and in patients with chronic obstructive pulmonary disease. Am Rev Respir Dis 1984; 129:460–464.

Wilson RS, Sullivan SF, Malm JR, et al. The oxygen cost of breathing following anesthesia and cardiac surgery. Anesthesiology 1973; 39:387–393.

Yang SC, Specht NL, Killeen T, et al. Comparison of intermittent mandatory ventilation and T-piece as a weaning method from mechanical ventilation. Am Rev Respir Dis 1988; 137:A66.

43

Assessment of Respiratory Sensation

MURRAY D. ALTOSE

Case Western Reserve University School of Medicine
Cleveland, Ohio

I. Introduction

Breathing differs from other homeostatic processes in that it both regulates the internal metabolic milieu of the body and also participates in a wide variety of volitional activities and behavioral acts of daily living. The coordination and integration of these wide-ranging and diverse functions requires a complex control system.

The control of breathing is fundamentally automatic and reflex. Networks of neurons in the brain stem receive input from chemoreceptors in the blood and brain that are activated by changes in oxygen and carbon dioxide levels in the body and in turn govern the activity of chest wall and upper airway muscles allowing ventilation (Mitchell and Berger, 1981). Additionally, respiratory neurons in the bulbopontine areas of the brain receive afferent impulses that arise during breathing from vagal receptors in the airways and lungs including pulmonary stretch receptors, irritant receptors around the epithelial cells of the bronchial walls, and C-fibers in the interstitium of the lung in proximity to the alveoli and pulmonary capillaries (Coleridge and Coleridge, 1986). Feedback from sensory receptors in the respiratory muscles also contributes to the automatic control of breathing (Shannon, 1986). Muscle spindles, predominantly in the intercostal muscles, monitor changes in muscle length and participate in both spinal and supraspinal reflexes. Tendon organs, primarily in the diaphragm but also in the intercostal muscles, are stimulated by increases in muscle tension and exert an inhibitory influence on medullary respiratory activity.

In addition to automatic reflex regulation at a brain stem level, breathing is also behaviorally controlled from higher brain centers (Plum, 1970). This behavioral control involving somatomotor and forebrain structures can, on a short-term basis, suppress or override automatic mechanisms, for example, with bending, lifting, or straining and during breath-holding and vocalization (Fowler, 1954; Bunn and Mead, 1971; Phillipson et al., 1978). Behavioral adjustments in breathing also accompany emotions like anger and fear and emotional expressions such as laughing or crying. In patients with chronic lung disease, volitional or behavioral influences may result in long-term or persistent changes in the level and pattern of breathing (Sorli et al., 1978; Oliven et al., 1985). These adaptive changes could serve to improve the efficiency of gas exchange in the lungs or minimize respiratory force output to relieve dyspnea.

Higher brain center influences on respiration have been discerned from changes in breathing activity including respiratory apraxia, posthyperventilation apnea, and enhanced respiratory responsiveness to chemical stimulation noted in patients with injuries or diseases of the cerebral hemispheres (Plum and Leigh, 1981). Additionally, neurophysiological and neuroanatomical studies in experimental animals have shown direct projections from the cerebral cortex to respiratory motoneuron pools in the spinal cord (Lipski et al., 1986). More recently motor cortical representation of the chest wall respiratory muscles has been demonstrated in humans using transcranial electrical or magnetic stimulation (Gandevia and Rothwell, 1987; Gandevia and Plassmann, 1988; Maskill et al., 1991). These pathways from the motor cortex are rapidly conducting and oligosynaptic, and innervation is contralateral.

The appropriate shaping of behavioral influences on breathing requires that higher brain centers be apprised of the state of the respiratory muscles, the condition of the lungs and chest wall, and the metabolic milieu. Indeed, sensory information from the ventilatory apparatus does project to the somatosensory cortex. Stimulation of afferents in the phrenic nerve and intercostal muscle mechanoreceptors evokes small short-latency focal cortical responses in the cat (Davenport et al., 1985; Davenport et al., 1993). In humans, sudden inspiratory airway occlusions produce evoked potentials over the somatosensory cortex (Davenport et al., 1986; Revelette and Davenport, 1990). The studies by Gandevia and Macefield (1989) provide clear evidence for a direct projection to the cerebral cortex of low threshold muscle afferents from the parasternal and lateral intercostal muscles of conscious humans.

The central processing of afferent projections from the ventilatory apparatus to higher brain centers appears to give rise to evoked sensations of the depth and force of breathing as well as the sensation of dyspnea. These perceptual responses may in turn play an important role in behavioral adjustments in the level and pattern of breathing. The study of respiratory sensation has enhanced our understanding of the mechanisms involved in the behavioral control of breathing and the adjustments in breathing patterns that accompany diseases of the lung. It has provided new insights into the basis of dyspnea and a framework for the medical management of this disabling symptom.

II. Sensory Mechanism

Sensations including those related to breathing originate with the stimulation of receptors. With respect to the respiratory system, receptors that may subserve respiratory sensation include mechanoreceptors in airways, lungs, respiratory muscles, or other chest wall structures and chemoreceptors that monitor blood gases or acid-base status (Altose, 1986). Receptor stimulation is transduced into neural electrical impulses that are transmitted along afferent pathways. The neural information is shaped by the firing frequency and the specific synapses being activated. Finally, central processing by higher brain centers involving recapitulation, abstraction, and interpretation results in some evoked expression (Livingstone, 1991).

In keeping with these physiological concepts, the study of respiratory sensation requires the identification and control of specific stimulus parameters related to the act of breathing and the development of quantitative measures of subjective response. Psychophysical techniques have provided a particularly useful and productive methodological approach.

III. Psychophysics

Psychophysics is the study of the functional relations between stimulus variables on a physical continuum and the corresponding conscious sensation. Measurements of sensation can be made indirectly by determining a stimulus threshold, i.e., the smallest intensity of a stimulus that can be reliably perceived, or a difference threshold, i.e., the magnitude of a change in stimulus intensity that is reliably perceived as a just noticeable difference. In direct measurements of sensation, subjects assign a value on a rating scale to the magnitude of the sensation evoked in response to the application of a stimulus (Kling and Riggs, 1971).

Because of the complexity of breathing, it is not possible to stimulate one type of receptor directly and exclusively. For example, during the act of taking a breath, the respiratory muscles develop tension and change their length, thereby activating tendon organs and muscle spindles. Additionally, the flow of air along the airways and expansion of the lungs simultaneously activate vagal receptors. Respiratory psychophysical studies have focused instead on several basic respiratory sensations. These include (1) the sensation of displacement that accompanies changes in lung volume, (2) the sensation of respiratory force associated with changes in airway, intrathoracic, or transdiaphragmatic pressure, and (3) the respiratory load sensation that follows the application of external ventilatory resistive or elastic loads. Psychophysical approaches have also been used to investigate the mechanisms of more complex sensations such as the sensation of effort and the sensation of discomfort as respiratory activity is changed volitionally, by exercise, during hypercapnia or hypoxia, or with progressive ventilatory loading.

IV. Threshold Discrimination

E. H. Weber, a nineteenth-century German physiologist, first showed that the amount by which the intensity of a stimulus must be changed in order for a sensory change to be detected ($\Delta\Phi$) is a constant fraction of the baseline stimulus intensity (Φ). In other words, a stimulus of high magnitude and one of low magnitude must undergo the same fractional change in intensity in order to produce a just noticeable difference in sensation. This relationship, expressed mathematically as $\Delta\Phi/\Phi = k$, where k is a constant, is known as Weber's law and remains a general statement of the discriminability of stimuli in all sensory modalities. Subsequently, G. T. Fechner used Weber's minimal detectable change or just noticeable difference as a unit of measurement of sensory intensity and formulated a basic logarithmic psychophysical law, $\Psi = k \log (\Phi/b)$, where Ψ is the sensation intensity, Φ is the physical magnitude of the stimulus, b is the stimulus magnitude at the absolute threshold, and k is a constant. According to this formulation, the sensation intensity resulting from a given physical stimulus is the sum of just noticeable differences from the absolute threshold, with each just noticeable difference considered to be of equal subjective magnitude (Boring, 1942).

There are several classical methods for determining absolute and difference thresholds. These include (1) the method of limits, (2) the method of adjustment, and (3) the method of constant stimuli (Craig and Metze, 1986).

In the method of limits, stimuli over a range of intensities from well below to well above threshold levels are presented in alternating ascending and descending order. In a series of trials, the magnitude of the stimulus is gradually increased or decreased in small discrete steps, and with each presentation subjects respond with a yes or a no depending on whether they perceive the stimulus. Difference thresholds can also be determined by pairing a standard stimulus with each variable target stimulus, and subjects are required to specify whether the two stimuli are different or the same. The threshold for each trial is determined from the stimulus magnitude at the point where the subjective response changes. The overall threshold is calculated from the mean of equal numbers of ascending and descending trial thresholds.

The method of limits can be used to determine the threshold for the detection of added ventilatory loads (Zechman and Burki, 1976). External resistive ventilatory loading that changes pressure-flow relationships during breathing can be produced by partially obstructing the breathing circuit. Commonly, a series of resistive loads is made up by securing screen discs with differing resistances at intervals of distance along a wide-bore tube (Fig. 1). By unplugging one of the lateral outlets along the wide-bore tube between the arrangement of screens, any one of a number of specific resistances can be applied. External elastic loading that changes pressure-volume relationships can be produced by having subjects breath from a sealed, rigid container. Graded elastic loads can be made up by arranging different-sized rigid containers in parallel (Fig. 2). Each container is separated from the common line by a stopcock, and by selectively opening the various stopcocks any one of a number specific elastic loads can be applied.

The method of limits has several potential sources of error. The starting point of each trial must be changed from series to series to prevent the development of a response pattern independent of stimulus conditions. In progressive ascending and descending trials, response habituation may occur where responses are shaped by those during the preceding presentation.

In the method of adjustment also known as the method of average error, the subject rather than the experimenter adjusts a variable stimulus so that it equals a standard stimulus. As in the method of limits, there are alternating ascending and descending trials with varying starting distances. The point at which the variable stimulus is felt subjectively to be equal to the standard stimulus is referred to as the point of subjective equality. The difference between the physical magnitude of the variable stimulus and the standard stimulus at the point of subjective equality is termed the constant error. The standard deviation of the constant error over repeated trials provides a measure of the difference threshold (Baird and Noma, 1978).

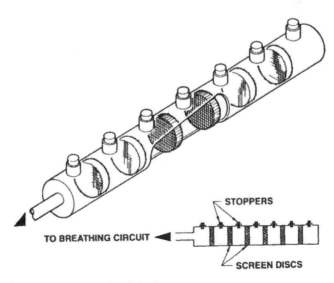

Figure 1 Apparatus for graded resistive loading.

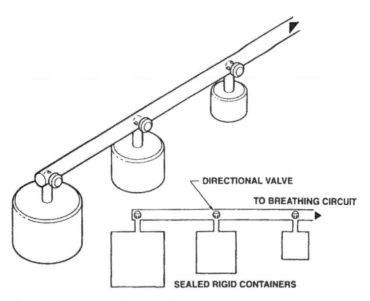

Figure 2 Apparatus for graded elastic loading.

The method of adjustment has been used to determine the threshold for detection of changes in inspired volume (Gliner et al., 1981; DiMarco et al., 1982). The subject first produces a target tidal volume either spontaneously or by following a tracing on an oscilloscope. Next, in the absence of any external feedback, the subject undertakes to duplicate the target volume. The procedure is repeated several times so that the constant error can be determined and the difference threshold calculated.

Because subjects are active in manipulating the variable stimulus in the method of adjustment, errors of habituation or anticipation are less likely compared to the method of limits. Subjects, however, must understand the task to be performed and must know how to manipulate the variable stimulus.

The most commonly used method in studies of ventilatory load detection is the method of constant stimuli, also known as the frequency method (Campbell et al., 1961; Bennett et al., 1962; Wiley and Zechman, 1967; Gottfried et al., 1978). A series of from five to nine discrete ventilatory loads that bracket the threshold for detection are selected. The range of loads should be such that at one end the stimulus is rarely perceived, while at the other end the stimulus is almost always perceived. Each of the loads is presented in a random order many times, and with each presentation the subject indicates whether the added load is perceived. In general the percentage of presentations that is detected increases progressively with the intensity of the stimulus. That load level that is detected during 50% of the presentations is considered the threshold for detection or the just noticeable difference.

During testing of threshold discrimination, subjects' responses may be biased by motivation, expectation, or attitude so that the results may not accurately reflect the actual sensitivity to physical stimuli. For example, an aggressive risk taker with lax decision criteria may maximize the number of correct detections of a stimulus, i.e., hits, by regularly signaling false alarms where the stimulus was not present but the subject indicated that it was. On the other hand, a cautious, conservative subject with the same perceptual sensitivity to the physical stimulus but with stringent decision criteria would have fewer false alarms but also a smaller proportion of hits. In the frequency method of testing threshold discrimination, response bias can be roughly assessed from the false alarm rate during catch trials where no stimulus is actually presented. Response bias can be minimized but not totally eliminated by training subjects to maintain a low, constant false alarm rate.

Sensory factors can be distinguished from decision criteria using formal signal detection theory techniques (Swets et al., 1968). Subjects are repeatedly presented with either a test stimulus or a blank control in a random order. With each presentation, subjects respond either affirmatively or negatively depending on whether they feel the test stimulus was present. In separate trials the decision criterion is changed either by instructing the subjects to be more lax or stringent or by changing the payoffs for different decisions. A receiver-operating-characteristic (ROC) curve is then constructed by plotting the hit rate on the vertical axis against the false alarm rate on the horizontal axis (Fig. 3). If the test stimulus is below the detection threshold, responses will be random and the ROC curve will fall along the diagonal from the lower left- to upper right-hand corners. The area between that diagonal and ROC curves situated upward and to the left is a measure of detectability

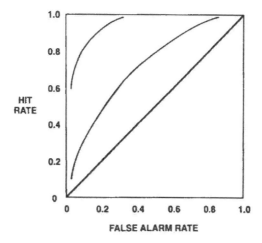

Figure 3   Receiver-operating-characteristic (ROC) curve.

that is independent of response bias. Signal detection theory techniques are theoretically and statistically sound, but experiments are long, arduous, and tedious. Consequently, they are used rarely in studies of respiratory sensation.

V. Detection of Ventilatory Loads

Campbell et al. (1961) and Bennett et al. (1962) were the first to use tests of threshold discrimination to measure the just noticeable difference for added resistive and elastic loads. Normally a 10–20% change in the elastic load to breathing is required before the added load is detected. Similarly, resistive load detection occurs only after a 25–30% change in resistance. In keeping with Weber's law, the just noticeable difference in airflow resistance increases proportionally with the baseline resistance (Gottfried et al., 1981). In asthmatics the just noticeable difference in airflow resistance is greater than normal, but this increase is accounted for by their elevated baseline airway resistance since the Weber fraction is the same as that in normal individuals. In contrast, the just noticeable difference in airflow resistance expressed as a fraction of the baseline resistance in patients with chronic obstructive pulmonary disease is greater than normal (Gottfried et al., 1981). This suggests an impairment in ventilatory load detection that could be the result of respiratory mechanoreceptor dysfunction or a defect in the central processing of mechanoreceptor inputs.

Numerous studies have investigated the mechanisms of ventilatory load detection. Guz et al. (1966) have reported that elastic load detection is unaffected by bilateral vagal blockade in normal subjects. The finding that airway anesthesia does not alter ventilatory load detection also suggests that sensory information arising in upper airway receptors is not important in mediating the sensation of ventilatory loads (Chaudhary and Burki, 1978, 1980). More recently it has been shown that the detection of resistive ventilatory loads in heart-lung transplant recipients is no different from that in normal control subjects, indicating that lower respiratory tract pulmonary afferents are not essential for load sensation (Tapper et al., 1992).

The observation that load detection is impaired during passive ventilation points to a key role for active respiratory muscle contraction (Killian et al., 1980). However, spinal anesthesia to the level of the first thoracic segment does not affect elastic load detection (Eisele et al., 1968). Some but not all studies also report that ventilatory load detection is no different from normal in patients with low cervical spinal cord transection that interrupts feedback from intercostal muscle receptors (Newsom Davis, 1967; Zechman et al., 1967; Noble et al., 1971).

There is a close temporal relationship between changes in transdiaphragmatic pressure and load detection, suggesting that information based on diaphragmatic tension is involved in the detection of added ventilatory loads (Zechman et al., 1985). Yet bilateral phrenic nerve block does not impair load detection (Noble et al., 1970). These conflicting experimental results point to great redundancy of signals during ventilatory loading. Following the loss of sensory information from one source, alternate sensory pathways remain available to signal the presence of an added ventilatory load.

VI. Detection of Changes in Breath Volume

Different investigators using a variety of psychophysical techniques have shown that the just noticeable difference in inspired volume during normal or near normal tidal breathing is about 100 ml (Gliner et al., 1981; Wolkove et al., 1981; DiMarco et al., 1982; Katz-Salamon, 1984). As the baseline inspired volume enlarges, the just noticeable difference in inspired volume increases in keeping with Weber's law. Benzett et al. (1987) have reported that tracheotomized, high-level (C1–C3) quadriplegics are able to detect changes in ventilator-delivered tidal volume as well as normal subjects. Since high cervical spinal cord transection eliminates feedback of sensory information from the chest wall, including the rib cage, intercostal muscles, and diaphragm, it seems that sensory information from intrathoracic airway or pulmonary receptors carried along the vagus nerve may project to higher brain centers and mediate the sensation of thoracic displacement. However, tidal volume reproduction studies where the load on the ventilatory muscles was changed between control and test breaths indicate that the sensation of changes in tidal volume is based not only on signals related to volume per se but also on information about the forces generated by the respiratory muscles (Stubbing et al., 1981; DiMarco et al., 1982).

The role of rib cage receptors in the sensation of inspired volume has been assessed by comparing the detection of changes in inspired volume during active breathing in normal subjects and in quadriplegics with low cervical spinal cord transection (DiMarco et al., 1982). There are no differences in the ability of normal subjects and quadriplegic patients to reproduce inspired volumes, suggesting that inputs from rib cage receptors are not essential to the sensation of inspired volume. However, it is possible that feedback from mechanoreceptors in the diaphragm or accessory muscles or the intensity of central motor command signals contribute to shaping respiratory volume sensation.

VII. Psychophysical Scaling

It has become widely accepted that the subjective sensation evoked by the presentation of a physical stimulus is measurable and can be quantitated by matching the perceived magnitude of the sensation to some other continuum such as a system of numbers. There are different types of scales depending on the rules for assigning a number to represent an attribute on a psychological dimension (Kling and Riggs, 1971).

Nominal scales use numbers to represent differences of kind rather than degree and to label different categories of objects, events, or phenomena. The relative size or value of a number on a nominal scale has no meaning. Ordinal scales rank objects, events, or phenomena according to the magnitude or degree of some particular attribute, but ordinal scale numbers do not reflect the magnitude of the differences between categories. Interval scales have all of the properties of an ordinal scale, but in addition the magnitude of differences between successive points on the scale is constant. For example, on a 10-point interval scale the difference between scale points 2 and 3 represents the same degree of change as the difference between scale points 8 and 9. Ratio scales differ from interval scales in that a ratio scale has a true zero point where none of the attributes being measured exists. Correspondingly, there is a proportional relationship between sensation intensity and scale numbers such that if one stimulus is perceived to be twice as large as another, it is assigned a number twice as big.

S. S. Stevens popularized the technique of ratio scaling to characterize the relationship between stimulus intensity and sensation magnitude when both are measured as qualities (Stevens, 1957, 1971, 1975). In the method of magnitude estimation, stimuli over a wide range of intensities are presented in random order and subjects assign a numerical value to each stimulus based on their perception of the intensity of that stimulus. Alternatively, using cross-modality matching, subjects can express the sensation response by generating a force on a handgrip dynamometer, for example, or by actively adjusting some other sensory signal such as the brightness of a light or the loudness of a sound to produce an intensity proportional to the perceived magnitude of the test stimulus. In magnitude production, subjects are provided with a numerical value of sensation magnitude and they adjust or produce a stimulus intensity to match the sensation level.

Stevens noted that a constant percentage change in stimulus intensity produced a constant percentage change in sensation magnitude. He proposed that the relationship between stimulus intensity (Φ) and sensation magnitude (Ψ) was not logarithmic, as previously suggested by Fechner, but rather exponential according to the equation $\Psi = k\Phi^n$, where k is a constant and n is the exponent of the power function. The value of the exponent, a measure of perceptual sensitivity, is readily determined from the slope of the straight line relationship between stimulus intensity and sensation response plotted on logarithmic coordinates. An exponent of greater than 1 indicates that the sensation grows more and more rapidly as the stimulus increases, while an exponent of less than 1 signifies that a wide range of stimulus intensities is compressed into a small range of subjective sensations.

The power function relationship between stimulus intensity and sensation magnitude has been shown to hold for many different sensory modalities, including loudness, brightness, sweetness, warmth, heaviness, and electric shock (Stevens, 1975). The exponents for magnitude scaling range from 0.33 for brightness to 1.5 for heaviness to 3.5 for electric shock. However, the exponent of the power function relationship for any given sensory modality varies depending on the specific set of experimental conditions. For example, exponents determined by magnitude production are higher than those obtained by magnitude estimation. This is explained by the tendency of subjects to constrict the range of that variable under their control. Similarly, there is a range effect whereby the exponents will vary depending on the range of stimulus intensities presented in an experimental session.

There are considerable interindividual differences in magnitude scaling exponents for a given sensory modality even when experimental conditions are tightly controlled. Consequently, exponents are determined from mean values in groups of 10 or more like subjects. In open magnitude scaling using ratio scales, values along the response continuum are proportional to the perceived intensity of the stimulus but in no way reflect absolute sensation magnitude. Thus, open magnitude ratio scale does not permit a comparison among individuals or groups of individuals of the absolute sensation magnitude produced by a given stimulus.

VIII. Magnitude Scaling of Ventilatory Loads

In ventilatory load scaling, loads over at least a 10-fold range are added to the breathing circuit for one or several consecutive breaths. With each presentation subjects respond by assigning a numerical value proportional to the perceived magnitude of the load. In normal subjects, the relationship between the physical magnitude of the ventilatory load and the resulting sensation follows the psychophysical power law (Altose and Cherniack, 1981; Killian et al., 1981). The exponent for the magnitude estimation of external elastic loads is approximately 1, indicating a near linear relationship between load intensity and sensation magnitude. The exponent for the magnitude estimation of resistive loads is about 0.8, indicating that the sensation magnitude grows less and less rapidly as the size of the load is increased. In an elegant series of experiments where subjects used a wide range of respiratory efforts and inspiratory durations during ventilatory load scaling, Killian et al. (1982) demonstrated that with both elastic and resistive loading there is a unique relationship between sensation magnitude (Ψ) and the product of peak airway pressure (P) and inspiratory duration (Ti), according to the equation $\Psi = kP^{1.3} \cdot Ti^{0.56}$, where k is a constant. These findings suggest that load sensation is preferentially shaped by the magnitude and the duration of the forces generated by the inspiratory muscles during the loaded breath. On the other hand, with explicit and detailed instructions subjects can also reliably scale resistance independent of the effort used in breathing (Altose et al., 1985). This appears to be the result of some complex integration by higher brain centers of separate pressure (muscle tension) and flow (rate of thoracic displacement) signals to procure a sensation proportional to resistance itself.

The exponents for the magnitude estimation of elastic and resistive ventilatory loads are reduced in the elderly (Tack et al., 1981, 1982). This impairment in ventilatory load sensation is part of age-related alterations in perceptual sensitivity and may be secondary to a generalized loss of kinesthetic sensibility with advancing age.

Compared to normal subjects, patients with chronic obstructive pulmonary disease also demonstrate impaired perceptual responses to resistive ventilatory loading and subnormal magnitude scaling exponents (Gottfried et al., 1985). The reduction in the perception of airway resistance is thought to be due to an impairment in the central nervous system integration of pressure and flow signals or possibly those signals related to respiratory muscle force and thoracic displacement.

IX. Magnitude Scaling of Respiratory Force and Displacement

The sensations of respiratory force and of thoracic displacement have been assessed by magnitude scaling of breath volume and of airway pressure during breathing maneuvers against a closed airway.

In magnitude estimation, subjects generate an inspired volume during a free inspiration or an inspiratory pressure during an effort against a closed airway from functional residual capacity and then assign a numerical value proportional to the perceived magnitude of the size of the breath or the level of force. In repeated trials inspired volumes are made to vary over the range of the inspiratory capacity and inspiratory pressures are made to vary up to the maximum inspiratory pressure.

Magnitude production involves providing the subject with numerical sensation targets ranging from zero to 100% of maximum. With each assigned numerical target, subjects are required to produce a corresponding inspired volume or inspiratory pressure in keeping with the rules of ratio scaling.

The results of magnitude scaling of breath volume were first reported by Bakers and Tenney (1970). Their findings have been reproduced on many occasions and indicate a power function relationship between inspired volume and sensation magnitude with an exponent of 1.3 (Stubbing et al., 1981; DiMarco et al., 1981). Katz-Salamon et al. (1976), however, subsequently demonstrated that magnitude scaling exponents differ systematically at lung volumes above and below functional residual capacity. This was explained by differences in the engagement of inspiratory and expiratory muscles during breathing above and below functional residual capacity. Sensory information from the respiratory muscles thus appears to be critical in shaping the sensation of thoracic displacement. This is also suggested by the observations that the perceived magnitude of breath volume varies with respiratory muscle tension and is greater during ventilatory loading and less during passive mechanical ventilation as compared to normal active breathing (Stubbing et al., 1981; DiMarco et al., 1981).

The sensation of respiratory force is quantitatively similar to the sensation of force in limb muscles and depends on both the magnitude and duration of muscle contraction (Altose et al., 1982; Stubbing et al., 1983). The exponent of the power function relationship between airway pressure and sensation magnitude is approximately 1.5. This exponent does not vary with age (Tack et al., 1983) and is no different from normal in patients with chronic obstructive pulmonary disease (Gottfried et al., 1985) or in quadriplegics in whom feedback from rib cage muscle receptors is disrupted (Gottfried et al., 1984).

Respiratory force sensation appears to have at least two components: a sense of tension related to feedback of afferent signals from muscle receptors and a sense of efforts based on central nervous system motor command signals. Sensations of muscle tension and effort are distinguishable and can be independently perceived (Altose et al., 1982). However, the sensation of respiratory force seems to be based preferentially on signals of motor command. This is suggested by the observations that when the respiratory muscles are weakened or fatigued so that a greater level of respiratory neuromotor output is required to achieve a given muscle tension, the sensation of respiratory force is intensified (Gandevia et al., 1981; Stubbing et al., 1981; Redline et al., 1991).

X. Mechanisms of Dyspnea

At least one aspect of the sensation of breathlessness or dyspnea is an expression of the sense of respiratory effort (Killian and Jones, 1988). The intensity of dyspnea increases progressively with the level of ventilation during exercise. With ventilatory loading, the intensity of dyspnea increases further at a given level of ventilation but continues to correspond to the level of respiratory motor output (Altose, 1992).

Chest wall receptors also appear to play a role in mediating the sensation of dyspnea. This is suggested by the observation that vibration of the chest wall to stimulate respiratory muscle mechanoreceptors reduces the severity of dyspnea (Homma et al., 1984; Manning et al., 1991; Sibuya et al., 1994). Changes in the firing of chest wall muscle mechanoreceptors may also explain the finding that the intensity of dyspnea increases when ventilation is voluntarily constrained below the spontaneously adopted breathing level even when chemical drive is held constant (Chonan et al., 1987; Chonan et al., 1990).

XI. Category Scaling

In open magnitude scaling subjects are free to use any range of numbers provided they adhere to the rule of ratios when comparing stimuli of different intensities. Because of differences in the range of numbers used by different subjects, open magnitude scaling does not provide any measure of absolute sensation magnitude to permit comparisons among individuals. This limitation can be overcome through the use of category scaling. Category scaling techniques are based on the assumption that the full extent of perceptual responses is encompassed within a closed range from a noise level at the threshold for detection to a maximum intensity level that is the same for all subjects. Category scales have interval properties and require the subject to partition a sensory continuum (Stevens, 1971). Scales such as the Borg scale (Table 1) may use numerical gradations and spaced verbal descriptors, e.g., mild, moderate, severe. The numbers and descriptions constitute the categories for partitioning the sensory continuum and provide a measure of absolute sensation magnitude (Borg, 1979, 1982). The visual analog scale, in contrast, is simply a line without numbers or descriptors (Fig. 4). One end of the line represents an absolute zero and may be labeled "none at all." The other end represents the maximum intensity level and may also be so labeled. The visual analog scale has an infinite number of intervals, and subjects, by making a point on the line, can establish their own interval size and absolute sensation magnitude (Aitken, 1969).

The characteristics of the visual analog scale, which include an absolute zero, an infinite number of potential categories, and the freedom to adjust interval size, may preserve the ratio properties of this scale and permit subjects to provide sensation responses that are proportional to the intensity of the stimulus. In contrast, the original Borg scale (Table 1), first developed for rating perceived exertion during exercise, was a 15-point graded category scale with numbers ranging from 6 to 20 and equally spaced verbal descriptors at every odd number (Borg, 1970). The scale ratings were set in such a way as to provide a linear relationship with exercise workload as work intensity varied from light to heavy work and to approximate one-tenth the expected heart rate of a middle-aged man at that work intensity (Borg, 1970). However, open magnitude scaling of perceived exertion revealed a power

Table 1 Borg Scales

Original		Revised	
No.	Descriptor	No.	Descriptor
6		0	nothing at all
7	very, very slight	0.5	very, very slight
8			
9	very slight	1.0	very slight
10			
11	slight	2.0	slight
12		3.0	moderate
13	somewhat severe	4.0	somewhat severe
14		5.0	severe
15	severe	6.0	
16		7.0	very severe
17	very severe	8.0	
18		9.0	very, very severe
19	very, very severe	10.0	maximal
20			

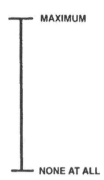

Figure 4 Visual analog scale.

function relationship between exercise workload and sensation magnitude with an exponent of 1.6, indicating that as work intensity doubles, the magnitude of the sensation of exertion increases threefold (Borg, 1970). Accordingly, the Borg scale has been modified in an attempt to provide it with ratio properties (Borg, 1982). The revised Borg scale is numbered from zero to 10, and the associated verbal descriptors are placed such that a doubling of the numerical rating corresponds to a twofold increase in sensation intensity (Table 1).

Using category scales such as visual analog scales or the modified Borg scale, the change in sensation magnitude for a given proportional change in stimulus intensity tends to be less than with open, magnitude scaling (Stevens and Galanter, 1957). Thus, these quasi-ratio scales may not provide an accurate measure of the true stimulus-response relationship. On the other hand, their advantage in providing an index of absolute sensation magnitude seems clear.

XII. Measurements of Dyspnea

Both visual analog and Borg scales have been widely used in the measurement of dyspnea during exercise (Stark et al., 1982; El-Manshawi et al., 1986; LeBlanc et al., 1986). These scales are easily applied and are easily understood and utilized by experimental subjects and patients. The Borg scale has the additional advantage of simple descriptive terms to define sensory magnitude, but it is not clear that this necessarily improves the validity of the scale.

Visual analog and Borg scale ratings both correlate closely with minute ventilation and with one another during exercise, and these relationships are equally strong in normal subjects and patients with lung disease (Adams et al., 1985; Wilson and Jones, 1989; Muza et al., 1990). There is a high degree of reproducibility in dyspnea responses during repeated trials whether measured with the visual analog or Borg scale (Mahler et al., 1991; Mador and Kufel, 1992).

Visual analog and Borg scale rating also provide sensitive measures of dyspnea. Dyspnea ratings are reduced by bronchodilation but increased by external ventilatory loading and by bronchoconstriction (Stark and Gambles, 1981; Stark et al., 1982, 1983; El-Manshawi et al., 1986; Mahler et al., 1991). The sensitivity of these tests has made visual analog and Borg scale rating useful in the evaluation of the efficacy of various therapeutic interventions.

XIII. Summary

Normal breathing is largely an automatic function that takes place without much awareness. However, distinct sensations associated with breathing can result in significant behavioral influences on respiration. The use of a variety of psychophysical techniques, including threshold discrimination and direct magnitude and category scaling, has enabled the assessment of the conscious experiences produced by changes in respiratory chemical drive, thoracic displacement, and respiratory muscle force. This has resulted in major advances in our understanding of the physiological mechanisms regulating breathing in conscious humans and has provided a means for evaluating the basis of dyspnea in patients with respiratory disease.

References

Adams, L., Chronos, N., Lane, R., and Guz, A. (1985). The measurement of breathlessness induced in normal subjects: validity of two scaling techniques. *Clin. Sci.*, 69:7–16.

Aitken, R. C. B. (1969). Measurement of feelings using visual analogue scales. *Proc. R. Soc. Med.*, 62:989–993.

Altose, M. D. (1986). Dyspnea. In *Current Pulmonology*. Vol. 7. Edited by D. H. Simmons. Chicago, Year Book Medical Publishers, pp. 199–226.

Altose, M. D. (1992). Respiratory muscles and dyspnea. *Semin. Resp. Med.*, 13:1–6.

Altose, M. D., and Cherniack, N. S. (1981). Respiratory sensation and respiratory muscle activity. *Adv. Physiol. Sci.*, 10:111–119.

Altose, M. D., DiMarco, A. F., Gottfried, S. B., and Strohl, K. P. (1982). The sensation of respiratory muscle force. *Am. Rev. Respir. Dis.*, 126:807–811.

Altose, M. D., Leitner, J., and Cherniack N. S. (1985). Effects of age and respiratory effort on the perception of resistive ventilatory loads. *J. Gerontol.*, 40:147–153.

Baird, J. C., and Noma, E. (1978). *Fundamentals of Scaling and Psychophysics*. New York, Wiley.

Bakers, J. H. M., and Tenney, S. M. (1970). The perception of some sensations associated with breathing. *Respir. Physiol.*, 10:85–92.

Banzett, R. B., Lansing, R. W., and Brown, R. (1987). High-level quadriplegics perceive lung volume changes. *J. Appl. Physiol.*, 62:567–573.

Bennett, E. D., Jayson, M. I. V., Rubenstein, D., and Campbell, E. J. M. (1962). The ability of man to detect added non-elastic loads to breathing. *Clin. Sci.*, 23:155–162.

Borg, G. (1970). Perceived exertion as an indicator of somatic stress. *Scand. J. Rehab. Med.*, 2–3:92–98.

Borg, G. A. V. (1973). Perceived exertion: a note on "history" and methods. *Med. Sci. Sports*, 5:90–93.

Borg, G. A. V. (1982). Psychophysical bases of perceived exertion. *Med. Sci. Sports Exercise*, 14:377–381.

Boring, E. G. (1942). *Sensation and Perception in the History of Experimental Psychology*. New York, Appleton-Century.

Bunn, J. C., and Mead J. (1971). Control of ventilation during speech. *J. Appl. Physiol.*, 31:870–872.

Campbell, E. J. M., Freedman, S., Smith, P. S., and Taylor, M. E. (1961). The ability of man to detect added elastic loads to breathing. *Clin. Sci.*, 20:223–231.

Chaudhary, B. A., and Burki, N. K. (1978). Effects of airway anesthesia on the ability to detect added inspiratory resistive loads. *Clin. Sci.*, 54:621–626.

Chaudhary, B. A., and Burki, N. K. (1980). The effects of airway anesthesia on detection of added inspiratory elastic loads. *Am. Rev. Respir. Dis.*, 122:635–639.

Chonan, T., Mulholland, M. B., Cherniack, N. S., and Altose, M. D. (1987). Effects of voluntary constraining of thoracic displacement during hypercapnia. *J. Appl. Physiol.*, 63:1822–1828.

Chonan, T., Mulholland, M. B., Altose, M. D., and Cherniack, N. S. (1990). Effects of changes in level and pattern of breathing on the sensation of dyspnea. *J. Appl. Physiol.*, 69:1290–1295.

Coleridge, H. M., and Coleridge, J. C. G. (1986). Reflexes evoked from the tracheobronchial tree and lungs. In: *Handbook of Physiology*. Sec. 3: Control of Breathing. Vol. 2. Part II. Edited by N.S. Cherniack and J. G. Widdicombe. Bethesda, MD, American Physiological Society, pp. 395–431.

Craig, J. R., and Metze, L. P. (1986). *Methods of Psychological Research*. 2nd ed. Monterey, CA, Brooks/Cole Publishing Co.

Davenport, P. W., Thompson, F. J., Reep, R. L., and Freed, A. N. (1985). Projection of phrenic nerve afferents to the cat sensorimotor cortex. *Brain Res.*, 328:150–153.

Davenport, P. W., Friedman, W. A., Thompson, F. J., and Franzen, O. (1986). Respiratory-related cortical potentials evoked by inspiratory occlusion in humans. *J. Appl. Physiol.*, 60:1843–1848.

Davenport, P. W., Shannon, R., Mercak, A., Reep, R. L., and Lindsey, B. G. (1993). Cerebral cortical evoked potentials elicited by cat intercostal muscle mechanoreceptors. *J. Appl. Physiol.*, 74:799–804.

DiMarco, A. F., Wolfson, D. A., Gottfried, S. B., and Altose, M. D. (1982). Sensation of inspired volume in normal subjects and quadriplegic patients. *J. Appl. Physiol.*, 53:1481–1486.

Eisele, J., Trenchard, D., Burki, N., and Guz, A. (1968). The effect of chest wall block on respiratory sensation and control in man. *Clin. Sci.*, 35:23–33.

El-Manshawi, A., Killian, K. J., Summers, E., and Jones, N. L. (1986). Breathlessness during exercise with and without resistive loading. *J. Appl. Physiol.*, 61:896–905.

Fowler, W. S. (1954). Breaking point of breathholding. *J. Appl. Physiol.*, 6:539–545.

Gandevia, S. G., Killian, K. J., and Campbell, E. J. M. (1981). The effect of respiratory muscle fatigue on respiratory sensation. *Clin. Sci.*, 60:463–466.

Gandevia, S. C., and Rothwell, J. C. (1987). Activation of the human diaphragm from the motor cortex. *J. Physiol.*, 384:109–118.

Gandevia, S. C., and Plassman, B. L. (1988). Responses in human intercostal and truncal muscles to motor cortical and spinal stimulation. *Respir. Physiol.*, 73:325–338.

Gandevia, S. C., and Macefield, G. (1989). Projection of low-threshold afferents from human intercostal muscles to the cerebral cortex. *Respir. Physiol.*, 77:203–214.

Gliner, J. A., Folinsbee, L. J., and Horvath, S. M. (1981). Accuracy and precision of matching inspired lung volume. *Percep. Psychophys.*, 29:511–515.

Gottfried, S. B., Altose, M. D., Kelsen, S. G., Fogarty, C. M., and Cherniack, N. S. (1978). The perception of changes in airflow resistance in normal subjects and patients with chronic airways obstruction. *Chest*, 73:286–288.

Gottfried, S. B., Altose, M. D., Kelsen, S. G., and Cherniack, N. S. (1981). Perception of changes in airflow resistance in obstructive pulmonary disorders. *Am. Rev. Respir. Dis.*, 124:566–570.

Gottfried, S. B., Leech, I., DiMarco, A. F., Zaccardelli, W., and Altose, M. D. (1984). Sensation of respiratory muscle force following low cervical spinal cord transection. *J. Appl. Physiol.*, 57:989–994.

Gottfried, S. B., Redline, S., and Altose, M. D. (1985). Respiratory sensation in chronic obstructive pulmonary disease. *Am. Rev. Respir. Dis.*, 132:954–959.

Guz, A., Noble, M. M., Widdicombe, J. G., Trenchard, D., Mushin, W. W., and Makey, A. R. (1966). The role of vagal and glossopharyngeal afferent nerves in respiratory sensation, control of breathing and arterial pressure regulation in conscious man. *Clin. Sci.*, 30:161–170.

Homma, I., Obata, T., Sibuya, M., and Uchida, M. (1984). Gate mechanism in breathlessness caused by chest wall vibration in humans. *J. Appl. Physiol.*, 56:8–11.

Katz-Salamon, M. (1984). The ability of human subjects to detect small changes in breathing volume. *Acta Physiol. Scand.*, 120:43–51.

Killian, K. J., Mahutte, C. K., and Campbell, E. J. M. (1980). Resistive load detection during passive ventilation. *Clin. Sci.*, 59:483–495.

Killian, K. J., Mahutte, C. K., and Campbell, E. J. N. (1981). Magnitude scaling of externally added loads to breathing. *Am. Rev. Respir. Dis.*, 123:12–15.

Killian, K. J., Bucens, D. D., and Campbell, E. J. M. (1982). Effects of breathing pattern on the perceived magnitude of added loads to breathing. *J. Appl. Physiol.*, 52:578–584.

Killian, K. J., and Jones, N. L. (1988). Respiratory muscles and dyspnea. *Clin. Chest Med.*, 9:237–248.

Kling, J. W., and Riggs, L. A., eds. (1971). *Woodworth and Schlosberg's Experimental Psychology*. 3rd ed. New York, Holt, Rinehart and Winston.

LeBlanc, P., Bowie, D. M., Summers, E., Jones, N. L., and Killian, K. J. (1986). Breathlessness and exercise in patients with cardiorespiratory disease. *Am. Rev. Respir. Dis.*, 133:21–25.

Lipski, J., Bektas, A., and Porter, R. (1986). Short latency inputs to phrenic motoruerons from the sensorimotor cortex in the cat. *Exp. Brain Res.*, 61:280–290.

Livingstone, R. B. (1991). Sensory processing. In *Best and Taylor's Physiological Basis of Medical Practical*. 12th ed. Edited by J. B. West. Baltimore, Williams and Wilkins, pp. 926–934.

Mador, M. J., and Kufel, T. J. (1992) Reproducibility of visual analog scale measurements of dyspnea in patients with chronic obstructive pulmonary disease. *Am. Rev. Respir. Dis.*, 146:82–87.

Mahler, D. A., Faryniarz, K., Lentme, T., Ward, J., Olmstead, E. M., and O'Connor, G. T. (1991). Measurement of breathlessness during exercise in asthmatics: predictor variables, reliability and responsiveness. *Am. Rev. Respir. Dis.*, 144:39–44.

Manning, H. L., Basner, R., Ringler, J., Rand, C., Fencl, V., Weinberger, S. E., Weiss, J. W., and Schwartzenstein, R. M. (1991). Effect of chest wall vibration on breathlessness in normal subjects. *J. Appl. Physiol.*, 71:175–181.

Maskill, D., Murphy, K., Mier, A., Owen, M., and Guz, A. (1991). Motor cortical representation of the diaphragm in man. *J. Physiol.*, 443:105–121.

Mitchell, R. A., and Berger, A. J. (1981). Neural regulation of respiration. In: *Regulation of Breathing*. Vol. 17, Part I. Edited by T. F. Hornbein. New York, Marcel Dekker, pp. 541–620.

Muza, S. R., Silverman, M. T., Gilmore, G. C., Hellerstein, H. K., and Kelsen, S. G. (1990). Comparison of scales used to quantitate the sense of effort to breathe in patients with chronic obstructive pulmonary disease. *Am. Rev. Respir. Dis.*, 141:909–913.

Newsom Davis, J. (1967). Contribution of somatic receptors in the chest wall to detection of added inspiratory airway resistance. *Clin. Sci.*, 33:249–260.

Noble, M. I. M., Eisele, J. H., Trenchard, D., and Guz, A. (1970). Effect of selective peripheral nerve blocks on respiratory sensations. In *Breathing: Hering-Breuer Centenary Symposium*. Edited by R. Porter. London, Churchill, pp. 233–246.

Noble, M. I. M., Frankel, H. L., Else, W., and Guz, A. (1971). The ability of man to detect added resistive loads to breathing. *Clin. Sci.*, 41:285–287.

Oliven, A., Kelsen, S. G., Deal, E. C., Jr., and Cherniack, N. S. (1985). Respiratory pressure sensation: relationship to changes in breathing pattern in patients with chronic obstructive lung disease. *Am. Rev. Respir. Dis.*, 132:1214–1218.

Plum, F. (1970). Neurological integration of behavioral and metabolic control of breathing. In: *Breathing: Hering-Breuer Centenary Symposium*. Edited by R. Porter. London, Churchill, pp. 168–171.

Plum, F., and Leigh, R. J. (1981). Abnormalities of central mechanisms. In *Regulation of Breathing*. Vol. 17, Part II. Edited by T. F. Hornbein. New York, Marcel Dekker, pp. 989–1067.

Phillipson, E. A., McClean, P. A., Sullivan, C. E., and Zamel, N. (1978). Interaction of metabolic and behavioral respiratory control during hypercapnia and speech. *Am. Rev. Respir. Dis.*, 117:903–909.

Redline, S., Gottfried, S. B., and Altose, M. D. (1991). Effects of changes in inspiratory muscle strength on the sensation of respiratory force. *J. Appl. Physiol.*, 70:240–245.

Revelette, W. R., and Davenport, P. W. (1990). Effects of timing of inspiratory occlusion on cerebral evoked potentials in humans. *J. Appl. Physiol.*, 68:282–288.

Salamon, M., Euler, C. von, and Franzen, O. (1976). Perception of mechanical factors in breathing. In *Physical Work and Effort*. Wenner-Gren Center International Symposium Series, Vol. 32. Edited by G. Borg. Oxford, Pergamon Press, pp. 101–113.

Shannon, R. (1986). Reflexes from respiratory muscles and costovertebral joints. In *Handbook of Physiology*. Sec. 3: Control of Breathing, Vol. 2, Part II. Edited by N. S. Cherniack and J. G. Widdicombe. Bethesda, MD, American Physiological Society, pp. 431–448.

Sibuya, M., Yamada, M., Kanamaru, A., Tanaka, K., Suzuki, H., Noguchi, E., Altose, M. D., and Homma I. (1994). Effect of chest wall vibration on dyspnea in chronic respiratory disease patients. *Am. Rev. Respir. Dis.* 149:1235–1240.

Sorli, J., Grassino, A., Lorange, G., and Milic-Emili, J. (1978). Control of breathing in patients with chronic obstructive lung disease. *Clin. Sci. Mol. Med.*, 54:295–304.

Stark, R. D., and Gambles, S. A. (1981). Effects of salbutamol ipratropium bromide and disodium cromoglycate on breathlessness induced by exercise in normal subjects. *Br. J. Clin. Pharmacol.*, 12:497–501.

Stark, R. D., Gambles, S. A., and Chaterjee, S. S. (1982). An exercise test to assess clinical dyspnea: estimation of reproducibility and sensitivity. *Br. J. Dis. Chest*, 76:269–278.

Stark, R. D., Morton, P. B., Sharman, P. Percival, P. G., and Lewis, J. A. (1983). Effects of codeine on the respiratory responses to exercise on healthy subjects. *Br. J. Clin. Pharmacol.*, 15:355–359.

Stevens, S. S. (1957). On the psychophysical law. *Psychol. Rev.*, 64:153–181.

Stevens, S. S., and Galanter, E. H. (1957). Ratio scales and category scales for a dozen perceptual continua. *J. Exp. Psychol.* (*Hum. Percept.*), 54:377–411.

Stevens, S. S. (1971). Issues in psychophysical measurement. *Psychol. Rev.*, 78:426–450.

Stevens, S. S. (1975). *Psychophysics: Introduction to Its Perceptual, Neural and Social Prospects*. New York, Wiley.

Stubbing, D. G., Killian, K. J., and Campbell, E. J. M. (1981). The quantitation of respiratory sensations by normal subjects. *Respir. Physiol.*, 44:251–260.

Stubbing, D. G., Ramsdale, E. H., Killian, K. J., and Campbell, E. J. M. (1983). Psychophysics of inspiratory muscle force. *J. Appl. Physiol.*, 54:1216–1221.

Swets, J. A., Tanner, W. P., Jr., and Birdsall, T. G. (1968). Decision process in perception. In *Contemporary Theory and Research in Visual Perception*. Edited by R. H. Haber. New York, Holt, Rinehart and Winston, pp. 78–101.

Tack, M., Altose, M. D. and Cherniack, N. S. (1981). Effect of aging on respiratory sensations produced by elastic loads. *J. Appl. Physiol.*, 50:844–850.

Tack, M., Altose, M. D., and Cherniack, N. S. (1982). Effects of aging on the perception of resistive ventilatory loads. *Am. Rev. Respir. Dis.*, 126:463–467.

Tack, M., Altose, M. D., and Cherniack, N. S. (1983). Effects of aging on sensation of respiratory force and displacement. *J. Appl. Physiol.*, 55:1433–1440.

Tapper, D. P., Duncan, S. R., Kraft, S., Kagawa, F. T., Marshall, S., and Theodore, J. (1992).

Detection of inspiratory resistive loads by heart-lung-transplant recipients. *Am. Rev. Respir. Dis.*, 145:458–660.

Wiley, R. L., and Zechman, F. W. (1966). Perception of added airflow resistance in humans. *Respir. Physiol.*, 2:73–87.

Wilson, R. C., and Jones, P. W. (1987). A comparison of the visual analog scale and modified Borg scale for the measurement of dyspnea during exercise. *Clin. Sci.*, 76:277–282.

Wolkove, N., Altose, M. D., Kelsen, S. G., Kondapalli, P. G., and Cherniack, N. S. (1981). Perception of changes in breathing in normal subjects. *J. Appl. Physiol.*, 50:78–83.

Zechman, F. W., and Burki, N. K. (1976). Tracking procedure to assess load detection threshold. *Chest*, 70:165–168.

Zechman, F. W., Muza, S. R., Davenport, P. W., Wiley, R. L., and Shelton, R. (1985). Relationship of transdiaphragmatic pressure and latencies for detecting added inspiratory loads. *J. Appl. Physiol.*, 58:236–243.

Zechman, F. W., O'Neill, R., and Shannon, R. (1987). Effect of low cervical cord transection on detection of increased airflow resistance in man. *Physiologist*, 10:356.

44

Ultrasonography of the Diaphragm

F. DENNIS McCOOL

Brown University Medical School
Providence
Memorial Hospital of Rhode Island
Pawtucket, Rhode Island

FREDERIC G. HOPPIN, Jr.

Brown University Medical School
Providence, Rhode Island

I. Introduction

The human diaphragm is relatively inaccessible to direct study. To assess its function, it would be desirable to know the pressure it develops, its position, and its motion. The pressure it develops (transdiaphragmatic pressure, P_{di}) can be measured relatively noninvasively with gastric and esophageal balloons. Its position and motion, however, generally require measurements that expose the subject to ionizing radiation (radiograms, fluoroscopy, computed tomography) and/or are limited to discrete moments (MRI). Ultrasonography, although it too has distinct limitations, provides an alternative; diaphragm thickness, configuration, and displacement can be evaluated without the use of ionizing radiation, noninvasively, continuously, and with a device that is relatively portable and can be applied to subjects in a variety of postures. This chapter briefly reviews the principles of ultrasonography, some practicalities of using ultrasound for study of the diaphragm, and some current examples of its use in studies of diaphragm function.

II. Principles and Practicalities

An ultrasound transmitter applied to the skin emits bursts of high-frequency focused sound. The sound waves propagate through the body tissues and are partially reflected back by boundaries at which there is an abrupt change of acoustic impedance. The acoustic impedance of a particular tissue is determined by its mass density and its elastance. These properties differ enough between muscle tissue, fat, and fluids such as blood that partial reflection occurs at boundaries between such tissues. The ultrasound receiver analyzes the returning echo for its delay and for the direction from which it comes. The delay and direction, respectively, indicate the depth and direction of the reflecting boundaries. Two strategies are commonly used to display this information. In the M-mode, the depths of reflecting boundaries along a selected soundpath (e.g., the diaphragmatic pleura) are recorded as a one-dimensional tracing against time (Fig. 1). In the B-sector mode, the soundpath

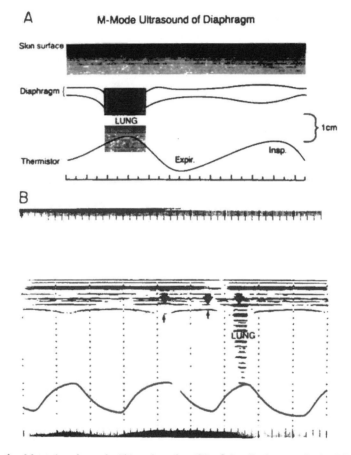

Figure 1 M-mode schematic (A) and tracing (B) of the diaphragm obtained in the zone of apposition. The tracing demonstrates time-based changes in diaphragm thickness during inspiration. Large arrows and small arrows depict the pleural and peritoneal surfaces of the diaphragm, respectively. When the lung enters the field of view, all echos are reflected and none of the deeper structures can be visualized. (From Wait et al., 1989.)

is swept through an arc, either mechanically or by an electronically controlled linear array of transmitter/receivers. The information is then displayed as a two-dimensional image (e.g., cross-section of the diaphragm, liver, and lung) with the brightness of the image representing the intensity of the reflected signal (Fig. 2).

The depth from which useful images can be recovered and the resolution of the image depend on the sound frequency used. Lower frequencies travel further but, because of their longer wavelength, have lesser resolution than higher frequencies. For abdominal imaging, 2.5 or 3.5 MHz is usually used and can resolve structures on the order of 0.3 mm. For superficial structures, higher frequencies (5–15 MHz) are ideal as they provide better resolution (0.1–0.05 mm, respectively). The texture of the structure of most organs (e.g., rib cage muscles) causes scatter, particularly at higher frequencies, and appears speckled on the image. By contrast, a fluid collection (e.g., pleural fluid), being homogeneous, has no internal boundary where acoustic impedance changes, is not echogenic, and appears featureless (black) on the B-mode scan. At many tissue interfaces, the change of acoustic impedance is small and sound is only partially reflected (~0.1%), and the primary soundwave continues beyond the interface only to be partially reflected from serially deeper boundaries. This property has been exploited to visualize the diaphragm and its adjacent structures [e.g., the serial boundaries at the parietal pleura, the diaphragmatic pleura, and the liver (Fig. 3)].

The lung, because it contains air, has a very different acoustic impedance from the analyzing tissues such as the diaphragmatic pleura, intercostal muscles, and liver. It reflects sound so effectively that the sound wave does not proceed well

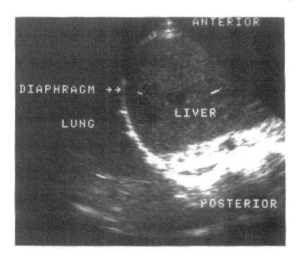

Figure 2 Sector scan (B-mode) of the right hemidiaphragm obtained using a right sagittal subcostal approach. This provides a two-dimensional view depicting the diaphragm and adjacent structures.

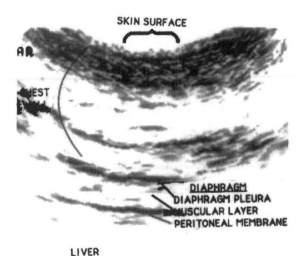

Figure 3 Sector scan of the right hemidiaphragm obtained in the zone of apposition of a cadaver. The diaphragm can be identified as a three-layered structure consisting of the pleural and peritoneal membranes and the muscle itself.

into the deeper structures and those structures do not appear on the image. This characteristic has been used to identify the location of the lower border of the air-containing lung (Loring et al., 1985). It also helps to identify the pleural boundary of the diaphragm as the echogenic boundary nearest the lung, which is masked by the lung as it descends (Wait et al., 1989; Cohn et al., 1992). Unfortunately, this property also obscures structures subjacent to the lung. To circumvent this problem (e.g., in order to visualize the configuration of the diaphragm) one can use a subcostal approach, placing the ultrasound transmitter/receiver on the right side well below the lower border of the lung and angling it upward, thus using the liver as an acoustic "window." Unfortunately, with the subcostal approach on the left, the view of the left hemi-diaphragm is much more limited because of gas in the gastrointestinal tract.

It should be noted, incidently, that multiple internal reflections from a curved boundary such as the diaphragm can generate phantom images, which may signify the existence of a true image elsewhere (Cosgrove et al., 1978; Gardner et al., 1980; Mayo and Cooperberg, 1984; Delattre et al., 1986). Phantom images include repetitive liver parenchyma echoes beyond the diaphragm, mirror images of subdiaphragmatic anatomical structures or pathological lesions, and duplication of the dome of the diaphragm. The presence of perihepatic ascites may also produce artifacts, which appear as a discontinuous diaphragm (Fig. 4) image, probably due to the pattern of sound beam refraction through the liver and perihepatic ascites (Middleton and Melson, 1988).

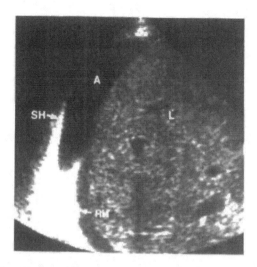

Figure 4 Right longitudinal subcostal view of the liver (L) and diaphragm in a patient with ascites (A). There is apparent discontinuity between the retrohepatic (RH) and suprahepatic (SH) segments of the diaphragm. (From Middleton and Melson, 1988.)

III. Specific Applications

A. Measurement of the Extent of Zone of Apposition: Correlation with Diaphragm Length

Although diaphragm displacement has been modeled for some purposes as a simple pistonlike descent, it interacts significantly with rib cage displacement. Ultrasonography has been used to evaluate that interaction. Loring et al. (1985) used ultrasound to track the upper margin of the diaphragmatic zone of apposition in a study of the relationship of diaphragm length, lung volume, and thoroabdominal configuration. They estimated the length of the diaphragm from insertion to insertion (L_{di}) from the vertical lengths of both zones of apposition (Lap_1 and Lap_2), the thickness of the chest wall on both sides (T_1 and T_2), the external diameters of the rib cage (D), and a shape constant (K_{dome}).

$$L_{di} = K_{dome} (D - T_1 - T_2) + Lap_1 + Lap_2 \qquad (1)$$

To obtain T and Lap, a real-time ultrasonic array scanner was applied to the chest. T was measured as the distance from the transmitter to the pleura on the ultrasound sector image. Lap was the axial distance between the margin of the zone of apposition (the lower border of the lung image) and the insertion of the diaphragm, which they took as the apparent location of the zone of apposition at relaxed total lung capacity (TLC) (Fig. 5). D was obtained with an anthropometric caliper. K_{dome} was obtained as the ratio of the length of the diaphragmatic profile to the inner

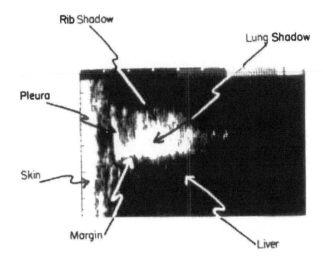

Figure 5 Ultrasonographic view through the lateral rib cage depicting the chest wall, pleura, liver, and lung. The lower margin of the zone of apposition is demarcated as the most caudal displacement of the lung at TLC. The distance traversed by the lung along the chest wall between FRC and TLC is the length of the zone of apposition of the diaphragm. (From Loring et al., 1985.)

diameter of the rib cage as seen on chest radiographs; as these varied nearly alike over a range of lung volumes, K_{dome} was nearly constant.

On the basis of comparisons with chest radiographs in dog and with measurements taken from humans, Loring et al. concluded that changes in diaphragmatic length can be usefully estimated from surface measurements (calipers and ultrasound). They then used such estimates to confirm earlier theoretical predictions that the length of the diaphragm was not simply related to displacements of the abdominal wall, but also to displacements of the rib cage.

B. Diaphragm Thickness: Correlation with Diaphragm Shortening

Wait et al. (1989) and we (Cohn et al., 1992, 1993) have used ultrasonography to noninvasively study the thickness of the muscular portion of the diaphragm. With the transducer placed over the lower rib cage, the diaphragm in the zone of apposition (ZOA) (Mead, 1979) appears as a three-layered structure comprised of two parallel echogenic lines (peritoneal and diaphragmatic pleura) sandwiching a relatively nonechogenic layer (the muscle itself) (Fig. 3). Wait et al. (1989) used a 15 MHz transducer in the M-mode to identify the relevant layers as the most superficial structures to be progressively obliterated by descent of the lung. We used similar criteria but found that the dynamic context of the real time B-mode sector scan was very helpful in securely identifying and tracking the diaphragm. Its thickness (t_{di}) can be measured as the separation of the two echogenic layers. This measurement is reproducible (coefficient of variation of 10%). Its accuracy is attested by comparison at autopsy of ultrasonographic and direct measurements of diaphragm thickness. Wait et al. (1989) found a high correlation ($r = 0.93$; $p < 0.001$) with a slope (ultrasound thickness/direct measure of thickness) that approximated a line of identity (0.97).

Wait et al. (1989) were interested in *changes* in diaphragm thickness, i.e., the thickening of the diaphragm as it shortens during inspiration. They reported a thickening fraction (TF), defined as the increment in thickness during inspiration divided by the initial thickness measured over a range of inspired volumes. Thickening fraction increased linearly with inspired volume. However, the slopes of the relationship between TF and inspired volume varied widely among subjects (from 0.7 to 4.3, where inspired volume is expressed as a fraction of inspiratory capacity V_I/IC). Studies in our laboratory (Cohn et al., 1992) also showed thickening with inspiration (Fig. 6), but differed from the results of Wait et al. (1989) in several respects. First, the increase in thickness appeared to be alinear, with the slope of the diaphragm thickness versus lung volume relationship increasing as lung volume increases (Fig. 7). Furthermore, there was much less variation of overall slope among our 10 subjects than among theirs, and the mean slope was lower (~ 1.56).

The significance of the slope lies in the information it contains about muscle shortening. Thickening of the diaphragm as viewed by ultrasound in the ZOA should be representative of general thickening of the diaphragm muscle. (As the inherent thickness of the diaphragm in this region varies only slightly from place to place at autopsy, the thickening noted on ultrasound should not be due to movement of an adjacent relatively thicker part of the diaphragm under the transducer.) Thickening in turn is related to shortening. The volume of the diaphragm muscle (v) is the product of its length (ℓ), width (w), and thickness (t_{di}). With the assumption that v is constant, ℓ will vary inversely with w · t_{di}. This relationship can be applied to the TF data as follows. A slope of TF versus V_I/IC of 4.3 implies a thickness at end-inspiration 5.3 times that at end-expiration. Because $\ell = w \cdot t_{di}$, if w were constant, the muscle would have shortened to 19% of its original length. More likely, w, which is related to the perimeter of the thoracic cavity, increases during inspiration and the calculated shortening would therefore be even greater. Such shortening is more than has been estimated for the diaphragm radiographically (Braun et al., 1982; Whitelaw, 1987) and from direct measures in animals (Decramer et al., 1987; Newman et al., 1984) and indeed is more than striated muscles are capable of shortening. Our own results suggest shortening from RV to TLC of lesser magnitude to 0.64 of rest length, a value similar to that reported radiographically (Braun et al., 1982; Whitelaw, 1987). The major difference between the studies of Wait et al. (1989) and Cohn et al. (1992) was that the former used the M-mode and the latter the B-sector scan. Direct comparison of these two techniques has not

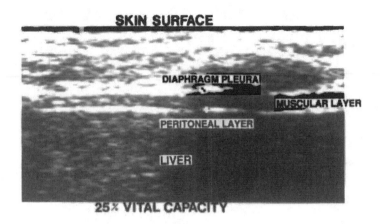

(a)

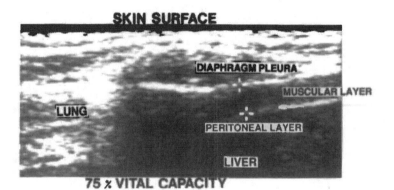

(b)

Figure 6 Sector scan of the right hemidiaphragm obtained in the zone of apposition at 25% (a) and 75% (b) of vital capacity. Note the thickening that occurs with inspiration.

been reported and must be done before the discrepancy can be resolved and the appropriate technology selected for studies of dynamic diaphragm thickness.

C. Diaphragm Thickness: Correlation with Inspiratory Muscle Strength

The pressure that is developed across the diaphragm (transdiaphragmatic pressure, P_{di}) can be related to the stress (specific force) developed by the contracting muscle itself and several readily measured dimensions as follows. First, assume that the muscle fibers in the ZOA are nearly parallel. The net diaphragm *force* that they develop along that axis, then, is the product of the muscle stress (specific force, σ)

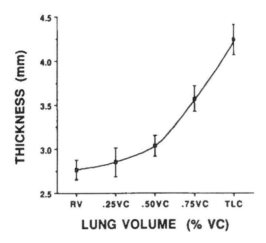

Figure 7 Diaphragm thickness (mean + SD for 10 subjects) measured in the zone of apposition at 25% increments of VC between RV and TLC. The diaphragm thickened as lung volume increased with a mean increase in t_{di} of 56% from RV to TLC.

and the net cross-sectional area of the muscle fibers themselves. The cross-sectional area of the diaphragm in the ZOA, in turn, is the product of the diaphragm muscle's width (w) and thickness (t_{di}). Transdiaphragmatic *pressure* can then be calculated as the net diaphragm force divided by the area spanned by the diaphragm at the level of the ZOA and measured normal to the axis of the fibers (A_{span}). Combining, we obtain the following:

$$P_{di} = \frac{\sigma \cdot t_{di} \cdot w}{A_{span}}$$

Note that w is the perimeter of the diaphragm's profile at the level of the ZOA. Both w and A_{span} can be reasonably and noninvasively estimated from caliper measurements of the chest wall diameters and ultrasonic measurements of chest wall thickness, and t_{di} can be accurately obtained from ultrasonic measurements. Inspiratory pressure, then, is predictable for a given level of diaphragm stress (a function largely of the level of neural activation) and in particular is directly proportional to diaphragm thickness.

Studies of diaphragm thickness at a standard configuration such as FRC from one time to another in a given individual or among individuals across a population should give insights into the sources of normal and pathologic variability of diaphragm strength, e.g., of inspiratory weakness in cachexia, of the effects of inspiratory muscle training, and of the mechanism and progression of the inspiratory impairment with hyperinflation in chronic lung diseases. It is conceivable that muscle stress itself could be usefully inferred from combining anthropometric measurements and ultrasonographic measurements of chest wall and diaphragm thickness. Furthermore, maximum P_{di} could be noninvasively predicted from measurements of t_{di} with the assumption that there is a characteristic maximal stress for healthy striated muscle.

We have some early data which tend to support this general approach (Cohn, et al., 1993). In a group of healthy subjects, we measured diaphragm thickness and maximum voluntary inspiratory pressures at FRC (PI_{max}). The range of maximum pressures was large. This has been long noted (Black and Hyatt, 1969; Koulouris, et al., 1989) but may have been too readily dismissed as reflecting variability of voluntary performance. The maximal pressure, however, was highly correlated with diaphragm thickness (Fig. 8) thereby suggesting that some of the variability of PI_{max} can be attributed to a range of thickness that can be seen in healthy adults.

D. Configuration and Displacement of the Diaphragm

Displacement During Breathing

Motion of the right hemidiaphragm can be assessed (Harber et al., 1975; Haller et al., 1980; Harris et al., 1983; Diament et al., 1985; Traver et al., 1989; Fedullo et al., 1992; DeVita et al., 1993) and followed from day to day (Ambler et al., 1985) without the risks of radiation inherent with fluoroscopy. Drummond et al. (1986) used ultrasound to evaluate diaphragm motion during quiet breathing. They selected the point on the diaphragm that showed the greatest movement along its local radius of curvature during quiet breathing. This point was always focused near the most

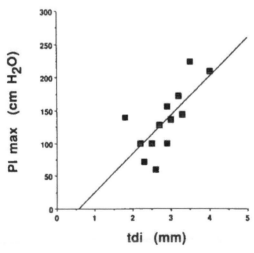

Figure 8   Measurements of PI_{max} and t_{di} obtained at FRC in 13 healthy subjects. The wide range of PI_{max} can be attributed in part to the variability of t_{di} in these subjects ($r^2 = 0.72$).

dependent part of the dome of the diaphragm, and its displacement during inspiration was directed anteriorly as well as caudad. The mean displacement among 20 subjects was 1.6 cm. Harris et al. (1983) recorded displacement of the diaphragmatic image somewhat differently, along rays drawn from the transducer/receiver to the diaphragmatic profile. The middle third of the diaphragm moved a mean of 4.8 cm (range 1.9–9.0 cm) along its ray from the resting expiratory position to full inspiration (Fig. 9). These data are in reasonable accord with those obtained with fluoroscopy (Wade, 1954; Alexander, 1966; Simon et al., 1969). Additionally, Harris et al. (1983) found that about two thirds of the diaphragmatic movement has occurred by the time midinspiratory capacity is reached in supine volunteers. Liang et al. (1988) extended ultrasound measurements of diaphragm motion to the study of infants. They divided the diaphragm in three in a manner similar to Harris et al. (1983) but then recorded the displacements of the midpoints of these segments along an axial direction parallel to the spine. Not surprisingly, the displacements during quiet breathing were much smaller than in adults (mean of 4.5 mm for the posterior segment).

Configuration

The movement of the diaphragm is not uniform from region to region. Harris et al. (1983) found greater displacement in the middle and posterior regions than in the anterior region in supine subjects during large inspirations. Liang et al. (1988) had similar findings in children. They both attributed this difference to the greater abdominal pressure acting on the posterior diaphragm; if the transdiaphragmatic pressure of the passive diaphragm is greater posteriorly, one would expect that at end-expiration the posterior hemidiaphragm intrudes further into the chest than the anterior portion. Consequently, the posterior portion would have to descend further during inspiration in moving toward the relatively flattened configuration of full inspiration. If this were the correct mechanism, one might predict the reverse finding

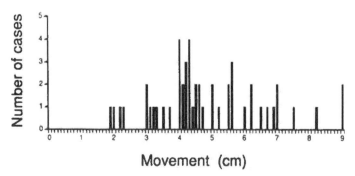

Figure 9 Histogram of movement of the middle third of the diaphragm in adult males and females. The range of motion was between 1.9 and 9.0 cm with a mean and SD of 4.8 + 1.6 cm. (From Harris et al., 1983.)

in the prone position, namely that the anterior region would move more than the posterior. A study in our laboratory (Eveloff and McCool, 1991), however, did not support this prediction. Changing body position had little effect on regional motion. This result downplays the importance of abdominal hydrostatic pressure in determining the pattern of diaphragm contraction.

Passive mechanical ventilation, on the other hand, did change the pattern of regional motion. In supine infants, Liang et al. (1988) found that diaphragm displacement was less and that the posterior displacement was no longer dominant over the anterior displacement. Similar findings were also noted in supine adults (Froese and Bryan, 1974). The lesser diaphragmatic displacement during passive in contrast to active inspiration may reflect (1) the more symmetrical action of the positive inflation pressure on rib cage/diaphragm partitioning and (2) the decreasing rather than increasing tension of the diaphragm during inflation.

In the above studies, several cautions are worth noting. First, the different strategies applied to the geometric analyses of the images could be expected to have systematic effects. The radii of Drummond et al. (1986) or the rays Harris et al. (1983) used to partition the diaphragm into different segments may lie at systematically different angles to the spine, causing displacements of the different regions to have different values. Second, some variability may be introduced by the choice of reference points. If the ultrasound head moves relative to the kidney during breathing, different results would be obtained when measurements were made relative to the ultrasound head or relative to the kidney. Third, variability may be introduced by changing the direction of the ultrasound head; any profile that departs from circularity as seen from the ultrasound head will appear to displace on the image screen simply as the head is rotated. Finally, it is important to recognize that the changes seen in a two-dimensional profile give no direct information regarding the movement of a given anatomical location of the diaphragm. In particular, a given displacement of the diaphragm profile could in theory be as easily generated by shortening of muscle fibers at one end of the diaphragm as the other. The anatomical movement would differ in the two cases, but the distinction would not be appreciated as the displacement of the profile in the source. Several of these cautions, of course, are shared in employing other approaches to diaphragm imaging.

Disordered Motion

A variety of processes may alter global or regional diaphragm motion, including developmental defects such as eventration, trauma resulting in diaphragm rupture, inflammatory processes such as subphrenic abscess, or any process that results in diaphragm paralysis.

Eventration is an abnormally thin part of the diaphragm due to an inadequate migration of myoblasts into the diaphragm resulting in incomplete muscularization of the membranous diaphragm (Wayne et al., 1974; Hesselink et al., 1987). It accounts for about 5% of diaphragm defects, may be partial or complete, and may involve one or both hemidiaphragms. This thin portion of the diaphragm is subject to upward displacement and stretching by the abdominal contents. Eventration presents most commonly on the left in children and on the right in adults (Hesselink et al., 1987). On ultrasound, a focal eventration appears as an abnormal bulge in an otherwise normally shaped diaphragm (Yeh et al., 1991) and motion of the affected area is disordered, with a lag in the downward motion of the affected part relative to the normal portion. However, after the initial inspiratory lag, the area of eventration will move caudally in concert with the remainder of the hemidiaphragm (Symbas et al., 1977). Ultrasound can identify an intact but thin diaphragm and the contents within it, thereby distinguishing eventration from hernia.

Ultrasound may have a limited role in the difficult diagnosis of diaphragm rupture. It occurs in approximately 4–8% of patients who sustain multiple trauma (Bekassy et al., 1972; McCune et al., 1976; Hegarty et al., 1978; Estrera et al., 1979; Adamthwaite, 1983) but may also occur following minor injuries (Ball et al., 1982). Some studies have shown predominance of left-sided injury varying from 90 to 98% (Hedblom, 1934; Bernatz et al., 1958; Ebert et al., 1967; Amman et al., 1983). However, a postmortem series by Estrera et al. (1979) showed an equal left-to-right ratio with an overall incidence of diaphragm rupture in deaths from multiple trauma of 5.2%. More recent studies report that the proportion of right-sided rupture may be as high as 22–46% (Somers et al., 1990). Thus, the liver may not be as protective in preventing diaphragm rupture than previously thought (Bekassy et al., 1972). Although the CT can be helpful when establishing the diagnosis of rupture of the left hemidiaphragm (Heiberg et al., 1980), it is limited in demonstrating pathology of the right hemidiaphragm (Nilsson et al., 1988). In this instance, ultrasound may be particularly useful. The ultrasound may show fluid above and below the diaphragm and the discontinuous free edge of the diaphragm may appear as a "flap" within the fluid (Fig. 10). Or the rupture may be identified by the appearance of a bare surface of the liver herniating through the defect of the diaphragm (Somers et al., 1990).

Fluid collections under the diaphragm affect its motion. In patients with ascites, diaphragm excursion is normal or decreased. With ascites due to malignant processes, diaphragm motion is more likely to be reduced secondary either to fixation of the diaphragm from a malignant process or to splinting. Subdiaphragmatic abscesses, which often cause elevation of a hemidiaphragm, are easily identified by ultrasonography. Abscesses appear as complex fluid collections, often with debris and septa (Haber et al., 1975). However, evaluating diaphragm motion may be of considerable diagnostic significance, since motion may become impaired, absent, or even paradoxical in the presence of inflammation. Restricted movement of the ipsilateral diaphragm was noted in 92% of 48 cases of subphrenic acid reported by Miller and Tallman (1967). This is a much higher prevalence than the finding of air-fluid levels in abscessed cavities [30% of the 48 cases of Miller and Tallman (1967)]. Similarly, Haber et al. (1975) studied diaphragm movement in 17 cases of subphrenic abscess and in 4 of these noted no air-fluid level but only localized

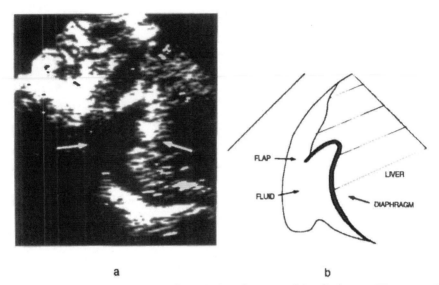

a   b

Figure 10   Ultrasound (a) and schematic (b) of rupture of the diaphragm. The ruptured diaphragm can be seen as a "flap" in the pleural fluid. (From Nilsson et al., 1988.)

restriction of movement of the diaphragm. Since fluoroscopy only visualizes the dome, it may miss processes that do not affect the central portion of the diaphragm. Since ultrasound can assess motion of anterior, middle, and posterior diaphragm segments and provides better definition of the fluid collection, it may be better suited than fluoroscopy to make this diagnosis.

Ultrasonography can be of diagnostic value when assessing hemidiaphragm paralysis. By placing the transducer over the xiphoid process and scanning in the transverse plane, both hemidiaphragms may be viewed simultaneously. Hemidiaphragm paralysis results in paradoxical upward motion of the affected hemidiaphragm during inspiration (Haber et al., 1975; Diament et al., 1985). The paradoxical motion is a consequence of the normal action of the contralateral hemidiaphragm raising intraabdominal pressure and thereby displacing the passive affected diaphragm cephalad. This paradoxical motion is best demonstrated by observing diaphragm movement during the sniff test or with forceful inspirations. Urmey et al. (1991) used ultrasound to demonstrate transient paralysis of the hemidiaphragm following interscalene brachial plexus anesthesia. A number of diseases can result in unilateral diaphragm paralysis including infectious, iatrogenic, malignant, and neurological processes. Fedullo et al. (1992) and DeVita et al. (1993) utilized ultrasound to demonstrate that disordered hemidiaphragm motion may commonly occur following coronary artery bypass surgery.

Surprisingly, bilateral diaphragm paralysis can be difficult to diagnose with ultrasound or fluoroscopy since there may be the misleading finding of downward motion during inspiration. To compensate for the loss of diaphragm activity (Mier-Jedrzejowicz et al., 1988; Loh et al., 1977; Wilcox and Pardy, 1989), a patient may actively contract the abdominal muscles during expiration in order to use the passive recoil of the respiratory system for inhalation. This breathing strategy results in passive inspiratory descent of a paralyzed diaphragm. Downward motion of the diaphragm during inspiration may also appear in erect patients who use their rib cage muscles to inhale. The mechanism is controversial but may be related to the generation of negative pressure in the subdiaphragmatic regions due to shifting the support of the abdominal contents from the abdominal wall to the diaphragm (McCool and Mead, 1989). If both hemidiaphragms move cephalad during inspiration, bilateral diaphragm paralysis is most likely present but should be confirmed by measuring transdiaphragmatic pressure. Gradual recovery of movement of the diaphragm has been documented using ultrasound in a term infant with bilateral diaphragm paralysis (Ambler et al., 1985).

IV. Conclusion

Ultrasound is a promising new approach for the study of the diaphragm. It is particularly attractive in that it is noninvasive, can be used at the bedside, delivers no ionizing radiation, provides a permanent record of function, provides a real-time image, and distinguishes the diaphragm from adjacent soft tissue or fluid. It can been applied to address questions of diaphragm structure, configuration, and motion in health and disease. Ultrasound may allow us to extend studies of mechanisms of muscle action on the respiratory system and to assess biological determinants of diaphragm structure and structural changes with disease.

References

Adamthwaite, D. N. (1983). Traumatic diaphragmatic hernia. *Surg. Ann.*, 15:73–97.

Alexander, C. (1966). Diaphragm movements and the diagnosis of diaphragmatic paralysis. *Clin. Radiol.*, 17:79–83.

Ambler, R., Gruenewald, S., and John, E. (1985). Ultrasound monitoring of diaphragm activity in bilateral diaphragmatic paralysis. *Arch. Dis. Child.*, 60:170–172.

Amman, A. M., Brewer, W. H., Mauld, K. I., and Walsh, J. W. (1983). Traumatic rupture of the diaphragm. Real time sonographic diagnosis. *Am. J. Roentgenol.*, 140:915–916.

Ball, T., McCrory, R., Smith, J. O., and Clements, J. L., Jr. (1982). Traumatic diaphragmatic hernia: errors in diagnosis. *AJR*, 138:633–637.

Bekassy, S. M., Dave, K. S., Wooler, G. H., and Ionescu, M. I. (1972). "Spontaneous" and traumatic rupture of the diaphragm. *Ann. Surg.* 177:320–323.

Bernatz, P. E., Burnside, A. F., and Clagett, O. T. (1958). Problems of the ruptured diaphragm. *JAMA*, 168:877–881.

Black, L. F., and Hyatt, R. E. (1969). Maximal respiratory pressures: normal values and relationship to age and sex. *Am. Rev. Respir. Dis.*, 99:696–702.

Braun, N. M. T., Arora, N. S., and Rochester, D. F. (1982). Force-length relationship of the normal human diaphragm. *J. Appl. Physiol.*, 53(2):405–412.

Cohn, D. B., Benditt, J. O., Eveloff, S. E., and McCool, F. D. (1992). Two-dimensional ultrasound assessment of diaphragm thickness. *Am. Rev. Respir. Dis.*, 145:A255.

Cohn, D. B., Benditt, J. O., Sherman, C. B., Hoppin, F. G., Jr., and McCool, F. D. (1993). Diaphragm thickness: an index of respiratory muscle strength. *Am. Rev. Respir. Dis.*, 147:A694.

Cosgrove, D. O., Garbutt, P., and Hill, C. R. (1978). Echoes across the diaphragm. *Ultrasound Med. Biol.*, 3:385–392.

Decramer, M., Jiang, T.-X., and Demendts, M. (1987). Effects of acute hyperinflation on chest wall mechanics in dogs. *J. Appl. Physiol.*, 63(4):1493–1498.

Delattre, J. F., Plainfosse, M. C., and Hernigou, A. (1986). Repetitive echoes in ultrasonography of the diaphragm demonstrated by cadaver studies. *Eur. J. Radiol.*, 6:218–211.

DeVita, M. A., Robinson, L. R., Rehder, J., Hattler, B., and Cohen, C. (1993). Incidence and natural history of phrenic neuropathy occurring during open heart surgery. *Chest*, 103:850–856.

Diament, M. J., Boechat, M., and Kangarloo, H. (1985). Real-time sector ultrasound in the evaluation of suspected abnormalities of diaphragmatic motion. *J. Clin. Ultrasound.*, 13:539–543.

Drummond, G. B., Allan, P. L., and Logan, M. R. (1986). Changes in diaphragmatic position in association with the induction of anaesthesia. *Br. F. Anaesth.*, 58:1246–1251.

Ebert, P. A., Gaertner, R. A., and Zuidema, G. D. (1967). Traumatic diaphragmatic hernia. *Surg. Gynaecol. Obstet.*, 125:59–65.

Estrera, A. S., Platt, M. R., and Mills, L. J. (1979). Traumatic injuries of the diaphragm. *Chest*, 75:306–313.

Eveloff, S. E., and McCool, F. D. (1990). Regional displacements of the diaphragm vary with posture. *Am. Rev. Respir. Dis.*, 141(4):A722.

Fedullo, A. J., Lerner, R. M., Gibson, J., and Shayne, D. S. (1992). Sonographic measurement of diaphragm motion after coronary artery bypass surgery. *Chest*, 102:1683–1686.

Froese, A. B., and Bryan, A. C. (1974). Effects of anesthesia and paralysis on diaphragmatic mechanics in man. *Anesthesiology*, 41:242–55.

Gardner, F. J., and Clark, R. N., and Kozlowski, R. (1980). A model of a hepatic mirror image artefact. *Med. Ultrasound*, 4:19–21.

Haber, K., Asher, W. M., and Freimanis, A. T. (1975). Echographic evaluation of diaphragmatic motion in intra-abdominal diseases. *Radiology*, 114:141–144.

Haller, J. O., Schneider, M., Kassner, E. G., Friedman, A. P., and Waldroup, L. D. (1980). Sonographic evaluation of the chest in infants and children. *Am. J. Roentgenol.*, 134:1019–1027.

Harris, R. S., Giovannetti, M., and Kim, B. K. (1983). Normal ventilatory movement of the right hemidiaphragm studied by ultrasonography and pneumotachography. *Radiology*, 146:141–144.

Hedblom, C. A. (1934). Diaphragmatic hernia. *Ann. Int. Med.*, 8:156–176.

Hegarty, M. M., Bryer, J. V., Angorn, I. B., and Baker, L. W. (1978). Delayed presentation of traumatic diaphragmatic hernia. *Ann. Surg.*, 188:229–233.

Heiberg, E., Wolverson, M. K., Hurd, R. N., Jagannadharao, B., and Sundaram, M. (1980). CT recognition of traumatic rupture of the diaphragm. *AJR*, 135:369–372.

Hesselink, J. R., Chung, K. J., Peters, M. E., and Crummy, A. B. (1978). Congenital partial eventration of the left diaphragm. *AJR*, 131:417–419.

Koulouris, N., Mulvey, D. A., Laroche, C. M., Sawicka, E. H., Green, M., and Moxham, J. (1989). The measurement of inspiratory muscle strength by sniff esophageal, nasopharyngeal, and mouth pressures. *Am. Rev. Respir. Dis.*, 139:641–646.

Laing, I. A., Teele, R. L., and Stark, A. R. (1988). Diaphragmatic movement in newborn infants. *J. Pediatr.*, 112:638–43.

Loh, L., Goldman, M. D., and Newson Davis, J. (1977). The assessment of diaphragm function. *Medicine* (Baltimore), 56:165–169.

Loring, S. H., Mead, J., and Griscom, N. T. (1985). Dependence of diaphragmatic length on lung volume and thoracoabdominal configuration. *J. Appl. Physiol.*, 59:1961–1970.

Mayo, J., and Cooperberg, P. L. (1984). Displacement of the diaphragmatic echo by hepatic cysts: a new explanation with computer simulation. *J. Ultrasound Med.*, 3:337–340.

McCool, F. D., and Mead, J. (1989). *Am. Rev. Respir. Dis.*, 139:275–276.

McCune, R. P., Roda, C. P., and Eckert, C. (1976). Rupture of the diaphragm caused by blunt trauma. *J. Trauma*, 16:531–537.

Mead, J. (1979). Functional significance of the area of apposition of diaphragm to rib cage. *Am. Rev. Respir. Dis.*, 119(2):31–52.

Middleton, W. D., and Melson, G. L. (1988). Diaphragmatic discontinuity associated with perihepatic ascites: a sonographic refractive artifact. *Am. J. Radiol.*, 151:709–711.

Mier-Jedrzejowicz, A., Brophy, C., Moxham, J., and Green, M. (1988). Assessment of diaphragm weakness. *Am. Rev. Respir. Dis.*, 137:877–883.

Miller, W. T., and Talman, E. A. (1967). Subphrenic abscess. *AJR*, 101:961–969.

Newman, S., Road, J., Bellmare, F., Clozel, J. P., Lavigne, C. M., and Grassino, A. (1984). Respiratory muscle length measured by sonomicrometry. *J. Appl. Physiol.*, 56:753–764.

Nilsson, P. E., Aspelin, P., Ekberg, O., and Senyk, J. (1988). Radiologic diagnosis in traumatic rupture of the diaphragm. *Acta Radiologica*, 29:653–655.

Simon, G., Bonnell, J., Kazantzis, G., and Waller, R. E. (1969). Some radiological observations on the range of movement of the diaphragm. *Clin. Radiol.*, 20:231–233.

Somers, J. M., Gleeson, F. V., and Flower, C. D. R. (1990). Rupture of the right hemidiaphragm following blunt trauma: the use of ultrasound in diagnosis. *Clin. Radiol.*, 42:97–101.

Symbas, P. N., Hatcher, C. R., and Waldo, W. (1977). Diaphragmatic eventration in infancy and childhood. *Ann. Thorac. Surg.*, 4:113–119.

Tarver, R. D., Conces, D. J., Cory, D. A., and Vix, V. A. (1989). Imaging the diaphragm and its disorders. *J. Thorac. Imag.*, 4(1):1–18.

Urmey, W. F., Talts, K. H., and Sharrock, N. E. (1991). One hundred percent incidence of hemidiaphragmatic paresis associated with interscalene brachial plexus anesthesia as diagnosed by ultrasonography. *Anesth. Analg.*, 72:498–503.

Wade, O. L. (1954). Movements of the thoracic cage and diaphragm in respiration. *J. Physiol.* (Lond), 124:193–212.

Wait, J. L., Nahormek, P. A., Yost, W. T., and Rochester, D. F. (1989). Diaphragmatic thickness-lung volume relationship in vivo. *J. Appl. Physiol.*, 67:1560–1568.

Wayne, E. R., Campbell, J. B., Burrington, J. D., and Davis, W. S. (1974). Eventration of the diaphragm. *J. Pediatr. Surg.*, 9:643–651.

Whitelaw, W. A. (1987). Shape and size of the human diaphragm in vivo. *J. Appl. Physiol.*, 62:180–186.

Wilcox, P. G., and Pardy, R. L. (1989). Diaphragmatic weakness and paralysis. *Lung*, 167:323–341.

Yeh, H. C., Halton, K. P., and Gray, C. E. (1990). Anatomic variations and abnormalities in the diaphragm seen with US. *Radiographics*, 10:1019–1030.

Part V

SPECIFIC APPLICATIONS

45

Speech

MARC ESTENNE

Erasme University Hospital
Brussels, Belgium

LUCIANO ZOCCHI

University of Milan
Milan, Italy

I. Introduction

Phonation is of particular interest in physiology because it requires a close coordination between the movements of the respiratory bellows, the vocal cords, and the supralaryngeal structures. Movements of the respiratory bellows provide the subglottic pressure and the expiratory airflow needed to drive the sound generator and determine the loudness of the voice. Movements of the vocal cords produce sound by transforming the pressurized airstream from the lungs into a series of air pulses. Contraction of intrinsic and extrinsic laryngeal muscles regulates the length, tension, and mass of the vocal cords and affects the pitch of the voice. Finally, movements of the supralaryngeal structures (pharynx, soft palate, tongue, lips), by acting as resonators, influence the loudness of the voice and modify the sound to obtain recognizable phonemes. These different processes need to be tightly adjusted to produce intelligible speech while minimizing the interference with the respiratory function of the system. In this chapter, we will focus on the mechanical events responsible for the generation and the control of subglottic pressure during normal speech at conversational sound level. We will also describe some features of special phonatory tasks like singing or producing a single tone at constant pitch and loudness. Finally, we will discuss speech production in patients with neuromuscular diseases involving the respiratory muscles and in patients with stuttering speech.

II. General Features of Sound Production

During speech, the pressure drop across the glottis provides the driving pressure for sound production, i.e., the force setting and maintaining the vocal cords into vibration (Bouhuys, 1974; Proctor, 1980, 1986; Otis, 1988). This pressure drop can be assumed to equal the difference between subglottic (P_{sg}) and atmospheric pressure since the main resistance to airflow during phonation is offered by the glottis. Furthermore, the pressure drop from the alveoli to the subglottic region is extremely small because low expiratory flow rates are used. As a result, alveolar pressure (P_{alv}) approximates P_{sg} during speech. At any lung volume, P_{alv} is determined by the elastic recoil pressure of the respiratory system [$P_{st(rs)}$] and the pressure exerted by the contracting respiratory muscles (the pressure related to the inertance of the system can be considered as negligible). Accordingly, the mechanisms producing P_{sg} are given by the following equation:

$$P_{sg} = P_{alv} = P_{st(rs)} + P_{mus} = P_{st(l)} + P_{st(w)} + P_{mus}$$

where $P_{st(rs)}$, $P_{st(l)}$, and $P_{st(w)}$ are the static recoil pressures of the respiratory system, lung, and chest wall, respectively, P_{alv} is alveolar pressure, P_{sg} is subglottic pressure, and P_{mus} is the pressure caused by contraction of the respiratory muscles (P_{mus} is negative during contraction of inspiratory muscles and positive during contraction of expiratory muscles.)

Subglottic pressure during phonation is nearly constant at a given pitch and loudness. To understand how the static recoil forces of the respiratory system and the forces generated by contraction of the respiratory muscles interact to attain this constancy of pressure, it is helpful to analyze how a tone of constant pitch and loudness can be maintained throughout the vital capacity (VC) (Bouhuys et al., 1966; Bouhuys, 1974). Figure 1A shows the static pressure-volume curve of the respiratory system obtained during voluntary relaxation against an occluded airway (rs) and the P_{sg} achieved while a constant tone is produced over most of the VC (arrow). At high lung volumes, $P_{st(rs)}$ is positive and is greater than P_{sg}. This indicates that the expiratory force provided by the lung and chest wall recoil is greater than that required to produce the target P_{sg}. Hence, at these lung volumes, the inspiratory muscles must contract to counteract $P_{st(rs)}$ and maintain a low P_{sg}. The horizontal distance between the P_{sg} and $P_{st(rs)}$ curves represents the pressure developed by the inspiratory muscles at each lung volume. As utterance proceeds, $P_{st(rs)}$ decreases and the inspiratory muscles gradually relax in order to keep P_{sg} constant. At about 50% VC, the P_{sg} and $P_{st(rs)}$ curves intersect, i.e., $P_{st(rs)}$ is equal to the intended P_{sg} and the net muscle force exerted by the respiratory muscles is zero ($P_{mus} = 0$). At lower lung volumes, $P_{st(rs)}$ is smaller than the target P_{sg} and contraction of the expiratory muscles is needed to maintain the tone. This is particularly true below functional residual capacity (FRC) because at these lung volumes the respiratory system tends to expand ($P_{st(rs)}$ is negative). At each lung volume below the intersection of the P_{sg} and $P_{st(rs)}$ curves, the horizontal distance between these curves corresponds to the pressure developed by the expiratory muscles. It thus appears that maintaining a P_{sg} approximately constant throughout VC

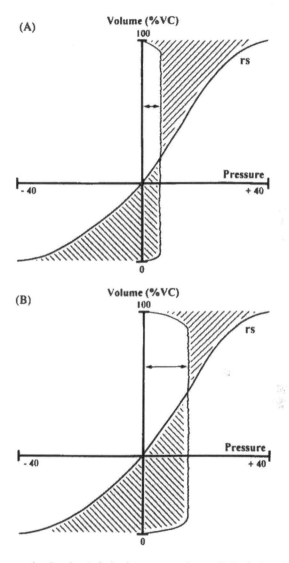

Figure 1 Changes in alveolar (subglottic) pressure (in cm H_2O) during the production of a tone of constant pitch and loudness over most of the vital capacity (VC). (A) Conversational loudness, $P_{alv} = 6$ cm H_2O (arrow). (B) Increased loudness, $P_{alv} = 15$ cm H_2O (arrow). The static pressure-volume curve of the respiratory system (rs) is also shown. In both panels, the triangular area above and below the point of intersection of the two curves represents the net inspiratory or expiratory muscle effort required to maintain alveolar pressure constant during phonation while elastic recoil is continuously changing.

requires a continuously changing degree of respiratory muscle effort. In general, inspiratory muscle contraction is required for the checking of P_{sg} at high lung volumes, while expiratory muscle contraction is required to achieve a similar P_{sg} level at low lung volumes. It should be stressed, however, that the magnitude of the net inspiratory or expiratory effort depends on the loudness of the tone. A louder tone requires a greater P_{sg}; as shown in Figure 1B, increasing P_{sg} will reduce the triangular area between the P_{sg} and $P_{st(rs)}$ curves above their point of intersection (net inspiratory muscle force) and increase the triangular area below their point of intersection (net expiratory muscle force). Conversational speech is usually performed at a P_{sg} of 3–7 cm H_2O, loud speech requires up to 20 cm H_2O, and P_{sg} in singing can be as high as 70 cm H_2O (Fig. 2) (Proctor, 1986). These pressures are well below the maximal expiratory pressures attainable over most of the VC range.

P_{sg} can be measured directly using needle puncture of the trachea (Draper et al., 1959, 1960; Strenger, 1960) or using a catheter introduced through the glottis (Van den Berg, 1956). Alternatively, P_{sg} can be derived from esophageal pressure measurements obtained with standard techniques. Because $P_{st(l)} = P_{alv} - P_{pl}$, where P_{pl} is pleural pressure,

$$P_{sg} = P_{alv} = P_{st(l)} + P_{pl}$$

Therefore, by measuring $P_{st(l)}$ separately, one can measure P_{sg} as the sum of $P_{st(l)}$ and esophageal pressure. When compared with the direct (tracheal puncture) method

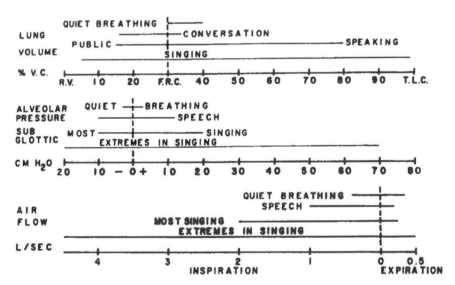

Figure 2 Relative changes in lung volume, subglottic pressure, and airflow rate in quiet breathing, speech, and song. VC, vital capacity; RV, residual volume; FRC, functional residual capacity; TLC, total lung capacity. (From Proctor, 1974. Reprinted by permission of Oxford University Press.)

during speech, the esophageal pressure method has proved to provide valid estimates of P_{sg} (Draper et al., 1959, 1960; Lieberman, 1968). Another indirect mesurement of P_{sg} is based on the compression of alveolar gas resulting from the increased alveolar pressure (Bouhuys et al., 1966).

III. Respiratory Mechanics

A. Pattern of Breathing

During speech and singing the majority of time is, from necessity, devoted to expiration (Fig. 3). Inspirations are more rapid than during quiet, quiet breathing at rest and expirations are longer; T_i/T_{tot} is 0.08–0.17 during reading (Bunn and Mead, 1971) and as low as 0.05 during singing (Proctor, 1980). Frequency is generally less than in nonphonated breathing, dependent on the material spoken, emphasis, and emotional factors.

B. Airflow Rates

During conversational speech, mean expiratory flow rate is generally low relative to nonphonated expirations, ranging from 0.1 to 0.4 liter/s (Fig. 2) (Cavagna and Margaria, 1965; Bouhuys et al., 1966; Bunn and Mead, 1971; Bouhuys, 1974; Proctor, 1980, 1986). However, because sound is produced by alternatively closing and opening the vocal cords and by periodic occlusions at other sites during articulated speech, instantaneous flow rate varies as a function of these rapid changes in the resistance of the vocal and supravocal tract. As a matter of fact, different phonemes have characteristic flow rate patterns, and rapid variations in flow rate are a prominent feature of articulated speech. The relationship between sound output on the one hand and P_{sg} and expiratory flows on the other, however, is complex. For example, at constant vocal-cord tension, pitch rises with increased P_{sg} (Cavagna and Margaria, 1965). Thus, if one increases P_{sg} and expiratory flow in order to produce a louder tone, vocal-cord tension must be adjusted to maintain a constant pitch. Furthermore, a wide range of flows can be used to produce a given tone at the same pitch and loudness by varying the amount of air shunted through the posterior segments of the vocal cords (Cavagna and Margaria, 1965; Cavagna and Camporesi, 1974).

During speech, the quick inspirations interspersed between phonated phrases occur through a widened oropharyngeal airway. Inspiratory flow rates as high as 4.5 L/s have been recorded in trained singers (Proctor, 1986).

C. Alveolar Ventilation

Despite extreme distortion in the pattern of breathing and relatively long periods without inspiration, hypoventilation does not occur during conversational speech and singing. In fact, alveolar ventilation slightly increases (by about 20%), in

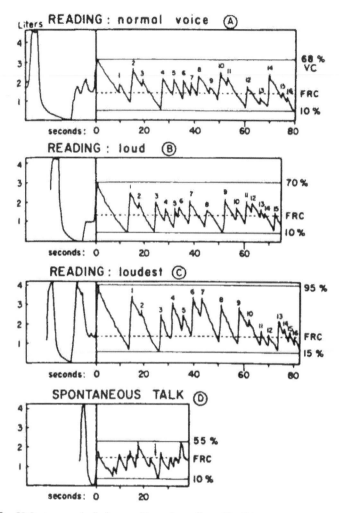

Figure 3 Volume events during reading of a written English text. (A) At normal voice; (B) at increased loudness; (C) at maximum loudness; (D) spontaneous talking at the end of the experiment. At arrow the subject laughed. (From Bouhuys et al., 1966.)

particular when the speech material includes high-flow consonants (e.g., letters "h" and "s"), and there is a slight reduction in end-tidal P_{CO_2} (Bunn and Mead, 1971; Phillipson et al., 1978). Hyperventilation also occurs during singing, and values of minute ventilation above 20 L/min have been reported (Bouhuys et al., 1966). Thus, normal, resting speech and singing are both compatible with the ventilatory requirements for gas exchange.

When the ventilatory demands are increased, as during exercise or CO_2

rebreathing, the airflow requirements for speech can no longer be reconciled with the ventilatory requirements for gas exchange, and speech decreases the average minute ventilation compared to the nonphonated condition (Bunn and Mead, 1971; Bouhuys, 1974; Phillipson et al., 1978). However, the speaker appears to achieve a compromise between the ventilatory and speech demands on flow rates. This is accomplished by increasing the mean expiratory flow rate during speech and by superimposing quick nonphonated expirations upon the speech-breathing pattern (Bunn and Mead, 1971; Bouhuys, 1974). When the ventilatory requirements are particularly high, as in heavy exercise, interference with speech becomes intolerable and the ventilatory function takes priority.

D. Lung Volume

Changes in lung volume during phonation have been assessed using spirometers (Hoshiko, 1965), body plethysmographs (Bouhuys et al., 1966), and volume-calibrated magnetometers (Hixon et al., 1973, 1976; Hoit and Hixon, 1986, 1987; Estenne et al., 1990a). The vast majority of these studies have demonstrated that during conversational speech and reading, phonation is initiated from within the tidal breathing range or from a slightly larger than usual tidal inspiration and that the ensuing expiration is often to a volume below FRC (Figs. 2 and 3). On the other hand, one detailed study by Hixon et al. (1973) has shown that speech-related changes in lung volume measured with magnetometers are in the midrange of the VC but mostly above FRC, both in the upright and the supine posture. Although the reason for this discrepancy is unclear, it should be stressed that the range of lung volume used during speech is affected by the linguistic content of the material spoken and the loudness of the voice. Longer phrases and louder utterances, as often used in singing, encompass a greater fraction of the VC (Hixon et al., 1973; Leanderson et al., 1987). In addition, the pattern of lung volume changes during the production of standardized speech activities also shows some intersubject variability (Hixon et al., 1973).

E. Rib Cage and Abdominal Volume

Six studies have used rib cage and abdominal magnetometers to assess the displacements of the two chest wall compartments during speech (Hixon et al., 1973, 1976; Sharp et al., 1975; Hoit and Hixon, 1986, 1987; Estenne et al., 1990a). Most measurements have been performed in the upright posture, but data have also been obtained with the subjects seated and supine. Comparison between postures indicates that postural changes have a major effect on the behavior of the thoracoabdominal system during speech.

Upright Posture

All the available data indicate that speech in the upright posture occurs to the left of the relaxed thoracoabdominal configuration. This is illustrated in Figure 4, which

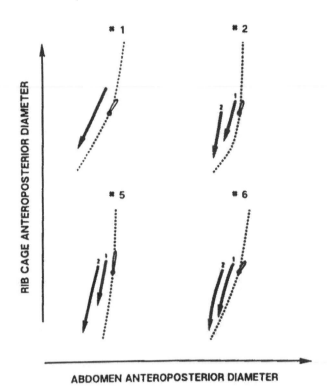

Figure 4 Changes in thoracoabdominal configuration during spontaneous speech or reading (solid lines) in four normal subjects in standing posture. Only expiratory limbs of speech motion loops are shown; arrows, direction of changes. In subjects 2, 5, and 6, two expiratory limbs recorded at the beginning (1) and at the end (2) of the run are shown. Relaxation characteristics (broken lines) and one tidal breathing loop obtained shortly after relaxation (loops) are also shown. Closed circles, spontaneous end-expiration. Note that all expiratory limbs are located to the left of relaxation characteristics and that both rib cage and abdominal dimensions are smaller at the end of utterances than at spontaneous end-expiration. (From Estenne et al., 1990a.)

shows the expiratory limbs of speech motion loops (solid lines) and the relaxation curves of the thoracoabdominal system (dashed lines) in four standing normal subjects. The figure clearly shows that at any given volume, the abdomen is confined to smaller dimensions during speech than during relaxation. Most phrases are initiated at abdominal volumes smaller than those corresponding to spontaneous end-expiration, while the volume of the rib cage is usually greater at the beginning of the phrase than at relaxed FRC (Fig. 5). The rib cage volume attained at the end of the phrase appears to be more variable; in some subjects it is close to the relaxed end-expiratory level (Hixon et al., 1973, 1976; Hoit and Hixon, 1986, 1987), while in others it is substantially below this level (Figs. 4 and 5) (Hoit and Hixon, 1986;

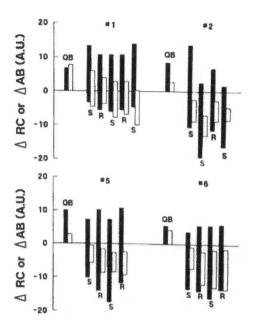

Figure 5 Average changes in rib cage (RC; closed bars) and abdominal (AB; open bars) dimensions during quiet breathing (QB) and successive runs of speech (S) and reading (R) in four normal subjects in standing posture. Positive and negative deflections denote displacements above and below end-expiratory levels for resting breathing. AU, arbitrary units. (From Estenne et al., 1990a.)

Estenne et al., 1990a). In the vast majority of upright subjects, changes in lung volume are primarily produced by emptying of the rib cage (Figs. 4 and 5), but the relative volume contribution of the two compartments may differ among subjects and speaking tasks and may even change within phrases (Hixon et al., 1973). Part of this intersubject variability might be accounted for by differences in body type (Hoit and Hixon, 1986). With increases in loudness, speech starts from higher rib cage but not from higher abdominal volumes (Hixon et al., 1973).

Supine Posture

Speech in the supine posture produces a different pattern of thoracoabdominal motion. Although there is a trend toward less rib cage displacement supine than upright (Hixon et al., 1973), the major difference is that speech motion loops are located to the right, rather than to the left, of the chest wall relaxation characteristics. That is, in supine posture the abdomen is confined to larger volumes during speech than during relaxation. At the start and at the end of the utterance, both rib cage and abdominal volumes are usually greater than at spontaneous end-expiration

(Hixon et al., 1973, 1976; Sharp et al., 1975). In addition the two compartments assume higher preutterance volumes with increases in loudness (Hixon et al., 1973).

Seated Posture

The pattern of thoracoabdominal motion in seated posture is intermediate between those prevailing in the upright and the supine posture. Speech motion loops are generally close to, or superimposed on, the chest wall relaxation characteristics (Sharp et al., 1975; Estenne et al., 1990a). A preponderance of rib cage displacement is observed in most subjects and most phrases are initiated at rib cage and abdominal volumes greater than those corresponding to spontaneous end expiration (Estenne et al., 1990a). In contrast, rib cage and abdominal volumes at the end of the phrases are smaller than the resting end-expiratory levels (Estenne et al., 1990a).

F.   Pressures

Figure 6 shows the changes in esophageal, gastric, and transdiaphragmatic pressures during two runs of quiet speech in one normal seated subject. The onset of phonation (marked by the arrow) is accompanied by an immediate increase in esophageal and gastric pressures 5–7 cm H_2O above the end-expiratory value. Esophageal pressure is remarkably stable during the successive utterances but tends to slightly increase toward the end of each phrase. This is required to keep P_{sg} constant because $P_{st(l)}$ decreases with lung volume as utterance proceeds (see Sec. II). Figure 6 also shows that inspirations interspersed between phrases are accompanied by sharp falls in esophageal pressure and increases in gastric and transdiaphragmatic pressures. At the end of inspiration, transdiaphragmatic pressure rapidly returns to zero, but a gradual increase in this pressure is occasionally observed toward the end of the utterance (Fig. 6A).

Detailed analysis of pressure-volume data for the rib cage and the abdomen has shown that during conversational speech in the upright posture, both compartments produce net expiratory muscular pressures, and do increasingly so as volume decreases (Hixon et al., 1976). On the other hand, the diaphragm is invariably inactive, and development of a small transdiaphragmatic pressure near the end of some phrases (Fig. 6A) only reflects passive stretching of the muscle. Increases in utterance loudness are accomplished by a predominant increase in the expiratory pressures contributed by the abdomen. In the supine posture, net expiratory muscular pressures are also produced by the rib cage but the abdomen is totally relaxed. As in the upright posture, the diaphragm is inactive during speech in the supine posture (Hixon et al., 1976). Although no pressure-volume data have been reported for speech in the seated posture, the position of speech motion loops relative to the relaxed chest wall configuration suggests that the level of abdominal muscle activation is intermediate between the upright and the supine posture.

During sustained vowel or syllable repetition throughout the VC, pressure-

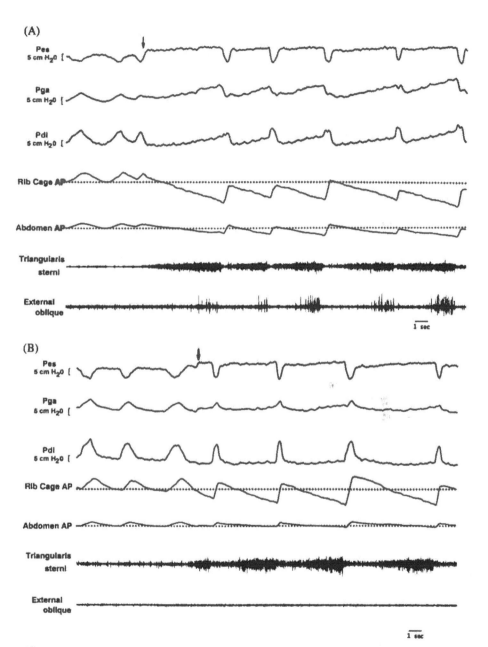

Figure 6 Recordings obtained during conversational speech in one normal subject in the seated posture. (A) Changes in esophageal (P_{es}), gastric (P_{ga}), and transdiaphragmatic (P_{di}) pressures; rib cage and abdominal anteroposterior (AP) diameters; and electromyograms of triangularis sterni and external oblique muscles. Arrow, onset of phonation. Upward

volume data indicate that, as anticipated (see Sec. II), net inspiratory muscular pressures are generated at high lung volumes. As phonation proceeds, the inspiratory effort gradually decreases to zero, and thereafter phonation is accompanied by expiratory efforts that continuously increase in magnitude until utterance termination. The inspiratory effort at high lung volumes is primarily provided by the rib cage muscles, but the diaphragm may also be active, in particular in the supine posture (Hixon et al., 1976). Similarly, active use of the diaphragm has been reported at high lung volumes during singing in professional singers (Leanderson et al., 1987).

G. Respiratory Muscle Activity

Seven studies have described the electromyographic (EMG) activity of various respiratory muscles during phonation (Draper et al., 1959, 1960; Hoshiko, 1960; Eblen, 1963; Newsom Davis and Sears, 1970; Hoit et al., 1988; Estenne et al., 1990a). Although these studies have used different utterance tasks, EMG techniques, and body positions, they provide a relatively consistent pattern of respiratory muscle use, which can be summarized as follows:

1. During conversational speech, EMG activity is invariably recorded from the internal intercostal and triangularis sterni muscles, which are both expiratory in their action on the lung (Fig. 6). This EMG activity starts 20–40 ms before esophageal pressure begins to rise, and it increases in magnitude as utterance proceeds. The internal intercostal EMG activity fluctuates during the phrases, suggesting that the small changes in P_{sg} that are superimposed on the mean P_{sg} level and correspond to the production of certain linguistic elements result from rapid and subtle changes in the activation of these muscles. In fact, because they are small and fast-acting muscles, richly supplied by muscle spindles (Duron, 1981; Farkas et al., 1985), they may be particularly well suited to produce rapid and precise adjustments in P_{sg}. Recruitment of the rib cage expiratory muscles is increased during louder utterances.

2. The abdominal muscles are invariably active during speech in the upright posture. The EMG activity present in the abdominal muscles during resting breathing

---

Figure 6   Continued

deflections are positive pressure changes and increases in thoracoabdominal dimensions. Horizontal dotted lines show spontaneous end-expiratory levels for rib cage and abdomen. Note that triangularis sterni and external oblique are activated with each phrase and that virtually all changes in rib cage and abdominal volume occur below spontaneous end-expiratory levels; slight increase in P_{di} is seen toward end of expiratory limbs, which reflects passive stretching of diaphragm. (B) Tracings obtained during another run of speech obtained in the same subject as in A. Compare with A (same conventions are used): external oblique only shows low-voltage tonic activity, abdominal dimension at end of expiratory limbs is approximately at spontaneous end-expiratory level, and P_{di} does not increase during speech. In contrast, a large amount of activity is present in triangularis sterni, in particular when rib cage dimension is below spontaneous end-expiratory level. (From Estenne et al., 1990a.)

in this posture is augmented during speech, increasingly so toward the end of the phrase. It is worth stressing, however, that the different abdominal muscles do not have a similar threshold of activation during speech. Whereas the rectus abdominis is generally inactive, the muscle layers that constitute the lateral walls of the abdomen are recruited. Although selective EMG recordings have not been obtained from these muscle layers during conversational speech, it is possible that the transversus abdominis is recruited preferentially to the external oblique and internal oblique muscles, as occurs during CO_2 rebreathing and inspiratory loading (De Troyer et al., 1990). Activation of the abdominal muscles is increased when louder utterances are produced; in contrast, it is markedly reduced during speech in the supine posture.

3. The diaphragm does not participate in the control of P_{sg}, becoming electrically silent just after the end of each interspersed inspiration.

4. During sustained vowel or syllable repetition throughout the VC, the external intercostals are active at high lung volumes, providing the inspiratory force required to balance the excess of $P_{st(rs)}$ (Fig. 7). As utterance proceeds, the EMG activity in the external intercostals decreases and eventually ceases when $P_{st(rs)}$ and P_{sg} are equal to each other. Thereafter, the rib cage and abdominal expiratory muscles start to contract and contribute to P_{sg} (Fig. 7). As during conversational speech, the diaphragm is electrically silent during syllable repetition in the upright posture.

These studies have thus demonstrated that the abdominal muscles actively contribute to speech production in the upright posture but are essentially relaxed in the supine posture. Contraction of the abdominal muscles may be required for optimal speech production in the upright posture for at least two reasons. First, it prevents the paradoxical expansion of the abdomen that isolated contraction of the rib cage expiratory muscles would otherwise produce. All other things being equal, such paradoxical expansion would tend to minimize the rise in pleural (and alveolar) pressure, that is, the driving force available for speech. Second, any increase in abdominal volume is expected to promote caudal displacement of the diaphragm and shortening of its muscle fibers. By contracting during speech, the abdominal muscles prevent shortening of the diaphragm, thereby optimizing its inspiratory muscle function. As suggested by Hixon et al. (1976), this mechanism may be of considerable relevance during conversational speech, where inspirations are needed at regular intervals to refill the respiratory system. These inspirations have to be as brief as possible so that interruption of speech is minimal. On the other hand, contraction of the abdominal muscles is not required during speech in the supine posture because the action of gravity prevents excessive shortening of the diaphragm.

IV. Speech in Diseases

A. Neuromuscular Diseases

Because phonation is an active muscular process, one would expect speech production to be altered in patients with weakness of the respiratory muscles. In

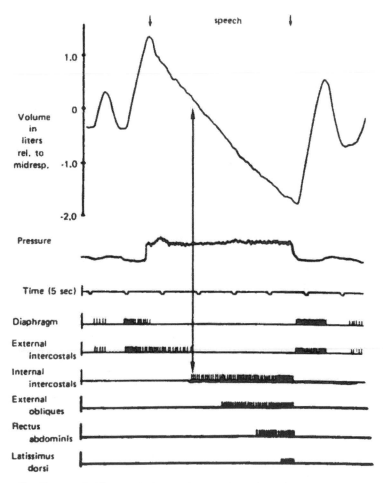

Figure 7   Top panel: Changes in lung volume and esophageal pressure during one tidal breath and during counting from 1 to 32 at conversational loudness. Lower panel: Diagrammatic representation of muscular activity. When the volume of air in the lung is slightly less than at the end of a tidal inspiration (arrow), external intercostal activity ceases and internal intercostal activity commences. (Adapted from Draper et al., 1959. Reprinted by permission of the American Speech-Language-Hearing Association.)

fact, the production of intelligible speech in these patients is usually maintained by compensatory adjustments in the pattern of respiratory muscle use. These adjustments, which vary according to the distribution and the severity of the muscle weakness, have been studied in patients with traumatic transection of the lower cervical cord who have complete paralysis of the intercostal and abdominal muscles but retain a normal diaphragmatic function (Draper et al., 1960; Estenne et al.,

1990b) and in a patient with paralytic poliomyelitis in whom the neck muscles were the only functioning respiratory muscles (Hixon et al., 1983).

Although patients with traumatic transection of the lower cervical cord have severely compromised expiratory muscle function, these patients are still able to empty their lungs actively by contracting the clavicular portion of the pectoralis major (De Troyer et al., 1986). This muscle bundle is invariably active during voluntary expiration below FRC and during cough (Estenne and De Troyer, 1990; Estenne and Gorini, 1992) and produces contraction of the upper portion of the rib cage. In a recent study of speech production in tetraplegic patients, we have demonstrated, in agreement with the suggestion made by Draper et al. (1960), that this muscle is also active during phonation, in particular toward the end of utterances (Estenne et al., 1990b). In addition, in contrast to normal subjects most tetraplegic patients use the diaphragm to brake expiratory flow at the onset of phonation. This checking action is required to maintain a low P_{sg} because at any given lung volume, $P_{st(rs)}$ is greater in tetraplegic patients than in normal subjects (Estenne and De Troyer, 1986), and it cannot be provided by the intercostal muscles, which are totally paralyzed. This combination of pectoralis and diaphragmatic muscle use produces an essentially normal pattern of esophageal pressure change and fully intelligible speech. These data thus indicate that adequate speech can still be produced in the absence of functional intercostal muscles. Most tetraplegic patients, however, cannot produce long sentences and are unable to stress the last word in a sentence or to speak at increased loudness (Draper et al., 1960).

Hixon et al. (1983) have studied one poliomyelitic patient who had paralysis of all respiratory muscles except the sternocleidomastoids, trapezii, and scalenes. Speech in this patient was a passive process, that is, inspiration was made by contraction of the neck muscles but the ensuing expiration was uniquely driven by $P_{st(rs)}$ and the speech motion loop was superimposed on the relaxation characteristics of the thoracoabdominal system. Because $P_{st(rs)}$ decreases with lung volume and no other expiratory force was available, speech had to be restricted to the first half of each expiratory excursion, and inspirations frequently occurred at inappropriate points. However, in order to maintain the fluency of speech, the patient interspersed glossopharyngeal inspirations between and even within words. This strategy enabled him to produce longer sentences without detectable interruptions. In addition to this mechanism, the volume of air consumed per syllable was reduced by increasing the laryngeal resistance to expiratory flow, which produced a strained-strangled quality of voice.

B. Stuttering Speech

Studies of speech production in stutterers have demonstrated that one salient feature of this disease is a failure to control P_{sg} that is too low or too high and fluctuates between these extremes. Abnormalities in the build-up of P_{sg} are observed both during the time period between a stimulus to speak and the onset of speech (Peters and Boves, 1987) and during attempts at phonation (Zocchi et al., 1990). These abnormalities result from incoordination of the respiratory muscles. The diaphragm may remain contracted tonically or speech may be interrupted by twitchlike diaphragmatic contractions that render P_{sg} too low for effective speech (Fig. 8). Expiratory muscle contraction may be absent, also resulting in low P_{sg}, or excessive, making P_{sg} too high (Fig. 8). P_{sg} may be too low even though the diaphragm is relaxed, indicating abnormal contraction of rib cage inspiratory muscles. These abnormalities may all be present in the same patient, but all stutterers do not show abnormalities of all three muscle groups.

Although it is not clear whether incoordination of the respiratory muscles is an integral part of the primary abnormality underlying stuttering speech or is a secondary struggle behavior, it is possible that programs to teach coordination of respiratory muscle activity may be beneficial. One possible approach would be to teach coordination with singing. A curious feature of stutterers is that they can sing perfectly normally (Proctor, 1980). It might therefore be beneficial if stutterers could

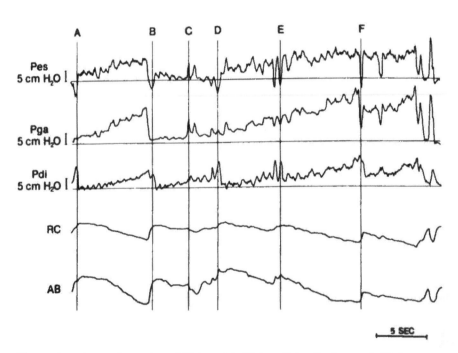

Figure 8 Changes in esophageal (P_{es}), gastric (P_{ga}), and transdiaphragmatic (P_{di}) pressures and in rib cage (RC) and abdominal (AB) dimensions during speech in a stutterer. Horizontal lines indicate end-expiratory pressure levels. Speech starts at A and continues throughout figure, with intercurrent brief inspirations. Several abnormalities are shown, marked by vertical lines: abnormally low P_{es} (B–D), twitchlike contraction of AB muscles (C) and of diaphragm (E), sudden AB muscle relaxation (F). (From Zocchi et al., 1990.)

be taught to carry over their normal respiratory muscle coordination during singing to speech. Alternatively, biofeedback therapy using P_{sg} as the biofeedback signal might help restore fluency.

V. General Conclusions

The pattern of breathing during speech consists of long expirations at low flow rates and quick interspersed inspirations. Alveolar ventilation is slightly increased compared to nonphonated breathing. Speech in the upright posture generally occurs about FRC, involves a predominance of rib cage displacement, and takes place to the left of the relaxed thoracoabdominal configuration. Both the rib cage and the abdomen generate net expiratory muscular pressures, and do increasingly so as utterance proceeds. The expiratory force is provided by contraction of the internal intercostals, the triangularis sterni, and the muscle layers of the lateral walls of the abdomen. In the supine posture, the rib cage is also active in the expiratory direction but the abdomen is essentially relaxed; as a result, speech motion loops are located to the right of the chest wall relaxation characteristics. The diaphragm does not participate in the control of P_{sg} in conversational speech.

Studies in patients with neuromuscular disorders involving the respiratory muscles illustrate the remarkable mechanical and linguistic adjustments that allow acceptable speech to be produced in patients with respiratory muscle dysfunction. To the best of our knowledge, speech production has not been studied in patients with chronic airflow obstruction or other parenchymal lung disease, but there is no doubt that these patients also develop sophisticated adjustments that help compensate for their mechanical impairment.

References

Bouhuys, A., Proctor, D. F., and Mead, J. (1966). Kinetic aspects of singing. *J. Appl. Physiol.*, 21:483–496.

Bouhuys, A. (1974). Voluntary breathing acts: speech, singing, and wind instrument playing. In *Breathing*. New York, Grune and Stratton, pp. 234–259.

Bunn, J. C., and Mead, J. (1971). Control of ventilation during speech. *J. Appl. Physiol.*, 31:870–872.

Cavagna, G. A., and Margaria, R. (1965). An analysis of the mechanics of phonation. *J. Appl. Physiol.*, 20:301–307.

Cavagna, G. A., and Camporesi, E. M. (1974). Glottic aerodynamics and phonation. In *Ventilatory and phonatory control systems*. Edited by B. Wyke. London, Oxford University Press, pp. 76–88.

De Troyer, A., Estenne, M., and Heilporn, A. (1986). Mechanism of active expiration in tetraplegic patients. *N. Engl. J. Med.*, 314:740–744.

De Troyer, A., Estenne, M., Ninane, V., Van Gansbeke, D., and Gorini, M. (1990). Transversus abdominis muscle function in humans. *J. Appl. Physiol.*, 68:1010–1016.

Draper, M. H., Ladefoged, P., and Whitteridge, D. (1959). Respiratory muscles in speech. *J. Speech Hear. Res.*, 2:16–27.

Draper, M. H., Ladefoged, P., and Whitteridge, D. (1960). Expiratory pressures and air flow during speech. *Br. Med. J.*, 1:1837–1843.

Duron, B. (1981). Intercostal and diaphragmatic muscle endings and afferents. In *Regulation of Breathing*. Edited by T. F. Hornbein. New York, Marcel Dekker, pp. 473–540.

Eblen, R. E. (1963). Limitations on use of surface electromyography in studies of speech breathing. *J. Speech. Hear. Res.*, 6:3–18.

Estenne, M., and De Troyer, A. (1986). Effects of tetraplegia on chest wall statics. *Am. Rev. Respir. Dis.*, 134:121–124.

Estenne, M., and De Troyer, A. (1990). Cough in tetraplegic subjects: an active process. *Ann. Intern. Med.*, 112:22–28.

Estenne, M., Zocchi, L., Ward, M., and Macklem, P. T. (1990a). Chest wall motion and expiratory muscle use during phonation in normal humans. *J. Appl. Physiol.*, 68:2075–2082.

Estenne, M., Kinnear, W., Gorini, M., and De Troyer, A. (1990b). Respiratory muscle use during speech in tetraplegia (Abstract). *Eur. Respir. J.*, 3:195S.

Estenne, M., and Gorini, M. (1992). Action of the diaphragm during cough in tetraplegic subjects. *J. Appl. Physiol.*, 72:1074–1080.

Farkas, G. A., Decramer, M., Rochester, D. F., and De Troyer, A. (1985). Contractile properties of intercostal muscles and their functional significance. *J. Appl. Physiol.*, 59:528–535.

Hixon, T. J., Goldman, M. D., and Mead, J. (1973). Kinematics of the chest wall during speech production: volume displacement of the rib cage, abdomen and lung. *J. Speech Hear. Res.*, 16:78–115.

Hixon, T. J., Mead, J., and Goldman, M. D. (1976). Dynamics of the chest wall during speech production: function of the thorax, rib cage, diaphragm, and abdomen. *J. Speech Hear. Res.*, 19:297–356.

Hixon, T. J., Putnam, A. H. B., and Sharp, J. T. (1983). Speech production with flaccid paralysis of the rib cage, diaphragm, and abdomen. *J. Speech Hear. Dis.*, 48:315–327.

Hoit, J. D., and Hixon, T. J. (1986). Body type and speech breathing. *J. Speech Hear. Res.*, 29:313–324.

Hoit, J. D., and Hixon, T. J. (1987). Age and speech breathing. *J. Speech Hear. Res.*, 30:351–366.

Hoit, J. D., Plassman, B. L., Lansing, R. W., and Hixon, T. J. (1988). Abdominal muscle activity during speech production. *J. Appl. Physiol.*, 65:2656–2664.

Hoshiko, M. S. (1960). Sequence of action of breathing muscles during speech. *J. Speech. Hear. Res.*, 3:291–297.

Hoshiko, M. S. (1965). Lung volume for initiation of phonation. *J. Appl. Physiol.*, 20:480–482.

Leanderson, R., Sundberg, J., and von Euler, C. (1987). Role of diaphragmatic activity during singing: a study of transdiaphragmatic pressures. *J. Appl. Physiol.*, 62:259–70.

Lieberman, P. (1968). Direct comparison of subglottal and esophageal pressure during speech. *J. Acoust. Soc. Am.*, 43:1157–1164.

Newsom Davis, J., and Sears, T. A. (1970). The proprioceptive reflex control of the intercostal muscles during their voluntary activation. *J. Physiol.* (London), 209:711–738.

Otis, A. B. (1988). Two functions of breathing: respiration and sound production. In *Respiratory Function of the Upper Airway*. Edited by O. P. Mathew and G. Sant'Ambrogio. New York, Marcel Dekker, pp. 519–534.

Peters, H. F. M., and Boves, L. (1987). Aerodynamic functions in fluent speech utterances of stutterers and non-stutterers in different speech conditions. In *Speech Motor Dynamics in Stuttering*. Edited by H. F. M. Peters and W. Halstign. New York, Springer-Verlag, pp. 229–244.

Phillipson, E. A., McLean, P. A., Sullivan, C. E., and Zamel, N. (1978). Interaction of metabolic and behavioral respiratory control during hypercapnia and speech. *Am. Rev. Respir. Dis.*, 117:903–909.

Proctor, D. F. (1974). Breathing mechanics during phonation and singing. In *Ventilatory and Phonatory Control Systems*. Edited by B. Wyke, London, Oxford University Press, pp. 39–57.

Proctor, D. F. (1980). *Breathing, Speech and Song*. New York, Springer-Verlag.

Proctor, D. F. (1986). Modifications of breathing for phonation. In *Handbook of Physiology*. Section 3. The Respiratory System. Mechanics of Breathing. Vol. 3. Edited by P. T. Macklem and J. Mead. Bethesda, Md., American Physiological Society, pp. 597–604.

Sharp, J. T., Goldberg, N. B., Druz, W. S., and Danon, J. (1975). Relative contributions of rib cage and abdomen to breathing in normal subjects. *J. Appl. Physiol.*, 39:608–618.

Strenger, F. (1960). Methods for direct and indirect measurement of the subglottic air pressure in phonation. *Studia Linguistica*, 14:98–112.

Van den Berg, J. (1956). Direct and indirect determination of the mean subglottic pressure. *Folia Phonat.*, 8:1–24.

Zocchi, L., Estenne, M., Johnston, S., Del Ferro, L., Ward, M. E., and Macklem, P. T. (1990). Respiratory muscle incoordination in stuttering speech. *Am. Rev. Respir. Dis.*, 141:1510–1515.

46

Cough

Physiological and Pathophysiological Considerations

**DEMOSTHENES BOUROS and
NIKOS SIAFAKAS**

University of Crete Medical School
Heraklion, Greece

MALCOLM GREEN

Royal Brompton Hospital
National Heart and Lung Institute
London, England

I. Introduction

Cough is a physiological mechanism that protects the lungs from the inhalation of foreign materials and clears them from excessive bronchial and other secretions in conjunction with other protective mechanisms, such as mucociliary clearance, bronchoconstriction, and phagocytosis. A number of patients have nonproductive cough, which is not associated with mucus clearance and may have a different stimulation (Empey et al., 1976; Fuller and Choudry, 1988). Cough may occur as a single event without any significance or as persistent or paroxysmal episodes reflecting the presence of underlying disease. It is the most common symptom of respiratory disease and a very common presenting symptom in general practice and in the pulmonary medicine. The prevalence of cough in the population depends on precipitating factors, such as smoking and environmental pollutants, and is said to be between 5 and 40% (Wynder et al., 1964; Cullen et al., 1968; Woolcock et al., 1987). In the United Kingdom it is estimated that there are over 75 million self-prescribed doses for cough per year (Higenbottam, 1984) and (Choudry and Fuller, 1992).

II. Description

The typical cough has four phases: inspiration, compression, expiration, and cessation (Fig. 1). Before the inspiratory phase the cough receptors must be stimulated.

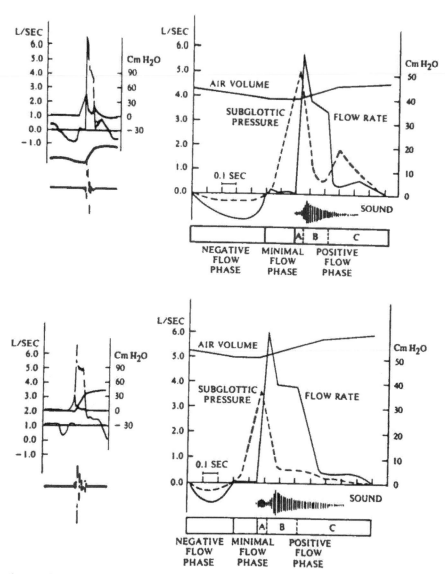

Figure 1 Diagrammatic illustration of two representative coughs with changes observed in flow rate, volume, subglottic pressure, and sound level. Recordings on the left are diagrammed on the right. The flow rate is negative during inspiration zero at glottic closure, and positive during expiration. Positive flow phase is divided into increasing (A), constant (B), and decreasing (C) phases. (Adapted from Yanagihara et al., 1966.)

A. Inspiratory Phase

Whether cough is initiated voluntarily or by stimulation of the cough receptors, the first action is usually inspiration of a variable volume of air. Active abduction of the glottis is caused by contraction of the abductor muscles of the arytenoid cartilage. The inspiratory muscles are also contracted, and inspiration occurs. The inspired volume varies from less than 50% of tidal volume to 50% of vital capacity (Yanagihara et al., 1966; Lawson and Harris, 1967; Harris and Lawson, 1968). Under controlled conditions in which the tested subjects made cough maneuvers through a spirometer, the volume at which cough began was 200–3500 ml above functional residual capacity (FRC) (Leith, 1977). In young adults with acute bronchitis tested with respiratory inductive plethysmography in the supine position, the mean lung volume above FRC before spontaneous coughing was 1250 ± 90 ml (SD) (Sackner, 1988).

Initiating the cough from a high lung volume has the advantage of improving the mechanical function of the expiratory muscles, as their length-tension relationships are optimized, allowing them to generate greater expiratory pressures. It may also allow the reopening of closed peripheral lung units, allowing potential clearance. Absence of the inspiratory phase has been reported in the case of inhaled foreign material, presumably in order to minimize the probability of deeper penetration into the airway (Korpas and Tomori, 1979).

B. Compressive Phase

During this phase, in contrast to the other forced expiratory maneuvers, the glottis is closed by contraction of the adductor muscles of the arytenoid cartilage. The thoracoabdominal expiratory muscles contract against the closed glottis, causing rapid rise in intraabdominal and intrathoracic pressures. Lung volume decreases due to gas compression. It has been found that the compression of the thoracic gas volume is less under hyperbaric conditions and greater at high altitude (Jaeger, 1972), obeying Boyle's law.

The glottis remains closed for about 0.2 s, during which time intrathoracic pressures may occasionally reach values as high as 300 cm H_2O. These pressures are 30–180% greater than those observed during forced expiratory maneuvers at the same lung volumes (Melissinos et al., 1976, 1977, 1978). This might be attributed to a greater neural drive and lower diaphragmatic opposition in the case of cough or to a pattern that optimizes the force-length-velocity relationships of the expiratory muscles (McCool and Leith, 1987). The very high pressures are consistent with complications such as rib fractures and muscle tears, which are not seen during forced expiration and Valsalva maneuvers.

Melissinos and Leith (1988) examined the relationship of peak pleural pressure at the point of laryngeal opening in 83 spontaneous or induced coughs from seven normal subjects and three bronchitics. They found that pleural pressure at the point of laryngeal opening in cough has no constant relationship to peak pleural pressure and ranges from near critical to extremely high values.

Glottic clossure is not necessary for the development of an effective cough. When the glottis is open during the compression phase, intrathoracic pressures are smaller but do not intervene importantly in the effectiveness of cough. Indeed, intubated patients and patients with tracheostomy may generate cough that effectively clears the lower airways (Rayl, 1965). Similarly, normal subjects and patients sometimes clear their airways by voluntary, short, and sharp forced expiratory maneuvers with the glottis open, sometimes called "huffing" (Negus, 1949; Rayl, 1965; Yanagihara et al., 1966, Rossman et al., 1982; Young et al., 1987).

C. Expiratory (Expulsive) Phase

The glottis is opened by active abduction about 0.1–0.4 second after its closure (von Leden and Isshiki, 1965; Lambert et al., 1982; Melissinos and Leith, 1988). Explosive flow follows, causing passive vocal cord and gas vibration with the characteristic noise (Yanagihara et al., 1966). This phase is divided into three parts according to flow rate: increasing, constant, and decreasing (Fig. 1).

When the glottis opens, the pressure in the large airways drops rapidly toward atmospheric, whereas the intraalveolar and intrathoracic pressures remain positive or continue to rise for about 0.5 s. The high intrapleural and intraalveolar pressures produce high expiratory flow rates and dynamic compression with collapse of the central airways. Both are essential for effectiveness of the cough.

Maximal peak flow at the mouth occurs early during this phase and is the product of two flow regimes; peak flow of gas is generated from the periphery of the lung with alveolar pressure as driving pressure. This can exceed 10 L/s, depending on the inspiratory lung volume in normal subjects. Limiting flow is generated by the abrupt collapse of the central airways due to their dynamic compression. Linear velocities for flow rates approaching 10 L/s in the regions of the central airway with a cross-section of about 2 cm^2 can equal to speed of sound (Leith et al., 1986).

Linear velocities are considerably higher in the central airways than peripheral airways because they have a lower total cross-sectional area and are dynamically compressed. The compressional collapse of large airways causes a 50- to 150-ml rapid volume decrement during the expiratory phase (Rayl, 1965, Mead et al., 1967; Knudson et al., 1974). Indeed a significant reduction in tracheal cross-sectional area, up to 80%, may be seen in a cough observed during fiberoptic bronchoscopy (Loudon, 1981). A transient spike of maximal flow occurs and is depicted as an abrupt decrease in volume on the spirogram (Fig. 1). Subsequently there is a short phase of sustained expiration, followed by a phase during which lung volume and flow rate decrease exponentially, as in the forced expiratory maneuver.

The total volume expired during a cough depends on inspired volume and the type of cough. It ranges from less than 100 ml up to 1 L. Loudon et al. (1985) found that peak flow rates and expired volume correlate better with the volume above FRC from which the cough started than the peak intrapleural pressure. Loudon and Shaw (1967) found that normal subjects expire a mean of 2.2 ± 0.46 L, while patients with airways obstruction expire 0.66 ± 0.22 L.

Melissinos et al. (1978) noted another pattern of expiration seen in 70% of the coughs they examined. Immediately after the glottis opened, expiratory muscle activity ceased abruptly, causing a 40% drop in intrathoracic pressure within 0.1 s after peak pressure was reached and earlier reduction of the maximum peak flow at the mouth (V_{ao}).

D. Relaxation Phase

In this phase expiratory muscles relax and intraabdominal, intrapleural, and alveolar pressures drop towards ambient. Transmural pressure of central intrathoracic airways returns to that of static conditions, i.e., it rises from highly negative to slightly positive due to elastic recoil of the lung (Leith et al., 1986). Figure 1 shows the changes in the cough-related parameters during the cough phases, and Figure 2 shows diagrammatically the phase sequence of coughing.

III. The Cough Pump

The cough pump has five components (Table 1, Fig. 3): (1) the cough receptors, (2) the afferent nerves, (3) the cough center (controller), (4) the efferent nerves, and (5) the effectors, i.e., inspiratory and expiratory muscles.

A. Airway Cough Receptors

Despite extensive study of the cough reflex in recent decades, the exact physiological and pathophysiological mechanisms have not been completely elucidated. Our knowledge of cough receptors is still incomplete, although the processes that elicit

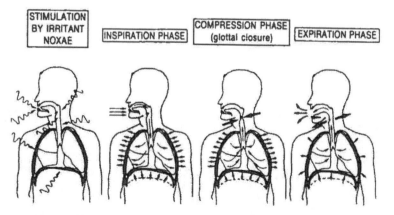

Figure 2 Diagrammatic representation of the sequence of cough phases. (Adapted from Braga, 1989a.)

Table 1 Cough Pump Components

Receptor site	Afferent pathway	Cough center	Efferent pathway	Effectors
Larynx	Superior and recurrent laryngeal nerves		Vagus nerve Phrenic nerve	Muscles of larynx, trachea, and bronchi
Trachea Bronchi	Vagus nerve	Dorsolateral area of the medulla oblongata of the descending nuclei of the vestibular tract and the tractus solitarius	Intercostal and lumbar nerves	Diaphragm
External auditory meatus				
Pleura				Intercostal, abdominal, and lumbar muscles
Stomach			Trigeminal, facial, hypoglossal, and accessory nerves	
Nose Paranasal sinuses	Trigeminal nerve			Upper airways and accessory respiratory muscles
Pharynx	Glossopharyngeal nerve			
Pericardium	Phrenic nerve			
Diaphragm				

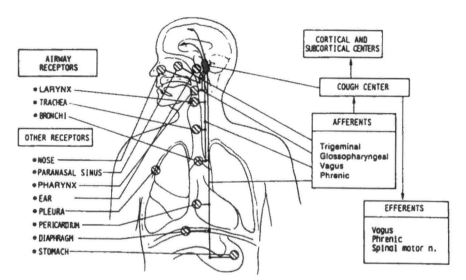

Figure 3 Diagrammatic representation of the components of the cough pump. (Adapted from Braga et al., 1989a.)

cough are better understood (Widdicombe, 1954a,b; Jain et al., 1972; Sampson and Vidruk, 1975; Coleridge et al., 1978; Korpas and Tomori, 1979; Widdicombe, 1985; Fuller, 1991).

There is some confusion concerning the nomenclature of cough receptors. Thus, C-fiber receptors have also been referred to as deflation receptors, high-threshold inflation receptors, J-receptors, and nociceptive lung receptors. Similarly, rapidly adapting pulmonary stretch receptors have also been referred to as irritant receptors and cough receptors (Korpas and Widdicombe, 1991). Indeed, Paintal (1983, 1986a,b) has suggested that rapidly and slowly adapting pulmonary stretch receptors may be the two extremes of one indistinct group.

B. Afferent Pathways

The afferent innervation of cough reflex involves the vagus, the glossopharyngeal, the trigeminal, and the phrenic nerves (Fig. 4; Table 1).

1. The vagus nerve (cranial nerve X) innervates trachea, bronchi, and lung parenchyma both by myelinated (rapidly and slowly adapting receptors) and unmyelinated (C-fiber) receptors.
2. The glossopharyngeal nerve (cranial nerve IX) is a mixed sensory and motor nerve. Its fibers innervate receptors located in the pharynx, including mechanoreceptors, thermoreceptors, and irritant receptors.
3. The trigeminal nerve (cranial nerve V) has three main branches: the

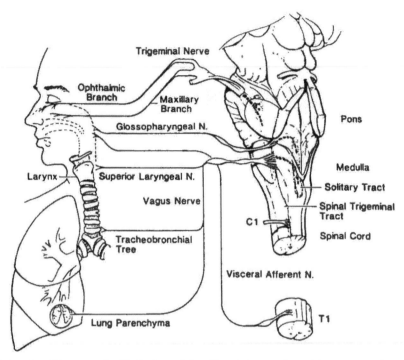

Figure 4 Diagrammatic illustration of the afferent innervation of the cough reflex. See text for details. (Adapted from van Lunteren and Dick, 1991.)

ophthalmic, the maxillary, and the mandibular branches. It divides into three nerves: (1) the ophthalmic nerve, the nasociliary branch of which supplies the mucous membrane of the nasal cavity, (2) the maxillary nerve, which supplies the mucous membrane of the nasopharynx, maxillary sinus, soft palate, tonsils, and the roof of the mouth, the upper gums, and teeth, and (3) the mandibular nerve, which is a mixed nerve. Its sensory fibers supply the auricula and the external meatus (Gray and Goss, 1976).

4. The phrenic nerve is the motor nerve to the diaphragm. It contains about half as many sensory as motor fibers. It originates mainly in the fourth cervical nerve and is afferent from the diaphragm and the upper parts of the pericardium and the pleura (Gray and Goss, 1976). Terminal branches pass through the diaphragm, distribute on the abdominal surface, and also supply the peritoneum.

C. Cough Center (Controller)

Although the term "cough center" (controller) is frequently used, its exact site in humans is unknown. In the best-studied animal, the cat, the site for the cough center has been identified in the medulla oblongata in an area adjacent to the nucleus of the tractus solitarius or the trigeminal tract and nucleus (Chou and Wang, 1975; Korpas and Tomori, 1979). Some antitussives, such as opiates, which are considered to act "centrally," seem to have their effect at this site (Braga, 1989b). Although afferent signals for the cough reflex travel via the vagal nerve fibers, their further connections to brain stem respiratory complex is not known in detail (Korpas and Tomori, 1979).

Likewise, transmitters of the cough stimulus in the central nervous system in humans are unknown (Fuller, 1991). In the cat, inhibitory serotoninergic nerves mediate the effect of opiate antitussives (Das et al., 1978; Davies et al., 1982) and catecholaminergic nerves that inhibit respiration may also inhibit cough. Gamma-aminobutyric acid (GABA) may be involved in the transmission of the cough reflex, since benzodiazepine has shown to inhibit it in the cat (Chou and Wang, 1975). Reduced cough predisposing to respiratory infections is present in some patients with stroke in whom the efferent pathway is intact and in postoperative patients, the mechanism of which is unknown (Fuller, 1991).

D. Efferent Pathway

The efferent pathway includes the vagus, and spinal motor, the phrenic, and the trigeminal, facial, hypoglossal, and accessory nerves (Fig. 3; Table 1).

1. The vagus nerve is both the afferent and efferent nerve of the cough reflex. It is the motor nerve for the muscles of the pharynx and the larynx.
2. The spinal motor nerves emerge from the ventral surface of the spinal cord. The thoracic nerves (intercostal and subcostal) and the lumbar nerves supply the thoracoabdominal muscles.
3. The phrenic nerve is the motor nerve to the diaphragm, but it should be noted that the lower thoracic nerves also contribute to the innervation of the diaphragm.
4. The trigeminal, facial, hypoglossal, and accessory nerves innervate the upper airway and accessory respiratory muscles, which may be activated during cough.

E. The Effectors

These include the muscles of the larynx, trachea, bronchi, diaphragm, intercostal, abdominal and lumbar muscles as well as upper airways and accessory respiratory muscles.

IV. Thoracoabdominal Mechanics During Cough

A. Electroneurograms (Efferent Pathway)

In contrast to forced expiration, which is a voluntary respiratory maneuver and cannot be reproduced in anesthetized humans, reflex cough can be elicited when the relevant afferent pathway is stimulated. Several studies have confirmed that phrenic nerve activity increases during the inspiratory phase of cough and that this increase is greater than during quiet breathing. In spontaneously breathing anesthetized cats, the spike frequency of multiple motor units of the phrenic nerve increases three- to fourfold relative to quiet breathing (Tomori and Widdicombe, 1969). Yanaura et al. (1982) confirmed that during the inspiratory phase of coughing, the discharge frequency of the active phrenic motor units increases and, in addition, new motor units are recruited. It was found that the value of the autocorrelation of coefficient of the phrenic electroneurogram was lower during coughing than during breathing in anesthetized dogs (Yanaura et al., 1982). Phrenic nerve electroneurogram in anesthetized cats showed that the activity of nerve persisted during the early expiratory phase of coughing (Tomori and Widdicombe, 1969; van Lunteren et al., 1989).

B. Electromyograms

Electromyographic studies of the costal and crural parts of the diaphragm showed increased activity during the inspiratory phase of cough compared with normal breathing. The peak electrical activity of the two parts of the diaphragm and that at the parasternal intercostal muscles was found to increase two- to fivefold during coughing in spontaneously breathing cats (van Lunteren et al., 1989). The same study showed that the activity of the crural diaphragm and the parasternal intercostal increased proportionately more than that of the costal diaphragm. Iscoe and Grelot (1992) found in decerebrate, spontaneously breathing cats that midthoracic external intercostal muscles discharged synchronously with the diaphragm, but caudal external and the internal intercostal muscles discharged synchronously with abdominal muscles. They concluded that there are differences in the control and functional roles of intercostal muscles at different thoracic levels during coughing.

However, the pattern of muscle recruitment during the inspiratory phase of cough does not vary greatly from the pattern seen in hypercapnea. In contrast, during the expiratory phase of coughing, the coordination and recruitment of the respiratory muscles is different from that seen in quiet expiration (van Lunteren et al., 1989).

Electromyographic studies show that the abdominal, intercostal, and triangularis sterni muscles are activated more during the expiratory phase of cough than during spontaneous breathing. Studies in humans (Floyd and Silver, 1950; Melissinos et al., 1976; Strohl et al., 1981) showed that upper and lower abdominal muscle activity during cough is vigorous in contrast to rectus abdominalis, which shows minimal activity. The triangularis sterni muscle is also active during coughing in humans (De Troyer et al., 1987). These findings have been confirmed in animal studies, from which it was apparent that the pattern of recruitment of different muscles during coughing may not be the same as that during breathing (van Lunteren et al., 1989).

Electromyographic studies showed inspiratory muscle activity during the early expiratory phase of cough. Tomori and Widdicombe (1969) reported that activity of the diaphragm during early expiration of cough exceeded that during the inspiratory phase. This activity during early expiration is not limited to the diaphragm, but is also present in the rib cage muscles and lasts even longer in the parasternal intercostals (0.3 s vs. 0.25 s for the diaphragm) (van Lunteren et al., 1989; 1991).

The upper airway muscles play an important role during cough. Faaborg-Anderson (1957) recorded the electrical activity of laryngeal adductor and abductor muscles during cough in human subjects with normal vocal cords and in patients with vocal cord paresis. They showed that the adductor muscles (cricothyroid, vocal, arytenoid) were maximally activated prior to the onset of sound produced by coughing and that this activity was greater than during quiet breathing or vocalization. The abductor muscle (posterior cricoarytenoid) activated in reciprocal order to that of the laryngeal adductors during cough. It is not clear if the activity seen in the genioglossus muscle of anesthetized cats is part of a coughing pattern or the consequence of mucosal stimulation (Tatar et al., 1988).

C. Chest Wall Motion and Pressure Changes During Coughing

Melissinos et al. (1978) studied thoracoabdominal mechanics in spontaneous cough in five normal subjects. They showed that esophageal pressure (P_{es}) reached a peak after glottis opening and exceeded by 32–70% the maximum P_{es} seen at the same lung volume during forced expiration. Throughout cough, the pressure in the thoracic cavity was higher than that needed for flow limitation to occur. In addition, they reported that the abdominal diameter increased during decompression but the rib cage diameter continuously decreased.

Morris et al. (1979) studied chest wall configuration during voluntary cough in seven normal subjects. They recorded chest wall motion using linearized magnetometers, monitoring anteroposterior diameter of the rib cage (RC_{a-p}) and abdomen (Abd_{a-p}) and lateral diameters of the rib cage at high (RC_{H-L}) and low (RC_{L-L}) levels. They made also simultaneous recording of gastric pressure (P_g) and P_{es} and transdiaphragmatic pressure (P_{di}), volume, and flow at the mouth. During the compressive phase, P_{es} and P_g rose abruptly and continued to be high approximately 100 ms after the opening of the glottis and the initiation of flow. Direct measurement of pleural pressures during cough in patients who have undergone thoracotomy showed that the pressures are higher in the sitting position than in the supine (Yamazaki et al., 1980). Pleural pressures during cough are also higher in patients after surgery using epidural analgesia.

During cough P_{di} was raised, indicating activity of the diaphragm during this violent expiratory maneuver, leading to the conclusion that the diaphragm is active and appears to modulate violent expiration during coughing. Chest wall diameters decreased abruptly during the compression phase (except RC_{A-P}). When the glottis opened RC_{A-P} and RC_{H-L} showed a rapid inward motion but RC_{LL} and Abd_{A-P} either held their positions constant or more commonly moved outwards in paradoxical function. As a consequence the two lateral diameters of the rib cage moved in opposite directions during cough. They postulated that this paradoxical movement may be the mechanism of cough fracture (Morris et al., 1979) reported previously by Savage (1956) and Pearson (1957).

Electromyographic and mechanical (pressure changes) evidence showed that both the diaphragm and other inspiratory muscles are active during the expiratory phase of cough. This agonist-antagonist relationship could exist to optimize the timing of pressure distribution between abdomen and thorax during the compressive phase of cough (van Lunteren et al., 1988). In addition, contracting the inspiratory muscles may maintain the expiratory muscles at a longer length and keep them in a more advantageous position of the length-tension curve at the onset of the expiratory phase of cough.

Morris et al. (unpublished data), comparing chest wall mechanics during cough in normal subjects and in patients with fibrosing alveolitis (FA) and emphysema, found that chest wall motion was similar in pattern and in range in normal males and females with predominant excursions in the rib cage diameters. In FA chest wall movements were smaller than in normals, with the diameters spanning the abdominal cavity most mobile. In emphysema the movements were all small and disorganized. The maximum intrathoracic pressures generated prior to airflow were similar in all groups despite marked differences in chest wall movements and overall lung volumes. The maximum flow, pressure, and total resistance after the glottis opened were similar in normals and FA, but in emphysema flow was lower and total pulmonary resistance higher (Fig. 5). Esophageal pressure and flow 0.2 s after the glottis opened was lowest in normals and highest in emphysema. The diaphragm was active through cough in all groups, as evidenced by the positive trasdiaphragmatic pressure. Patients with FA have high and curved diaphragms and had the highest P_{di}. Patients with emphysema, who have low and flat diaphragms, had P_{di} no lower than the normals.

V. Cough and Airway Clearance

Cough is considered to be more effective at high lung volumes, where high expiratory flows can be reached, and at high flow velocities during the expulsory phase of cough. The necessary flow velocities to shear mucus from the tracheo-bronchial walls is thought only to be achieved down to the sixth or seventh generation of bronchi (Langlands, 1967; Leith, 1968), although Scherer (1981) suggests that under conditions of excess mucus production cough is efficient down to the respiratory bronchioles (17th airway generation). He suggested that there is no need for dynamic compression for the increase in flow velocity and that the effectiveness of cough is dependent on a complex interaction of viscosity, elasticity, and surface

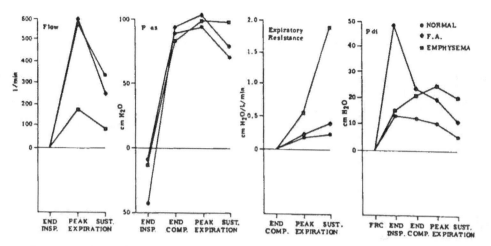

Figure 5 Mean changes in flow, pressure, and resistance during cough. "Peak" values were 0.04 s and "sustained" values 0.2 s after glottis opening. (From Morris et al., unpublished data.)

tension of the mucus. Pavia et al. (1987) concluded that cough efficiency in the proximal airways depends on the presence of increased mucus secretions, while Clarke et al. (1970) showed that the thickness of the mucus layer is critical; too thick or too thin a layer (normal = 5–10 μm) is cleared inefficiently by cough.

The mechanism of airway clearance by cough is best explained by the two-phase gas-liquid flow or interaction (Leith, 1977; Clarke, 1988). According to this theory there are four primary types of airflow in liquid: bubble, slug, annular, and misty (Fig. 6). When the airflow rate is low (<60 cm/s) air flows through mucus as small bubbles. Bubble flow is not relevant to cough and does not effect significant removal of mucous plugs. At flow rates between 60 and 1000 cm/s bubbles increase in size and coalescence occurs to form slug flow, which appears to be very effective in removing large plugs of semisolid sputum. Gas velocities between 1000 and 2500 cm/s form a continuous gas channel through the mucus secretions. The mucus occupies an annular sleeve along the sides of the airways and is transported with a wavelike motion in an annular gas-liquid flow.

At very high flow rates (velocities exceeding 2500 cm/s), as happens in large airways during cough, a misty flow occurs, i.e., the mucus may be blown off the surface as plugs or forms droplets as an aerosol. There is a broad transition between annular and misty flows, and atypical patterns occur (Leith, 1968, 1977, 1985, 1986). Normally, gas velocity exceeding 1000 cm/s is necessary for annular or mist flow at the level of the eighth-generation of airways (Sackner, 1988).

Removal of secretions can be accomplished at relatively low airflow obtained in tidal breathing and in smaller airways because, under proper conditions, annular flow of secretions can be achieved (Leith, 1977; Loudon, 1981; Sackner, 1988).

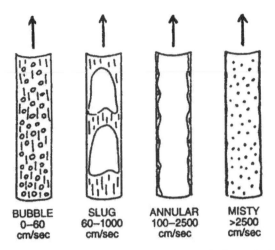

Figure 6 Two-phase gas-liquid flow. The primary types of airflow in liquid are shown, together with the associated gas velocities for large rigid conduits and ordinary Newtonian liquids. Lower velocities may apply in the lung. Arrows indicate the flow direction. (Adapted from Leith, 1968.)

Two-phase gas-liquid efficiency depends on surface velocity, liquid layer thickness, and the type of airflow (continuous or to-and-fro, as during breathing), as well as on the rheological properties of the secretions, so increased viscosity of mucus decreases its clearance when coughing. However, lower airflows such as those during huffing (expiring from midlung volumes to low lung volumes, followed by a period of relaxed diaphragmatic breathing) can also be effective in removing secretions. This technique may avoid bronchospasm, especially in asthmatics.

VI. Cough Pump Failure

Inefficient cough may have deleterious effects on the respiratory system. Accumulation of mucus secretions may lead to atelectasis, infection, and gas exchange abnormalities. Ineffective cough means inappropriate function of one or more of the constituents of the cough pump. Cough pump failure is attributed to three causes: drive failure, feed failure, and structural failure (Table 2).

A. Pump Drive Failure

Pump drive failure may be attributed to abnormalities located in any level of the reflex path from the cough receptors, the afferent nerves, the cough center, the efferent pathways, and the expiratory muscles. The result is a reduction in expiratory pressures and flows attained during cough.

Table 2 Causes of Cough Pump Failure

I. Pump Drive Failure
1. Central nervous system
Depressants (narcotics, sedatives, alcohol)
Injury
Pain
2. Afferent/Efferent neural pathways
3. Neuromuscular synapsis
Myasthenia gravis
Curarelike drugs
Cholinesterase inhibitors(?)
4. Muscular disorders
5. Low sensitivity of cough receptors
Anesthesia
Inflammation
Irritation
II. Pump Feed Failure
Mucus secretion abnormalities
Viscid mucous
Cystic fibrosis, COPD, asthma
III. Pump Structure Failure
Flow limitation (airway obstruction)
COPD, asthma, bronchiectasis, cystic fibrosis
High closing volume
Mucus plugging
Cough collapse of large airways
Tracheobronchomalacia
Emphysema
Stenosis of large airways
Intraluminal lesions, e.g., tumor
Mural lesions, e.g., Swyer-James syndrome
Extramural lesions, e.g., tumor, vascular structures

The central nervous system may be affected by neurological disease, hyperthermia, depressants (e.g., narcotics), sedatives, alcohol, or injury to the level of medulla. Cough drive may be diminished or abolished voluntarily or when pain of, e.g., rib fractures or surgery, is aggravated by coughing (Dilworth et al., 1990; Dilworth and Pounsford, 1991). Epidural analgesia diminishes the reduction in postoperative peak expiratory flow rate after cesarian section (Gamil, 1989) and increases the force of cough after thoracic surgery (Yamazaki et al., 1980).

Neuromuscular junction disorders, such as myasthenia gravis, curarelike drugs, and cholinesterase inhibitors may all affect the cough drive. Muscular disorders, such as myotonia or muscular dystrophy, may also impair cough drive, reducing expiratory pressures and flows attained during cough.

Muscle weakening by these diseases may reduce expiratory flows by limiting lung volume during the inspiratory phase of cough. In this case the length of the expiratory muscles is suboptimal, the elastic recoil of the lung is reduced, and the resultant flows are diminished. Arora and Gal (1981), studying coughs at different lung volumes (TLC, FRC) in healthy, partially curarized subjects, found a reduced expiratory muscle strength and maximal pleural pressures, but not reduced flow rates, with curare. However, an absence of spikes of flow were observed. They suggested that expiratory muscle weakness might reduce cough effectiveness, with a reduction in the dynamic compression and reduced linear gas velocities.

Cough receptor sensitivity may be diminished by local anesthesia and long-standing inflammation and irritation. Diminished sensitivity may be due to rapid adaptation to stimuli with gradual loss of cough, so that patients undergoing fiberoptic bronchoscopy who initially present with paroxysmal cough during insertion of bronchoscope in the glottis gradually lose the cough. Patients with nonproductive cough, as in viral infections and after administration of angiotensin-converting enzyme inhibitors (Empey et al., 1976; Fuller and Choudry, 1987), have increased sensitivity of cough reflex (Choudry and Fuller, 1992).

B. Pump Feed Failure

Effective cough needs normal mucociliary activity to feed secretions into the central airways (Leith, 1977). Feed failure occurs with alterations in mucus components and rheological properties, resulting in viscid, tenacious secretions that are hard to expectorate, as may occur in chronic bronchitis, cystic fibrosis, asthma, bronchiectasis, ciliary dyskinesia, or severe dehydration. The lower the water content of mucus, the higher the viscosity (Lifschitz and Denning, 1970) and elasticity (Shih et al., 1977). Hydration of mucus depends on the relative humidity in the airways and activity of chloride and ion transport in the epithelium (Yeates, 1991). A defect in the latter could be the cause of increased mucus viscosity in cystic fibrosis (Sackner, 1988).

A number of investigators have studied the rheological behavior of mucus, although it is difficult to evaluate accurately because biofluids have unsteady rheological properties with time and flow (shear-thinning effect). Shear-dependent properties of mucus associated with repetitive coughing may increase the efficiency of mucus clearance (Zahm et al., 1991). King et al. (1985) found that clearance was increased by increasing the depth of mucus and decreased by increasing the degree of mucus viscosity and elasticity.

C. Pump Structure Failure

Abnormalities of the pump structure or configuration may reduce cough efficiency by a variety of mechanisms, including increasing closing volume, mucus plugging, and cough collapse of large airways as in tracheobronchomalacia (Leith, 1977) and emphysema. Stenosis of the large airways by intraluminal, mural, or extramural lesions may impair cough. Macklem (1974) has speculated that coughs initiated from lower lung volumes may be more effective in clearing the secretions from bronchiectatic areas, since the choke point moves upstream at the beginning of expiratory phase perhaps as far as lobar or segmental bronchi (Smaldone et al., 1979). In bronchiectasis the lesions are usually located in the peripheral airways upstream of the choke point, so it may be difficult to clear them adequately by coughing. Chest physiotherapy and postural drainage may help. Alterations in mucociliary clearance has been suggested as the possible explanation for the observed ineffectiveness of cough in asymptomatic smokers (Bennett et al., 1992).

In patients with chronic obstructive pulmonary disease (COPD), flow rates during cough are lower than that needed for an effective removal of the increased secretions. An additional factor in these patients is the site of the choke point, which determines the length of the downstream airways dynamically compressed (Macklem, 1974). The site of choke point in COPD is determined by two opposing factors. First, the increased resistance of the airways results in early diminishing of the intraluminal pressure from the alveolus to the mouth and choke point movement closer to alveolus (upstream) than in normal subjects. Second, the large airways of COPD patients (especially emphysematous) are more compliant and become more narrowed for a given transmural pressure. This results in a more central (downstream) movement of the choke point, resulting in limited length of the airway undergoing compression and high gas velocities (Macklem, 1974; Smaldone et al., 1979).

VII. Conclusions

Cough is a complex parameter of the protective system of the respiratory tract involving many neuromuscular and respiratory structures. Coordination between muscle groups has, as a result, a four-phase motor activity consisting of inspiration, compression, expulsion, and relaxation. The maximal mechanical efficiency of cough through the expulsive phase is a result of the first two phases, inspiration and compression.

Ineffective cough is the result of the inappropriate function of one or more of the constituents of the cough pump and can be interpreted as drive, feed, or structure failure. Despite progress in recent years in the understanding of the mechanics of cough, especially of flow limitation during forced expiration, the two-phase gas-liquid flow, and the many causes of cough pump failure, many areas need further investigation. The exact physiological and pathophysiological mechanisms are not completely understood. Similarly, our knowledge of cough receptors is still incomplete. Furthermore, the mechanisms of airway clearance by cough are also still unclear.

References

Arora N. S., and Gal, T. J. (1981). Cough dynamics during progressive expiratory muscle weakness in health curarized subjects. *J. Appl. Physiol.*, 51:494–498.

Braga, P. C., Legnani, D., and Allegra, L. (1989). Clinical aspects of cough. In *Cough*. Edited by P. C. Braga and L. Allegra. New York, Raven Press, pp. 47–105.

Braga, P. C. (1989). Centrally acting opioid drugs. In *Cough*. Edited by P. C. Braga and L. Allegra. New York, Raven Press, pp. 47–105.

Bennett, W. D., Chapman, W. F., and Gerritty, T. R. (1992). Ineffectiveness of cough for enhancing mucus clearance in asymptomatic smokers. *Chest*, 102:412–416.

Chou, D. T., and Wang, S. C. (1975). Studies on the localization of central cough mechanism: site of action of antitussive drugs. *J. Pharmacol. Exp. Ther.*, 194:499–505.

Choudry, N. B., and Fuller, R. W. (1992). Sensitivity of the cough reflex in patients with chronic cough. *Eur. Respir. J.*, 5:296–300.

Clarke, S. W., Jones, J. G., and Oliver, D. R. (1970). Resistance to phase gas-liquid flow in airways. *J. Appl. Physiol.*, 29:464–471.

Clarke, S. W. (1988). Two-phase gas-liquid flow. In *Methods in Bronchial Mucology*. Edited by P. C. Braga and L. Allegra. New York, Raven Press, pp. 125–133.

Coleridge, H. M., Coleridge, J. C. G., Baker, D. G., Ginzel, K. H., and Morrison, M. A. (1978). Comparison of the effects of histamine and prostaglandin on afferent C-fiber endings and irritant receptors in the intrapulmonary airways. *Med. Biol.*, 99:291–305.

Cullen K. J., Stienhouse, N. S., Welborn, T. A., McCall, M. G., and Curnow, D. H. (1968). Chronic respiratory disease in a rural community. *Lancet*, ii:657–660.

Das, R. M., Jeffery, P. K., and Widdicombe, J. G. (1978). The epithelial innervation of the lower respiratory tract of the cat. *J. Anat.*, 126:123–131.

Davies, B., Roberts, A. M., Coleridge, H. M., and Coleridge, J. C. G. (1982). Reflex tracheal gland secretion evoked by stimulation of bronchial c-fibres in dogs. *J. Appl. Physiol.*, 53:985–991.

De Troyer, A., Ninane, V., Gilmartin, J. J., Lemerre, C., and Estenne, M. (1987). Triangularis sterni muscle use in supine humans. *J. Appl. Physiol.*, 62:919–925.

Dilworth, J. P., Pounsford, J. C., and White, R. J. (1990). Cough threshold after upper abdominal surgery. *Thorax*, 45:207–209.

Dilworth, J. P., and Pounsford, J. C. (1991). Cough following general anaesthesia and abdominal surgery. *Respir. Med.*, 85(suppl):13–16.

Empey, D. W., Laitinen, L. A., Jacobs, L., Gold, W. M., and Nadel, J. A. (1976). Mechanism of bronchial hyperreactivity in normal subjects after upper respiratory tract infection. *Am. Rev. Respir. Dis.*, 113:131–139.

Faaborg-Anderson, K. (1957). Electromyographic investigation of intrinsic laryngeal muscles in humans. *Acta Physiol. Scand.*, 41:1–148.

Floyd, W. F., and Silver, P. H. S. (1950). Electromyographic study of patterns of activity of the anterior abdominal wall muscles in man. *J. Anat.*, 84:132–145.

Fuller, F. W. (1991). Cough. In *The Lung*. New York, Raven Press, pp. 61–67.

Fuller, F. W., and Choudry, N. B. (1987). Patients with a non-productive cough have increased cough reflex (abstract). *Thorax*, 43:255.

Gamil, M. (1989). Serial peak expiratory flow rates in mothers during cesarian section under extradural anaesthesia. *Br. J. Anaesth.*, 62:415–418.

Gray, H. G., and Goss, C. M. (1976). *Anatomy of the Human Body*. Philadelphia, Lea & Febiger.

Green, M., Siafakas, N., Morris, A. J. R., and Brennan, N. (1979). Respiratory muscles in health and disease. *Bull. Eur. Physiopath. Resp.*, 15:97–103.

Harris, R. S., and Lawson, T. V. (1968). The relative mechanical effectiveness and efficiency of successive voluntary coughs in healthy young adults. *Clin. Sci.*, 34:569–577.

Higenbottam, T. (1984). Cough induced by changes of ionic composition of airway surface liquid. *Bull. Eur. Physiopathol. Respir.*, 20:553–562.

Iscoe, S., and Grelot, L. (1992). Regional intercostal activity during coughing and vomiting in decerebrtate cats. *Can. J. Physiol. Pharmacol.*, 70:1195–1199.

Jaeger, M. J. (1972). Coughing and forced expiration at reduced barometric pressure (abstract). *Fed. Proc.* 31:322.

Jain, S. K., S. Subramanian, D. B. Julka, and Guz, A. (1972). Search for evidence of lung chemoreflexes in man: study of respiratory and circulatory effects of phenyldiguanide and lobeline. *Clin. Sci. (Lond.)*, 42:163–177.

King, M., Brock, G., and Lundell, C. (1985). Clearance of mucus by simulated cough. *J. Appl. Physiol.*, 58:1776–1782.

Knudson, R. J., Mead, J., and Knudson, D. E. (1974). Contribution of airway collapse to supramaximal expiratory flows. *J. Appl. Physiol.*, 36:653–667.

Korpas, J., and Tomori, Z. (1979). *Cough and Other Respiratory Reflexes*. Basel, Karger.

Korpas, J., and Widdicombe, J. G. (1991). Aspects of the cough reflex. *Respir. Med.*, 85 (supplement A): 3–5.

Lambert, R. K., Wilson, T. A., Hyatt, R. E., and Rodarte, J. R. (1982). A computational model for expiratory flow. *J. Appl. Physiol.*, 52:44–56.

Langlands, J. (1967). The dynamics of cough in health and in chronic bronchitis. *Thorax*, 22:88–96.

Lawson, T. V., and Harris, R. S. (1967). Assessment of the mechanical efficiency of coughing in healthy young adults. *Clin. Sci.*, 33:209–224.

Leith, D. E. (1977). Cough. In *Respiratory Defense Mechanisms*, Vol. 5. Edited by J. D. Brain, D. Proctor, and L. M. Reid. New York, Marcel Dekker, pp. 545–592.

Leith, D. E. (1968). Cough. *Phys. Ther.*, 48:439–447.

Leith, D. E. (1985). The development of cough. *Am. Rev. Respir. Dis.*, 131(suppl):39–42.

Leith, D. E., Butler, J. P., Sneddon, S. L., and Brain, J. D. (1986). Cough. In *Handbook of Physiology 3*. Edited by P. T. Macklem. American Physiological Society, pp. 315–336.

Lifschitz, M. I., and Denning, C. R. (1970). Quantitative interaction of water and cystic fibrosis sputum. *Am. Rev. Respir. Dis.*, 102:456–458.

Loudon, R. G., Rashkin, M., and Jackson, J. L. (1985). The effect of starting volume on cough mechanisms (abstract). *Chest*, 88:175.

Loudon, R. G. (1981). A symptom and a sign. *Basics R. D.*, 9:1–6.

Macklem, P. T. (1974). Physiology of cough. *Ann. Otol. Rhinol. Laryngol.*, 83:761–768.

McCool, F. D., and Leith, D. E. (1987). Pathophysiology of cough. *Clin. Chest Med.*, 8:189–195.

Mead, J., Turner, J. M., Macklem, P. T., and Little, J. B. (1967). Significance of the relationship between lung recoil and maximum expiratory flow. *J. Appl. Physiol.*, 22:95–108.

Melissinos, C., Bruce, E. N., and Leith, D. (1976). Factors affecting pleural pressure during cough in normal man (abstract). *Clin. Res.*, 25:421A.

Melissinos, C., Bruce, E. N., Leith, D., and Mead, J. (1977). Flow and pressure during cough in normal subjects (abstract). *Clin. Res.*, 25:421A.

Melissinos, C., Leith, D. E., Brody, J. S., Bruce, E., and Mead, J. (1978). Thoracoabdominal mechanics in spontaneous cough (abstract). *Am. Rev. Respir.*, 117:372.

Melissinos, C., and Leith, D. (1988). Pleural pressure at the point of laryngeal opening in spontaneous and induced cough. *Eur. Respir. J.*, 1:286s.

Morris, A. J. R., Siafakas, N., and Green, M. (1979). Thoracoabdominal motion and pressures during coughing. *Thorax*, 34:421.

Negus, V. E. (1949). *The Comparative Anatomy and Physiology of the Larynx*. New York, Grune & Stratton.

Paintal, A. S. (1983). Reflex effects of J-receptors. Central neuron environment. Berlin, Springer-Verlag, pp. 134–141.

Paintal, A. S. (1986a). The visceral sensations—some basic mechanisms. In *Progress in Brain Research*. Edited by F. Gervero and J. F. B. Morrisson. Amsterdam, Elsevier Scientific Publishers, pp. 3–19.

Paintal, A. S. (1986b). The significance of dry cough, breathlessness and muscle weakness. *Ind. J. Tuberc.*, 33:51–55.

Pavia, D., Agnew, J. E., and Clark, S. W. (1987). Cough and mucociliary clearance. *Clin. Respir. Physiol.*, 23(suppl):41–45.

Pearson, J. E. G. (1957). Cough fractures of the ribs. *Br. J. Tub. Dis. Chest*, 51:251–254.

Rayl, J. E. (1965). Tracheobronchial collapse during cough. *Radiology*, 85:87–92.

Rossman, C. M., Waldes, R., Sampson, D., and Newhouse, M. T. (1982). Effect of chest physiotherapy on the removal of mucus in patients with cystic fibrosis. *Am. Rev. Respir. Dis.*, 126:131–135.

Sampson, S. R., and Virduk, E. H. (1975). Properties of irritant receptors in canine lung. *Respir. Physiol.*, 25:9–22.

Savage, D. (1956). Stress fractures of the ribs in pregnancy. *Lancet*, 1:420–421.

Scherer, P. W. (1981). Mucus transport by cough. *Chest* 80(suppl):830–833.

Slih, C. K., Litt, M., Kan, M. A., and Wolf, D. P. (1977). Effect of nondialyzable solids concentration and viscoelasticity on ciliary transport of tracheal mucus. *Am. Rev. Respir. Dis.*, 115:989–995.

Smaldone, G. G., Itoh, H., Swift, D. L., and Wagner, H. N. (1979). Effect of flow limiting segments and cough on particle deposition and muciociliary clearance in the lung. *Am. Rev. Respir. Dis.*, 120:747–758.

Strohl, K. P., Mead, J., Banzett, R. B., et al. (1981). Regional differences in abdominal muscle activity during various maneuvers in humans. *J. Appl. Physiol.*, 51:1471–1476.

Tatar, M., Webber, S. E., and Widdicombe, J. G. (1988). Lung c-fibre receptor activation and defensive reflexes in anesthetised cats. *J. Physiol.*, 402:411–420.

Tomori, Z., and Widdicombe, J. G. (1969). Muscular, bronchomotor and cardiovascular reflexes elicited by mechanical stimulation of the respiratory tract. *J. Physiol.*, 200:25–49.

Van Lunteren, E., Haxhiu, M. A., Cherniack, N. S., and Arnold, J. S. (1988). Role of triangularis sterni during coughing and sneezing in dogs. *J. Appl. Physiol.*, 65:2440–2445.

Van Lunteren, E., Daniels, R., Deal, E. C., Jr., and Haxhiu, M. A. (1989). Role of costal and crural diaphragm and parasternal intercostals during coughing in cats. *J. Appl. Physiol.*, 66:135–141.

Van Lunteren, E., and Dick, T. E. (1991). Neuromuscular physiology of cough and other respiratory tract reflexes. In *Chronic Obstructive Pulmonary Disease*. Edited by N. Cherniack. Philadelphia, W.B. Saunders Co., pp. 157–164.

Von Leden, H., and Isshiki, N. (1965). An analysis of cough at the level of the larynx. *Arch. Otolaryngol.*, 81:616–625.

Widdicombe, J. G. (1954a). Respiratory reflexes from the trachea and bronchi of the cat. *J. Physiol. (Lond.)*, 123:55–70.

Widdicombe, J. G. (1954b). Receptors in the trachea and bronchi of the cat. *J. Physiol. (Lond.)*, 123:71–104.

Widdicombe, J. G. (1985). Innervation of the airways. *Progr. Respir. Res.*, 19:8–16.

Widdicombe, J. C. (1982). Pulmonary and respiratory tract receptors. *J. Exp. Biol.*, 100:41–57.

Widdicombe, J. G. (1989). Physiology of cough. In *Cough*. Edited by P. C. Braga and L. Allegra. New York, Raven Press, pp. 3–25.

Woolcock, A. J., Peat, J. K., and Salone, C. M. (1987). Prevalence of bronchial hyperresponsiveness and asthma in a rural adult population. *Thorax*, 42:361–368.

Wynder, E. L., Lemon, F. R., and Mantel, N. (1964). Epidemiology of persistent cough. *Am. Rev. Respir. Dis.*, 91:679–700.

Yamazaki, S., Ogawa, J., Shohzu, A., and Yamazaki, Y. (1980). Intrapleural cough pressure in patients after thoracotomy. *J. Thorac. Cardiovasc. Surg.*, 80:600–604.

Yanagihara, N., von Leden, H., and Werner-Kukuk, E. (1966). The physical parameters of cough: the larynx in a normal single cough. *Acta Otolaryngol.*, 61:495–510.

Yanaura, S., Kamei, J., Goto, K., et al. (1982). Analysis of the efferent discharges of the phrenic nerve during the cough reflex. *Jap. J. Pharmacol.*, 32:795–801.

Yeates, D. B. (1991). Mucus rheology. In *The Lung: Scientific Foundations*. Edited by R. G. Crystal et al. New York, Raven Press, pp. 197–203.

Young, S., Abdul-Sattar, N., and Caric, D. (1987). Glottic closure and high flows are not essential for productive cough. *Bull. Eur. Physiopathol.*, 23(suppl. 10):115–175.

Zahm, J. M., King, M., Duvivier, C., Pierrot, D., Girod, S., and Puchelle, E. (1991). Role of simulated repetitive coughing in mucus clearance. *Eur. Respir. J.*, 4:311–315.

47

The Thorax in Exercise

KIERAN J. KILLIAN, MARK DAVID INMAN, and NORMAN L. JONES

McMaster University
Hamilton, Ontario, Canada

I. Introduction

In the previous edition of this book, we included in our review the factors setting the demand for ventilation during exercise, including metabolism, the control of breathing, and the efficiency of gas exchange. For the present edition we feel that this material is redundant because these factors have been reviewed in many chapters of the present volume and others published in the intervening 10 years (Jones, 1991). This allows us to concentrate on the other aspects of the behavior of the thorax during exercise, some of which we believe are not generally appreciated. Specifically, we will explore the notion that respiratory muscle fatigue frequently limits exercise in both health and disease. The demonstration by Roussos and Macklem (1977) that the respiratory muscles, specifically the inspiratory muscles, are prone to fatigue has changed the way we look at ventilation during exercise even in normal subjects. The time to partial failure of force generation decreases as the demand on striated muscle approaches capacity. The demand on the respiratory muscles during exercise is generally felt to be nonfatiguing because the forces involved are thought to be submaximal and because the respiratory muscles are thought to be less fatiguable than other skeletal muscles.

Because, unlike in many skeletal muscles, it may be difficult or impossible to establish fatigue in terms of an inability to generate force, respiratory muscle fatigue will be defined as an increase in the effort required to generate force to a point where the sensation becomes intolerable and the person stops exercise.

II. The Traditional Approach to Respiratory Muscles in Exercise

The forces generated by the respiratory muscles and the forces opposing their contraction are the two independent contributors to ventilation. Because ventilation is more easily measured than force, the balance between demand and capacity has been traditionally approached by expressing ventilation relative to ventilatory capacity, which conceptually expresses the stress on the respiratory muscle. The idea that ventilation should be considered in relationship to capacity was introduced by Means in the 1920s because logically dyspnea should intensify as ventilation progressively encroaches on ventilatory capacity. Over the years the ventilatory index became a conceptual cornerstone to the understanding of dyspnea (Hugh-Jones and Lambert, 1952) and was expressed as a percentage of the maximal voluntary ventilation (MVV) observed over 10–15 s at rest, or estimated from measurements of FEV_1 or the flow-volume loop by spirometry. Because in maximum progressive exercise in healthy subjects ventilation reaches 50–60% of 15-s MVV (a ventilatory index of 50–60%), ventilatory limitation, and by inference respiratory muscle limitation, is considered unlikely in these circumstances. Limitation only emerges as ventilatory capacity decreases as a consequence of pulmonary disease. Because ventilation, in these terms, is not limiting in normal subjects, limitation to exercise is broadly attributed to an inability of the heart and circulation to support oxygen delivery to exercising muscle (cardiovascular limitation).

III. Some Problems Related to the Ventilatory Index

A. Measurement of Ventilatory Capacity

Maximum Breathing Capacity (MBC). When directly evaluated, ventilatory capacity is usually measured using the maximal voluntary ventilation (MVV) achieved over 10–15 s. Ventilation at maximal exercise is referenced to this value. However, MVV measured over 4 min is approximately 70% of that observed over 15 s. Furthermore, the 4-min measurement may be as little as 40% or as much as 90% of that measured over 15 s in individual subjects (Freedman, 1970) (Fig. 1). While motivation and toleration are factors contributing to the variation, fatigue is the central and most important factor contributing to the decline in performance. Because of this, measurement of resting MVV is not a reliable indication of the capacity available during exercise lasting several minutes.

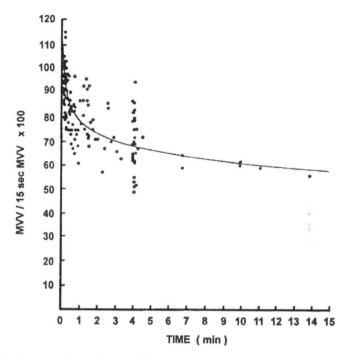

Figure 1   Maximal isocapnic ventilation plotted against the time it can be sustained; ventilation is expressed as a percentage of the 15-s maximal voluntary ventilation. (From Freedman, 1971.)

B.   Prediction of Ventilatory Capacity

Ventilatory capacity is commonly predicted and the prediction equations are largely based on the ventilation observed at maximal exercise in patients with impaired function yielding such relationships as ventilatory capacity = $35*FEV_1$ (Hugh-Jones and Lambert, 1952). However, when such relationships are used to examine the ventilatory index in impaired subjects thought to be limited by a reduced ventilatory capacity, highly variable results have been obtained, and often patients with severe airflow limitation achieve a ventilation in exercise that is well in excess of the predicted MVV. This has led to other predictive equations such as $MVV = 20 + 20*FEV_1$ (Clark et al., 1969). Thus the traditional evidence used to support the idea that ventilation is limiting in patients with impaired pulmonary function is tautological.

C.   Maximal Achievable Ventilation (MAV)

Maximal ventilation is effort dependent, conditional on the tidal volume and frequency adopted and on the fatiguability of the respiratory muscles. To avoid confusion as to the factors contributing to the measurement of maximal voluntary ventilation it is more rational to measure the maximal achievable ventilation (MAV) and standardize ventilation at maximal exercise relative to it.

Estimations of MAV (Killian et al., 1992) can be made by placing breaths of various tidal volumes at various operating lung volumes within the easily measured maximal flow-volume envelope (Fig. 2). The maximal achievable ventilation would obviously be greatest with small tidal volumes operating at a volume where inspiratory and expiratory flow rates are maximal (thick dashed line, Fig. 2), but this would lead to breathing at a high lung volume with a respiratory frequency of several hundred breaths/minute. This pattern is never observed probably because fatigue would be rapid and severe. During exercise, the tidal volume at maximal exercise lies consistently between 50–60% of the vital capacity and respiratory rates between 30–50 breaths per minute and the operating lung volume ranges from 40–90% of TLC in normal subjects (thin solid line, Fig. 2). Estimation of the MAV at this operating lung volume and tidal volume could be made using this approach (thin dashed line, Fig. 2). A less complicated means of making this estimation is to calculate ventilation using tidal volumes observed during exercise, the average flow during an FEV_1 (the most reliable expiratory flow measurement because of its repeatability and the volume dependence of expiratory flow) and the inspiratory flow at 50% of the vital capacity. Using this approach, ventilation during maximal exercise on a cycle ergometer was

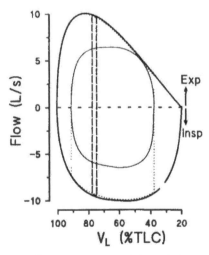

Figure 2 Stylized maximal flow:volume curve (thick solid line) compared to the flow-volume relationship during maximal exercise (thin solid line) in healthy subjects. Maximum possible minute ventilation could be achieved with the flow-volume relationship shown by the thick dashed line. The thin dashed line indicates the flow-volume relationship that would produce the maximum level of ventilation at the same operating volume as adopted during exercise.

52% (SD 14) of maximal achievable ventilation ($\dot{V}E/MAV$) in normal subjects ($n =$ 503); it was 53% (SD 15.4) in those with mild ventilatory impairment (FEV$_1$ 60–80%; $n = 513$), 65% (SD 26.3) in those with moderate impairment (FEV$_1$ 40–60%; $n =$ 105), and 71% (SD 18.4) in those with severe pulmonary impairment (FEV$_1$ <40%; $n = 53$). While the mean data may be used to support the idea of a ventilatory limitation, it should be recognized that variability is great in all groups and that many normal subjects and patients with pulmonary impairment are subjectively limited by dyspnea even when the $\dot{V}E/MAV$ is low, and conversely are limited mainly by leg fatigue even when $\dot{V}E/MAV$ is high. A judgment regarding a ventilatory limit to exercise cannot be made from measurement of $\dot{V}E/MAV$ alone.

IV. Symptoms Limiting Exercise

To anyone who has exercised to their capacity it is self-evident that people stop exercise at the point of limitation because the discomfort of continuing is intolerable. This reality is seldom directly acknowledged by physiologists because discomfort is seen as the product of more fundamental physiological constraints. Nonetheless the discomfort experienced and associated with the exercising muscle and/or dyspnea are the specific sensations commonly cited as limiting exercise during formal exercise testing. Furthermore these symptoms are common to both health and disease, although occurring at a reduced working capacity in the presence of disease. However, the relationship between the symptoms limiting exercise and the underlying disease state is variable and in reality far more variable than commonly appreciated. Patients with pulmonary disease are often limited by leg muscle fatigue whereas normal subjects may be limited by dyspnea (Killian et al., 1992). The behavior of the respiratory muscles during exercise has become far more relevant since limiting symptoms have been formally evaluated.

The intensity of dyspnea and leg effort experienced during incremental exercise in normal subjects increases systematically as exercise increases, reaching similar perceptual magnitude for both sensations at capacity (Fig. 3). The current physiological definition of fatigue has excluded its sensory consequences but a relationship between effort, motor drive, and fatigue is not seriously disputed. In everyday communication the discomfort associated with intense effort is loosely labeled fatigue. This discomfort is the ultimate limiting factor to incremental and sustained exercise performance.

There is a large array of unit processes required to sustain exercise, and they influence sensory responses directly and indirectly, alone and in combination. Hence, symptoms reflect the stimulation of sensory systems and are physiological in nature, and the resulting perceptual responses modify exercise performance and eventually limit maximal performance. Exercise is a volitional event and the final factor limiting exercise is a neural event which is sensory and perceptual in nature. Formal evaluation of the sensory system during exercise has been conspicuously

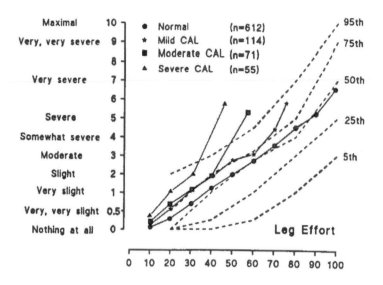

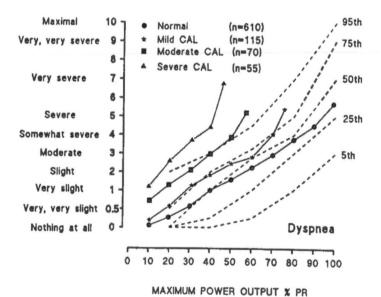

MAXIMUM POWER OUTPUT X PR

Figure 3 Mean intensity of leg effort and dyspnea experienced during incremental exercise to capacity by four groups of subjects categorized in terms of airflow limitation (AL): normal AL ($FEV_1 > 80\%$ predicted), mild AL ($FEV_1 = 60–80\%$), moderate AL ($FEV_1 = 40–60\%$), and severe AL ($FEV_1 < 40\%$). Percentile responses in normal subjects shown as dotted lines. Note similar sensory intensities in all groups at maximum.

overlooked in favor of the more fundamental physiological changes, probably because of prejudice against measurement of sensory phenomena as being subjective and quantitatively unreliable. However, the use of psychophysical techniques has advanced to such a degree that we can formally identify the perceptual limitation to exercise (Killian, 1992). The approach and its validation is dealt with in more detail elsewhere in this volume, but we have demonstrated that measurements of sensory intensity may be used to explore quantitatively the physiological factors contributing to symptoms during exercise.

The intensity of dyspnea and leg effort have been formally evaluated during incremental exercise to limitation (Kearon et al., 1991a, 1991b). Both increase as exponential functions of exercise intensity and duration as expressed in the following equations:

$$\text{Perceived leg effort} = k \cdot \%\text{Wcap}^{2.13} \cdot \text{Time}^{0.39}$$
$$\text{Perceived dyspnea} = k \cdot \%\text{Wcap}^{2.41} \cdot \text{Time}^{0.47}$$

These relationships demonstrate that doubling work intensity results in approximately fourfold increases in effort and dyspnea, whereas doubling the duration of work increases effort and dyspnea only by approximately 30%. Reducing intensity and increasing the duration of activity is thus very effective in maximizing comfort during muscular exercise.

The measurement of symptom intensity at maximal exercise has provided results that are surprising and unexpected when viewed from a traditional understanding of limiting factors to exercise. First, the average healthy subject stops exercise at a symptom intensity rated "very severe" (7 on the Borg psychophysical rating scale). Only 20% of subjects exercise until symptom intensity is rated "maximal" (10 on the Borg scale). The average tolerance appears to be "very severe" but tolerance varies from "somewhat severe" (4) to "maximal" (10). We asked 200 normal subjects to answer a questionnaire about why they stopped exercise during incremental exercise to capacity: 8% claimed that dyspnea alone limited exercise; 61% claimed dyspnea and leg fatigue were equally limiting whereas only 25% claimed limitation due to leg fatigue alone (Hamilton et al., 1993). In a normal elderly population, 42% rated dyspnea and leg effort the same; 22% rated dyspnea greater than leg effort; 36% rated leg effort greater than dyspnea at maximal exercise (Killian et al., 1992). Dyspnea is a common factor limiting exercise alone or in combination with leg fatigue and raises questions about the validity that ventilation is never limiting in normal subjects.

Dyspnea may be defined as an appreciation of increased effort and discomfort associated with the act of breathing (see also Chap. 60). Increases in ventilation contribute to dyspnea through increases in pleural pressure swings (P_{pl}), inspiratory flow ($\dot{V}_I$), tidal volume (V_T), breathing frequency (f_b), and the muscle duty cycle (T_I/T_{TOT}) (El-Manshawi et al., 1986; Leblanc et al., 1986). These factors respectively are related to respiratory muscle force, velocity of contraction, extent of shortening, frequency of contraction, and duration of contraction. Reductions in muscle strength (MIP) and increases in lung volume also contribute to dyspnea through increases in perceived effort (Killian et al., 1984). When effort is quantified by the Borg (1980) scale in normal subjects and patients with a wide variety of cardiopulmonary disorders, the interaction of contributory factors may be expressed quantitatively:

$$B = k_1 P_{pl}/MIP + k_2 \dot{V}_I + k_3 V_T/VC + k_4 f_b + k_5 T_I/T_{TOT} + k_6$$

where B is breathlessness rated on the Borg scale (Leblanc et al., 1986). These findings suggest that dyspnea, and thus a ventilatory limitation to exercise, have to be considered in relation to a number of properties of the respiratory muscles and their operating characteristics, and not solely in relation to ventilation expressed as a ratio of the ventilatory capacity.

V. Forces and Power Developed by Respiratory Muscles During Exercise

Mechanics is the study of the relationships between force and displacement. In the case of respiratory mechanics, the force generator is the mass of respiratory muscle, the displacement involves flow, volume, and breathing frequency, requiring appropriate velocity, extent, and frequency of muscle contraction. The forces, or tensions generated, are reflected in changes in intrathoracic pressure.

A. Flow

The resting maximal flow-volume curve in healthy subjects is unchanged by exercise (Stubbing et al., 1980a) and defines the limits of the tidal volumes and flows which may be recruited to meet ventilatory demands. Because of the linkage between variables contributing to ventilation, it also defines the maximal ventilatory capacity, frequency of breathing, T_I, and T_E. In normal subjects (Fig. 4), inspiratory and expiratory flows increase, and approach maximal levels for a given lung volume; in highly trained subjects, Grimby et al. (1971a) showed that the expiratory flow-volume envelope may be reached at maximal ventilations of 130–170 liters/min. Inspiratory flow increases in a similar manner, but the maximum flow (measured at rest) is not reached; maximum exercise inspiratory flow seldom exceeds 75% of the flow capacity measured at rest.

In patients with severe airflow limitation, the maximal expiratory flow may be reached at low exercise levels, and maximal ventilation is mainly dependent on achieving high inspiratory flows (Grimby and Stiksa, 1970; Leaver and Pride, 1971; Stubbing et al., 1980b), leading to a pattern of breathing with a short T_I, and prolonged T_E.

B. Volume

Stubbing and co-workers (1980a) performed studies in a body plethysmograph and Inman et al. (1991, 1992) used helium dilution to measure lung volume at higher

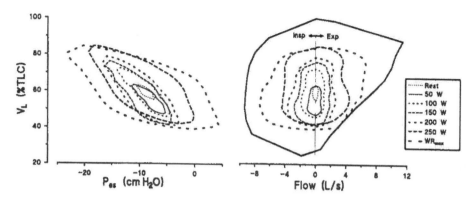

Figure 4 Flow-volume and pressure-volume relationships during tidal breathing in normal subjects breathing freely (without mouthpiece) at rest and during increasing exercise.

levels of exercise, thus validating the assumption by Olafsson and Hyatt (1969), Grimby et al. (1971b), and Hesser et al. (1981) that absolute lung volumes could be standardized by total lung capacity (TLC) maneuvers during exercise. These studies also suggested that variation in volume changes in exercise may be normalized by expressing volume changes in terms of %TLC. Increases in tidal volume in healthy subjects are achieved by gradual increases in end inspiratory volume to about 80% of TLC, and reductions in end expiratory volume to about 40% TLC (Fig. 4). The ability to reduce end-expiratory lung volume is severely limited in patients with airway obstruction, due to flow limitation and hyperinflation.

Hey et al. (1966) analyzed the increase in V_T with exercise in terms of two intersecting straight lines, representing an early linear increase in V_T followed by a plateau at a V_T of about 50% of VC. However, in most normal subjects, the relationship is a curve in which V_T increases asymptomatically. The maximal observed exercise tidal volume ($V_{T_{max}}$) in healthy subjects usually amounts to 55–60% of the VC (Åstrand, 1952), but is proportionally smaller in subjects with smaller VC, as described by the equation (Jones and Rebuck, 1979):

$$V_{T_{max}} = 0.67VC - 0.64 \text{ liters}$$

Patients with restrictive pulmonary disorders breathe with a limited tidal volume, but the reduction in V_T is less than expected from the above relationship (Burdon et al., 1983).

C. Intrapleural Pressures

Increasingly negative esophageal pressures are generated during increasing exercise to achieve increases in tidal volume and inspiratory flow against the impedance imposed by the elastic recoil of the lungs and thorax, and by resistive forces. During expiration pressures become more positive in generating high expiratory flow and in reducing end-expiratory lung volume to below resting FRC (Leblanc et al., 1988). Measurements of esophageal pressure during exercise in healthy subjects (Milic-Emili et al., 1960; Grimby et al., 1971b; Hesser et al., 1981; Inman et al., 1991, 1992) indicate that the high flow rates achieved in heavy exercise by healthy subjects, in whom VT may exceed 4 liters, and VT/TI 6 liters/s, are accompanied by intrapleural pressure swings of –20 to +5 cm H_2O (Fig. 4). The studies of Inman et al. (1991, 1992) have enabled a partitioning of the inspiratory and expiratory pressures into their respective components- against the elastic recoil of the lungs and thorax, and against flow resistive forces (Fig. 5); in addition they showed that the pressures developed seldom exceed the maximum effective pressure that is required to achieve maximum flow.

D. Forces

The mechanical forces opposing displacement are partitioned into static and dynamic components (Campbell, 1958). For the static component (elastance, P/V), as thoracic volume increases, the chest cage becomes more compliant and the lung becomes stiffer; as the thoracic volume decreases the chest cage becomes stiffer and the lung becomes more compliant. Hence, the elastance of the total system is approximately linear over the range used during exercise and approximates 14 cm H_2O/L. The dynamic components are resistance (P/$\dot{V}$), inertance (P/$\dot{V}^2$), and viscoelastance. Inertial pressure accounts for a relatively small fraction of total pressure generation during physiological breathing patterns and traditionally has been ignored in mechanical analyses. Resistive pressure increases in an accelerating

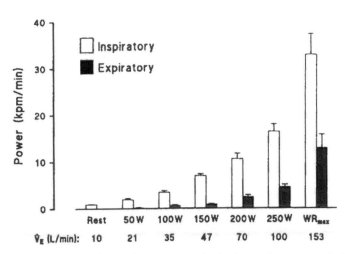

Figure 5   Power developed in inspiration and expiration by respiratory muscles in exercise of increasing intensity. (From Inman et al., 1991, 1992.)

manner relative to flow, and after the classical approach introduced by Rohrer (1925) is expressed as a polynomial function having coefficients related to flow ($\dot{V}$) and $\dot{V}^2$. The approximate values of the components related to resistive pressure (P_r) are expressed in:

$$P_r = 1.9 * \dot{V} + 0.52 * \dot{V}^2.$$

The magnitude of viscoelastance is also small during exercise as frequency of breathing is high (Milic-Emili, 1991) (see below).

E. Estimates of Respiratory Muscle Power

The power output of the inspiratory muscles in normal subjects can be estimated using these values for the resistive and elastic impedances, and the volume, flow, and timing patterns observed during exercise using a simple graphical approach (Otis, 1954). As detailed recently by Milic-Emili (1991), power output may also be calculated by a complex expression which takes into account the viscoelastic properties of the lungs and chest wall during sinusoidal cycling of breathing, in addition to elastance (E), frequency (f), resistive forces (R), and flow ($\dot{V}$):

$$\text{Power} = 0.5E\dot{V}^2/f + 0.25\pi^2K_1\dot{V}^2 + 0.67\pi^2K_2\dot{V}^3 \\ + 0.25\pi^2R\dot{V}^2/(1 + 4\pi^2\tau f^2)$$

where τ is the time constant of viscoelastic behavior and K_1 and K_2 represent the resistive properties of the airways. Such expressions indicate the changing components of the power requirements of breathing with different patterns of breathing. Although the contribution of viscoelastic forces increases at low frequency of breathing, they are negligible at frequencies of more than 20 breaths/min, and thus are not an important contributor to exercise requirements.

The calculated total power output of the respiratory muscles at maximal exercise is approximately 40–80 kpm/min with 75% of the power produced by the inspiratory muscles and 25% by the expiratory muscles (Figs. 5 and 6) (Margaria et al., 1960; Goldman et al., 1976; Thoden et al., 1969; Inman, 1992).

F. Respiratory Muscle Capacity

The area under the esophageal pressure volume loop expresses the work performed on the lungs and thoracic air volume (cm $H_2O*L/100 = 1$ kpm/min) and is a relatively easy measurement (Fig. 5). The power-generating capacity of the respiratory muscles is the product of tension and the velocity of contraction. The maximal values for tension and velocity are crudely reflected by the maximal dynamic pressure and maximal flow rates. These vary widely even in a normal population, mainly due to the variation in respiratory muscle strength. Both maximal inspiratory pressures (MIP) and maximal inspiratory flow rates vary widely in normal subjects.

The maximal power that can be generated depends on the contractile capacity

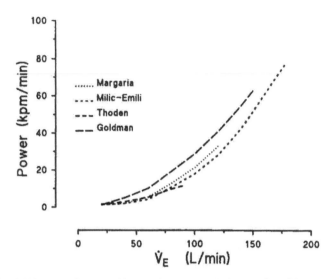

Figure 6 Total power developed by respiratory muscle in exercise of increasing intensity recorded by several investigators. (From Margaria et al., 1960; Milic-Emili et al., 1960; Thoden et al., 1969); Goldman et al., 1976.)

of the respiratory muscles. However, the maximal power output progressively decreases as inspiratory resistance increases and the maximal velocity of respiratory muscle contraction decreases. Hence, the capacity of the inspiratory muscles to perform work is dependent both on the contractile characteristics of the muscles and on the characteristics of the mechanical impedance. Thus the inspiratory power output during incremental exercise progressively falls with increasing inspiratory resistance.

Patients with pulmonary disorders, in addition to generating increased pressures against resistive and elastic impedances, additionally face reductions in respiratory muscle strength related to chronic shortening of muscle secondary to hyperinflation, and to increased velocity and frequency of shortening secondary to changes in the pattern of breathing.

VI. Coordination of Respiratory Muscle Activity

Konno and Mead (1967, 1968) paved the way for the study of coordination of respiratory muscle activity by studying changes in the diameters of the rib cage and abdomen. From these analyses they inferred that the diaphragm is responsible for virtually all ventilation at rest. During exercise Grimby and co-workers (1968) showed that there was an increase in the volume of the rib cage and a fall in abdominal volume suggesting that the diaphragm moved upward, increasing its length at the start of inspiration. The activity of the abdominal and rib cage muscles is timed so that their contraction accounts for chest and abdominal wall movement leaving the diaphragm free to drive the lungs. Goldman et al. (1976) also showed that the rib cage and abdominal contributions to volume deviated from their relaxation characteristics during exercise, indicating additional work which is referred to as distortion (Grimby et al., 1976). The work done related to distortion cannot be precisely measured but in one estimate, it approached 20% of the measured respiratory work at maximal exercise. Hence, the estimates of work addressed above are likely to be underestimates.

VII. Measurements of the Oxygen Cost of Breathing

There have been many attempts to quantify the oxygen cost and "efficiency" of breathing. However, these studies have been dogged by difficulties related to the measurement of work and the errors in measuring oxygen consumption of respiratory muscles. Measurements of the increase in O_2 consumption which accompanies increases in $\dot{V}E$ have yielded widely varying results and these in turn yield varying estimates for mechanical efficiency, from 1% (Cain and Otis, 1949) to 25% (Milic-Emili et al., 1960). Estimates of oxygen cost per liter $\dot{V}E$ have usually varied between 0.5 and 1 ml/min for levels of $\dot{V}E$ below 100 liters/min, with greater variation being observed at higher $\dot{V}E$, where values from 1 ml/min (Milic-Emili et al., 1960) to 8 ml/min (Shephard, 1966) have been reported. On the basis of these estimates the O_2 cost of breathing at maximal exercise has been estimated to vary between 3% (Milic-Emili et al., 1962) and 25% (Fritts et al., 1959; Levison and Cherniack, 1968) of the total O_2 consumption. Liljestrand in 1918 highlighted the basis of many errors in the measurement of the oxygen cost of breathing. Many of these errors have contributed to the variability in oxygen costs subsequently measured. His estimates remain the most reliable and indicate an accelerating oxygen cost of breathing from 0.5 ml O_2/L/min at low ventilations up to values of 1.5 ml O_2/L/min at the ventilations usually seen at maximal exercise. Considering that 75% of the work of breathing is performed by the inspiratory muscles, with a mass of 0.5–1 kg (Arora and Rochester, 1982) these estimates have face validity, but the idea that the needs of the respiratory muscles for oxygen could become a factor limiting maximal $\dot{V}_{O_2}$ (Otis, 1954) has not been widely accepted. The maximal oxygen consumption of these muscles could not realistically exceed 200–400 ml/min given the highest estimates of sustainable muscle oxygen consumption per unit mass. Using conventional steady-state measurements the sustainable oxygen consumption of the respiratory muscles is between 200–300 ml in healthy young subjects following incremental addition of dead space to toleration (Villafranca et al., 1991). With incremental resistive loading the oxygen consumption at maximal sustainable respiratory muscle activity is approximately half this value (Jones et al., 1985). Given that no discrete oxygen consumption is seen across different contractile activities at maximal performance, one must conclude that limitation of respiratory muscle activity is sensory in nature.

In patients with lung or chest wall diseases, the oxygen cost of breathing is increased but, in general, the oxygen consumption at limitation is not larger than that seen in normal subjects (Jones et al., 1971), although the oxygen cost per unit ventilation is increased; as pointed out above limitation is sensory (Fig. 3).

VIII.   Respiratory Muscle Fatigue During Exercise

A.   Identification of Fatigue

The definitive demonstration of respiratory muscle fatigue requires a reduction in force output for a given level of neural activation. This is best done using force:frequency response curves to recognize both high and low frequency fatigue. This is simply not possible during exercise because there are multiple muscles and the isolation of the nerve supply for electrical stimulation is difficult. Indirect approaches such as spectral frequency analysis of the Fourier transform of the diaphragmatic EMG record have been used but the information obtained falls short of formal force:frequency response curves. In recent years mechanical analysis has reemerged in the hope that the mechanical performance of the respiratory muscles may be predictive of fatigue and explain the variable deterioration in the performance of the respiratory muscles seen across subjects.

B.   Tension-Time Index as an Indicator of Fatigue

For practical purposes, the muscles and mechanical constraints which apply during inspiration and expiration must be approached separately. The power output of the inspiratory muscles is considerably greater than that of the expiratory muscles during exercise (Fig. 5). Particular attention has been paid to the diaphragm in the belief that as the force output of the diaphragm approaches capacity, the probability and the severity of diaphragmatic fatigue increases. The tension time index for the diaphragm (TTdi) was introduced by Bellemare and Grassino (1982) as a method for recognizing potentially fatiguing from nonfatiguing contractions and a threshold TTdi (Ti/Ttot $*$ Pdi/Pdi$_{max}$) of 0.15 was established during loaded breathing. The rate at which the diaphragm fatigues increases as the TTdi increases. There are difficulties with the TTdi when applied to exercise compared to respiratory loading. The Pdi is an easy and reliable measurement but the Pdi$_{max}$ is a difficult measurement. Pdi$_{max}$ depends on the conditions in both the chest and abdominal cavities at the time of measurement. If the abdomen is relaxed Pdi$_{max}$ approximates maximal inspiratory pressure measured at the mouth or in the esophagus. Contraction of the abdominal muscles increases Pdi by generating a positive pressure in the abdomen. Maximal Pdi depends on the simultaneous activation of both inspiratory and expiratory muscles (abdominal muscles). During this maximal static effort, the diaphragm holds the transdiaphragmatic pressure but does not generate the pressure (i.e., it may even contract in an eccentric fashion after an initial concentric contraction). Hence, there are conceptual difficulties with TTdi during exercise in that the Pdi is a dynamic measurement expressed relative to a static measurement of Pdi_{max}. The Pdi measured during exercise should be referenced to the maximal Pdi achievable under the same dynamic conditions (Leblanc et al., 1988). Lastly, any differences in the decline in force-generating capacity at the same relative performance of the diaphragm is not measured, even though variability almost certainly exists.

C. Pressure Versus Capacity to Generate Pressure

A simpler technique can be adopted by examining esophageal pressure during maximal exercise in relationship to the esophageal pressure measured during a maximal inspiratory/expiratory maneuver measured immediately following exercise. Relatively greater stress is placed on the inspiratory muscles, with inspiratory pressures during maximal exercise being approximately 60% of those during the maximal inspiratory maneuver, while pressures during expiration reach only 20–30% of those during the maximal effort.

The potential for respiratory muscle fatigue is high during exercise where the ventilatory demands may result in fatiguing tensions. This potential is even greater when the impedance to breathing is increased with airflow limitation or restrictive disorders. The occurrence of fatigue is so life threatening that one might argue teleologically that fail-safe mechanisms to prevent the occurrence of fatigue must exist. For example, fatigue in a given muscle may be lessened through distribution of the load to a greater bulk of muscle. Alternatively, when a muscle generates forces of fatiguing intensity, the subject's perception of effort is greatly increased and is usually sufficiently distressing for the subject to stop exercising before fatigue occurs. During exercise, the sense of effort is primarily reduced by distributing a greater proportion of the load to the rib cage and accessory muscles.

The possibility that respiratory muscle fatigue may become a limiting factor to further increases in exercise has been raised by a number of authors. The hypothesis is usually tested by examining the relationship between Pmus during exercise and the maximum inspiratory force that can be generated voluntarily (Pmax,insp). However, this limiting value is never reached because the subject's tolerance for the associated discomfort is simply not achievable.

The maximal ventilation which may be sustained for more than 4 min is about 75% of the 15-s maximal voluntary ventilation (Freedman, 1970; Leith and Bradley, 1976), and Roussos and Macklem (1977) have shown that the diaphragm fatigues rapidly when generating a transdiaphragmatic pressure of only 40% of the maximum static value. Given these facts and considering the high V_T and f_b employed in heavy exercise, it seems possible that respiratory muscle fatigue may limit ventilation. Loke et al. (1982) demonstrated small falls in maximum transdiaphragmatic pressures at the end of a marathon run, and Hesser and colleagues (1981) showed that maximal inspiratory work declines at exhaustion during maximal exercise.

Similar arguments may apply to the consideration of respiratory muscle fatigue in limiting the time for which a given level of exercise may be maintained. A crucial factor in this consideration is the ventilation required for a given proportion of $\dot{V}O_2$ max. If exercise is performed at a level of $\dot{V}O_2$ associated with lactate production and concomitant increases in $\dot{V}O_2$ and $\dot{V}E$, the intensity, duration, and frequency of respiratory muscle force development may be in a critical region which cannot be maintained for more than a few minutes. The "anaerobic threshold" and respiratory fatigue (i.e., symptom limitation of exercise) may occur at much lower levels of exercise in sedentary than trained subjects.

As pointed out elsewhere in this book, the factors which lead to fatigue in respiratory muscles are the same as in other skeletal muscles, and are presumably determined by the availability of fuel substrates, oxygen delivery by arterial blood flow, efficiency of oxygen extraction, and acid–base status.

IX. Summary

The sense of effort in breathing is at, or close to, maximal tolerable magnitude at the limitation of sustained exercise performance, and the same is true for the active peripheral skeletal muscle. As failure is approached, discomfort increases and the tolerance of the individual is exceeded, before depletion of ATP, with its associated irreversible actin and myosin interaction. Exercise is terminated before such irreversible failure. Thus, while one may question the validity of using the term fatigue in this situation, in everyday language it does represent the intolerable discomfort that accompanies muscle contraction as it nears limiting conditions.

Acknowledgments

We are grateful for the help of Edie Summers in the preparation of the manuscript. Our research is supported by the Medical Research Council of Canada.

References

Arora, N. S., and Rochester, D. F. (1982). Respiratory muscle strength and maximal voluntary ventilation in undernourished patients. *Am. Rev. Respir. Dis.*, 126:5–8.

Åstrand, P. O. (1952). *Experimental Studies of Physical Working Capacity in Relation to Sex and Age*. Copenhagen, Munksgaard.

Bellemare, F., and Grassino, A. (1982). Effect of pressure and timing of contraction on human diaphragm fatigue. *J. Appl. Physiol.*, 53:1190–1195.

Borg, G. A. V. (1980). A category scale with ratio properties for intermodal and interindividual comparisons. In *Psychophysical Judgment and the Process of Perception*. Proceedings of the 22nd International Congress of Psychology. Edited by H. G. Geissler and P. Petzold. Amsterdam, North Holland Publishing Co., pp. 25–34.

Burdon, J. G. W., Killian, K. J., and Jones, N. L. (1983). Pattern of breathing during exercise in patients with interstitial lung disease. *Thorax*, 38:778–784.

Cain, C. C., and Otis, A. B. (1949). Some physiological effects resulting from added resistance to respiration. *J. Aviation Med.*, 20:149–160.

Campbell, E. J. M. (1958). *The Respiratory Muscles and the Mechanics of Breathing*. London, Lloyd-Luke (Year Book Medical Publishers) Ltd.

Clark, T. J. H., Freedman, S., Campbell, E. J. M., and Winn, R. R. (1969). The ventilatory capacity of patients with chronic airway obstruction. *Clin. Sci.*, 36:307–316.

El-Manshawi, A., Killian, K. J., Summers, E., and Jones, N. L. (1986). Breathlessness during exercise with and without resistive loading. *J. Appl. Physiol.*, 61:896–905.

Freedman, S. (1970). Sustained maximum voluntary ventilation. *Respir. Physiol.*, 8:230–244.

Fritts, H. W., Filler, J., Fishman, A. P., and Cournand, A. (1959). The efficiency of ventilation during voluntary hyperpnea: studies in normal subjects and in dyspneic patients with either chronic pulmonary emphysema or obesity. *J. Clin. Invest.*, 38:1339–1348.

Goldman, M. D., Grimby, G., and Mead, J. (1976). Mechanical work of breathing derived from rib cage and abdominal V-P partitioning. *J. Appl. Physiol.*, 41:752–763.

Grimby, G., Bunn, J., and Mead, J. (1968). Relative contribution of rib cage and abdomen to ventilation during exercise. *J. Appl. Physiol.*, 24:159–166.

Grimby, G., and Stiksa, J. (1970). Flow-volume curves and breathing patterns during exercise in patients with obstructive lung disease. *Scand. J. Clin. Lab. Invest.*, 25:303–313.

Grimby, G., Saltin, B., and Wilhelmsen, L. (1971a). Pulmonary flow-volume and pressure-volume relationship during submaximal and maximal exercise in young well trained men. *Bull. Eur. Physiopathol. Respir.*, 7:157–172.

Grimby, G., Goldman, M., and Mead, J. (1971b). Rib cage and abdominal volume partitioning during exercise and induced hyperventilation. *Scand. J. Respir. Dis.* (Suppl.), 77:4–7.

Grimby, G., Goldman, M., and Mead, J. (1976). Respiratory muscle action inferred from rib cage and abdominal V-P partitioning. *J. Appl. Physiol.*, 41:739–751.

Hamilton, A., Summers, E., Jones, N. L., and Killian, K. J. (1993). Symptom limitations during a progressive incremental exercise test. *Am. Rev. Respir. Dis.* (in press).

Hesser, C. M., Linnarsson, D., and Fagraeus, L. (1981). Pulmonary mechanics and work of breathing at maximal ventilation and raised air pressure. *J. Appl. Physiol.*, 50:747–753.

Hey, E. M., Lloyd, B. B., Cunningham, D. J. C., Jukes, M. G. M., and Bolton, D. P. G. (1966). Effects of various respiratory stimuli on the depth and frequency of breathing in man. *Respir. Physiol.*, 1:193–205.

Hugh-Jones, P. and Lambert, A. V. (1952). A simple standard exercise test and its use for measuring exertion dyspnea. *Br. Med. J.*, 1:65–71.

Inman, M. D., Campbell, E. J. M., and Killian, K. J. (1991). Work performed by expiratory muscles during exercise. *Am. Rev. Respir. Dis.* 143(4) (suppl):A346.

Inman, M. D. (1992). *The Role of Expiratory Muscle Activity in Ventilation During Exercise*. Ph.D. thesis, McMaster University.

Jones, G. L., Killian, K. J., Summers, E., and Jones, N. L. (1985). Inspiratory muscle forces and endurance in maximum resistive loading. *J. Appl. Physiol.*, 58:1608–1615.

Jones, N. L., Jones, G., and Edwards, R. H. T. (1971). Exercise tolerance in chronic airway obstruction. *Am. Rev. Respir. Dis.*, 103:477–491.

Jones, N. L., and Rebuck, A. S. (1979). Tidal volume during exercise in patients with diffuse fibrosing alveolitis. *Bull. Eur. Physiopathol. Respir.*, 15:321–327.

Jones, N. L. (1991). Determinants of breathing pattern. In *Exercise*. Edited by B. J. Whipp and K. Wasserman. New York, Marcel Dekker, Inc.

Kearon, M. C., Summers, E., Jones, N. L., Campbell, E. J. M., and Killian, K. J. (1991a). Breathing during prolonged exercise in man. *J. Physiol.*, 442:477–487.

Kearon, M. C., Summers, E., Jones, N. L., Campbell, E. J. M., and Killian, K. J. (1991b). Effort and dyspnoea during work of varying intensity and duration. *Eur. Respir. J.*, 4:917–925.

Killian, K. J., Gandevia, S. C., Summers, E., and Campbell, E. J. M. (1984). Effect of increased lung volume on perception of breathlessness, effort, and tension. *J. Appl. Physiol.*, 57:686–691.

Killian, K. J., Leblanc, P., Martin, D. H., Summers, E., Jones, N. L., and Campbell, E. J. M. (1992). Exercise capacity, ventilatory, circulatory, and symptom limitation in patients with chronic airflow limitation. *Am. Rev. Respir. Dis.*, 146:935–940.

Killian, K. J. (1992). The nature of breathlessness and its measurement. In *Breathlessness 1991*. Proceedings of the Campbell Symposium, Hamilton, Ontario, May 1991. Edited by N. L. Jones and K. J. Killian. Hamilton, Decker Medical Publications, pp. 74–87.

Konno, K., and Mead, J. (1967). Measurement of the separate volume changes of rib cage and abdomen to ventilation during exercise. *J. Appl. Physiol.*, 22:407–422.

Konno, K., and Mead, J. (1968). Static volume pressure characteristics of rib cage and abdomen. *J. Appl. Physiol.*, 24:544–548.

Leaver, D. G., and Pride, N. B. (1971). Flow-volume curves and expiratory pressures during exercise in patients with chronic airflow obstruction. *Scand. J. Respir. Dis.* (suppl.), 177:23–28.

Leblanc, P., Bowie, D. M., Summers, E., Jones, N. L., and Killian, K. J. (1986). Breathlessness and exercise in patients with cardiorespiratory disease. *Am. Rev. Respir. Dis.*, 133:21–25.

Leblanc, P., Summers, E., Inman, M. D., Jones, N. L., Campbell, E. J. M., and Killian, K. J. (1988). Inspiratory muscles during exercise: a problem of supply and demand. *J. Appl. Physiol.*, 64:2482–2489.

Leith, D. E., and Bradley, M. (1976). Ventilatory muscle strength and endurance training. *J. Appl. Physiol.*, 41:508–516.

Levison, H., and Cherniack, R. M. (1968). Ventilatory cost of exercise in chronic obstructive pulmonary disease. *J. Appl. Physiol.*, 25:21–27.

Liljestrand, G. (1918). Studies of the work of breathing. *Skand. Arch. Physiol.*, 35:199–293.

Loke, J., Mahler, D. A., and Virgulto, J. A. (1982). Respiratory muscle fatigue after marathon running. *J. Appl. Physiol.*, 52:821–824.

Margaria, R., Milic-Emili, J., Petit, J. M., and Cavagna, G. (1960). Mechanical work of breathing during muscular exercise. *J. Appl. Physiol.*, 15:354–358.

Means, J. H. (1924). Dyspnoea. *Med. Monograph*, 5:309–416.

Milic-Emili, J., Petit, J. M., and Deroanne, R. (1960). The effects of respiratory rate on the mechanical work of breathing during exercise. *Int. Z. Angew. Physiol.*, 18:330–340.

Milic-Emili, J., Petit, J. M., and Deroanne, R. (1962). Mechanical work of breathing during exercise in trained and untrained subjects. *J. Appl. Physiol.*, 17:43–46.

Milic-Emili, J. (1991). Work of breathing. In *The Lung. Scientific Foundations*. Vol. I. Edited by J. B. West and R. G. Crystal. New York, Raven Press, pp. 1065–1075.

Olafsson, S., and Hyatt, R. E. (1969). Ventilatory mechanics and expiratory flow limitation during exercise in normal subjects. *J. Clin. Invest.*, 48:564–573.

Otis, A. B. (1954). The work of breathing. *Physiol. Rev.*, 34:449–458.

Rohrer, F. (1925). The physiology of respiratory movements. *Handbuch Norm. Path. Physiol.*, 2:70–127.

Roussos, C. S., and Macklem, P. T. (1977). Diaphragmatic fatigue in man. *J. Appl. Physiol.*, 43:189–197.

Shephard, R. J. (1966). Oxygen cost of breathing during vigorous exercise. *Q. J. Exp. Physiol.*, 51:336–350.

Stubbing, D. G., Pengelly, L. D., Morse, J. L. C., and Jones, N. L. (1980a). Pulmonary mechanics during exercise in normal males. *J. Appl. Physiol.*, 49:506–510.

Stubbing, D. G., Pengelly, L. D., Morse, J. L. C., and Jones, N. L. (1980b). Pulmonary mechanics during exercise in subjects with chronic airflow obstruction. *J. Appl. Physiol.*, 49:511–515.

Thoden, J. S., Dempsey, J. A., Reddan, W. G., Birnbaum, M. L., Forster, H. V., Grover, R. F., and Rankin, J. (1969). Ventilatory work during steady state response to exercise. *Fed. Proc.*, 28:1316–1321.

Villafranca, C. C., Casan, P., Summers, E., Jones, N. L., and Campbell, E. J. M. (1991). Metabolic cost of breathing and dyspnea. *Am. Rev. Respir. Dis.*, 143(4):A592.

48

Respiratory Muscle Activity During Sleep

AILIANG XIE and T. DOUGLAS BRADLEY

University of Toronto
Toronto, Ontario, Canada

I. Introduction

Sleep is a reversible behavioral state of perceptual disengagement from the environment. The general depression of respiration, circulation, and other vital activity during this period has long been recognized. However, sleep is not a homogeneous phenomenon but is, rather, a physiologically heterogeneous condition characterized by frequent transient alterations in the state of consciousness. It can be subdivided into two fundamentally distinct neurophysiological states based on behavioral and electrographic characteristics: non–rapid-eye-movement (NREM), or quiet sleep, and rapid-eye-movement (REM), or active sleep (Carskadon and Dement, 1989). The effects of NREM and REM sleep on physiological processes are very different. In NREM sleep, mental activity is minimal or absent and respiration is controlled mainly by chemical-metabolic factors. In contrast, REM sleep is characterized by central nervous system activation associated with a variety of phasic events, which seem to be under behavioral influence. Similarly, respiration during REM sleep, especially phasic REM sleep, is largely independent of chemical-metabolic control but is influenced more predominantly by non–metabolic-behavioral factors (Phillipson and Bowes, 1986; Douglas, 1989).

Since the recognition that sleep-related breathing disorders, such as the sleep apnea syndromes, are common and that hypoxia is a frequent occurrence during sleep in a number of respiratory diseases, the study of respiration during sleep has become a crucial area of investigation in the field of respiratory medicine. Since the respiratory muscles comprise the force generator that moves the respiratory pump to subserve ventilation and since they must remain rhythmically active at all times, their behavior and regulation during sleep are critically important. Structurally and functionally, the respiratory muscles are part of the musculoskeletal system, and, therefore, their activity during sleep must be considered in light of the motor system in general. In fact, it has been recognized that tonic inhibition of some respiratory muscles occurs in association with the generalized muscle atonia of REM sleep (Kline et al., 1990).

As our main interest is the influence of sleep on the respiratory muscles that generate airflow, the following discussion will be confined to the chest wall muscles. The activity of the muscles of the upper airway during sleep will not be considered in any detail.

II. Control of Skeletal Muscles During Sleep

During wakefulness, most skeletal muscles are constantly active due to the asynchronous, sustained firing of motoneurons in response to reflex activation, maintenance of posture, and behavioral functions. The transition from wakefulness to sleep is generally associated with a gradual decline in muscle tone (Kleitman, 1963; Pompeiano, 1967; Chase, 1972), yet, spinal reflex activity is preserved in NREM sleep (Giaquinto et al., 1963; Kubota et al., 1965). Hence, the tonic EMG activity of the postural muscles persists, although at a lower level (Jouvet, 1967). During REM sleep tonic postural muscle activity is almost abolished (Kleitman, 1963; Jouvet, 1967; Chase, 1972). In addition, monosynaptic and polysynaptic reflexes are depressed (Giaquinto et al., 1963; Gassel et al., 1964; Kubota et al., 1965; Lenzi et al., 1968). Furthermore, an additional phasic inhibition of spontaneous and reflex motor activity is superimposed on the tonic depression of motor activity coincident with bursts of REM sleep (Morrison and Pompeiano, 1965a,b). REM sleep is, therefore, partly characterized by muscle atonia. Despite the prevailing muscle atonia during REM sleep, irregular phasic motor discharges occur, creating scattered bursts of activity upon a quiescent tableau. The amount of phasic motor discharge is proportional to the density of REMs (Pompeiano, 1978).

The mechanisms by which sleep affects motor control are not well understood. Intracellular neural recordings have shown that during sleep, particularly REM sleep, there is a hyperpolarization of motoneuron membrane potential both in the brain stem (Chandler et al., 1980) and in the lumbar spinal cord (Glenn and Dement, 1981). Recent studies of the interaction between sleep and neuromotor action have been focused largely on the skeletal muscular atonia in REM sleep. Available evidence indicates that the influence of REM state on motoneuron membrane potential results from direct postsynaptic inhibition (Chandler et al., 1980; Glenn and Dement, 1981). In addition, presynaptic dysfacilitation has been proposed as another possible mechanism of REM sleep atonia, which, with postsynaptic inhibition, may operate in concert or independently for restricted periods (Chase and Morales, 1982, 1983; Morales et al., 1988). In any case, postsynaptic inhibition is the principal, and probably sufficient, mechanism responsible for the atonia of the somatic musculature during active sleep (Chase and Morales, 1989). Polysynaptic reflex activity is also tonically depressed in REM sleep, though the mechanism of inhibition is not the same as for monosynaptic responses (Lenzi et al., 1968).

III. Control of Respiratory Muscles During Sleep

Although respiratory muscles are skeletal muscles, they are distinct in displaying constant coordinated rhythmic activity. This rhythmic activity is a manifestation of their vital role as force generators to move the respiratory pump for the maintenance of ventilation. However, unlike the other vital muscular pump, the heart, the respiratory muscle system itself does not have a built-in pacemaker. Instead, rhythmic activity of the respiratory muscles is governed by a network of respiratory neurons in the medulla. This respiratory center generates the respiratory rhythm and respiratory drive either through intrinsic cellular mechanisms or through interconnections among different neurons. The earliest studies of medullary respiratory activity during sleep were carried out by Puizillout and Ternaux (1974) and Orem and colleagues (1974). The former recorded multiunit respiratory activity in the medulla of the encephalon-isolated cat during sleep, and the latter recorded single medullary respiratory neurons in the chronic intact cat. Both found that respiratory-related activity decreased in sleep. Furthermore, in the course of a series of microelectrode penetrations through the brain stem at the level of the facial nucleus, Orem et al. (1974) found that neurons that exhibited mainly respiratory activity during wakefulness continued to display respiratory activity in NREM and, to a lesser extent, in REM sleep. However, neurons that demonstrated both respiratory and nonrespiratory activity had a marked decrease in respiratory activity in NREM and almost complete abolition of respiratory activity in REM sleep. Taken together, these findings indicated a reduction in central respiratory drive during sleep, which was most pronounced in those respiratory-related neurons that displayed significant nonrespiratory activity. These observations imply that sleep-related withdrawal of central respiratory drive to respiratory muscles, such as the intercostal and scalene, which have substantial postural activity, would be more pronounced than to the diaphragm, whose activity is predominantly respiratory in nature.

All types of skeletal motor acts are modulated by sensory feedback from proprioceptors, and breathing is no exception to this rule. In order to maintain breathing at levels adequate to support a wide range of metabolic and behavioral requirements, the medullary respiratory center regulates the respiratory muscles on the basis of continuously altering feedback from chemoreceptors and proprioceptors.

In addition, the activity of the respiratory motoneuron is influenced by input from the cerebral cortex in order to override metabolic influences to subserve behavioral respiratory activity such as phonation and breath-holding. However, owing to their vital role in maintaining ventilation, rhythmic discharge to the respiratory pump muscles, but not to other skeletal muscles, during sleep is essential to the maintenance of life. It is therefore obvious that sleep acts on the activity of respiratory muscles in a much more complicated way than on general skeletal muscles. Sleep not only has a direct impact on respiratory muscles per se but also exerts some indirect impact through affecting the sensitivity of the chemoreceptors and respiratory motoneurons. Although the primary focus of this chapter is not control of breathing during sleep, a brief review of this subject will shed light on the influence of sleep on respiratory muscle activity. Readers wishing a more in-depth review of respiratory control during sleep are referred elsewhere (Phillipson and Bowes, 1986).

A. Mechanical Factors

During sleep, several important changes in lung mechanics occur that have potential effects on the action of respiratory muscles. Sleep usually occurs in the horizontal position, which increases upper airway resistance (R_{UAW}), reduces respiratory compliance, reduces functional residual capacity (FRC), and changes chest wall configuration and thus alters the anatomical linkage of the respiratory muscles to the rib cage (Mortola et al., 1978). Duggan et al. (1990) found that in the supine position R_{UAW} increased by 30% compared to the upright position. During sleep R_{UAW} increases further due to hypotonia of the upper airway dilating muscles and the altered distribution of respiratory motor output to upper airway versus chest wall musculature (Lopes et al., 1983; Hudgel and Devadatta, 1984; Henke et al., 1991, 1992). The magnitude of this resistive load varies markedly across the normal healthy population and within subjects across sleep states and sometimes even from breath to breath. The increase of R_{UAW} and reduction of respiratory compliance have a fundamental influence on the activity of respiratory muscles and respiration during sleep, which will be discussed later. FRC is reduced approximately 20% in normal humans while supine compared to upright while awake (Moreno and Lyons, 1961) and decreases even further during sleep due to inspiratory muscle hypotonia (Hudgel and Devadatta, 1984). The fall in FRC during sleep may affect breathing in three ways. First, it increases diaphragmatic length and, therefore, optimizes its contractile efficiency in normal people. However, the gravitational effects of the abdominal contents may increase the mechanical load on the diaphragm to the extent that it may play a role in precipitating sleep-induced alveolar hypoventilation in the obesity-hypoventilation (Pickwickian) syndrome (Lopata and Onal, 1982). Second, the fall in FRC facilitates both large and small airway collapse, thereby increasing respiratory resistance (Hoffstein et al., 1984). Third, reduction in FRC reduces O_2 stores in the body, consequently predisposing to oxygenhemoglobin desaturation during apneas (Bradley et al., 1985).

In addition to the above, the alteration of anatomical linkage of the respiratory muscles to the respiratory pump in the recumbent position and especially the distortion of the chest wall configuration due to inhibition of the rib cage muscles during REM sleep may influence reflex drives originating from muscle spindle afferents and chest wall receptors (Henke et al., 1988).

B. Chemical Factors

The chemical drives from peripheral and central chemoreceptors exert their actions on respiratory motoneurons via the respiratory center. Hypoxia affects the respiratory system in a complex way. First, it stimulates respiration through its effects on the carotid body. Because of the nonlinear relationship between Pa_{O_2} and ventilation, ventilation usually increases appreciably only when Pa_{O_2} is less than 60 mm Hg. On the other hand, when hypoxia is sustained or when Pa_{O_2} drops acutely below 30–40 mm Hg, it may cause central nervous system depression. As a result, the activity of medullary respiratory neurons may also be inhibited, resulting in a reduction in respiratory muscle activity and a consequent depression of ventilation (Fitzgerald and Lahiri, 1986; Douglas, 1989). An important interaction of Pa_{O_2} with Pa_{CO_2} exists such that elevation of Pa_{CO_2} increases the ventilatory response to hypoxia. Under these conditions, which prevail in many respiratory diseases, small reductions in Pa_{O_2} can cause relatively large increases in ventilation. Conversely, reductions in Pa_{O_2} increase the ventilatory response to an increase in Pa_{CO_2}.

Under normal conditions, small changes in Pa_{CO_2} result in significant alterations of ventilation which are linearly related to the increase or decrease in Pa_{CO_2} (Fitzgerald and Lahiri, 1986). Pa_{CO_2} is sensed in both the carotid body and the medullary chemoreceptor. Thus, alteration in Pa_{CO_2} is probably the main metabolic factor affecting ventilation during wakefulness, keeping in mind that nonmetabolic factors also affect respiration in this state. During NREM sleep, respiration is critically dependent on chemical-metabolic factors so that Pa_{CO_2} assumes the principal role in regulating respiration (Bradley and Phillipson, 1992). Upon the withdrawal of the nonchemical wakefulness drive to breathe, Pa_{CO_2} increases 2–7 mm Hg and Sa_{O_2} decreases 2–3% during NREM sleep (Phillipson and Bowes, 1986). At the same time, the slope of the ventilatory responses to CO_2 and hypoxia are decreased. These findings indicate that the thresholds for ventilatory responses to CO_2 and hypoxia are increased and the sensitivities of the central and peripheral chemoreceptors are decreased at the transition from wakefulness to NREM sleep (Douglas, 1989). The fall of basal metabolic rate during sleep (Brebbia and Altshuler, 1965; White et al., 1985) also has an effect in reducing ventilation, therefore, lessening the demand on the respiratory muscles (Zwillich et al., 1977).

C. Higher Central Neural Factors

Although the automatic respiratory control system can function independently, it is subject to higher neural influences, which are largely nonrespiratory and nonchemical in nature (Hugelin, 1986). This nonrespiratory, nonchemical drive arises from cortical and subcortical centers. As one sleeps quietly, arouses abruptly, or dreams intensely, there may be dramatic changes in the inputs from higher nervous centers. For instance, cerebral metabolic rate and cerebral blood flow in humans during slow wave sleep are reduced significantly compared to wakefulness, reflecting a low overall level of cerebral activity. In contrast, during REM sleep, cerebral metabolic rate and blood flow are as high as or higher than in the awake state (Townsend et al., 1973, Madsen et al., 1991). McGinty et al. (1974) also found a dramatic increase in cerebral blood flow that was associated with increases in cerebral neuronal activity during REM sleep. Although there are no direct data available to demonstrate cortical neural interactions of sleep and breathing, it seems that the hypoventilation and decreased responses to chemical and mechanical stimuli in NREM sleep partially reflect a loss of the nonchemical wakefulness drive to respiratory motoneurons, which may arise from cortical and subcortical centers (Phillipson and Bowes, 1986; Douglas, 1989). Nevertheless, respiration in NREM sleep is highly regular and is governed predominantly by chemical-metabolic stimuli. On the other hand, the relatively irregular pattern of breathing characteristic of REM sleep may reflect the influence of nonchemical, dream-related cortical or subcortical output on the respiratory system.

Despite the fundamental importance of the wakefulness drive to breathe, its anatomical source has remained obscure. Recently, however, Manaker and Fogarty (1992) observed that the caudal raphe nuclei contained many neurons projecting to respiratory motoneurons. They demonstrated that these nuclei had, as one of their functions, the integration of inputs originating from various neural centers and, in turn, affected respiration apparently independent of chemical respiratory stimuli. This finding suggested an anatomical basis for the wakefulness drive to breathe.

With respect to the overall effects of sleep on the activity of respiratory muscles, it is apparent that there is a dichotomy between the reticular (inhibitory) and the respiratory (excitatory) descending influences that control the spinal motoneurons, the final common pathway to the respiratory muscles (Duron and Marlot, 1980). As indicated above, the interpretation of the behaviors of respiratory muscles during sleep is complicated by alterations in chemical respiratory drive and sensory feedback from the respiratory apparatus and by alteration in the mechanics of breathing as well as by the intervention of nonrespiratory influences on muscle activity during REM sleep.

IV. Functions of Respiratory Muscles During Sleep

A. Respiratory Motoneural and Muscular System

In general, the respiratory pump muscles can be classified as either inspiratory muscles (diaphragm, scalene, sternocleidomastoid, external intercostal muscles, and parasternals) or expiratory muscles (internal intercostal muscles, triangularis sterni, and abdominal muscles). The contribution of these muscles to ventilation varies according to their anatomical structure, location, and functional characteristics as well as their afferent and efferent innervation. The influence of sleep on these muscles does not appear to be uniform.

B. Function of Respiratory Muscles During NREM Sleep

There is general agreement that the transition from wakefulness to NREM sleep is associated with a reduction in the activity of the upper airway dilator muscles (Orem and Lydic, 1978; Sauerland et al., 1981; Phillipson and Bowes, 1986). Physiologically, this is associated with an increase in R_{UAW} (Lopes et al., 1983; Hudgel and Devadatta, 1984), which has important effects on the respiratory system such as causing distortion of the rib cage, retention of CO_2 and recruitment of the respiratory pump muscles, especially the nondiaphragmatic muscles (Skatrud and Dempsey, 1985). In contrast, there is controversy regarding the effect of NREM sleep on the actions of the respiratory pump muscles.

As the diaphragm is the principal inspiratory muscle, its behavior during sleep has been extensively studied. Based on the observations of electromyographic activity of the diaphragm (EMG_{di}), the motor control of the diaphragm is believed to be relatively spared from the direct inhibitory influence of sleep. The pattern of EMG_{di} activity during NREM sleep in humans has been reported to be similar to that during quiet wakefulness or may even be slightly increased (Parmeggiani and Sabattini, 1972; Tusiewicz et al., 1977; Tabachnik et al., 1981a; Henke et al., 1992; Kimoff et al., 1992).

In agreement with findings in humans, the general pattern of intercostal muscle activity in the course of NREM sleep was reported as being similar to that found during quiet wakefulness in cats (Duron and Marlot, 1980). In addition, phasic intercostal EMG activity has been shown to increase up to 34% above the wakefulness level during NREM sleep in normal adults (Tabachnik et al., 1981a; Lopes et al., 1983). Furthermore, another primary inspiratory muscle, the scalene, is active both tonically and phasically during NREM sleep (Sherrey and Megirian, 1987). Thus it seems that respiratory muscle activity is preserved or even increased in NREM sleep compared to quiet wakefulness.

On the surface, these observations are difficult to understand because a sleep-induced inhibition of the central nervous system and reduced motor output from medullary respiratory neurons should lead to lower EMG activity of the respiratory pump muscles in NREM sleep compared to wakefulness. Increased respiratory muscle EMG activity might be related to CO_2 retention during sleep, causing an increase in chemoreceptor stimulation resulting in increased activation of respiratory muscles. However, this feedback alone could not explain the increase in respiratory muscle activity above awake levels, otherwise Pa_{CO_2} should decrease rather than increase (Skatrud et al., 1988). Accordingly, NREM sleep must induce additional changes that augment respiratory muscle activity.

In view of the possible effects of increased R_{UAW} on respiratory muscle activity, the activity of the respiratory muscles has been studied while the upper airway has been bypassed during NREM sleep. Orem et al. (1985) found that most ventral medullary respiratory cells in the tracheotomized cat were less active in NREM sleep than in relaxed wakefulness, which would reduce EMG activity of respiratory muscles and ventilation during NREM sleep. In contrast, where respiration occurs through the upper airway, respiratory muscle EMG activity in intact humans and animals is unchanged or increased during NREM sleep (Parmeggiani and Sabattini, 1972; Tabachnik et al., 1981a; Lopes et al., 1983; Wiegand et al., 1988; Henke et al., 1992). These observations imply that a sleep-induced increase in R_{UAW} could account for higher EMG activity of the respiratory muscles during NREM sleep.

Indeed, Skatrud et al. (1985) showed that inhalation of a low-density helium-O_2 mixture in healthy nonobese male snorers, a case of markedly exaggerated R_{UAW}, reduced both inspiratory and expiratory muscle activities in association with a reduction of airflow resistance and Pa_{CO_2}. Similarly, when R_{UAW} was reduced to the waking level via continuous positive airway pressure (CPAP), the EMG activity of the respiratory pump muscles was significantly reduced (Fig. 1) (Henke et al., 1988, 1991). Moreover, by comparing EMG_{di} activity, EMG activity of the scalene (EMG_{sc}), and EMG activity of the abdominal muscles (EMG_{ab}) with and without CPAP and with and without isocapnia, these authors found that the scalene and abdominal muscles were more sensitive than the diaphragm to changes in state and airways resistance. Furthermore, these findings indicated that some of the increase in respiratory muscle activity during NREM sleep was secondary to load-compensating activity over and above that due to CO_2 retention. Finally, these findings suggested that nondiaphragmatic respiratory muscles played a greater role in compensating for increases in mechanical loads to breathing than did the diaphragm. Similar observations have been made in awake humans where the activities of the abdominal muscles and scalenes increase to a much greater extent than the diaphragm to compensate for diaphragmatic shortening in the upright position during CO_2 rebreathing. Increased activity of the scalene and abdominal muscles would tend to passively lengthen the diaphragm so as to optimize its mechanical efficiency (Xie et al., 1991). During sleep, increased intercostal and accessory muscle activity would prevent rib cage distortion and contribute to the generation of tidal volume in the presence of increased R_{UAW}. This would also have the effect of unloading the diaphragm.

In contrast to findings in humans, however, there is evidence in cats breathing through intact upper airways that respiratory muscle activity is reduced in NREM sleep. Sieck and colleagues (1984) investigated the motor unit recruitment in the diaphragm of the cat during different sleep-waking states and demonstrated that fewer motor units of the diaphragm were recruited compared to during wakefulness. In those motor units still active, the discharge frequency typically slowed in the course of NREM sleep (Fig. 2). Unfortunately, V_T, V_I, and Pa_{CO_2} were not measured, so that the chemical stimulus and respiratory output could not be

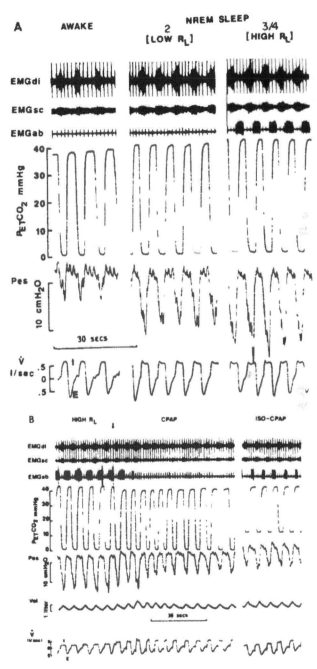

Figure 1 Respiratory muscle activity in a snorer. Channels show electromyographic activity of diaphragm (EMG$_{di}$), scalene (EMG$_{sc}$) and abdomen (EMG$_{ab}$), end-tidal P$_{CO_2}$ (P$_{ET}$CO$_2$), esophageal pressure (P$_{es}$), and airflow ($\dot{V}$). In (A) the subject was breathing

correlated to respiratory muscle activity. In addition, it may be that in the cat, R_{UAW} does not increase to the same extent during NREM sleep as in snoring humans. Nevertheless, they attributed the slight increase in the peak amplitude of the diaphragmatic EMG during NREM sleep to a prolongation of inspiratory duration in this stage. Although respiration was not measured, their findings suggested a primary reduction in respiratory muscle activity in NREM sleep compared to wakefulness. This concept was supported by Remmers and colleagues (1976), who proposed that the only change that occurred in diaphragmatic activity during NREM sleep was a delay in the transition from inspiration to expiration. A reduction in diaphragm muscle tone during NREM sleep provides further evidence for inhibited diaphragm activity during by NREM sleep (Parmeggiani and Sabattini, 1972; Duron & Marlot, 1980).

Orem et al. (1985) found that sleep affected some but not other respiratory neurons, suggesting there may be a sleep-specific inhibition of some respiratory muscles. Therefore, a different degree of inhibition of respiratory pump muscles during NREM sleep is expected. Although the compensatory adjustment of the respiratory center for the increase of respiratory impedance may selectively recruit some nondiaphragmatic muscles, a lower V_I and higher Pa_{CO_2}, Pa_{CO_2} are universally seen during NREM sleep. This observation indicates that the depression of the respiratory center renders the muscles incapable of completely compensating for the sleep-related increase in R_{UAW}. Some would argue that the reduction of V_I in NREM sleep may result purely from the increase in R_{UAW}. However, when adding external inspiratory resistances to the same degree, $P_{0.1}$ markedly increased (Iber et al., 1982) and V_I was maintained (Daubenspeck, 1981) during wakefulness but not during NREM sleep.

The reasons for the variable observations of the effect of NREM sleep on respiratory muscle activity are not entirely clear. However, several possibilities that might explain these discrepancies can be entertained. First, NREM sleep is a general term used to describe four sleep stages. For instance, the lighter stages of NREM sleep (i.e., stages 1 and 2) are a transitional period between wakefulness and the deeper stages of NREM sleep (i.e., stages 3 and 4, or slow-wave sleep). During

---

Figure 1 Continued
spontaneously. Note the progressive increase in P_{es} excursions indicative of increasing R_{UAW} from wakefulness to stage 2 to stage 3/4 NREM sleep accompanied by progressive increases in EMG activity of the respiratory muscles. (B) Application of CPAP in stage 3/4 sleep [high lung resistance (R_L) state] was associated with a reduction in R_L to waking levels with an accompanying reduction in the EMG activities of the respiratory muscles. Note the more pronounced reduction in EMG_{sc} and EMG_{ab} than in EMG_{di} activity. This was associated with an increase in $\dot{V}$ and a reduction in $P_{ET}CO_2$. However, when $P_{ET}CO_2$ was raised to eupneic sleeping levels, EMG activity of the respiratory muscles increased but not back to spontaneous sleeping levels. This indicated that some of the EMG activity of the respiratory muscles was related to load compensation for increased R_{UAW} associated with snoring. (From Henke et al., 1991.)

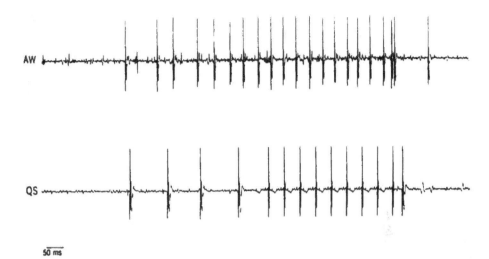

Figure 2 Discharge pattern of a diaphragmatic motor unit recorded from an intact cat while awake (AW) and in NREM sleep (QS). The motor unit demonstrated an augmenting pattern during inspiration in both states. Note, however, that during QS the discharge frequency is markedly slowed compared to AW. (From Sieck et al., 1984.)

this period of transition, breathing is inherently unstable and is frequently interrupted by arousals from sleep. Accordingly, data observed during NREM may be variable according to the choice of the NREM sleep period used for analysis. Second, methodological differences may exist which affect results. For example, surface recordings of EMG activity may provide only a rough approximation of neuronal activation of a particular muscle due to lack of proximity to the muscle and to contamination by electrical activity from neighboring muscles. In addition, absence of respiratory output measurements has been a problem in some studies. Third, since both the diaphragm and intercostal muscles are composed of several separate muscles—for instance, the crural and costal parts of the diaphragm have different embryological development, different segmental innervation, and different mechanical actions (DeTroyer et al., 1981)—the effect of NREM sleep on the pattern EMG activities may be different according to the precise location of EMG recordings. For these reasons, when describing the activity of respiratory muscles body position should be controlled and the particular location of EMG electrodes should be specified. Finally, caution must be exercised when extrapolating from findings in various animal preparations to the intact sleeping human.

    Taken together, the above studies indicate that where the upper airway is bypassed or where its flow resistance is reduced during NREM sleep, the activities of the respiratory muscles are generally decreased compared to wakefulness. Even where respiratory muscle activity increases in the face of an increase in R_{UAW}, the increase is not sufficient to maintain $\dot{V}_I$ and Pa_{CO_2} at the wakefulness level.

Furthermore, reduced load compensation in response to added loads to breathing compared to wakefulness point to a generalized reduction in the activity of the respiratory muscles during NREM sleep.

C. Function of Respiratory Muscles During REM Sleep

In comparison to NREM sleep, state-specific effects on respiratory muscle activity are more pronounced in REM sleep even though R_{UAW} remains elevated compared to wakefulness. To complicate matters, REM sleep can be divided into tonic and phasic components defined by the absence or presence of phasic eye movements, respectively (Carskadon and Dement, 1989). During tonic REM sleep, breathing seems still to be under mainly chemical control, as it is in NREM sleep. However, in phasic REM sleep, breathing becomes largely dissociated form chemoreceptor or vagal afferent influences (Sullivan, 1980; Phillipson and Bowes, 1986). Non-chemical, behavioral-related activity appears to be the main influence on breathing during phasic REM sleep. The following discussion will focus on the effects of phasic REM sleep on respiratory muscle activity.

Studies in humans have demonstrated that tonic EMG_{di} activity is abolished during REM sleep (Phillipson and Bowes, 1986). More detailed studies on cats revealed a progressive reduction in activity for some motor units in both costal and crural regions of the diaphragm during the transition from NREM to REM (Sieck et al., 1984). However, phasic diaphragmatic bursts may or may not be subject to generalized inhibition during REM sleep. Despite the variations in frequency and size of EMG bursts, phasic EMG_{di} activity is relatively spared from REM-related inhibition (Tusiewicz et al., 1977; Duron and Marlot, 1980; Tabachnik et al., 1981a) and sometimes even shows an increase in both humans and other animals (Phillipson and Bowes, 1986). The persistence of rhythmic diaphragmatic function is obviously critical to survival. Moreover, in the presence of sleep-related increases in R_{UAW}, increases in phasic diaphragmatic activity in REM sleep may represent an essential compensatory response to loss of nondiaphragmatic muscle activity (Pack et al., 1987).

On the other hand, inhibition of isolated diaphragmatic EMG bursts has also been observed. Polygraphic recordings sometimes show suppressed or fractionated diaphragmatic activity coincident with pontogeniculooccipital (PGO) waves or REMs. PGO waves are rhythmic synchronous discharges in pontine neurons that trigger discharges in the lateral geniculate nucleus and occipetal cortex. They are one of the basic electrophysiological phenomena of REM sleep that presumably give rise to the occular activity characteristic of this state (Parmeggiani and Sabattini, 1972; Duron and Marlot, 1980). When the time course of the EMG_{di} moving time average in REM sleep is analyzed, two types of inhibition are found (Fig. 3). One is the "intermittent inhibition" phenomenon, which persists throughout the duration of inspiration (Kline et al., 1986). As a result, the rate of rise of the EMG_{di} of an individual breath may be reduced during flurries of REMs. The other is the

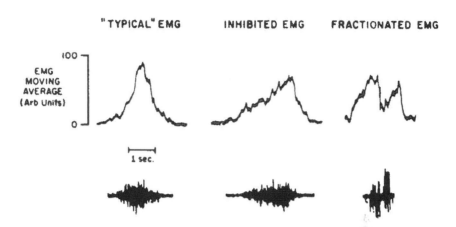

Figure 3 Two different types of inhibition of EMG$_{di}$ found during REM sleep. "Typical" EMG is that seen during tonic REM sleep and is similar to that seen during wakefulness and NREM sleep. In one type of inhibition (middle panel), the EMG shows inhibition throughout inspiration with a slower rate of rise in comparison to the "typical" diaphragmatic EMG pattern. This indicates a prolonged inspiratory time associated with an overall reduction in inspiratory drive. In the second type of inhibition, fractionated (right panel), there is a brief intense inhibition. (From Pack et al., 1987.)

"fractionation" phenomenon, that is, a brief intense inhibition of diaphragmatic activity (Orem, 1980b). Kline and colleagues (1990) recently reported that these spontaneously occurring periods (20–100 ms) of cessation of diaphragmatic activity sometimes caused decreases in airflow and tidal volume. Hence, this inhibition probably reflects the additional phasic component of supraspinal inhibition of muscle activity. In contrast to phasic REM sleep, during tonic REM sleep, the pattern of diaphragmatic activity is highly consistent from breath to breath and the variability is similar to that in slow-wave sleep (Kline et al., 1986).

The mechanism through which phrenic motoneuron activity is modified during phasic REM sleep is unclear. Based on the observation that medullary respiratory neurons were not depressed but activated with PGO activity, Orem (1980a,b) proposed that respiratory neurons of the dorsal and ventral medullary groups are excited by phasic REM influences. This excitation is then secondarily relayed to phrenic motoneurons. At the same time there is a direct phasic REM inhibitory influence on phrenic motoneurons. The result of these opposing forces may be either an increase or a decrease in EMG$_{di}$ activity, depending upon the balance of excitatory versus inhibitory influences.

In contrast to NREM sleep, there is evidence that postural tonic activity of the intercostal and neck muscles disappears or is markedly attenuated during REM sleep (Figs. 4, 5) (Tusiewicz et al., 1977; Tabachnik et al., 1981a; Sherrey and Megirian, 1987). In addition, phasic intercostal EMG activity is also markedly

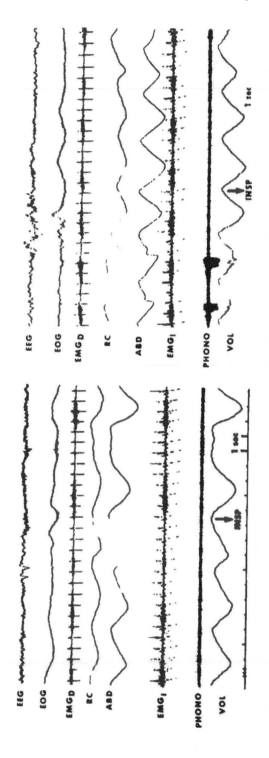

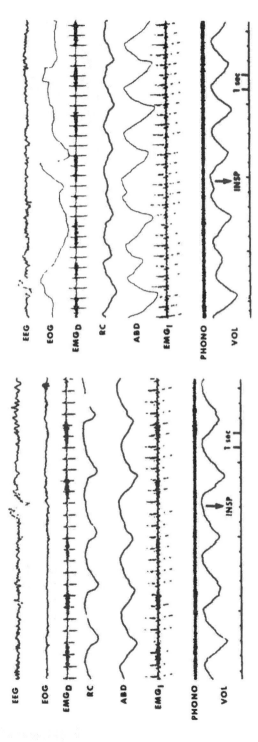

Figure 4 Upper left, wakefulness; lower left, NREM sleep without snoring; upper right, NREM sleep with snoring as evidenced by out-of-phase rib cage (RC) and abdominal (ABD) motion; lower right, REM sleep. Note general progressive reduction of intercostal EMG (EMG_I) activity from wakefulness to NREM to REM sleep. However, the upper right panel illustrates that when inspiratory flow resistance increases in association with snoring, EMG_I increases in response. Diaphragmatic EMG activity, however, does not display so obvious a state-related alteration in activity, although there is some reduction in activity from wakefulness to NREM sleep without snoring. (From Tusiewicz et al., 1977.)

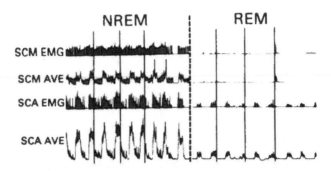

Figure 5 Recordings of EMG activity of sternocleidomastoid (SCM EMG) and scalene (SCA EMG) muscles from a subject with severe chronic obstructive pulmonary disease during NREM and REM sleep, respectively. Solid vertical lines delineate transition from inspiration to expiration. Compared to NREM sleep, both tonic and phasic activity of SCM EMG and SCA EMG were significantly attenuated during REM sleep. (From Johnson and Remmers, 1984.)

reduced (Tusiewicz et al., 1977; Duron and Marlot, 1980; Tabachnik et al., 1981a; Dick et al., 1982) or completely absent (Henderson-Smart and Read, 1976). Sherrey and Megirian (1987) found that although tonic activity of the scalene disappeared, its inspiratory activity persisted. This marked reduction in phasic and tonic intercostal muscle activity during REM sleep may be considered as part of a generalized supraspinal inhibition of motor-neuron drive and selective depression of fusimotor function (Tabachnik et al., 1981a). The cessation of both postural and phasic respiratory activity in the intercostal muscles during REM sleep might cause a reduction of the rib cage contribution to Vт in this sleep stage. In newborn infants the inhibition of intercostal EMG might result in a paradoxical motion of the rib cage, which is quite often seen in REM sleep (Tusiewicz et al., 1977).

The differential effect of REM sleep on the diaphragmatic activity versus the activity of other respiratory muscles has been widely noted (Parmeggiani and Sabattini, 1972; Tusiewicz et al., 1976; Duron and Marlot, 1980; Sherrey and Megirian, 1980). A review of the mechanisms through which REM sleep directly influences the activity of these muscles as well as of the varying structural and functional properties of individual respiratory muscles provides a useful framework for understanding these disparities in respiratory muscle activity.

REM sleep may affect the activity of respiratory muscles via inhibition of the respiratory center or through direct depression of the spinal motoneurons. As mentioned above, sleep-related depression of respiratory-related neurons that demonstrate both respiratory and nonrespiratory activity is more pronounced than is that of the neurons that exhibit mainly respiratory activity (Orem et al., 1974). In addition, the effect of REM, especially phasic REM, on the respiratory center is complicated by the release of the respiratory center from hypothalamic control and by the influence of dream-related behavior. The direct effect of REM on skeletal muscles is a tonic presynaptic inhibition of group I_A afferents. The consequence of depression of both gamma and alpha motoneurons is related to the spindle density of individual muscles (Duron and Marlot, 1980). The diaphragm has relatively few spindles and some tendon organs and is, therefore, less sensitive to nonrespiratory influences mediated via muscle spindle feedback (Corda et al., 1965; Xie et al., 1991a). Hence, the diaphragm may be less subject to the direct inhibitory influence of REM sleep than are other muscles. In contrast, the intercostal and the scalene have more prominent posturally related activity than the diaphragm and are well endowed with muscle spindles. More interestingly, the muscle spindles of intercostal muscles are supplied by two distinct fusimotor systems: one under the control of the medullary center and the other under the control of the cerebellum (Corda et al., 1966). Phasic activity is more closely related to medullary influences, whereas tonic activity is more closely related to cerebellar influences. Thus, inhibition of intercostal activity may involve phasic or tonic activity or both. Generally, the posturally related tonic activity is subjected to greater inhibition during REM sleep. Furthermore, the descending influence from the respiratory center and the descending influence from the cerebellar-reticular projections may act separately on different motor units of the same muscles, or, alternatively, the descending motor pathways may suppress the action command of the medullary respiratory center at the level of the spinal motoneuron (Duron and Marlot, 1980). These complex influences may explain why, during REM sleep, (1) the activity of the intercostals and scalenes is generally reduced compared to NREM sleep, whereas the activity of the diaphragm is only marginally reduced in comparison and (2) tonic versus phasic activity of the intercostal muscles and scalenes may be affected unequally, with more pronounced reductions in tonic activity (Johnson and Remmers, 1984).

Two suprasegmental regions may produce postural muscle inhibition: the region around the caudal locus ceruleus and the nucleus reticularis magnocellularis. This conclusion is based on the following observations. If there are lesions in the former area, atonia is not seen during REM sleep (Henley and Morrison, 1969); conversely, if the latter area is stimulated, an inhibition of motoneuron activity will be produced (Jankowska et al., 1968). The precise role of either region in the generalized atonia has not been demonstrated.

The investigation of the effect of sleep on the abdominal muscles has been observed mainly under loaded conditions, because in supine humans the abdominal muscles are generally inactive during quiet breathing (De Troyer, 1983; Takasaki et al., 1989) but are active during chemically stimulated or mechanically loaded breathing. Where rhythmically active during NREM sleep, the onset of REM sleep causes complete inhibition of their activity (Fig. 6) (Hutt et al., 1991). Because abdominal expiratory activity is generally recruited by loading, the abdominal muscles will be discussed in the next section, where the response of respiratory muscles to various loads during sleep will be considered.

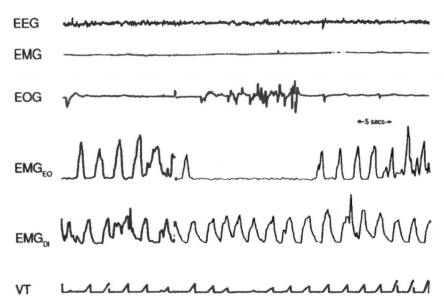

Figure 6   Recordings of external oblique EMG (EMG$_{eo}$) and diaphragmatic EMG (EMG$_{di}$) during REM sleep in an intact goat. During tonic REM, EMG$_{eo}$ and EMG$_{di}$ are both phasically active. Note during phasic eye movements, as shown by electrooculogram (EOG) activity, that although EMG$_{di}$ activity is relatively unaffected, there is complete inhibition of EMG$_{eo}$. EEG, electroencephalogram; EMG, submental EMG; V$_T$, tidal volume. (From Hutt et al., 1991.)

V.   Response of Respiratory Muscles to Loads During Sleep

Responses that tend to preserve adequate ventilation are referred to as load-compensating mechanisms. Henke et al. (1992) suggested that during sleep, the requirements for load compensation are similar to those during wakefulness, except for two constraints: upper airway patency must be maintained and the response must not stimulate arousal from sleep so that the sleep state is maintained undisturbed.

Sleep imposes an internal flow-resistive load on the chest wall muscles due mainly to increased R$_{UAW}$. This load may be minimal as in a healthy nonsnorer, moderate as in a habitual snorer, or infinite as in the case of someone with obstructive sleep apnea. In addition, the respiratory pump muscles may be exposed to the chronically elevated airways resistance associated with chronic obstructive airway disease or asthma or to increased elastic loads associated with fibrotic lung diseases and chest wall restriction. Although the respiratory muscles respond to these loads by increasing their EMG activity (Tabachnik et al., 1981b; Issa and Sullivan, 1983; Johnson and Remmers, 1984; Badr et al., 1990; Wilcox et al., 1990), it is not clear whether this increased activity is mediated mainly by reflexes provoked by the mechanical load or by the increased chemical drive associated with sleep-related hypoventilation. As mentioned above, respiratory muscles do not compensate for this load completely, resulting in lower ventilation and higher Pa_{CO_2}. Thus the evaluation of the responses of respiration system to added loads is crucial to understanding the tendency to CO_2 retention during sleep.

When adding an inspiratory flow-resistive load during NREM sleep, unlike during wakefulness, the load does not elicit an immediate increase in EMG_{di} or expiratory abdominal activity within the first or second breath (Fig. 7) (Badr et al., 1990; Hutt et al., 1991). Although the immediate EMG_{di} response to loading was diminished during sleep, the prolongation of inspiratory duration (T_i) was preserved, with the result that V_T was unchanged just as during wakefulness. As a result, the rate of rise of the EMG_{di} was reduced during all sleep stages compared to wakefulness for the same added load (Hutt et al., 1991). On the other hand, during sustained inspiratory resistive loading, both inspiratory and expiratory muscles exhibited a corresponding augmentation of activity (Fig. 8) (Badr et al., 1991), which was in concert with an increase in Pa_{CO_2} (Henke et al., 1992). In addition, the increase in $P_{0.1}$ that occurs when breathing against external loads in conscious

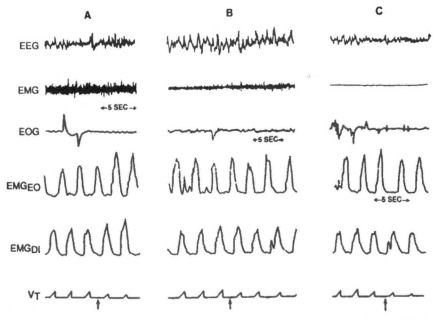

Figure 7 Respiratory muscle response to an inspiratory flow-resistive load (arrow) during wakefulness (A), NREM (B), and tonic REM sleep (C) in an intact goat. The channels are the same as for Figure 6. During wakefulness there was an immediate increase in EMG_{eo} and EMG_{di} activity in response to the added load. In contrast, in both NREM and tonic REM sleep, no immediate load-compensating response was apparent. (From Hutt et al., 1991.)

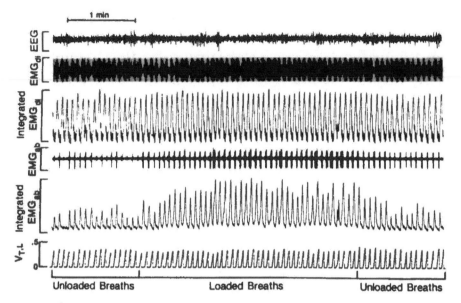

Figure 8 Respiratory muscle response to a sustained inspiratory flow-resistive load during NREM sleep in a healthy human. Diaphragmatic EMG (EMG_{di}) showed a slight increase while the abdominal EMG (EMG_{ab}) demonstrated a more pronounced augmentation. (Badr et al., 1990.)

humans is not apparent when loads are applied during sleep (Iber et al., 1982). These findings indicate that reflex neuromuscular responses to added resistive loads to breathing during NREM sleep are diminished compared to wakefulness.

Occlusion of the airway during sleep elicits an attempt to overcome the infinite resistance by generating progressively greater respiratory drive (Vincken et al., 1987). It is unclear whether this increased drive is primarily a result of a proprioceptor-mediated response to airway occlusion or to increasing chemical drive or both. In any case, eventually a behavioral response ensues characterized by an arousal from sleep within the first few occluded breaths in normal subjects and after several respiratory efforts in patients with OSA (Issa et al., 1983). Respiratory efforts are associated with a coincident augmentation of chest wall and upper airway muscle activity. This behavioral response is appropriate when one considers that the most effective means of ensuring continued ventilation is to remove the source of obstruction rather than to struggle fruitlessly against it. Indeed, it has recently been shown that mechanical factors play an important role in eliciting arousal from sleep during chemical respiratory stimulation (Vincken et al., 1987; Gleeson et al., 1990; Yasuma et al., 1991). Activity arising from respiratory muscle receptors probably contributes to the arousal response from sleep under these conditions just as it contributes to the sensation of dyspnea during wakefulness (Bradley et al.,

1986). The possibility that respiratory muscle fatigue secondary to generation of effort against the occluded upper airway during obstructive apnea might play a role in triggering arousal from sleep has been suggested (Vincken et al., 1987).

The immediate response of the respiratory muscles to elastic loads seen during wakefulness is also absent during NREM sleep, as reflected by an unchanged $P_{0.1}$ during the first two loaded breaths. Consequently, the V_T and V_I over the first five breaths are reduced (Wilson et al., 1984). However, during sustained loading ventilatory responses in NREM sleep are similar to those during wakefulness (Phillipson et al., 1976; Wilson et al., 1984). This apparent similarity is probably secondary to a rise in Pa_{CO_2}, which causes a chemical stimulus. Responses to elastic loading during REM sleep have not been well studied, but Knill and Bryan (1976) demonstrated that the increase in intercostal muscle EMG activity during elastic loading in infants was less in REM sleep than in NREM sleep, suggesting a further degree of depression of respiratory load-compensating responses during REM sleep.

Both sleeping humans (Begle et al., 1987) and anesthetized animals (Cheesman and Revelette, 1990) preserve their operational length-compensating reflex in response to experimentally induced shortening of diaphragmatic length during NREM sleep. However, although phasic expiratory abdominal muscle activity is usually activated by the pulmonary stretch receptors responding to a mechanical distention of the lungs (Bishop, 1973; Farkas et al., 1988), augmentation of expiratory muscle activity seen during wakefulness was less pronounced during NREM sleep in the presence of hyperinflated lungs (Fig. 9) (Begle et al., 1987; Begle and Skatrud, 1990). REM sleep further suppressed abdominal muscle recruitment in dogs in response to increased lung volume (Yasuma et al., 1990).

The importance of diaphragmatic activity during REM sleep was demonstrated by Stradling and associates (1987). They showed in dogs that during wakefulness or NREM sleep, ventilation was not impaired following acute bilateral phrenic nerve paralysis, presumably owing to increased compensatory activity of the intercostal and accessory muscles of respiration. During REM sleep, ventilation did fall but only to a minor extent. The addition of deadspace with a resultant increase in deadspace ventilation still did not adversely affect gas exchange during wakefulness or NREM sleep. In contrast, during REM sleep, the addition of deadspace caused a marked reduction in alveolar ventilation with a resultant rise in Pa_{CO_2}. These data emphasize the critical role of the diaphragm in maintaining adequate gas exchange during REM sleep and also indicate that load-compensating mechanisms involving the intercostal and accessory muscles of respiration are impaired during REM sleep compared to wakefulness and NREM sleep. These factors undoubtedly play an important role in the decompensation of the respiratory system during REM sleep, as evidenced by marked increases in Pa_{CO_2} and reductions in Pa_{O_2} in patients with respiratory muscle compromise due to hyperinflation (Goldstein et al., 1984), diaphragmatic paralysis, generalized respiratory muscle weakness (Newsom Davis et al., 1976), or chest wall deformities (Goldstein et al., 1987).

Taken together, the above indicates that the response of the respiratory muscles

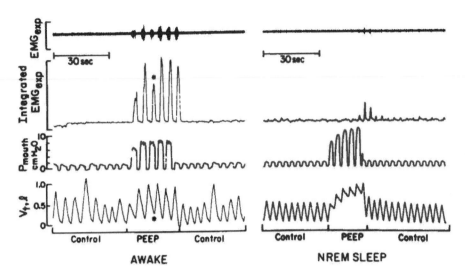

Figure 9   The effect of hyperinflation on expiratory muscle recruitment in a healthy human. Brief hyperinflation with positive end expiratory pressure (PEEP) caused activation of expiratory abdominal muscle EMG activity (EMG_{exp}) during wakefulness but not during NREM sleep despite the fact that lung volume was increased to the same extent. P_{mouth}, mouth pressure. (From Begle and Skatrud, 1990.)

to added loads to breathing is reduced during both NREM and REM sleep compared to wakefulness. In normal humans, this does not adversely affect gas exchange. However, if the load is great enough, as it may be in such diseases as obstructive sleep apnea or in the presence of respiratory muscle weakness, gas exchange deteriorates. Under these conditions, arousal from sleep becomes a critical defense mechanism wherein the greater ventilatory and load-compensating responses inherent during wakefulness are recruited in order to defend ventilation. Because the effects of sleep on respiratory muscle function and gas exchange in patients with respiratory or neuromuscular disease involving the respiratory muscles are discussed in detail elsewhere in this volume, this subject will not be reviewed here.

VI.   Response of the Respiratory Muscles to Chemical Stimuli During Sleep

Ventilatory responsiveness to CO_2 has been shown to fall during transition from wakefulness to NREM sleep in both animals (Phillipson et al., 1977; Sullivan et al., 1979; Santiago et al., 1981; Phillipson and Bowes, 1986) and humans (Birchfield et al., 1959; Gothe et al., 1981; Douglas et al., 1982; Berthon-Jones and Sullivan, 1984) and falls even further during REM sleep, especially phasic REM sleep

(Phillipson et al., 1977; Sullivan et al., 1979; Santiago et al., 1981; Netick et al., 1984). The ventilatory response to hypoxia during NREM is reduced compared to wakefulness (Phillipson et al., 1978; Douglas, 1982b). Whether hypoxic ventilatory responsiveness falls further during REM sleep remains controversial, with some studies indicating a further reduction (Douglas et al., 1982b; White et al., 1982) while others show no change (Phillipson et al., 1978; Jeffery and Read, 1980; Berthon-Jones and Sullivan, 1982; Hedemark and Kronenberg, 1982). Considering the evidence in both animals (Sears et al., 1982; Fregosi et al., 1987) and intact humans (Takasaki et al., 1989) that hypoxia inhibits expiratory muscle activity, it may be that withdrawal of expiratory activity during REM sleep has no effect on hypoxic ventilatory responses since the expiratory muscles may not have been recruited in any case. In contrast, REM sleep–related withdrawal of expiratory muscle activity during hypercapnia may partly account for the reduction in ventilatory response to CO_2 because the expiratory muscles contribute significantly to the generation of ventilation during hypercapnia in wakefulness (Takasaki et al., 1989; Xie et al., 1991).

These observations have generated interest in determining recruitment patterns of respiratory muscle activity in response to chemical stimuli. Figure 10 comes from work in our laboratory in which the activity of the respiratory muscles was studied in response to hyperoxic, progressive hypercapnic rebreathing in a nonsnoring human subject. It illustrates marked tonic activity with less obvious phasic activity of the scalene at a low level of $ETCO_2$ during wakefulness. In addition, expiratory external oblique activity, which was not apparent during quiet breathing, was recruited as $ETCO_2$ rose to about 6.5%. During NREM sleep, where inspiratory impedence was higher than during wakefulness, tonic-postural activity of the scalene was markedly reduced. Although external oblique activity was observed at the same level of $ETCO_2$ as during wakefulness, the amplitude of the EMG signal was reduced in comparison. However, phasic activity of the scalene was more pronounced, while diaphragmatic activity was less pronounced in association with a smaller V_T, indicating lower ventilatory responsiveness to CO_2 during NREM sleep than during wakefulness. These findings suggested that overall ventilatory drive was reduced in NREM sleep compared to wakefulness as exemplified by lower EMG_{di} activity. Nevertheless, phasic activity of the scalene was more pronounced, probably owing to a sustained loading response. External oblique activity was present at the same $ETCO_2$ as during wakefulness, also suggesting a sustained loading response but not sufficient to maintain ventilation at the same level as during wakefulness for the same $ETCO_2$. Furthermore, these data suggested a more pronounced inhibition of abdominal expiratory muscle activity than scalene activity because external oblique activity did not increase above the waking level despite an increase in impedance, whereas scalene activity did.

Figure 10C illustrates that even at a higher level of $ETCO_2$ than during NREM sleep, REMs were associated with marked suppression of phasic scalene and diaphragmatic activity in association with a reduction in V_T. Furthermore, external

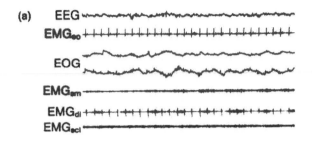

Figure 10 Respiratory muscle recruitment during hyperoxic progressive hypercapnic rebreathing in a normal human in wakefulness (a), stage 2 NREM sleep (b), and REM sleep (c). During wakefulness, phasic external oblique EMG (EMG$_{eo}$) activity has its onset at an end-tidal P$_{CO2}$ of 6.5–6.7%. Note also phasic diaphragmatic EMG (EMG$_{di}$) activity and marked tonic activity of scalene EMG (EMG$_{scl}$) with less obvious phasic activity. During NREM sleep, phasic expiratory EMG$_{eo}$ activity is just discernible at an ETCO$_2$ of 6.5–6.7%, as shown here. Higher inspiratory flow resistance was observed during NREM sleep than during wakefulness as evidenced by greater inspiratory esophageal pressure (P$_{es}$) swings. Note also the marked reduction in tonic EMG$_{scl}$ activity while pronounced phasic activity is apparent. EMG$_{di}$ activity is less than that seen during wakefulness and V$_T$ is lower at the same ETCO$_2$, indicating a reduction in ventilatory drive. During REM sleep, at an ETCO$_2$ of 7.5%, there is a complete absence of EMG$_{eo}$ activity during both tonic (REM$_T$) and phasic (REM$_P$) components of REM sleep. In addition, phasic EMG$_{scl}$ activity is present during REM$_T$ but is reduced compared to NREM sleep. Tonic EMG$_{scl}$ activity is absent. EMG$_{di}$ activity is similar to NREM sleep during REM$_T$. However, during REM$_P$ there is a sudden suppression of both EMG$_{scl}$ and EMG$_{di}$ activity associated with a reduction in V$_T$.

(b)   EEG

       EMG₍ₑₒ₎

       EOG

       EMG₍ₛₘ₎

       EMG₍dᵢ₎

       EMG₍ₛcᵢ₎

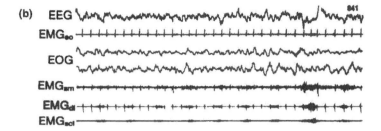

V_T (ℓ) 2 [

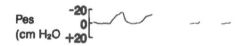

Pes
(cm H_2O)

-20
0
+20

(c)   EEG

       EMG₍ₑₒ₎

       EOG

       EMG₍ₛₘ₎

       EMG₍dᵢ₎

       EMG₍ₛcᵢ₎

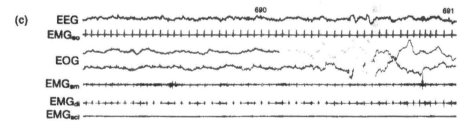

REM_T └────────────┘ REM_T
            REM_P

V_T (ℓ) 2 [

Pes
(cm H_2O)

-20
0
+20

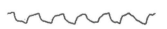

oblique activity was never seen during REM sleep even when $ETCO_2$ became as high as 9.0%. These observations were consistent with the notion that REM sleep inhibits the activity of all the respiratory muscles in response to hypercapnia. However, the nondiaphragmatic respiratory muscles experience greater suppression, and, among these, the abdominal expiratory muscles are particularly prone to inhibition. These findings in REM sleep paralleled those of other investigators under a variety of conditions (Johnson and Remmers, 1984; Parisi et al., 1987; Hutt et al., 1991).

There are only a few studies on the response of respiratory muscles to hypoxia during sleep. Among them the most interesting finding was that the EMG_{di} response to hypoxia during REM sleep was comparable to (Phillipson et al., 1990) or greater than (Megirian et al., 1980) that during the antecedent NREM period. This stands in contrast to the behavior of the diaphragm during REM sleep in response to hypercapnia (Parisi et al., 1987). These observations might be related to diaphragmatic compensation for reduced intercostal and accessory muscle activities, which are typically inhibited in REM sleep (Sherrey et al., 1987). Another possibility is that the diaphragm is more sensitive to hypoxia than hypercapnia (Takasaki et al., 1989; Phillipson et al., 1990) so that stimulation of the peripheral chemoreceptors may overcome the inhibitory influence of the REM state. Moreover, REM sleep may exert less inhibitory effects on inspiratory than on expiratory muscles in general (Kimoff et al., 1992).

VII. Summary

As the above review indicates, sleep has a generally depressant effect on respiratory muscle activity compared to wakefulness. The factors that contribute to this depression of muscular activity are complex and are not uniform throughout all stages of sleep, nor do they uniformly affect all respiratory muscles. In general, there is a progressive fall in the activity of the respiratory muscles from wakefulness to NREM to REM sleep, especially among those that have a relatively greater degree of posturally related activity than the diaphragm. On the other hand, the diaphragm is to a large extent spared from this NREM and REM sleep–related depression of skeletal muscle inhibition. In addition, there is a progressive reduction in the ability of the respiratory muscles to compensate for added mechanical loads to breathing due to inhibition of spinal reflex activity as well as to progressive presynaptic inhibition of respiratory motoneurons from wakefulness to NREM to REM sleep. These phenomena assume particular significance when sleep-related inhibition of respiratory muscle activity is superimposed upon abnormal mechanics related to respiratory or chest wall disease or to weakened respiratory muscles secondary to neuromuscular disease. Under these conditions, gas exchange may worsen during sleep, especially REM sleep. Arousal from sleep to wakefulness then becomes a critical defense mechanism to prevent progressive asphyxia.

Although a good deal of work has been done on the activity of the respiratory muscles during sleep, many questions remain unanswered. For instance, it is unclear whether all intercostal muscles are equally affected by REM sleep inhibition. The degree to which the sleep-related withdrawal of respiratory muscle activation affects lengthening and shortening of these muscles has not been explored in any detail. Furthermore, the extent to which sensations arising in the respiratory muscles contribute to arousal from sleep has received little attention. Since these questions bear on the clinical problem of sleep-related worsening of gas exchange and the high incidence of nocturnal death among patients with respiratory disease, all are worthy of further investigation.

References

Badr, M. S., Skatrud, J. B., Dempsey, J. A., and Begle, R. L. (1990). Effect of mechanical loading on expiratory and inspiratory muscle activity during NREM sleep. *J. Appl. Physiol.*, 68:1195–1202.

Begle, R. L., Skatrud, J. B., and Dempsey, J. A. (1987). Ventilatory compensation for changes in functional residual capacity during sleep. *J. Appl. Physiol.*, 62(3):1299–1306.

Begle, R., and Skatrud, J. B. (1990). Hyperinflation and expiratory muscle recruitment during NREM sleep in humans. *Respir. Physiol.*, 82:47–64.

Berthon-Jones, M., and Sullivan, C. E. (1982). Ventilatory and arousal responses to hypoxia in sleeping humans. *Am. Rev. Respir. Dis.*, 125:632–639.

Berthon-Jones, M., and Sullivan, C. E. (1984). Ventilatory and arousal responses to hypercapnia in normal sleeping humans. *J. Appl. Physiol.*, 57:59–67.

Birchfield, R. L., Sieker, H. O., and Heyman, A. (1959). Alterations in respiratory function during natural sleep. *J. Lab. Clin. Med.*, 54:216–222.

Bishop, B., and Bachofen, H. (1973). Comparative influence of proprioceptor and chemoreceptors in the control of respiratory muscles. *Acta Neurobiol. Exp.*, 33:381–390.

Bowes, G., Woolf, G. M., Sullivan, C. E., and Phillipson, E. A. (1980). Effect of sleep fragmentation on ventilatory and arousal responses of sleeping dogs to respiratory stimuli. *Am. Rev. Respir. Dis.*, 122:899–908.

Bradley, T. D., Chartrand, D. A., Fitting, J. W., Killian, K. J., and Grassino, A. (1986). The relation of inspiratory effort sensation to fatiguing patterns of the diaphragm. *Am. Rev. Respir. Dis.*, 134:1119–1124.

Bradley, T. D., Martinez, D., Rutherford, R., Lue, F., Grossman, R. F., Moldofsky, H., Zamel, N., and Phillipson, E. A. (1985). Physiological determinants of nocturnal arterial oxygenation in patients with obstructive sleep apnea. *J. Appl. Physiol.*, 59:1364–1368.

Bradley, T. D., and Phillipson, E. A. (1992). Central sleep apnea. *Clin. Chest Med.*, 13:493–505.

Brebbia, D. R., and Altshuler, K. Z. (1965). Oxygen consumption rate and electroencephalographic stage of sleep. *Science*, 150:1621–1623.

Carskadon, M. A., and Dement, W. C. (1989). Normal human sleep: an overview. In *Principles and Practice of Sleep Medicine*. Edited by M. H. Kryger, T. Roth, and W. C. Dement. Philadelphia, W. B. Saunders, pp. 3–13.

Chandler, S. H., Chase, M. H., and Nakamura, Y. (1980). Intracellular analysis of synaptic mechanisms controlling trigeminal motoneuron activity during sleep and wakefulness. *J. Neurophysiol.*, 44:359–371.

Chase, M. H. (1972). *The Sleeping Brain. Perspectives in the Brain Sciences*. Vol 1. Los Angeles, Brain Information Service/Brain Research Institute, UCLA, p. 537.

Chase, M. H., and Morales, F. R. (1982). Phasic changes in motoneuron potential during REM periods of active sleep. *Neurosci. Lett.*, 34:177–182.

Chase, M. H., and Morales, F. R. (1983). Subthreshold excitatory activity and motoneuron discharge during REM periods of active sleep. *Science*, 221:1195–1198.

Chase, M. H., and Morales, F. R. (1989). The control of motoneurons during sleep. In *Principles and Practice of Sleep Medicine*. Edited by M. H. Kryger, T. Roth, and W. C. Dement. Philadelphia, W. B. Saunders, pp. 74–85.

Cheesman, M., and Revelette, R. (1990). Phrenic afferent contribution to reflexes elicited by changes in diaphragm length. *J. Appl. Physiol.*, 69:640–647.

Corda, M., Von Euler, C., and Lennerstrand, G. (1965). Proprioceptive innervation of the diaphragm. *J. Physiol.* (London), 178:161–177.

Corda, M., Von Euler, C., and Lennerstrand, G. (1966). Reflex and cerebellar influences on alpha and on "rhythmic" and "tonic" gamma activity in the intercostal muscles. *J. Physiol.* (London), 184:898–923.

Daubenspeck, J. A. (1981). Influence of small mechanical loads on variability of breathing pattern. *J. Appl. Physiol.*, 50:299–306.

De Troyer, A. (1983). Mechanical role of the abdominal muscles in relation to posture. *Respir. Physiol.*, 53:341–353.

De Troyer, A., Sampson, M., Sigrist, S., and Macklem, P. T. (1981). The diaphragm: two muscles. *Science*, 213:237–238.

Dick, T. E., Parmeggiani, P. L., and Orem, J. (1982). Intercostal muscle activity during sleep in the cat: an augmentation of expiratory activity. *Respir. Physiol.*, 50:255–265.

Douglas, N. J. (1989). Control of ventilation during sleep. In *Principles and Practice of Sleep Medicine*. Edited by M. H. Kryger, T. Roth, and W. C. Dement. Philadelphia, W. B. Saunders, pp. 249–256.

Douglas, N. J., White, D. P., Weil, J. V., Pickett, C. K., and Zwillich, C. W. (1982a). Hypercapnic ventilatory response in sleeping adults. *Am. Rev. Respir. Dis.*, 126:758–762.

Douglas, N. J., White, D. P., Weil, J. V., Pickett, C. K., Martin, R. J., and Zwillich, C. W. (1982b). Hypoxic ventilatory response decreases during sleep in normal men. *Am. Rev. Respir. Dis.*, 125:286–289.

Duggan, C. J., Watson, A., and Pride, N. B. (1990). Increases in nasal and pulmonary resistance in the supine posture in asthmatic and normal subjects. *Am. Rev. Respir. Dis.*, 141:A716.

Duron, B., and Marlot, D. (1980). Intercostal and diaphragmatic electrical activity during wakefulness and sleep in normal unrestrained adult cats. *Sleep*, 3:269–280.

Farkas, G. A., Baer, R. E., Estenne, M., and De Troyer, A. (1988). Mechanical role of expiratory muscles during breathing in upright dogs. *J. Appl. Physiol.*, 64:1060–1067.

Fitzgerald, R. S., and Lahiri, S. (1986). Reflex responses to chemoreceptor stimulation. In *Handbook of Physiology*. Sec. 3, Vol. II. Part 1. The Respiratory System. Control of Breathing. Edited by N. S. Cherniack and J. G. Widdicombe. Bethesda, Md., American Physiological Society, Williams & Wilkins, pp. 313–361.

Fregosi, R. F., Knuth, S. L., Ward, D. K., and Bartlett, D., Jr. (1987). Hypoxia inhibits abdominal expiratory nerve activity. *J. Appl. Physiol.*, 63:211–220.

Gassel, M. M., Marchiafava, P. L., and Pompeiano, O. (1964). Tonic and phasic inhibition of spinal reflexes during deep, desynchronized sleep in unrestrained cats. *Arch. Ital. Biol.*, 102:471–499.

Giaquinto, S., Pompeiano, O., and Somogyi, I. (1963). Supraspinal inhibitory control of spinal reflexes during natural sleep. *Experientia*, 19:652–653.

Gleeson, K., Zwillich, C. W., and White, D. P. (1990). The influence of increasing ventilatory effort on arousal from sleep. *Am. Rev. Respir. Dis.*, 142:295–300.

Glenn, L. L., and Dement, W. C. (1981). Membrane potential, synaptic activity, and excitability of hindlimb motoneuron during wakefulness and sleep. *J. Neurophysiol.*, 46:839–854.

Goldstein, R. S., Ramcharan, V., Bowes, G., McNicholas, W. T., Bradley, T. D., and Phillipson, E. A. (1984). Effect of supplemental nocturnal oxygen on gas exchange in patients with severe obstructive lung disease. *N. Engl. J. Med.*, 310:425–429.

Goldstein, R. S., Molotiu, N., Skrastins, R., Long, S. De Rosie, J. Contreras, M., Popkin, J., Rutherford, R., and Phillipson, E. A. (1987). Reversal of sleep-induced hypoventilation and chronic respiratory failure by nocturnal negative pressure ventilation in patients with restrictive ventilatory impairment. *Am. Rev. Respir. Dis.*, 135:1049–1055.

Gothe, B., Altose, M. D., Goldman, M. D., and Cherniack, N. S. (1981). Effect of quiet sleep on resting and CO_2-stimulated breathing in humans. *J. Appl. Physiol.*, 50:724–730.

Henderson-Smart, D. J., and Read, D. J. C. (1976). Depression of respiratory muscles and defective responses to nasal obstruction during active sleep in the newborn. *Aust. Pediatr. J.*, 12:261–266.

Henke, K. G., Arias, A., Skatrud, J. B., and Dempsey, J. A. (1988). Inhibition of inspiratory muscle activity during sleep. *Am. Rev. Respir. Dis.*, 138:8–15.

Henke, K. G., Dempsey, J. A., Badr, M. S., Kowitz, J. M., and Skatrud, J. B. (1991). Effect of sleep-induced increases in upper airway resistance on respiratory muscle activity. *J. Appl. Physiol.*, 70:158–168.

Henke, K. G., Badr, M. S., Skatrud, J. B., and Dempsey, J. A. (1992). Load compensation and respiratory muscle function during sleep. *J. Appl. Physiol.*, 72:1221–1234.

Henley, K., and Morrison, A. R. (1969). Release of organized behaviour during desynchronized sleep in cats with pontine lesion. *Psychophysiology*, 6:245.

Hoffstein, V., Zamel, N., and Phillipson, E. A. (1984). Lung volume dependence of pharyngeal cross-sectional area in patients with obstructive sleep apnea. *Am. Rev. Respir. Dis.*, 130:175–178.

Hudgel, D. W., and Devadatta, P. (1984). Decrease in functional residual capacity during sleep in normal humans. *J. Appl. Physiol.*, 57:1319–1322.

Hugelin, A. (1986). Forebrain and midbrain influence on respiration. In *Handbook of Physiology*. Sec 3. Vol II. Edited by N. S. Cherniack and J. G. Widdicombe. Bethesda, Md., American Physiological Society, Williams & Wilkins, pp. 69–91.

Hutt, D. A., Parisi, R. A., Edelman, N. H., and Santiago, T. V. (1991). Responses of diaphragm and external oblique muscles to flow-resistive loads during sleep. *Am. Rev. Respir. Dis.*, 144:1107–1111.

Iber, C., Berssenbrugge, A., Skatrud, J. B., and Dempsey, J. A. (1982). Ventilatory adaptations to resistive loading during wakefulness and non-REM sleep. *J. Appl. Physiol.*, 52(3):607–614.

Issa, F. G., and Sullivan, C. E. (1983). Arousal and breathing response to airway occlusion in healthy sleeping adults. *J. Appl. Physiol.*, 55:1113–1119.

Issa, F. G., and Sullivan, C. E. (1985). Respiratory muscle activity and thoracoabdominal motion during acute episodes of asthma during sleep. *Am. Rev. Respir. Dis.*, 132:999–1004.

Jankowska, E., Lund, S., Lundberg, A., and Pompeiano, O. (1968). Inhibitory effects evoked through ventral reticulospinal pathways. *Arch. Ital. Biol.*, 106:124–140.

Johnson, M. W., and Remmers, J. E. (1984). Accessory muscle activity during sleep in chronic obstructive pulmonary disease. *J. Appl. Physiol.*, 57:1011–1017.

Jouvet, M. (1967). Neurophysiology of the states of sleep. *Physiol. Rev.*, 47:117–177.

Kimoff, R. J., Kozar, L., Bradley, T. D., and Phillipson, E. A. (1992). Differential effects of REM sleep on inspiratory and expiratory muscle activity. *Am. Rev. Respir. Dis.*, 45:A404.

Kleitman, N. (1963). Sleep and wakefulness. Chicago, University of Chicago Press, pp. 8–14.

Kline, L. R., Hendricks, J. C., Davies, R. O., and Pack, A. I. (1986). Control of activity of the diaphragm in rapid-eye-movement sleep. *J. Appl. Physiol.*, 61:1293–1300.

Kline, L. R., Hendricks, J. C., Silage, D. A., Morrison, A. R., Davies, R. O., and Pack, A. I. (1990). Startle-evoked changes in diaphragmatic activity during wakefulness and sleep. *J. Appl. Physiol.*, 68:166–173.

Knill, R., and Bryan, A. C. (1976). An intercostal-phrenic inhibitory reflex in newborn infants. *J. Appl. Physiol.*, 40:352–356.

Kubota, K., Iwamura, Y., and Niimi, Y. (1965). Monosynaptic reflex and natural sleep in the cat. *J. Neurophysiol.*, 28:125–138.

Lenzi, G. L., Pompeiano, O., and Rabin, B. (1968). Supraspinal control of transmission in the polysynaptic reflex pathway to motoneurons during sleep. *Pfluegers Arch.*, 301:311–319.

Lopata, M., and Onal, E. (1982). Mass loading, sleep apnea, and the pathogenesis of obesity hypoventilation. *Am. Rev. Respir. Dis.*, 126:640–645.

Lopes, J. M., Tabachnik, E., Muller, N. L., Levison, H., and Bryan, A. C. (1983). Total airway resistance and respiratory muscle activity during sleep. *J. Appl. Physiol.*, 54:773–777.

Madsen, P. L., Schmid, J. F., Wildschiodtz, G., Friberg, L., Holm, S., Vorstrup, S., and Lassen, N. A. (1991). Cerebral O_2 metabolism and cerebral blood flow in humans during deep and rapid-eye-movement sleep. *J. Appl. Physiol.*, 70:2597–2601.

Manaker, S., and Fogarty, P. E. (1992). Raphespinal neurons project axon collaterals to the nucleus of the solitary tract. *Am. Rev. Respir. Dis.*, 145:A408.

McGinty, D. J., Harper, R. M., and Fairbanks, M. K. (1974). Neuronal unit activity and the control of sleep states. In *Advances in Sleep Research*. Vol. 1. Edited by E. D. Weitzman. New York, Spectrum, pp. 173–216.

Megirian, D., Ryan, A. T., and Sherrey, J. H. (1980). An electrophysiological analysis of sleep and respiration of rats breathing different gas mixtures: diaphragmatic muscle function. *Electroenceph. Clin. Neurophysiol.*, 50:303–313.

Morales, F. R., Boxer, P., and Chase, M. H. (1988). Behavioral state-specific inhibitory postsynaptic potentials impinge on cat lumbar motoneuron during active sleep. *Exp. Neurol.*, 100:583–595.

Moreno, F., and Lyons, H. A. (1961). Effect of body posture on lung volumes. *J. Appl. Physiol.*, 16:27–29.

Morrison, A. R., and Pompeiano, O. (1965a). An analysis of the supraspinal influences acting on motoneuron during sleep in the unrestrained cat: responses of the alpha motoneuron to direct electrical stimulation during sleep. *Arch. Ital. Biol.*, 103:497–516.

Morrison, A. R., and Pompeiano, O. (1965b). Central depolarization of group Ia afferent fibers during desynchronized sleep. *Arch. Ital. Biol.*, 103:517–535.

Mortola, J. P., and Anch, A. M. (1978). Chest wall configuration in supine man: wakefulness and sleep. *Respir. Physiol.*, 35:201–213.

Netick, A., Dugger, W. L., and Symmons, R. A. (1984). Ventilatory response to hypercapnia during sleep and wakefulness in cats. *J. Appl. Physiol.*, 56:1347–1354.

Newsom Davis, J., Goldman, M., Loh, L., and Casson, M. (1976). Diaphragm function and alveolar hypoventilation. *Q. J. Med.*, 45:87–100.

Orem, J. (1980a). Neuronal mechanisms of respiration in REM sleep. *Sleep*, 3:251–267.

Orem, J. (1980b). Medullary respiratory neuron activity: relationship to tonic and phasic REM sleep. *J. Appl. Physiol.*, 48:54–65.

Orem, J., Montplaisir, J., and Dement, W. C. (1974). Changes in the activity of respiratory neurones during sleep. *Brain Res.*, 82:309–315.

Orem, J., Osorio, I., Brooks, E., and Dick, T. (1985). Activity of respiratory neurons during NREM sleep. *J. Neurophysiol.*, 54:1144–1156.

Orem, J., and Lydic, R. (1978). Upper airway function during sleep and wakefulness: experimental studies on normal and anaesthetized cats. *Sleep*, 1:49–68.

Pack, A. I., Kline, L. R., Hendricks, J. C., and Davies, R. O. (1987). Control of the diaphragm during rapid eye movement sleep (REM). In *Respiratory Muscles and Their Neuromotor Control*. Edited by G. C. Sieck. New York, Alan R. Liss, pp. 437–441.

Parisi, R. A., Neubauer, J. A., Santiago, T. V., and Edelman, N. H. (1987). Determination of respiratory neuromotor control during rapid eye movement (REM) sleep. In *Respiratory Muscles and Their Neuromotor Control*. Edited by G. C. Sieck. New York, Alan R. Liss, pp. 443–447.

Parmeggiani, P. L., and Sabattini, L. (1972). Electromyographic aspects of postural, respiratory and thermoregulatory mechanisms in sleeping cats. *Electroenceph. Clin. Neurophysiol.*, 33:1–13.

Phillipson, E. A., and Bowes, G. (1986). Control of breathing during sleep. In *Handbook of Physiology*. Sec. 3. Vol II. Edited by N. S. Cherniak and J. G. Widdicombe. Bethesda, Md., American Physiological Society, Williams & Wilkins, pp. 649–849.

Phillipson, E. A., Kozar, L. F., and Murphy, E. (1976). Respiratory load compensation in awake and sleeping dogs. *J. Appl. Physiol.*, 40:895–902.

Phillipson, E. A., Kozar, L. F., Rebuck, A. S., and Murphy, E. (1977). Ventilatory and waking responses to CO_2 in sleeping dogs. *Am. Rev. Respir. Dis.*, 115:251–259.

Phillipson, E. A., Sullivan, C. E., Read, D. J. C., Murphy, E., and Kozar, L. F. (1978). Ventilatory and waking responses to hypoxia in sleeping dogs. *J Appl. Physiol.*, 44:512–520.

Phillipson, E. A., Yasuma, F., Kozar, L. F., and England, S. J. (1990). Respiratory muscle activation by chemical stimuli in awake and sleeping dogs. In *Sleep and Respiration*. Edited by F. G. Issa, P. M. Suratt, and J. E. Remmers. New York, Wiley-Liss, pp. 201–213.

Pompeiano, O. (1967). The neurophysiological mechanisms of the postural and motor events during desynchronized sleep. In *Sleep and Altered States of Consciousness*. Edited by S. S. Kety, E. V. Evarts, and H. L. Williams. Baltimore, Md., Williams & Wilkins, pp. 351–423.

Pompeiano, O. (1978). The generation of rhythmic discharges during bursts of REM. In *Abnormal Neuronal Discharges*. Edited by N. Chalazonitis and M. Boisson. New York, Raven, pp. 75–89.

Puizillout, J. J., and Ternaux, J. P. (1974). Variations d'activites toniques, phasiques et respiratoire au niveau bulbaire pendant l'endormement de la preparation encephale isole. *Brain Res.*, 66:67–83.

Remmers, J. E., Bartlett, D., and Putnam, M. D. (1976). Changes in the respiratory cycle associated with sleep. *Respir. Physiol.*, 28:227–238.

Santiago, T. V., Sinha, A. K., and Edelman, N. H. (1981). Respiratory flow-resistive load compensation during sleep. *Am. Rev. Respir. Dis.*, 123:382–387.

Santiago, T. V., Guerra, E., Neubauer, J. A., and Edelman, N. H. (1984). Correlation between ventilation and brain blood flow during sleep. *J. Clin. Invest.*, 73:497–506.

Sauerland, E. K., Orr, W. C., and Hairston, L. E. (1981). EMG patterns of oropharyngeal muscles during respiration in wakefulness and sleep. *Electromyogr. Clin. Neurophysiol..*, 21:307–316.

Sears, T. A., Berger, A. J., and Phillipson, E. A. (1982). Reciprocal tonic activation of inspiratory and expiratory motoneurons by chemical drives. *Nature*, 299:728–730.

Sherrey, J. H., and Megirian, D. (1980). Respiratory EMG activity of the posterior cricoarytenoid, cricothyroid and diaphragm muscles during sleep. *Respir. Physiol.*, 39:355–365.

Sherrey, J. H., and Megirian, D. (1987). Respiratory activity of some extralaryngeal muscles during sleep: depression by hypoxia. In *Respiratory Muscles and Their Neuromotor Control*. Edited by G. C. Sieck. New York, Alan R. Liss, pp. 429–436.

Sieck, G. C., Trelease, R. B., and Harper, R. M. (1984). Sleep influences on diaphragmatic motor unit discharge. *Exp. Neurol.*, 85:316–335.

Skatrud, J. B., and Dempsey, J. A. (1985). Airway resistance and respiratory muscle function in snorers during NREM sleep. *J. Appl. Physiol.*, 59:328–335.

Skatrud, J. B., and Dempsey, J. A., Badr, S., and Begle, R. (1988). Effect of airway impedance on CO_2 retention and respiratory muscle activity during NREM sleep. *J. Appl. Physiol.*, 65:1676–1685.

Stradling, J. R., Kozar, L. F., Dark, J., Kirby, T., Andrey, S. M., and Phillipson, E. A. (1987). Effect of acute diaphragm paralysis on ventilation in awake and sleeping dogs. *Am. Rev. Respir. Dis.*, 136:633–637.

Sullivan, C. E. (1980). Breathing in sleep. In *Physiology in Sleep*. Edited by J. Orem and C. D. Barnes. New York, Academic Press, pp. 214–272.

Sullivan, C. E., Murphy, E., Kozar, L. F., and Phillipson, E. A. (1979). Ventilatory responses to CO_2 and lung inflation in tonic versus phasic REM sleep. *J. Appl. Physiol.*, 47:1304–1310.

Tabachnik, E., Muller, N. L., Bryan, A. C., and Levison, H. (1981a). Changes in ventilation and chest wall mechanics during sleep in normal adolescents. *J. Appl. Physiol.*, 51:557–564.

Tabachnik, E., Muller, N. L., Levison, H., and Bryan, A. C. (1981b). Chest wall mechanics and pattern of breathing during sleep in asthmatic adolescents. *Am. Rev. Respir. Dis.*, 124:269–273.

Takasaki, Y., Orr, D., Popkin, J., Xie, A., and Bradley, T. D. (1989). Effect of hypercapnia and hypoxia on respiratory muscle activation in humans. *J. Appl. Physiol.*, 66:381–391.

Townsend, R. E., Prinz, P. N., and Obrist, W. D. (1973). Human cerebral blood flow during sleep and waking. *J. Appl. Physiol.* 35:620–625.

Tusiewicz, K., Moldofsky, H., Bryan, A. C., and Bryan, M. H. (1977). Mechanics of the rib cage and diaphragm during sleep. *J. Appl. Physiol.*, 43:600–602.

Vincken, W., Guilleminault, C., Silvestri, L., Cosio, M., and Grassino, A. (1987). Inspiratory muscle activity as a trigger causing the airways to open in obstructive sleep apnea. *Am. Rev. Respir. Dis.*, 135:372–377.

White, D. P., Douglas, N. J., Pickett, C. K., Weil, J. V., and Zwillich, C. W. (1982). Hypoxic ventilatory response during sleep in normal premenopausal women. *Am. Rev. Respir. Dis.*, 126:530–533.

White, D. P., Weil, J. V., and Zwillich, C. W. (1985). Metabolic rate and breathing during sleep. *J. Appl. Physiol.*, 59:384–391.

Wiegand, L., Zwillich, C. W., and White, D. P. (1988). Sleep and the ventilatory response to resistive loading in normal man. *J. Appl. Physiol.*, 64:1186–1195.

Wilcox, P. G., Pare, P. D., Road, J. D., and Fleetham, J. A. (1990). Respiratory muscle function during obstructive sleep apnea. *Am. Rev. Respir. Dis.*, 142:533–539.

Wilson, P. A., Skatrud, J. B., and Dempsey, J. A. (1984). Effects of slow wave sleep on ventilatory compensation to inspiratory elastic loading. *Respir. Physiol.*, 55:103–120.

Xie, A., Takasaki, Y., and Bradley, T. D. (1991a). Influence of body position on diaphragmatic and scalene activation during hypoxic rebreathing. *Am. Rev. Respir. Dis.*, 141:A721.

Xie, A., Takasaki, Y., Popkin, J., Orr, D., and Bradley, T. D. (1991b). Chemical and postural influence on scalene and diaphragmatic activation in humans. *J. Appl. Physiol.*, 70:658–664.

Yasuma, F., Kozar, L. F., Kimoff, R. J., Bradley, T. D., and Phillipson, E. A. (1991). Interaction of chemical and mechanical respiratory stimuli in the arousal response to hypoxia in sleeping dogs. *Am. Rev. Respir. Dis.*, 143:1274–1277.

Yasuma, F., Kimoff, R. J., Kozar, L. F., Bradley, D. B., England, S. F., and Phillipson, E. A. (1990). Chemical and non-chemical control of abdominal muscle activation. *Clin. Invest. Med.*, 13:B122.

Zwillich, C. W., Sahn, S., and Weil, J. V. (1977). Effects of hyper-metabolism on ventilation and chemosensitivity. *J. Clin. Invest.*, 60:900–906.

49

Respiratory Muscle Fatigue

CHARIS ROUSSOS

National and Kapodistrian University
    of Athens Medical School
Athens, Greece
McGill University
Montreal, Quebec, Canada

FRANCOIS BELLEMARE

University of Montreal
Hôtel-Dieu Hospital
Montreal, Quebec, Canada

JOHN MOXHAM

King's College School of Medicine and Dentistry
London, England

I. Introduction

The word fatigue has several meanings; in daily life "fatigue" is often used to express tiredness or weakness, whereas in technical discussion fatigue may include impaired intellectual or motor performance, increased electromyographic (EMG) activity for a given performance, shift of the EMG power spectrum to lower frequencies, or inability of muscle to generate force. A recent NHLBI Workshop defined fatigue as the loss of capacity to develop force and/or velocity in response to a load that is reversible by rest (NHLBI, 1990). As a first approximation, fatigue of the respiratory muscles may be defined as an inability to continue to generate sufficient pressure to maintain alveolar ventilation. Fatigue should be distinguished from weakness, in which reduced force generation is fixed and not reversed by rest, although the presence of muscle weakness may itself predispose to muscle fatigue (Table 1).

Fatigue can occur as a result of failure at any one of the many steps in the command chain of voluntary muscular activity (Fig. 1). Thus, the site of fatigue may theoretically be anywhere from the brain to the peripheral contractile machinery. However, it is reasonable to consider fatigue as a class of acute effects that can impair motor performance, and not as a single mechanism (Enoka and Stuart, 1992).

The precise site or sites of fatigue remains controversial. It is not certain

Table 1 Factors Predisposing to Inspiratory Muscle Fatigue

Excessive Load:
 Increased work of breathing (minute ventilation, frequency, tidal volume,
  inspiratory time, compliance, resistance)
Reducing Capacity:
 Weakness (nutritional status, atrophy, neuromuscular disease, prematurity,
  lung volume)
 Limited energy supply and stores:
  Reduced muscle blood flow (cardiac output, distribution of perfusion,
   intensity of contraction)
  Reduced content of arterial blood (O_2 saturation, Hb concentration)
  Reduced blood substrate concentration (glucose, free fatty acids)
  Reduced ability to utilize oxygen and substrates (sepsis)
  Reduced energy stores (muscle glycogen, ATP, phosphocreatine)

whether failure to generate force follows reduced motor output from the central nervous system ("central fatigue") or failure at the neuromuscular junction or within the muscle machinery ("peripheral fatigue"). For the respiratory system, the question arises as to whether the respiratory controllers become too "tired" to continue to command the thorax to fulfill its role as a pump to ventilate the lung or whether the peripheral apparatus becomes unable to generate appropriate force despite an adequate neural drive. These questions were first considered early in the century by Davies et al. (1919, 1925). These investigators were the first to study respiratory muscle fatigue, and they deduced that both types of fatigue—central and peripheral—may exist. Furthermore, central and peripheral fatigue may be closely interrelated, with adaptive reduction of central output following excessive loading of peripheral muscles (see below).

II. Muscle Function and Fatigue

A. Force Generation

For voluntary contractions there is a long chain of command from the motor cortex to the eventual interaction of actin and myosin within the muscle fiber. These events can be broadly divided into three categories: (1) those concerned with delivering sufficient electrical activation from the central nervous system to the muscle, (2) the metabolic and enzymatic processes providing energy to the contractile mechanism, and (3) the excitation-contraction coupling processes that link these two.

Muscle tension can be altered either by varying the firing frequency of each of the active motor units or by varying the number of motor units that are active. At low intensities of muscle contraction, force is developed largely by recruitment of motor units; at moderate and high levels of voluntary contraction the number of additional motor units recruited during a given increment in force decreases sharply,

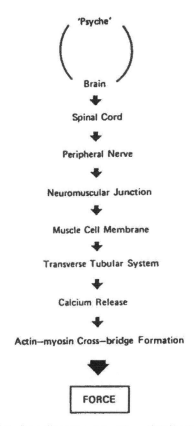

Figure 1 Command chain for voluntary contraction of skeletal muscle. (From Edwards, 1978.)

and force is generated by increasing the firing frequency of each motor unit (Milner-Brown et al., 1973a,b).

Motor units are generally recruited according to size principle (Henneman and Mendell, 1981). The size principle has also been shown to apply equally well to respiratory and phrenic motor neurons (Dick et al., 1987). However, Hilaire et al. (1983) using a cross-correlation analysis showed a specificity between early and late premotoneurons and early- and late-recruited phrenic motoneurons, thus suggesting the possibility of selective recruitment of specific motor units. Changes in the order of motor unit recruitment have been documented during rapid ballistic contractions of human limb muscles (Desmedt and Godaux, 1977). In the respiratory system, changes in order of recruitment of intercostal muscle motor units have been documented when breathing frequency is increased by raising body temperature (Citterio et al., 1983). In these circumstances, motor units are recruited that are best suited in relation to the velocity of shortening of the muscle. During fatigue of sustained maximum voluntary contractions lasting up to 3 min, all motor units appear to remain recruited even in extreme fatigue (Merton, 1954; Bigland-Ritchie et al., 1979, 1983; Belanger and McComas, 1981; Bellemare and Garzaniti, 1988). However, during fatigue of constant-force submaximal voluntary contractions there is alternation in the recruitment of motor units, with some dropping out while others are being recruited to maintain constant force (Person and Kudina, 1972; Grimby et al., 1981). By providing absolute rest to fatigued motor units, this alternation of recruitment may optimize performance by delaying task failure. A similar mechanism has been suggested to explain the alternation between different synergistic inspiratory muscles in the presence of fatiguing loads (see below).

Experimentally, it is possible to determine the effect of firing rates on force generation using electrical stimulation techniques, which have the advantage of being effort independent (Milner-Brown et al., 1973a; Edwards et al., 1977b). As the frequency increases from a single stimulus to a high-frequency train, the muscle responds with a brief twitch (unitary activity), then as an unfused (oscillatory) contraction, and finally a fused tetanus. The force-frequency characteristics of a muscle can be conveniently and precisely recorded by programmed electrical stimulation in an isolated muscle preparation (Moulds et al., 1977), in human limb muscles (Edwards et al., 1977b), and in the muscles of respiration (Moxham et al., 1980; Aubier et al., 1981a; Moxham et al., 1981b) (Fig. 2).

The shape of the force-frequency curve of skeletal muscle is determined by

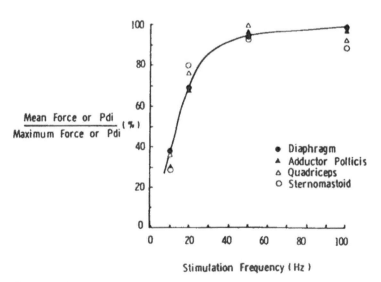

Figure 2 Frequency: P_{di} curve of the diaphragm and frequency-force curves of sternomastoid, quadriceps, and adductor pollicis, expressed as a percentage of the stimulated maximum for each muscle. The solid line is drawn through the diaphragm data. (From Moxham et al., 1982.)

the constituent fiber types (i.e., the proportion of fast and slow twitch fibers), and the shape of any given fiber type is species specific (Close, 1972). Because of its sigmoid shape, the low-frequency region, which has the steepest slope, is crucial for force modulation. For most human muscles of mixed fiber type composition or with intermediate contractile speed, such as most limb and respiratory muscles, as frequency increases above the critical fusion frequency of 5–7 Hz, there is a rapid increase in tension up to 30–40 Hz, after which tension rises much more slowly to reach a plateau at 70–100 Hz. The natural frequencies of motor units for most everyday muscular activities of 5–30 Hz are thus restricted to the optimal regulatory range for force production (Kukulka and Clamman, 1981; Thomas et al., 1991a). During brief (10 s) maximum voluntary contractions, maximum discharge rates vary over about a fourfold range among different motor units of the same muscle, in spite of evidence that all motor units are then maximally activated to respond with maximum force production (Bellemare et al., 1983). These rates are well suited to match the range in contractile speed of the constituent motor unit types of each muscle, which also vary over a fourfold range (Buchthal and Schmalbruch, 1970; Bellemare et al., 1983; Thomas et al., 1991b). Mean maximum discharge rates are thus about 30 Hz for the biceps brachii and adductor pollicis muscles but only about 11 Hz for the much slower soleus muscle (Bellemare et al., 1983). Thus under normal conditions, the maximum discharge rates of motor units appear to be limited not to exceed those just required for maximum force production in relation to speed of the constituent motor units. This may serve to optimize motor control while minimizing energy cost and reducing the chances of electrical transmission failure.

The position of the force-frequency curve and the slope of its steepest portion are not fixed but can be modified by cooling, fatigue, conditioning, reinnervation, pharmacological agents, and changes in muscle length. There can be selective loss of force at high and at low frequencies, referred to as high- and low-frequency fatigue. The former is associated with a fall in the size of the surface recorded action potentials as a consequence of defective neuromuscular transmission (Edwards, 1978) and/or impaired surface membrane excitation (Jones et al., 1979). Low-frequency fatigue is not accompanied by a decrease in the size of the surface action potential and is thought to be due to impaired excitation-contraction coupling, secondary to failure of propagation of the action potential in the tubular system (Westerblad et al., 1991) or insufficient release of calcium from the sarcoplasmic reticulum (Edwards et al., 1977a).

Following changes in the position of the steep section of the force-frequency curve, changes in motor unit discharge rates would be anticipated if optimal control of force modulation and economy of force maintenance are to be maintained. A progressive decrease in motor unit discharge rates from about 32 to 20 Hz has been documented during fatigue of sustained maximum voluntary contractions of adductor pollicis muscle involving a 50% reduction in force (Bigland-Ritchie et al., 1983). Because of a concomitant slowing in muscle contraction speed with such fatigue, changes in firing rates need not result in a decrease in muscle force output. Whether appropriate changes in motor unit discharge rate also occur with other forms of fatigue (high- and low-frequency fatigue) to optimize muscle force output is not known. A notable exception, now well documented, concerns the effect of cooling, which, although producing marked changes in the shape and position of the force-frequency relationship of adductor pollicis muscle, is not accompanied by any change in the rate of discharge of motor units (Marsden et al., 1983; Bigland-Ritchie et al., 1992a). It is possible, however, that cooling also blocks afferent activity from muscle that is involved in the adjustment of motor unit discharge to contractile speed. During fatigue of sustained submaximal contractions, the mean motor unit firing rates do not appear to change (Person and Kudina, 1972; Grimby et al., 1981). As mentioned above, this type of fatigue is characterized by alternation in motor unit recruitment.

B. Central Fatigue

In the past, fatigue has frequently been attributed to failure of central neural processes (Waller, 1891; Mosso, 1914; Reid, 1928). By comparing the forces generated by maximum voluntary and maximum electrically stimulated contractions, an assessment of central fatigue is possible (Merton, 1954; Ikai et al., 1967; Bigland-Ritchie et al., 1978). If maximal electrical stimulation is superimposed on a maximum voluntary contraction and force generation is thereby increased, a component of central fatigue can be said to exist. Some studies (Ikai et al., 1967; Bigland-Ritchie et al., 1978) have shown that forces generated with maximal electrical stimulation can exceed those of voluntary contractions, whereas others (Merton, 1954) have found no differences in the forces of voluntary and electrically stimulated contractions.

Merton's views have been widely accepted, and his findings confirmed in several studies of the same (Bigland-Ritchie et al., 1983) and other limb muscles using similar techniques (Belanger and McComas, 1981). More recently, similar conclusions have also been reached for fatigue of periodic submaximal constant force contractions of the quadriceps muscle, a pattern of contraction that more closely mimicks that of the respiratory muscles (Bigland-Ritchie et al., 1986). In this study, however, a component of central fatigue was found for similar contractions of the soleus muscle.

The technique of twitch interpolation or occlusion described by Merton (1954) was first applied to the human diaphragm by Bellemare and Bigland-Ritchie (1984) to evaluate the extent of diaphragm activation during maximum voluntary efforts in the fresh state. It was subsequently used, in combination with electromyographic recordings, to investigate changes in diaphragm and rib cage muscle activation during fatiguing tasks to exhaustion in normal volunteers (Bellemare and Bigland-Ritchie, 1987). For inspiratory resistive breathing tasks where all functional synergists could be recruited, as well as during tasks using diaphragmatic expulsive maneuvers in which the diaphragm contraction was largely isolated from the other muscles, considerable submaximal activation of the diaphragm was demonstrated at the limit of endurance and beyond, from which it was concluded that much of the observed fatigue was central in origin (Fig. 3). The central fatigue observed with both forms of exercise was associated with a corresponding decrease in the natural electromyogram of the diaphragm (Fig. 4) recorded with an esophageal electrode and, in the case of inspiratory resistive breathing tasks, by a compensatory recruitment of the intercostal and neck accessory muscles, as demonstrated by surface electromyographic recordings (Fig. 5). The progressive decrease in the level of diaphragm activation during fatigue, as well as the compensatory recruitment of the rib cage and accessory muscles, was confirmed for different breathing strategies by Ward et al. (1988) using EMG techniques. Ward's study also established that the increase in breathing effort sensation and dyspnea with fatigue of this type was more closely related to the recruitment of the rib cage/accessory muscles than to the decrease in diaphragm contractility as assessed by the E/T (EMG activity/transdiaphragmatic pressure) ratio of the diaphragm.

Hershenson and collaborators have shown that during inspiratory efforts performed without increasing abdominal pressure (i.e., without abdominal muscle recruitment), the transdiaphragmatic pressure, and by inference the level of diaphragm activation, is less than when the abdominal muscles are simultaneously recruited. They reasoned that under those conditions the rib cage inspiratory muscles and the abdominal muscles are both antagonists of the diaphragm and that the pleural pressure generated during the inspiratory effort is largely determined by the strength of the weaker rib cage muscles (Hershenson et al., 1988). They subsequently extended this analysis to the study of inspiratory muscle fatigue (Hershenson et al., 1989) and showed that inspiratory resistive breathing tasks, carried to the point of fatigue and beyond and in which abdominal pressure does not rise or even decreases, cause fatigue of the rib cage muscles without fatiguing the diaphragm. Thus, central fatigue of the diaphragm during inspiratory resistance breathing tasks may not be caused by a reduction in the capacity to maximally activate it but by a preferential fatigue of the weaker muscles of the rib cage.

Central fatigue of the diaphragm of the same magnitude as that found by Bellemare and Bigland-Ritchie (1987) was reported by McKenzie et al. (1992) for fatigue induced by diaphragmatic expulsive maneuvers. Their study also showed that central fatigue was more important in the diaphragm than in limb muscles. This difference was explained on the basis that, in the case of the diaphragm study, the diaphragm and abdominal muscles had to contract antagonistically to increase abdominal pressure. Because under such circumstances the abdominal pressure would be expected to be limited by the weaker muscle (Hershenson et al., 1986), they hypothesized that more rapid fatigue of the abdominal muscles than of the diaphragm would lead to submaximal activation of the latter during this type of contraction. This mechanism is, however, unlikely to account for the findings of Bellemare and Bigland-Ritchie (1987), since in their study of diaphragm expulsive maneuvers the abdomen was tightly bound with a nonelastic corset, which should have loaded the diaphragm sufficiently to produce maximum abdominal pressure.

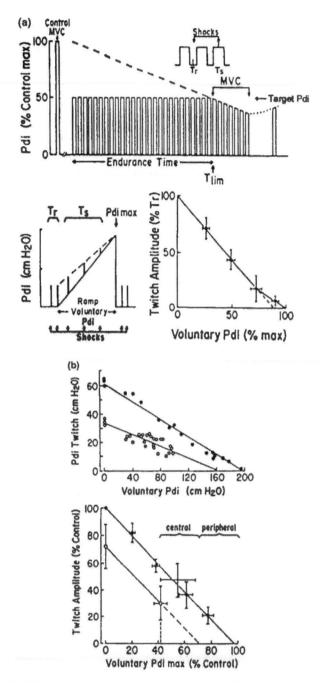

Figure 3 (a) Schematic representation of the twitch occlusion test to evaluate central and peripheral diaphragmatic fatigue and changes in the level of diaphragm activation during

That central fatigue of the diaphragm, and compensatory recruitment of rib cage/accessory muscles, need not necessarily result from fatigue of the weaker antagonist is supported by the study of Supinski et al. (1989). They used an isolated in situ perfused diaphragm muscle strip preparation. Fatigue was induced by selectively inducing ischemia of the diaphragm strip, while perfusion of the contralateral diaphragm and the rib cage/accessory muscles was maintained intact. As in human studies, the force developed by the diaphragm strip declined more rapidly in response to spontaneous efforts than in response to artificial nerve stimulation. Ischemia and fatigue was associated with a selective decrease in diaphragm strip EMG activity and with a progressive increase in the EMG activity of the contralateral hemidiaphragm and the inspiratory intercostal muscles. All these changes were reversible after removal of ischemia. As for the human studies mentioned above (Bellemare and Bigland-Ritchie, 1987; McKenzie et al., 1992), the decline in diaphragm strip EMG could not be accounted for by failure of neuromuscular transmission, since the size of the action potential in response to a constant nerve stimulation did not change. Hence the EMG changes probably reflected changes in central activation.

The importance of central fatigue in clinical ventilatory failure remains uncertain, and studies on patients are difficult to perform. It is possible that the recently described technique of magnetic phrenic nerve stimulation may facilitate progress in this area (Simolowski et al., 1989). Central fatigue may be caused by a reduction in the number of motor units that can be recruited by the motor drive or by a decrease in motor unit discharge rates or both. Derecruitment of previously active motor units has been reported during sustained maximal voluntary contractions of the big toe extensor muscles (Grimby et al., 1981).

If the firing frequency of a single motor unit is measured, the mean firing frequency characteristically falls throughout a strong contraction (Marsden et al., 1971; Grimby et al., 1981). This should not be regarded as "central fatigue," because in the conditions in which this was described, if the muscle is electrically stimulated at a higher frequency, the force response was not increased. Thus, although much of the loss of force observed during some types of fatigue may result directly from

---

fatigue of repeated submaximal voluntary contractions repeated until beyond the limit of endurance (T_{lim}) where all require a maximal effort (top). Top inset: Periodic stimulation to elicit twitches between contractions (Tr) and superimposed (Ts) on target voluntary Pdi. Bottom left: Ts superimposed on increasing voluntary ramp Pdi contractions. Bottom right: Relationship between Ts and the voluntary Pdi upon which they are superimposed. MVC: Maximal voluntary contraction. (b) Top: Changes in the relationships between twitch amplitude and voluntary transdiaphragmatic pressure (Pdi) obtained from one experiment before exercise (filled circles) and after the limit of endurance (open circles) during ramp to maximum voluntary Pdi contractions. Bottom: Pooled data from all subjects showing central and peripheral components of fatigue. Pdi_{max}, Maximum Pdi. Note that after fatigue the maximal Pdi that can be generated voluntarily is smaller than Pdi_{max}, calculated by extrapolation of the twitch occlusion diagram. (Adapted from Bellemare and Bigland-Ritchie, 1987.)

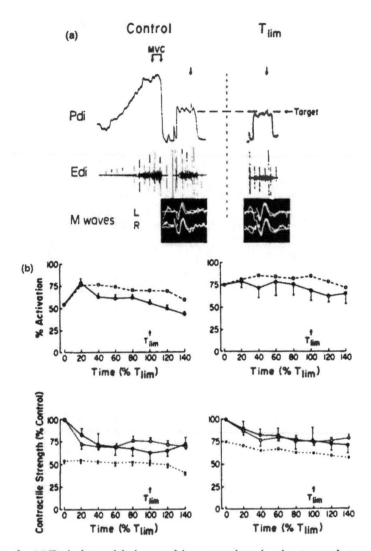

Figure 4 (a) Typical record during expulsive contractions showing a control ramp-to-maximum contraction, a contraction early in the fatiguing task and after the limit of endurance (T_{lim}) when target transdiaphragmatic pressure (Pdi) can no longer be reached. Maximal shocks were delivered to both phrenic nerves at arrows. Traces from top: Pdi, Edi (diaphragm electromyogram recorded with surface electrodes from left and right hemidiaphragms in response to single nerve shocks). MVC: Maximum voluntary contractions. (b) Top: Changes in muscle activation assessed from twitch occlusion (open circles) and from smoothed rectified diaphragm electromyogram recorded with esophageal electrode (filled circles) during expulsive contractions (left) and resistance breathing (right). Bottom: Corresponding changes in muscle contractile strength estimated by twitch occlusion (open circles) and from the amplitude of twitches between breaths (filled circles). Each is compared with mean fatiguing voluntary transdiaphragmatic pressure achieved (dotted lines). (Adapted from Bellemare and Bigland-Ritchie, 1987.)

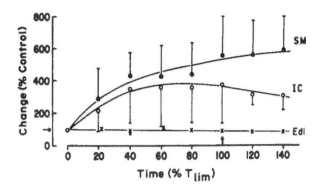

Figure 5 Comparison of the changes in diaphragm electromyogram recorded with esophageal electrodes (Edi) with those recorded simultaneously from the intercostal (IC) and sternomastoid (SM) muscles during fatigue-resistive breathing tasks. T_{lim}: Limit of endurance. (From Bellemare and Bigland-Ritchie, 1987.)

reduction in the rate of firing of motor units, it is not clear whether the decline in firing frequency is always the cause of force loss or a response to impaired contractility of peripheral muscle.

Several mechanisms have been suggested to explain the slowing of motor unit discharge rate with fatigue. At the extreme, the same mechanisms may cause motor unit to stop firing and be derecruited. During high force contractions, in which high threshold motor units are recruited, it may be the result of motor neuron adaptation, despite maintained synaptic excitation, as shown by Kernel and Monster (1982). Alternatively, a slowing in discharge rate may result from mounting reflex inhibition from group 3 and 4 muscle afferents, as suggested by Bigland-Ritchie et al. (1986) and Garland and McComas (1990), or a decrease in motor neuron excitability due to mounting Renshaw cell inhibition (Kukulka et al., 1986). However, both Bongiovanni et al. (1990) and Macefield et al. (1991) have shown a reduction in autogenic facilitation from spindle primary afferents during fatigue of sustained maximal voluntary contractions, which could account for the reduced motor unit discharge rate. A slowing in motor unit discharge rate may also occur as a result of neuromuscular propagation failure, as demonstrated by Krnjevic and Miledi (1959a). They showed that when single phrenic motoneurons are stimulated with a constant low frequency of 40 Hz, the muscle fibers fail to respond to every stimulus in the first few seconds of the stimulation, and the muscle fiber firing rate progressively declines thereafter, following a time course almost identical to that of the human motor units studied by Marsden et al. (1983) and Bigland-Ritchie et al. (1983).

Experimentally, the gradual loss of force following a prolonged maximum voluntary contraction can be accurately mimicked with electrical stimulation if the stimulation frequency is progressively reduced, whereas if high stimulation frequencies are maintained for too long, force loss is more rapid (Bigland-Ritchie, 1981) (Fig. 6). It could be that the central nervous system reflexively adjusts its outgoing signal as the contractile machinery of the muscle fails; such an adaptation would avoid the failure of electrical propagation associated with high-frequency fatigue as well as the complete depletion of vital chemicals within the muscle cell, which might occur if high firing rates were maintained (Fig. 6). In this context, it is of note that Hannertz and Grimby (1979) have presented evidence that motor neurons receive a tonic inhibitory drive from peripheral sources and that during a maximum

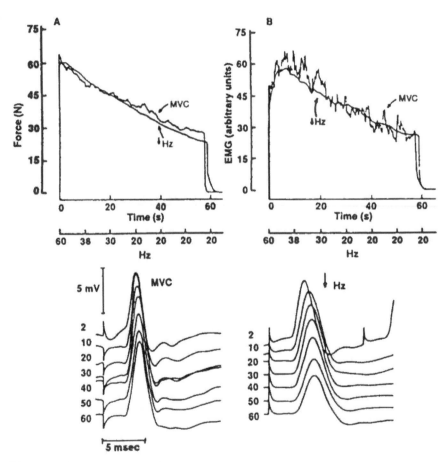

Figure 6 Top: Maximum voluntary contractions (MVC) of the adductor pollicis muscle sustained for 60 s. (A) During an electrically stimulated contraction, the force of the MVC is matched by initial stimulation at 60 Hz, followed by progressive reduction of the stimulation frequency to 20 Hz. (B) The surface EMGs for voluntary and stimulated contractions are closely matched. Bottom: The EMG M-waves during MVC and stimulated contractions are well maintained. (From Bigland-Ritchie, 1981.)

voluntary contraction (MVC), the motor neuron discharge rate increases if the muscle afferents are partially blocked. In this context it is of interest that in the respiratory system, Scardella and coworkers (1986, 1989, 1990) have now shown in awake goats subjected to severe inspiratory resistive loading an increase in diaphragm and abdominal muscle EMG activity after naloxone infusion (Fig. 7), suggesting that the endogenous opioid system was activated under those conditions and that it limited the extent to which the diaphragm and abdominal muscles could be recruited. (For a review see Chaps. 29 and 31.) They subsequently showed that this effect of naloxone was blocked when the animals were pretreated with dichloroacetate, which also prevented the rise in respiratory muscle lactate (Petroz-zino et al., 1992). They reasoned that the opioid system could have been activated by respiratory muscular afferents sensitive to metabolic changes in the muscle, such as group III and IV muscle afferents (Mense and Stahnke, 1983; Jammes et al., 1986; Graham et al., 1986; Hussain et al., 1990). Whether similar responses also underlie the central fatigue observed in limb muscles and the diaphragm remains to

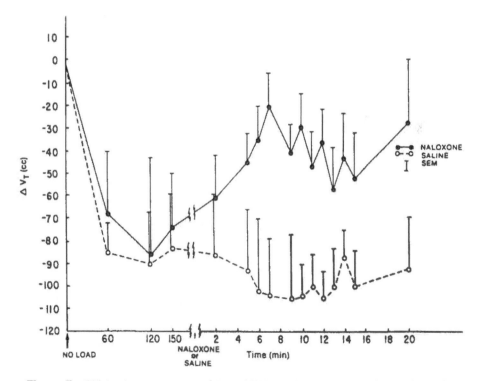

Figure 7 Tidal volume response to 2.5 h of high inspiratory flow-resistive loading prior to and following the administration of naloxone. The tidal volume decrease associated with loading is partially reversed by naloxone. (Note the change in time scale on the x-axis.) Closed circles = naloxone; open circles = saline control.

be established. In the studies of Scardella et al., the presence or absence of respiratory muscle fatigue was not documented, but the finding of high levels of lactate under their experimental conditions suggest that these muscles were driven hard and could be fatiguing (see Sec. II.D). Activation of the opioid system under those conditions could serve to protect the muscles from excessive metabolic deterioration, thereby minimizing peripheral fatigue while increasing central fatigue.

It must be pointed out, however, that the central nervous system may not always have the wisdom to adapt its motor neuron discharge rate to optimize performance in fatigue. Marsden et al. (1983) have shown that when the adductor pollicis muscle is cooled, maximum force during a sustained contraction is better maintained during an artificial tetany, during which the stimulation frequency is progressively decreased, than during maximum voluntary contractions.

The reduction in force associated with the progressive fall in motor neuron firing frequency is partially offset by the slowing of muscle contraction that occurs with fatigue (Jones, 1981). With fatigue, both the contraction and relaxation time are prolonged (Hill, 1913; Abbott, 1951), and tetanic fusion can therefore occur at lower stimulation frequencies.

The relaxation characteristics of skeletal muscle can be documented by measuring the maximum relaxation rate (MRR), defined as the percentage loss of maximum or plateau force in 10 ms. For the respiratory muscles MRR can be measured from pressures recorded at the mouth, in the esophagus, or across the diaphragm, and slowing of MRR following inspiratory resistive loading can be used as an index of excessive loading and an early indication of fatigue (Fig. 8) (see Sec. IV).

Esau et al. (1983a) have shown that MRR and EMG power spectrum changes of the diaphragm parallel each other during inspiratory resistive breathing tasks, and Moxham et al. (1982) have shown the EMG power spectrum changes to be more closely associated with high-frequency than with low-frequency fatigue of human diaphragm and quadriceps muscle. In the study of Bellemare and Bigland-Ritchie (unpublished observations, 1987), the changes in contraction and relaxation rates measured from single twitches between breaths closely followed the changes in the level of diaphragm activation; after an initial slowing in the first 5 min of the fatiguing tasks, both the contraction and the relaxation rates returned toward control values by the time the subjects reached their limit of endurance and beyond, a time when low-frequency fatigue was likely to be present. Similarly, in a more recent study, Yan et al. (1992) found no changes in the contraction and relaxation rates of single twitches at any given lung volume during recovery from fatigue despite a 40% reduction in the amplitude of single twitches. McKenzie and Gandevia (1991), studying the biceps brachii during periodic maximal voluntary contractions, found changes in the contraction and relaxation rates of single twitches with fatigue that were more pronounced when the duty cycle was high.

All of the above evidence points to the conclusion that changes in MRR and EMG power spectrum are more closely associated with fatigue of high-intensity contractions, such as maximum voluntary ventilation trials (Mulvey et al., 1991b).

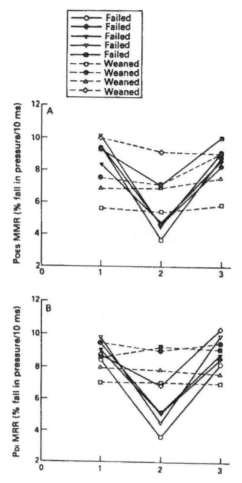

Figure 8 (A) Sniff esophageal and (B) transdiaphragmatic pressure maximum relaxation rates (MRR) in nine patients undergoing a weaning trial. MRR was measured before (1), during (2), and after (3) the weaning trial. MRR slowed in the five patients who failed to wean, returning to normal when mechanically ventilated. In the four patients who weaned successfully, MRR remained unchanged. (From Goldstone et al., 1994.)

It is possible that the same mechanism(s) may underlie the changes in both. The findings that the EMG power spectrum shifts (Cohen et al., 1982) and MRR measured during a sniff slows (Goldstone et al., 1990) in patients failing to wean from mechanical ventilation suggest that, in this particular clinical situation, respiratory muscle fatigue may be factor and that the respiratory muscles are being driven hard. This conclusion is consistent with the earlier findings of Aubier et al. (1980) of high occlusion pressures in such patients. Because the level of respiratory muscle activation appears to remain high in these patients during weaning trials, central fatigue is unlikely to be responsible for weaning failure.

Changes in the EMG power spectrum consistent with diaphragmatic fatigue have recently been documented in pregnant women during delivery (Nava et al., 1992), and a slowing in MRR during a sniff has been observed in patients with obstructive sleep apnea (Griggs et al., 1989).

With submaximal isometric contractions generating a given force, the EMG increases with time, thereby resulting in an increase in the ratio of EMG activity to mechanical response—the "E/T ratio" of Lippold et al. (1960). The phenomenon is considered to reflect an increase in the firing frequency and/or the number of active motor units recruited. An increase in the E/T ratio during fatigue of the strenomastoid muscle (Moxham et al., 1980), the parasternal intercostal muscles (Hershenson et al., 1989), and the diaphragm (Bellemare and Bigland-Ritchie, 1987) have also been reported in normal human volunteer subjects. Thus central and peripheral fatigue are not mutually exclusive, and both may be present simultaneously, as was shown for both limb (Bigland-Ritchie et al., 1977, 1986) and diaphragm (Bellemare and Bigland-Ritchie, 1987) muscles.

A similar response has been observed in the diaphragm of dogs breathing spontaneously during a low-cardiac-output state (Aubier et al., 1981b) (Fig. 9). As the diaphragm fails as a force generator, the output of the central nervous system increases, followed by a parallel increase in EMG, while the transdiaphragmatic pressure falls. However, there is a substantial decrease in the frequency of breathing

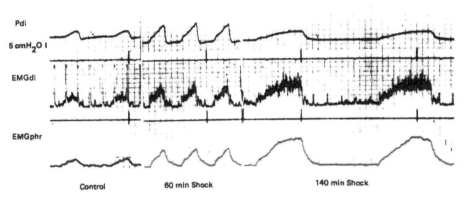

Figure 9 Typical record of one dog showing evolution during cardiogenic shock of transdiaphragmatic pressure (Pdi) (top trace), electrical integrated activity of diaphragm (Edi) (middle trace), and electrical integrated activity of phrenic nerve (Ephr) (bottom trace). Left panel, during control; middle panel, 60 min after onset of cardiogenic shock; right panel, 140 min after onset of cardiogenic shock prior to death of animal. Decrease in size of electrocardiographic artifact on Edi trace is a consequence of injection of saline into pericardium. (From Aubier et al., 1981b.)

toward the end of the experiment. Similarly, in patients with an excessive inspiratory load, an initial increase in respiratory frequency is followed by a decrease in the rate of breathing (Cohen et al., 1982). One hypothesis to explain this modulation of frequency is that it represents an adaptation of the central respiratory controllers to excessive load, which minimizes fatigue and serves to optimize respiratory muscle performance (Roussos, 1984).

It must be pointed out, however, that in another study of dogs in shock induced by other means using an inflated balloon in the inferior vena cava, decrease in breathing frequency and ensuing apnea was described, but no evidence of diaphragmatic fatigue could be demonstrated (Nava and Bellemare, 1989). Thus, although increased breathing frequency in the face of excessive inspiratory loads may be an appropriate strategy to minimize fatigue, the final decrease in breathing frequency may be related more to central respiratory depression, caused by hypercapnia and hypoxia, and may be unrelated to the contractile state of the respiratory muscles.

C. Peripheral Fatigue

Electrical stimulation techniques, which are used to activate muscle directly or via the intramuscular nerves, are available for the in vivo and in vitro study of human and animal skeletal muscle. It thus becomes possible to identify and study peripheral muscle fatigue under precise experimental conditions.

During maximum voluntary contractions of adductor pollicis and first dorsal interosseous, EMG amplitude, after an initial increase in the first 10 s, declines in proportion to the maximum force in the following 50–60 s (Stephens and Taylor, 1972; Bigland-Ritchie et al., 1979). Beyond 60 s, the maximum force declines more rapidly than the EMG amplitude, giving rise to a high E/T ratio (Stephens and Taylor, 1972). The decline in EMG in the first 60 s does not appear to contribute to the decrease in force because the latter cannot be increased by artificial nerve stimulation (Merton, 1954; Stephens and Taylor, 1972; Bigland-Ritchie et al., 1979, 1981). This could reflect an adaptive reduction in motor output of the central nervous system (see above) or a failure of neuromuscular transmission or action potential propagation. To distinguish between these possibilities, Stephens and Taylor (1972) recorded the action potentials evoked by ulnar nerve stimulation delivered in pairs with an interpulse interval to 20 ms and a stimulation frequency of 50 Hz. The surface-recorded muscle action potentials in response to the second impulse of each pair started to decline after 30 s and were reduced by about 65% of control value after 60 s. The authors concluded that failure of neuromuscular transmission was sufficient to account for the force loss observed in the first 60 s of a sustained MVC. Marsden et al. (1983) also using paired shocks at 33-ms intervals and, studying the abductor digiti minimi, reported a smaller decline of the second action potential, but only after 60 s of sustained MVC, which led them to conclude that this type of failure was insufficient to account for all of the force fatigue observed during the contractions. More recently, Bellemare and Garzaniti (1988), working with adductor pollicis, found a rapid decline in the size of action potentials in response to brief trains of tetanic stimulation at 70 Hz after only 5 s of MVC. They further showed that the amplitude of the smoothed rectified EMG, of both the voluntary motor drive and the artificial tetany, declined in parallel and in proportion to the maximum force, thus showing that the decline in natural EMG need not result from a corresponding decline in central nervous system output. A close correspondence between the size of the action potentials and the maximum force was also found throughout recovery. They found no decline in the size of the action potentials recorded from a similarly innervated muscle, the abductor digiti minimi, a muscle not involved in the voluntary adduction of the thumb, thereby showing that the decline was specific to the muscle being fatigued. The delayed occurrence of action potential failure in the studies of Stephens and Taylor (1972) and Marsden et al. (1983) was attributed to the lower stimulation frequency used.

In contrast to the studies mentioned above, Merton et al. (1954, 1981) and Bigland-Ritchie et al. (1979, 1981, 1986) have drawn opposite conclusions from their studies of adductor pollicis. They found no decline in the size of action potentials in response to single nerve shocks, even in extreme fatigue. The most striking experiment were one in which the motor cortex was directly stimulated with electrodes placed over the scalp (Merton et al., 1981), which showed that the entire motor pathway, as tested, functioned normally after 4 min of sustained MVC. However, as mentioned previously, action potential failure is most likely to occur in the first 60 s of a sustained MVC when the output from the central nervous system is high. Furthermore, the use of a single impulse to test the integrity of neuromuscular propagation can be misleading (Marsden et al., 1983; Bellemare and Garzaniti, 1988). The resulting action potential may be reduced artificially if the stimulus coincides with a burst of natural activity. If the underlying natural activity is insufficient to produce a maximum force, the single action potential can appear quite normal despite a severe reduction in the capacity to carry impulses at a sufficiently high frequency to produce maximum force. In the experiments of Merton (1954) and of Bigland-Ritchie et al. (1979, 1981), the voluntary effort was judged to be maximal on the basis that it matched that of an artificial 50 Hz tetanus. Subsequent studies, however, showed that 70–100 Hz are required to produce maximum force, the response at 50 Hz being 10–15% smaller (Marsden et al., 1983; Bellemare and Garzaniti, 1988). Thus, much of the controversy regarding the contribution of action potential failure in human muscle fatigue may result from different methodologies.

Bellemare and Bigland-Ritchie (1987) and McKenzie et al. (1992) found no evidence of action potential failure in normal subjects during repeated submaximal contractions of the diaphragm carried to the limit of endurance and beyond. However, they used single shocks, and since the diaphragm was submaximally activated even in extreme fatigue, the response may not have given a reliable picture of the state of action potential propagation. Nevertheless, faithful transmission of nerve activity through the neuromuscular junction of the diaphragm has been found in experiments in dogs in cardiogenic shock (Aubier et al., 1981b). In these experiments, as the E/T ratio of the diaphragm rose, the relationship between nerve and muscle electrical activity remained unchanged. In contrast, Aldrich (1987), studying ventilatory failure in rabbits breathing against resistive loads, was able to demonstrate a decline in the EMG response from phrenic nerve stimulation, supporting the contention that fatigue was in part due to failure of excitation. These results were recently extended to awake sheep, studied under similar conditions by Bazzy and Donnelly (1993), thus providing strong evidence that action potential failure can occur in the respiratory system. However, the differences between human and animal experiments on the diaphragm remain to be elucidated.

The mechanism(s) underlying the fall in action potential amplitude in human muscle fatigue, and in the spontaneously breathing rabbits and sheep, is not known. Propagation failure could occur at any site distal to the point of nerve stimulation: in the central nervous system (in the case of cortical stimulation), in the main nerve trunk itself, at the branch points of fine nerve terminals, at the neuromuscular junction, or along the muscle fiber surface membrane. For the in situ rat diaphragm preparation, stimulated via the phrenic nerve, action potential failure was found by Krnjevick and Miledi (1959a) to occur at both pre- and postsynaptic sites. Presynaptic failure, which tended to occur at the branch points of fine nerve terminals, was later found to be sensitive to hypoxia and low muscle temperature (Krnjevick and Miledi, 1959b). Postsynaptic failure resulted from a decreased end-plate potential and an increased muscle fiber threshold to direct muscle stimulation, and the probability of this type of failure was shown to increase with increasing stimulation frequency above 15 Hz (Krnjevick and Miledi, 1959a). The frequency dependence of this type of failure suggested that it may result from an increase in potassium or a decrease in sodium concentration of the extracellular interfiber space (Jones et al., 1979). This possibility was also considered by Krnjevic and Miledi (1959a) but thought unlikely to account for the slow recovery of the muscle fiber threshold to direct stimulation. Furthermore, the results of Marsden et al. (1983) in human adductor pollicis showed that action potential failure is more closely related to the number of impulses delivered than to the stimulation frequency. This finding, together with the long recovery time, is more consistent with the idea proposed some time ago by Luttgau (1965) that action potential failure is related to some aspect of muscle metabolism. He showed that action potential failure does not occur in metabolically poisoned isolated single muscle fibers. The results of Wiles et al. (1981) in patients with metabolic myopathy point to the same conclusion. In their study, action potential failure during constant low frequency stimulation (20 Hz) was precipated in patients with impaired glycolysis (myophosphorylase and phosphofructokinase deficiency) and delayed in hypothyroid patients when compared with normal subjects. Since all tests were carried out under anaerobic conditions and a constant frequency of stimulation, hypoxia or changes in electrolyte concentration gradients were unlikely to account for the different rates of action potential failure. These results rather strongly argue in favor of a metabolic hypothesis. It is also clear from the patients with impaired glycolysis that acidosis and lactate accumulation need not be involved in this type of failure. In this context it is worthy to note that the time course of action potential failure in normal human subjects, and its subsequent recovery (Bellemare and Garzaniti, 1988), is very similar to that of phosphocreatine breakdown and resynthesis during the following fatigue of human quadriceps (Bergstrom et al., 1971; Harris et al., 1976; Hultman et al., 1981).

Although controversy continues as to whether failure of neuromuscular transmission actually occurs during fatigue or whether it would occur if there were not an adaptive reduction in motor neuron firing frequency, such an impairment could nonetheless serve to limit the incoming signals that activate the muscle peripherally. As suggested by Nassar-Gentina et al. (1975), Kugelburg and Lindegren (1969), and Wilkie (1981), in this way the muscle is protected against excessive depletion of its ATP stores, which would ultimately lead to rigor.

All processes that link the electrical activation of the muscle cell to the metabolic and enzymatic processes providing energy to the contractile machinery are called excitation-contraction coupling processes. Perhaps the most convincing evidence that force loss is not principally the result of failure of action potential propagation also comes from the work of Merton et al. (1981), demonstrating that the loss of force following a sustained maximum voluntary contraction cannot be restored by massive direct stimulation of the adductor pollicis muscle fibers themselves. They therefore concluded that the site of fatigue was peripheral and within the contractile apparatus of the muscle fibers (Fig. 10). Conventionally, if force loss is not accompanied by a parallel decline of electrical activity, impaired excitation-contraction coupling is thought to be responsible (Merton, 1954). Characteristically, this type of fatigue may be produced by successive submaximal contractions, particularly if performed under anaerobic conditions. Such fatigue is characterized by a selective loss of force at low frequencies of stimulation (low-frequency fatigue), whereas force generation at high frequencies is well maintained (Fig. 11). Underlying and responsible for the reduced force at low-stimulation frequency is the diminished twitch response. This type of fatigue is not associated with depletion of ATP or phosphocreatine (PCr) and is characteristically long-lasting, taking several hours to recover, thus suggesting that it may be related to structural damage that requires repair (Jones, 1981).

Eccentric quadriceps contractions have been shown to produce more low-frequency fatigue than do concentric contractions, even though less chemical energy is required, again suggesting that the fatigue may be related to damage of muscle fibers (Edwards et al., 1981). Following eccentric contractions, electron microscopy of muscle biopsy specimens shows structural damage (Newham et al., 1982).

Low-frequency fatigue occurs during high-force contractions and is less likely to develop when the forces generated are smaller, even if these are maintained for longer time periods, thereby achieving the same total work. It thus appears likely

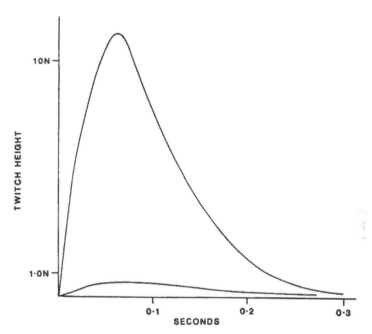

Figure 10 Control and fatigue twitches in adductor pollicis—the fatigued twitch was reduced 18 times. Twitch responses elicited by direct stimulation of muscle with a shock strength of 1440 volts. (From Merton et al., 1981).

that muscle ischemia and reliance on anaerobic metabolism are important factors in the generation of low-frequency fatigue. Certainly, patients with mitochondrial myopathies who are obliged to utilize energy anaerobically are particularly vulnerable to this type of fatigue (Wiles et al., 1981).

The mechanism by which force production is impaired is thought to implicate a reduced release of calcium or a change in the affinity of the troponin binding site for calcium. Both defects would effectively reduce the twitch response and hence reduce force at low stimulation frequencies, thereby shifting the steep section of the force frequency curve to the right. An alteration in the compliance of the series elastic component of the muscle may also play a part (Vigreux et al., 1980). In contrast, at higher stimulation frequencies, the interior of the fiber is saturated with calcium and hence relatively normal forces are produced (Edwards et al., 1977a; Jones, 1981).

Figure 9 shows that impaired excitation-contraction coupling also occurs in the diaphragm where, despite a threefold increase in the integrated EMG, the transdiaphragmatic pressure (P_{di}) decreases. Low-frequency fatigue has been demonstrated in the diaphragm and the sternomastoid muscles of normal subjects breathing against high resistive loads (Moxham et al., 1980; Aubier et al., 1981a;

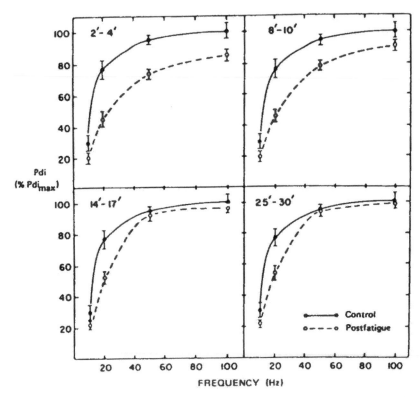

Figure 11   Time course of changes in pressure-frequency curves of the diaphragm of four subjects 2–4, 8–10, 14–17, and 25–30 min after fatigue. Solid curves represent average of three curves before fatigue (control). Dotted curves represent average of three curves at different times during recovery period. Pdi expressed as percent of Pdi generated for a stimulation frequency of 100 Hz (Pdi_{max}). Bars indicate 1 SE. (From Aubier et al., 1981.)

Moxham et al., 1981a (Fig. 11). Low-frequency fatigue also develops in the diaphragm of normal subjects who sustain maximum voluntary ventilation for 2 min (Wragg et al., 1992), and low-frequency fatigue develops in the sternomastoid at 50% of sustained maximum voluntary ventilation (MVV) (Wilson et al., 1984) (Fig. 12). Patients with chronic airways obstruction develop low-frequency fatigue of the sternomastoid muscle following sustained maximum voluntary ventilation (Moxham et al., 1981b; Wilson et al., 1984).

     Since low-frequency fatigue impairs force generation at physiological firing frequencies, ventilation may be reduced. To compensate for low-frequency fatigue, motor neuron firing frequency must be increased or additional contractile units must be recruited by an increase in central respiratory drive. This can be demonstrated by recording the smoothed and rectified EMG (SREMG) from the sternomastoid during the production of standard forces when the muscle has low-frequency fatigue

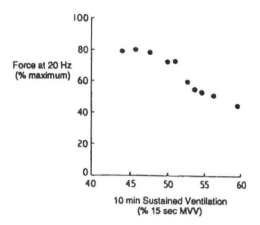

Figure 12 The effect of sustained maximal (MVV) and submaximal voluntary ventilation on the contractile properties of the sternomastoid muscle in a normal subject. The force generated by stimulation a5 20 Hz/maximum stimulated force (%) is a measure of the shape of the frequency-force curve, and a fall in this value reflects a shift to the right of the curve and is an index of low-frequency fatigue. Low-frequency fatigue develops at a sustained ventilation greater than 50% of the 15 sec MVV, which in absolute terms was 105 liters/min. (From Wilson et al., 1984.)

compared to the response obtained for fresh muscle (Moxham et al., 1980) (Fig. 13). Depression of respiratory drive by hypoxia or drugs could therefore impair compensatory responses, and ventilation would then become inadequate.

A similar shift to the right of the force-frequency curve can occur without fatigue as a consequence of muscle shortening (Farkas and Roussos, 1984); thus, low-frequency fatigue and muscle shortening, resulting from hyperinflation, may interact to compromise respiratory muscle force generation and predispose to ventilation failure. Recent studies have shown that for the normal human diaphragm in vivo (Yan et al., 1992), as well as for the isolated rat diaphragm studied in vitro (Gauthier et al., 1993), fatigue causes a greater decrease in transdiaphragmatic pressure or force when measured at a high lung volume or at a short muscle length than when measured at lower lung volumes or longer lengths.

D. Metabolic Considerations in Muscle Fatigue

Skeletal muscle is analogous to an engine: it converts chemical energy to heat and work. If the chemical energy available becomes limited or the ability of the muscle to utilize chemical energy is impaired, the muscle will fail as a force generator.

Muscle Fiber Types and Fatigue

Human muscles consist of fiber types with distinct metabolic and contractile characteristics. In particular, there are differences in fatiguability. The fast-twitch

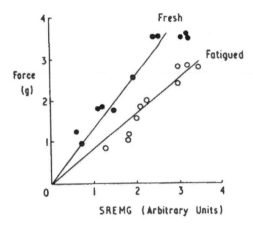

Figure 13 The smooth rectified electromyogram (SREMG) recorded from the skin surface over the sternomastoid muscle for normal subjects showing the effect of low-frequency fatigue. The SREMG for graded isometric voluntary contractions in fresh and fatigued muscle is plotted. For a given SREMG, the force produced is less with fatigue. (From Moxham et al., 1980.)

glycolytic fibers (type IIa) are more easily fatiguable than the fast-twitch oxidative (type IIb) and the slow-twitch oxidative (type I) fibers (Burke et al., 1971). A predominance of slow fibers effectively shifts the force-frequency curve to the left and potentiates force production at low physiological firing frequencies (Faulkner et al., 1980), and slow muscle is less susceptible to developing low-frequency fatigue (Kugelberg and Lindegren, 1969).

The endurance of a muscle is largely dependent on its oxidative capacity, which prompted Lieberman et al. (1973) to suggest that the endurance of the respiratory muscles is determined by the proportion of oxidative to glycolytic fibers. It is known that 55% of the fibers of the diaphragm in adults are type I fibers and that 50% of the type II fibers are of the high oxidative type. Hence, about 75–80% of the fibers of the adult diaphragm are fatigue resistant. In accord with their hypothesis, Liberman et al. (1973) found that maximum voluntary ventilation, after an initial rapid decline in the first few minutes, tended to stabilize after 10 min of sustained hyperpnea at around 80% of the initial maximal value. The human adult fiber type composition of the diaphragm and intercostal muscles is fully established at the age of one year (Keens et al., 1978). In full-term infants, about 25% of the diaphragm fibers and 45% of intercostal muscle fibers are type I fatigue-resistant fibers. The respiratory muscles of the newborn should be more susceptible to fatigue than those of the adult (Keens et al., 1978), but the fatiguability of the respiratory muscles in the neonatal period may not be correctly predicted from muscle fiber types, since endurance can be greater in the neonate than in the adult (Sieck et al., 1991).

The close relationship between the fiber composition of the diaphragm and its endurance may not apply in some circumstances. For the high oxidative capacity of the diaphragm to be fully expressed, a correspondingly high blood supply or high oxygen extraction is required. This has been shown to be the case (see Chap. 23). At normal perfusion pressure, maximum oxygen extractions of the order of 16 vol% and maximum blood flows of about 300 ml/min/100 g or higher have been reported in the diaphragm, values approaching those for the heart. However, conditions that interfere with blood supply or oxygen extraction may be expected to cause fatigue of the otherwise fatigue-resistant fiber types. In the respiratory system, Roussos and Macklem (1977) showed that during inspiratory resistive loading, with ordinary patterns of breathing, about 40% of the maximum voluntary Pdi can be sustained indefinitely, and Bellemare and Grassino (1982a) have shown that the Pdi that can be sustained indefinitely is inversely related to the inspiratory duty cycle (i.e., the fraction of time during which pressure is sustained). For sustained contractions, fatigue occurred at Pdi values as low as 20% of maximal. Bellemare et al. (1983) subsequently showed in the dog that for Pdi levels and duty cycle combinations known to cause diaphragm fatigue in humans, the blood flow to the diaphragm becomes limited, as evidenced both by a decreased blood flow with increasing pressure and/or duty cycle and by the occurrence of a blood flow debt that must be paid during recovery. The blood flow limitation was attributed to the high intramuscular tension during contractions. Intramuscular pressure has been measured directly in the diaphragm and found to increase in proportion to the force developed (Hussain and Magder, 1991). Under conditions of blood flow limitation, the relationship between the proportion of fatigue-resistant fibers and the load that can be sustained breaks down. By contrast, a close relationship between the fiber composition of the diaphragm and the maximum level of ventilation that can be sustained without fatigue was found by Lieberman et al. (1973), suggesting that blood flow and oxygen delivery to the diaphragm was not limited under the conditions of their study. Studies that measured blood flow to and oxygen consumption of the diaphragm during hyperventilation in dogs (Robertson et al., 1977), and horses (Manahar et al., 1990, 1991) found no limitation with increasing ventilation.

Alterations in Muscle Chemistry

The substances most directly involved in the transformation of chemical free energy into mechanical work in skeletal muscle are ATP, ADP, orthophosphate (Pi), hydrogen ion (H^+), magnesium ion (Mg^{2+}), and phosphocreatine (PCr). Experiments performed in anaerobic frog gastrocnemius muscle using the technique of nuclear magnetic resonance (nmr) show that phosphocreatine breaks down progressively and creatine, ADP, and H^+ levels rise (Dawson et al., 1978). Similarly, Nichols et al. (1993) have shown that fatiguing diaphragm contractions induced by phrenic nerve pacing lead to PCr depletion and Pi production, resulting in a Pi/PCr ratio of 1. A Pi/PCr ratio of 1 has been associated with complete muscle ischemia and reflects the threshold at which the muscle has become metabolically unstable because of excessive workload or inadequate fatigue (Chance, 1985; Gutierrez, 1988). These unstable changes in high-energy phosphate concentrations occur extremely rapidly (within 2–10 min) (Nichols, 1993). However, if fatiguing diaphragmatic contractions continue for a prolonged period of time (>45 min), PCr rises again and Pi falls coincident with the fall in activation of the diaphragm (transmission fatigue). This return to the resting metabolic state suggests that diaphragm metabolism may be linked to diaphragm activation to limit work output to a level that can be supported by aerobic metabolism. The mechanisms of such a link are incompletely understood. The intriguing observation is that ATP concentration—the direct source of energy for the cyclical attachment and detachment of myosin cross-bridges to and from active sites on actin filaments—remains constant until fatigue is very advanced, when it diminishes by about 25%. Similar results have been reported by Hultman et al. (1967) in normal subjects during dynamic exercise until exhaustion. These authors found that at a high workloads, when phosphocreatine was practically depleted, ATP decreased to about 40% of the control value. A large reserve of ATP at the end of static fatiguing exercise has also been found in several other studies using artificial (Hultman et al., 1981) and voluntary contractions (Bergstrom et al., 1971; Vollestad et al., 1988). Thus, the crucial question is why the muscle fails to generate force despite adequate sources of ATP. Although the answer may lie in the failure of muscle activation discussed above, it is nevertheless useful to look at changes in the chemistry that takes place in the muscle fibril.

The potential explanations for preservation of ATP levels in diaphragm during fatigue are best considered by appreciating the reactions that govern energy metabolism.

$$\text{ATP} \quad \xrightarrow{\text{myosin ATPase}} \quad \text{ADP} + \text{Pi} + \text{H}^+ + \text{work} \quad\quad (1)$$

$$\underline{\text{PCr} + \text{ADP} + \text{H}^+ \quad \overset{\text{creatine kinase}}{\rightleftarrows} \quad \text{ATP} + \text{Cr}} \quad\quad (2)$$

Net reaction:

$$\text{PCr} \rightarrow \text{Cr} + \text{Pi} + \text{work}$$

Myosin ATPase catalyzes the hydrolysis of ATP to ADP and Pi, yielding the energy necessary for muscle work [Eq. (1)]. Any change in ATP levels is immediately buffered by the high activity of the creatine kinase reaction [Eq. (2)], in which the phosphorus moiety of PCr combines with ADP to replenish to ATP and release free creatine (Cr). ATP content is well buffered by PCr hydrolysis as long as conditions of severe hypoxemia or tetanic contractions with very high stimulation frequency (100 Hz) are not employed (Kushmerick, 1985; Gutierrez, 1988). The second potential explanation for ATP preservation lies in the fact that the product of the myosin ATPase reaction, ADP, regulates the synthesis of ATP during oxidative phosphorylation. In this "classical" energetic model, increasing ADP concentrations from muscle work lead to increased ATP synthesis within the mitochondria (Jacobus, 1985; Balaban, 1990). Although the regulatory role of ADP is reasonably well established in limb skeletal muscle (Chance, 1985), its role in regulating oxidative phosphorylation in organs with very high aerobic capacity such as the heart (and potentially the diaphragm) is less clear (Katz, 1989). Finally, the apparent preservation of ATP levels during fatiguing contractions may represent a measurement artifact since samples are obtained from muscle homogenates or a whole muscle, which may obscure the fact that local ATP concentrations in the vicinity of the actin-myosin filaments could be severely depleted in some motor units, but not in others.

During an increase in the metabolic rate of skeletal muscle, including respiratory muscle, the consumption of oxygen and metabolic substrates increases to provide the ATP necessary for the contractile process. Fat (stored as triglycerides in adipose tissue), blood glucose from the liver, and glycogen from working muscle are the main fuels. The glycogen of nonworking muscle cannot be utilized because muscle lacks the enzyme glucose-6-phosphatase and therefore cannot contribute directly to blood glucose. The usefulness of protein as a fuel is limited because its consumption necessitates dissolution of muscle or parenchymal tissues.

During submaximal prolonged heavy exercise, exhaustion coincides with depletion of muscle glycogen, and exercise capacity is enhanced when the storage of muscle glycogen is increased (Bergstrom et al., 1967). Reduced energy sources are also found in biopsies of respiratory muscle of patients with respiratory failure (Gertz et al., 1977). Similar observations have been made for the diaphragm in dogs hyperventilating in response to low cardiac output. Diaphragmatic glycogen decreased to 40% of control values in animals breathing spontaneously, while animals with the same low cardiac output but mechanically ventilated had minimal reduction in diaphragmatic muscle glycogen (Roussos and Aubier, 1981; Aubier et al., 1982).

A close relationship between diaphragm glycogen depletion or lactate accumulation on the one hand and the E/T ratio or %fall in diaphragm strength on the other has also been documented in the rabbit during inspiratory threshold loading to the point of respiratory failure (Furguson et al., 1990). By contrast, no changes in diaphragmatic glycogen, ATP, and PC were found in one-month-old piglets after 6 h of inspiratory resistive loaded breathing, in spite of a 40% reduction in diaphragm strength (Mayock et al., 1991), thereby suggesting that substrate depletion may not be the only factor in fatigue of the respiratory muscles. One problem with this type of study is the possibility that the decline in diaphragm strength may be a reflection of hypercapnic acidosis, as opposed to fatigue processes in the muscle (Shee and Cameron, 1990; Vianna et al., 1990).

Why glycogen depletion coincides with fatigue is not clear. It is apparent that during prolonged intermittent heavy exercise, which depends upon aerobic metabolism, the rate of utilization of fatty acids and glucose is high, and despite the fact that these substances circulate in large amounts in the bloodstream, they cannot provide sufficient energy to meet the demand. Hence, muscle glycogen must be used to supplement bloodborne fuels, and fatigue will occur when it is depleted. In contrast, a genuine shortage of either glucose or free fatty acids is unlikely to be the cause of respiratory muscle fatigue in view of the small mass of the respiratory muscles and therefore their relatively small requirements for either glucose or free fatty acids and the large amounts of stored fat (140,000 kcal) and liver glycogen (80–90 g) forming a vast pool of substrate readily convertible to glucose.

A great deal of attention has been focused on the role that lactic acid plays in the development of fatigue. Hill and Kupalov (1929) were the first to relate fatigue and lactic acid accumulation, although Berzelius in 1807 had suggested "that the amount of free lactic acid in skeletal muscle is proportional to the extent to which this muscle has been previously exercised" (Lehman, 1851). There exists a firm correlation between lactic acid accumulation in muscle and its contractile force (Fitts and Holloszy, 1976; Dawson et al., 1978). An increase in blood lactate concentration has also been found in normal subjects breathing through high inspiratory loads to exhaustion (Jardim et al., 1981; Freedman et al., 1983). Although lactic acid accumulation in human experiments probably results from the anaerobic metabolism of respiratory muscles, no direct proof thereof is yet available. Animals in cardiogenic shock develop lactic acidosis to a substantially lesser extent if they are ventilated than when they are breathing spontaneously (Aubier et al., 1981b), and in these experiments diaphragmatic lactic acid is greater in the spontaneously breathing animals (these animals also developed diaphragmatic fatigue) than in the ventilated ones. Contractions that generate sufficient force to render the muscle ischemic, thus using anaerobic pathways and producing lactate, greatly predispose to the development of low-frequency fatigue (Wiles et al., 1981).

The effect of lactic acid on force generation is believed to be mediated by a lowering of pH. Human performance on a bicycle ergometer is impaired at low pH compared to high blood pH (Jones et al., 1979). Acute hypercapnia, probably through the mechanism of acidosis, impairs contractility. Hypercapnic acidosis (Pa_{CO_2} 70 mm Hg, arterial pH 7.25) reduces the twitch tension of adductor pollicis by 25% and substantially increases the fatiguability of the muscle (Vianna et al., 1990). Human diaphragm contractility is substantially reduced by hypercapnia (Juan et al., 1984). The mechanisms by which acidosis might exert its negative effect on force generation is still unclear, but certain observations are worthy of mention. It has been shown that at low pH, Ca^{2+} is sequestered in the sarcoplasmic reticulum (Nakamura and Schwartz, 1970), and at low pH a larger amount of Ca^{2+}, and thus increased excitation, is needed to produce a given tension (Robertson and Kerrick, 1976). Furthermore, there is clear evidence that an increased concentration of hydrogen ions will exert a direct negative influence on the contractile process itself (Katz and Hecht, 1969; Fabiato and Fabiato, 1978). Hydrogen ion and lactate accumulation are important in fatigue, but many other factors are involved; patients with myophosphorylase deficiency who are unable to produce lactate develop fatigue (Wiles et al., 1981), and if muscle is experimentally kept alkaline, fatigue still occurs (Needham, 1971).

E. An Integrated View of Respiratory Muscle Fatigue

It is clear from the above discussion that fatigue may take place at any level between the central nervous (CNS) and the contractile machinery. It is also possible that more than one site could fail simultaneously, depending on the motor unit type or if synergistic muscles with different properties and level of activation are being recruited. The site in the motor pathway most likely to fail may also vary, depending on the conditions under which the muscle is functioning (e.g., type of contraction, arterial perfusion pressure, hypoxemia, electrolyte composition, sleep/wake states).

Because fatigue is generally closely associated with a limitation of blood flow to muscle, metabolic factors may be particularly important. A restriction of muscle blood flow will force the muscle fibers to derive part or all of their energy demands from intramuscular energy stores and anaerobic metabolic pathways. The depletion of these energy stores or the excessive accumulation of metabolites may set a lower ceiling to the force the muscle is able to generate without causing fatigue. With long-lasting exercise (>60 min) at low intensity there is almost complete depletion of muscle glycogen, coincident with exhaustion. However, in most circumstances where fatigue is observed, such as during high-intensity exercise, a limit to performance is reached before glycogen stores are depleted. Furthermore, in no forms of exercise has complete depletion of muscle ATP stores been observed, even in extreme fatigue. Therefore, mechanism(s) must be present that prevent the crisis that would otherwise occur if these ATP stores were depleted.

The fall in intracellular pH caused by the production of lactic acid might directly interfere with maximum force production by preventing calcium binding to troponin. However, the experiments of Donaldson et al. (1978) suggest that this would only cause a modest 20% reduction in maximum force, the effect being more pronounced at subsaturating calcium concentrations. A fall in intracellular pH can also interfere with membrane depolarization and action potential propagation, further limiting maximum force production and energy store depletion. Thus the more severe the intracellular acidosis, the less severe the glycogen depletion, and this could vary in different fiber types of the same muscle. Substantial potassium loss from exercising muscle has also been documented during fatiguing exercise (Juel et al., 1990). The decline in intracellular K^+ concentration and possibly the accumulation of K^+ in the extracellular space, and particularly in the T-tubules, could also impair or even block membrane conduction, preventing activation of the sarcoplasmic reticulum. These changes in intracellular pH and K^+ concentration are more likely to occur in muscle fibers of fast twitch motor units, as these are more dependent on anaerobic metabolism and require higher discharge rates for maximum force production.

There is also accumulating evidence that the neural output to the muscle may slow during fatigue even though the subject perceives otherwise and increases effort. The most simple explanation of this phenomenon is the mechanism of motoneuron discharge adaptation, described by Kernel and Monster (1982), in response to a constant intracellular current injection. To keep motoneuron discharge constant under this condition, the injected current and hence the excitatory drive must increase, thereby giving rise to increased effort sensation. However, other mechanisms, such as a decreased facilitation from muscle spindles and primary afferents or a mounting inhibition from Renshaw cells or reflex pathways, are equally plausible, as these would also require an increased excitatory input to keep motoneuron discharges constant. When the excitatory drive reaches a limit, or if the motoneuron adaptation proceeds more rapidly than the increasing drive, or if the inhibitory influences exceed the excitatory ones, motor neuron discharge will decline. This could explain the rapid decline of motor unit discharge rate observed during sustained maximal voluntary contractions, as the excitatory drive and the effort by the subject are already maximal from the onset of the contraction. During submaximal constant force contractions, however, motoneuron adaptation, disfacilitation, or inhibition can be overcome by increasing the excitatory drive until this reaches a maximum. This could explain the nearly constant motor unit discharge rate observed under those conditions in spite of the subject progressively increasing the effort. However, whenever the effort becomes maximal, the motoneuron discharge will be expected to fall, as during maximum voluntary contractions. Whether a reduction in motoneuron discharge will also cause a decrease in muscle force output will depend on the concomitant slowing in muscle speed that occurs with fatigue. The slowing in muscle contractile speed with fatigue is proportional to the intensity of the contraction. Hence during relatively short (1 min) but intense maximum voluntary contractions, the slowing in motor unit discharge rate may not cause any decrease in force. In fact, by spreading out the action potentials the maximum force may be maintained at its best longer (Marsden et al., 1983). However, with less pronounced changes in contractile speed, such as with initially submaximal contractions, a decline in discharge rate may be expected to directly cause a corresponding decline in muscle force, in addition to any force loss caused by the derecruitment of motor units and by metabolic or electrolytic changes in the muscle.

Because the respiratory muscles are skeletal muscles, their response to fatiguing loads may be expected to be similar to limb muscles. In most conditions in which they have been examined, a peripheral component to respiratory muscle fatigue has been demonstrated. However, because of their higher blood supply and oxidative capacity, the respiratory muscles, and in particular the diaphragm, may not rely as much as the limb muscles on intramuscular energy stores and anaerobic pathways. Thus in the normal sheep or piglet subjected to inspiratory flow resistive loading, glycogen depletion does not occur (Mayock et al., 1991) or is restricted to type II fibers (Bazzy et al., 1988). Similarly, lactic acid and potassium accumulation are less likely to interfere with the mechanism of force production or action potential propagation than in limb muscles. All these factors could account for the reportedly higher endurance of the respiratory muscles when measured in vitro or in response to volitional efforts. However, under conditions of low cardiac output, or when breathing is under automatic control, metabolic or respiratory acidosis and hypoxemia might eventually interfere with respiratory muscle force production. Under such conditions, an increase in chemical stimuli appears to be the major mechanism by which excitatory input to respiratory motoneurons can be increased to compensate for any decline in the force-generating capacity caused by fatigue. These could also account for the conflicting evidence that neuromuscular transmission failure, which appears to contribute to diaphragmatic fatigue in spontaneously breathing rabbit and sheep, has not been found in normal human subjects breathing against severe inspiratory resistive loads. Central factors appear to play a more important role in the respiratory than in the limb motor systems. Central fatigue is a prominent feature of diaphragmatic fatigue, at least when fatigue is circumscribed to this muscle. This may in part be related to the lack of autogenic facilitation that seems to characterize the diaphragm, thereby permitting other mechanisms such as motoneuron adaptation or inhibition to manifest themselves more readily. The phenomenon of motoneuron adaptation appears to be present in phrenic motoneurons (Jodkowski et al., 1988). Furthermore, the chemical activation of thin fiber phrenic nerve afferents by capsaicin (Hussain et al., 1990; Supinski et al., 1993) and by potassium injection (Supinski et al., 1993) in the arterial supply to the diaphragm has been shown to have an excitatory and not an inhibitory effect (see Chap. 29). These afferents at first glance are therefore unlikely to be involved in central fatigue of this or any other muscle. However, they may play a role in optimizing the breathing pattern in order to avoid fatigue (Roussos, 1984). When the recruitment of other functional synergists is also permitted, the level of activation of the different muscles may also be determined by their relative strength and fatiguability, increasing the contribution of central factors to the fatigue observed.

The situation in the respiratory system is particularly complex because of the many muscles that can be involved during breathing, both inspiratory and expiratory, thus alternating the load on each. Furthermore, which muscle will fail first and the cause of respiratory muscle fatigue may differ depending on whether ventilation is under the control of the respiratory centers in the medulla or under volitional control, as this may also affect the recruitment pattern of different muscles. Furthermore, in conditions likely to cause respiratory muscle fatigue, awake subjects may become aware of their breathing, and this sensation may alter the response of the respiratory controllers.

Alterations in the pattern of breathing may also occur as a result of loading (Tobin et al., 1987) or fatigue, which may represent attempts by the respiratory controller to reduce the load or alleviate fatigue. Patients in acute and chronic respiratory failure, patients with severe respiratory muscle weakness, and normal subjects or animals subjected to fatiguing respiratory loads tend to adopt a rapid shallow pattern of breathing, consisting of an increase in breathing frequency and a decreased tidal volume, whereas minute ventilation remains constant or increases slightly. Although this pattern may not be efficient in terms of gas exchange, it may reduce the load on the muscle by decreasing the mean pressure developed, thereby preventing fatigue from occurring (Roussos, 1984; Tobin et al., 1986; Milic-Emili, 1986; Bellemare, 1989). In stable patients with chronic obstructive lung disease and CO_2 retention, this pattern of breathing may be sufficient to keep the diaphragm contraction below the fatigue threshold (Bellemare and Grassino, 1983; Roussos, 1984). The limit of this strategy, however, resides in the increased deadspace to tidal volume ratio, with worsening of hypercapnia and hypoxemia, which, in addition to their detrimental effects on the respiratory muscles themselves, may also interfere with the respiratory controllers, causing respiratory depression and eventually respiratory arrest.

The task facing the individual subjected to a large respiratory load in relation to ventilatory capacity is to optimize respiratory muscle force generation and minimize fatigue while maintaining gas exchange. Central excitation must be sufficient to minimize suboptimal activation (central fatigue), but not be so high as to precipitate excitation failure (high-frequency fatigue). Work on limb muscle contractions in normal subjects supports the hypothesis that the central nervous system is capable of modulating central output to optimize force generation. During a short fatiguing maximum voluntary effort, there is a progressive gradual reduction in central firing frequency, which optimizes force generation and minimizes fatigue (Fig. 6). If central nervous system output rises, high-frequency fatigue is precipitated. If central nervous system output falls inappropriately, central fatigue occurs with force loss. The central nervous system exerts a "central wisdom," which minimizes both central fatigue and high-frequency fatigue. There are no data from patients to substantiate the existence of central wisdom in ventilatory failure. Respiratory drive is high in such patients (Aubier et al., 1980; Gribben et al., 1983) and is influenced by Pa_{O_2}, Pa_{CO_2}, and pH. Whether respiratory muscles are optimally driven under these conditions is not known. Evidence from patients undergoing weaning trials suggests that central fatigue does not occur (Goldstone et al., 1994). Because the onset of high-frequency fatigue leads to catastrophic and rapid force loss, it is an inappropriate strategy for patients in ventilatory failure to drive peripheral respiratory muscle into high-frequency fatigue, although they could be forced into such a strategy by rapidly deteriorating blood gas values. When muscle develops low-frequency fatigue, the force-frequency curve is shifted to the right. In these circumstances to sustain a given ventilatory load there must be an increase in motor neuron firing frequency, which would then lead to greater fatigue, necessitating a further increase in firing frequency and causing an intensification of fatigue. The progressive increase in motor neuron firing frequency could also precipitate high-frequency fatigue, whereas failure to increase stimulation frequency results in task failure. Low-frequency fatigue is likely therefore to be relatively unstable.

Respiratory muscle fatigue is thus best considered as an integrated response of the respiratory system to excessive loading. It is unlikely that fatigue is due to a failure in any one particular link in the complex chain of events of voluntary contraction. It is more likely that when the respiratory muscles are excessively loaded, feedback mechanisms modify central drive, which reduces ventilation and serves to avoid overt peripheral fatigue and excessive force loss. In this way ventilation is best maintained. The integrated system serves to maximize ventilatory performance while minimizing overt fatigue. If loading is excessive, the optimization of ventilation will nevertheless be insufficient to avoid ventilatory failure and even death.

F. Respiratory Muscle Fatigue in Chronic Ventilatory Failure

Do patients with chronic ventilatory failure have chronic fatigue of the respiratory muscle? From all that is known about the nature of central fatigue and peripheral high-frequency fatigue, it is very unlikely that these fatigue states persist in a stable form. Chronic fatigue in the form of low-frequency fatigue is possible, albeit unlikely, as this recovers slowly and is relatively more stable. Some investigators have observed that when patients with chronic ventilatory failure are treated with assisted ventilation, the strength of the respiratory muscles improve. This improvement has been attributed to resting the respiratory muscles, and therefore reversing chronic muscle fatigue (Gutierrez et al., 1988b). However, the improved performance following assisted ventilation could represent improved effort by the patients. Some studies of chronic assisted ventilation in patients with hypercapnic respiratory failure have failed to demonstrate improvement in respiratory muscle strength, despite good evidence that the respiratory muscles were rested (Elliott et al., 1991). Further investigation of chronic respiratory muscle fatigue would be best undertaken using the nonvolitional techniques of phrenic nerve stimulation to assess diaphragm contractility before and after respiratory muscle rest. The newer technique of magnetic stimulation could be useful in this context (Simolowski et al., 1989). Additional studies are required; the data currently available give little support to the concept of chronic respiratory muscle fatigue. It seems more likely that hypercapnia develops as a consequence of the relative hypoventilation of the respiratory system in response to excessive respiratory loading, the central nervous system modifying its output to avoid overt fatigue (central wisdom).

G. Respiratory Muscle Fatigue in Acute Ventilatory Failure

Data on respiratory muscle function and fatigue in acute ventilatory failure are sparse. A useful clinical model of acute ventilatory failure is that of patients who are undergoing weaning trials on the intensive care unit. It has proved possible in these patients to measure the load imposed on the respiratory muscle pump and also the capacity of the respiratory muscles. In this way the ratio of load to capacity has been documented, and when the load is high in relation to capacity, weaning fails (Cohen et al., 1982; Tobin et al., 1986; Goldstone et al., 1994). During such weaning failure, the pattern of breathing alters (Cohen et al., 1982) and the EMG high/low ratio falls. However, weaning failure does not necessarily imply respiratory muscle fatigue, and it is possible that the alteration in breathing pattern is simply a response to excessive loading (Tobin et al., 1987). Both the alteration in breathing pattern and the respiratory muscle EMG high/low ratio may reflect alterations in central drive.

What evidence is there of respiratory muscle fatigue per se during weaning failure? Few data on this problem exist. Respiratory muscle maximum relaxation rate (MRR) has been measured during the weaning process and has been demonstrated to slow in those patients failing to wean and to remain unchanged in those weaning successfully (Goldstone et al., 1994) (Fig. 14). These data suggest that, in this model of acute ventilatory failure, a fatigue process is initiated peripherally in the respiratory muscles. Associated with the slowing of MRR, it is likely that central drive is modulated (Bigland-Ritchie et al., 1981) (see above).

III. Pathophysiology of Respiratory Muscle Fatigue

A. Energy Balance: Theoretical Considerations

The rate of energy supply to the respiratory muscles can directly or indirectly determine their performance. For the sake of simplicity, we shall consider the respiratory muscles to be an engine that consumes chemical energy and performs external work—the work of breathing. Respiratory muscle fatigue can occur when the rate of energy consumption by the muscle is greater than the energy supplied by the blood; under these circumstances, the muscle draws upon energy stores, which, when depleted, could result in failure of the muscle as a generator of force. Thus, when a muscle becomes fatigued, total energy consumed (U_t) is the sum of the energy stores, a, plus the total amount of energy extracted from blood by the muscle. This can be expressed in very general terms by a modification of the equation developed by Monod and Scherrer (1965):

$$U_t = \frac{W}{E} = a + Bt_{lim} \tag{3}$$

where W is the total external work performed by the respiratory muscles, E is efficiency, a is the energy stores, B is the rate of energy supply to the muscle, and t_{lim} is the endurance time. Solving for t_{lim}:

$$t_{lim} = \frac{aE}{W - BE} \tag{4}$$

where $\dot{W}$ is mean muscle power (W/t_{lim}). Equation (4) reveals that when $BE > \dot{W}$, the muscle can continue to work indefinitely, but that when $BE < \dot{W}$, there will be a finite endurance time. Thus, a decrease in either efficiency or B will predispose to fatigue, as will an increase in muscle power. Experimentally, it has been shown

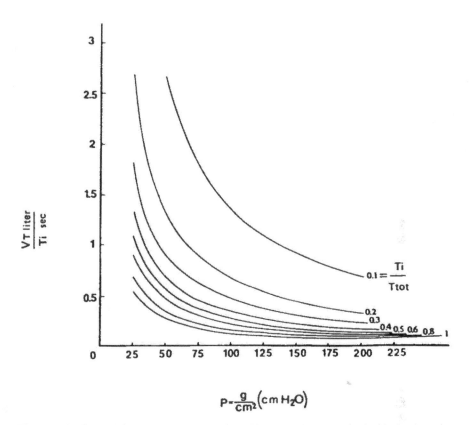

Figure 14 Interrelation of pressure (P), flow (VT/Ti), and duty cycle (Ti/Ttot) when the power of breathing and the maximum energy uptake are equal to 8 kg/min, thus rendering endurance time infinite.

that for the inspiratory muscles, during inspiratory resistive breathing with mouth pressure developed in a square-wave manner, the denominator becomes zero and therefore t_{lim} becomes infinite when $\dot{W} = 6\text{–}8$ kg/min (Roussos et al., 1979); this implies that BE is also 6–8 kg/min, and we therefore name these values critical power, critical product of efficiency, and rate of energy supply, respectively.

Assuming a square-wave form for the pressure generated by the inspiratory muscles, the first term of the denominator in Eq. (4) becomes:

$$\dot{W} = P \cdot V_T \cdot f = P \cdot \frac{1}{Ttot} \tag{5}$$

Where V_T is tidal volume, f is frequency of breathing, and Ttot is duration of breathing cycle. (Note that $V_T \cdot f$ or $V_T \cdot 1/Ttot$ equals minute ventilation.) Multiplying numerator and denominator by inspiratory time (TI), Eq. (5) becomes:

$$\dot{W} = P \cdot V_T/T_I \cdot T_I/T_{tot} \tag{6}$$

where V_T/T_I is mean inspiratory flow, T_I/T_{tot} is the ratio of inspiratory time to total duration of breathing cycle (duty cycle), and their product denotes minute ventilation. The term T_I/T_{tot}, as a first approximation, expresses the proportion of the total duration of the breathing cycle during which the inspiratory muscles contract. Combining Eqs. (5) and (6):

$$t_{lim} = \frac{aE}{PV_T/T_I \cdot T_I/T_{tot} - BE} \tag{7}$$

With the exception of a, the effect of all terms on the right of Eq. (7) on t_{lim} have now been tested. The metabolic demands of the respiratory muscles are largely determined by the pressure they develop and the pattern of breathing. Roussos and Macklem (1977) have shown that for a given duty cycle and mean inspiratory flow, t_{lim} of the diaphragm is inversely related to the transdiaphragmatic pressure developed once a critical threshold value is reached. With the pattern of breathing used in their studies, this threshold value corresponded to 40% of the maximal transdiaphragmatic pressure the subjects could develop. Bellemare and Grassino (1982a) subsequently showed that, for a given Pdi, t_{lim} is inversely related to the duty cycle or T_I/T_{tot}. The critical threshold value of Pdi that could be sustained indefinitely was also found to be inversely related to the duty cycle. In their experimental conditions, the fatigue threshold of the diaphragm was best described by the product of Pdi/Pdi_{max} and T_I/T_{tot}, which they termed the diaphragmatic tension-time index (TTdi), a value of 0.15 corresponding to the fatigue threshold. McCool et al. (1986) subsequently measured the esophageal pressure-time index (PTes) as a measure of inspiratory muscle pressure output and showed that for a given PTes, t_{lim} was inversely related to the mean inspiratory flow, or V_T/T_I, over a wide range of flows. The critical value of PTes that could be sustained for prolonged periods of time (>10 min) was also found to be inversely related to mean inspiratory flow. The interrelationship between pressure, V_T/T_I, T_I/T_{tot} and t_{lim} are represented graphically in Figure 14.

The value of B in Eq. (7) is determined by the blood flow to the muscle and by the oxygen and substrate content of the blood. In accordance with the predictions of Eq. (7), reduction of B, achieved by having normal subjects breath hypoxic gas mixtures, has been shown to reduce t_{lim} (Roussos and Macklem, 1977; Jardim et al., 1981). Similarly, decreasing the blood flow to the diaphragm of dogs has been shown to cause fatigue of this muscle, which was reversible by restoring normal perfusion (Supinski et al., 1989; Comtois et al., 1991). Supinski et al. (1988) have also shown in the dog that diaphragmatic fatigue can be reversed by hyperperfusion, achieved by increasing arterial blood pressure, thereby increasing t_{lim}. In spontaneously breathing dogs in cardiogenic shock, diaphragmatic fatigue can occur at relatively low levels of ventilation, which are not normally expected to cause fatigue of the respiratory muscles (Aubier et al., 1981b).

The efficiency of the respiratory muscles in performing external work is low compared to limb muscles (~5%), presumably because much of the consumed energy is expended in stabilizing and/or deforming the chest wall or because of the simultaneous recruitment of antagonist muscles. It is therefore a difficult parameter to isolate and study. Nevertheless, there is general agreement that E is reduced when breathing takes place at high lung volumes, presumably because the inspiratory muscles that perform most of the work are shorter (Collet and Engle, 1986; McCool et al., 1989). At half inspiratory capacity, E can be reduced by as much as 50% (Collett and Engle, 1986). Using inspiratory resistance breathing, Roussos et al. (1979) demonstrated that t_{lim}, for a given inspiratory mouth pressure or power output, was markedly reduced in their normal subjects when breathing at half inspiratory capacity as compared to FRC. The critical fatigue threshold was also reduced by hyperinflation. In that study, hyperinflation was achieved by the sustained activity of the inspiratory muscles, which itself could have hastened fatigue. However, McCool et al. (1989) used positive pressure to increase lung volume and obtained similar results. In addition, they showed that t_{lim}, for the various patterns of breathing they studied, over a wide range of flows and pressures, and at two different lung volumes, was uniquely related to the oxygen cost of breathing. Their data provide strong support for Eq. (3) and the notion that respiratory muscle fatigue occurs when energy demands exceed the rate of energy supply and that t_{lim} is reached when the intramuscular energy stores are depleted.

In summary, from Eq. (4), endurance is determined by energy demands (namely power, $\dot{W}$, and efficiency, E) and available energy (stored energy, a, and rate of energy supply, B). The critical power ($\dot{W}_{crit}$) may vary and increases with the rate of energy supply and efficiency. Finally, a given power and endurance of respiratory muscle may be achieved at different levels of pressure if the duty cycle (TI/Ttot) and/or the mean velocity of shortening (VT/TI) are altered (Fig. 15).

B. Respiratory Muscle Fatigue and Ventilatory Failure

When an individual breathes against a fatiguing load, an important question is whether the central controllers push the muscles to exhaustion or whether the muscles are protected by decreased drive (Roussos, 1982, 1984). In either case, of course, the end result is the same, namely, hypercapnic ventilatory failure.

Hypercapnic ventilatory failure for a given level of CO_2 production results from an inadequate alveolar ventilation ($\dot{V}_A$). The relation of $\dot{V}_A$ to Pa_{CO_2} is given by:

$$Pa_{CO_2} = K \frac{\dot{V}_{CO_2}}{\dot{V}_A} \tag{8}$$

where Pa_{CO_2} is arterial carbon dioxide tension, $\dot{V}_{CO_2}$ is the rate of carbon dioxide production, and K is the constant of proportionality. Since $\dot{V}_A = \dot{V}_E - \dot{V}_D$, where $\dot{V}_E$ is minute ventilation and $\dot{V}_D$ is deadspace ventilation, this equation can be expressed as

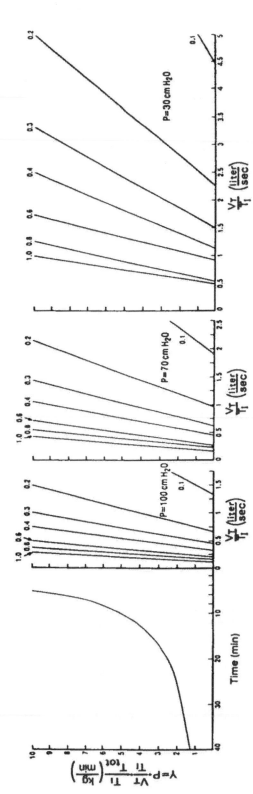

Figure 15 Relation of breathing power (ordinate) to endurance time at different combinations of pressure, inspiratory duty cycle (T_I/T_{tot}), and mean inspiratory flow (V_T/T_I) when the power of breathing is equal to or greater than a maximum rate of energy uptake of about 6–8 kg/min. Note that a given endurance is achieved with different critical pressures as the V_T/T_I and/or T_I/T_{tot} change.

$$Pa_{CO_2} = \frac{K\dot{V}_{CO_2}}{(\dot{V}_T - \dot{V}_D)} = \frac{K\dot{V}_{CO_2}}{(1-\dot{V}_D/\dot{V}_T)\,\dot{V}_Tf} = X \cdot \frac{\dot{V}_{CO_2}}{(1-\dot{V}_D/\dot{V}_T) \cdot \dot{V}_T/T_I \cdot T_I/T_{tot}} \quad (9)$$

where $\dot{V}_D$ is deadspace volume. Pa_{CO_2} will increase at a given level of $\dot{V}_{CO_2}$ and $\dot{V}_D$ by decreasing the mean inspiratory flow ($\dot{V}_T/T_I$) and/or the duty cycle (T_I/T_{tot}). The duty cycle and inspiratory time are entirely controlled by the central controllers, whereas $\dot{V}_T/T_I$ is controlled both centrally by altering the outgoing signals and peripherally by the resulting force of contraction. During fatigue, the primary site of force loss may frequently be peripheral, followed by secondary central modulation of CNS output, possibly so that the muscle may be protected against self-destruction. Therefore, when the respiratory muscles perform fatiguing work, the controllers may reduce their command per unit time to the thorax. This may serve to save energy and avoid exhaustion, but only at the expense of ventilation (Roussos, 1979, 1984).

The interrelation between the system's energetics and its central control was first suggested by Otis (1954), who concluded that for given alveolar ventilation and mechanical properties of the system there is an optimal frequency (f_{opt}) at which minimal work is performed. Thus, for a given deadspace and alveolar ventilation:

$$f_{opt} = \frac{\dot{V}_A}{\dot{V}_D} \quad (10)$$

This equation indicates that minimal work is achieved for a given alveolar ventilation if the $\dot{V}_A$ equals deadspace ventilation ($\dot{V}_A = \dot{V}_D \cdot f$) or, to put it differently, if minute ventilation is twice deadspace ventilation.

It is interesting that for normal subjects breathing at constant $\dot{V}_A$ and varying frequency, the rate of work is minimal at a frequency close to that adopted by subjects breathing spontaneously (McIlroy et al., 1954). During exercise, the frequency at which minimal work occurs increases progressively with increased alveolar ventilation and corresponds closely at each level of alveolar ventilation with the frequency spontaneously chosen by the subject (Milic-Emili and Petit, 1959). Similar results are found in animals of different species (Agostoni et al., 1959; Crosfill and Widdicombe, 1961). Finally, Mead (1960) found that in guinea pigs and in humans there is, for a given set of conditions, a frequency that is optimal in the sense that the average force required from the respiratory muscles is minimized. Available data thus suggest that the energetics of muscle is an important factor in determining respiratory rate.

Assuming that for a given impedance, mean flow is proportional to the pressure that the muscles generate, substituting $K^1 \cdot P$ for $\dot{V}_T/T_I$ in Eq. (9) yields:

$$Pa_{CO_2} = \frac{K\dot{V}_{CO_2}}{f(K^1PT_I - \dot{V}_D)} \quad (11)$$

where P is the mean driving pressure and K^1 is a constant.

The significance of this equation lies in the fact that the pressure and the pressure-time index $P \cdot T_I$ is related to Pa_{CO_2}. The pressure-time index is an approximate measure of the energy demands per breath of the inspiratory muscles. If energy supplies are inadequate to meet demands, $P \cdot T_I$ will decrease, and if other variables remain constant, Pa_{CO_2} must increase. In fact, what usually occurs is that a reduction in $P \cdot T_I$ is counterbalanced by an increase in frequency, a strategy that, while keeping $\dot{V}_A$ and Pa_{CO_2} constant, fails because f is no longer optimal and the work required to maintain $\dot{V}_A$ must increase. While the energy demands per breath decrease, the energy demands per unit time increase. Eventually, f decreases and f_{opt} may be achieved, but at the cost of increased $PaCO_2$ (Aubier et al., 1981b; Cohen et al., 1982).

The reduction in PTI per breath [Eq. (11)] can be either the result of muscle failure, i.e., decrease in contractility (Fig. 4), which will result in a reduction in P, or an adaption of the central nervous system, either by reducing the outgoing signal, thus reducing P, or by shortening T_I. In animals breathing against high loads, any of these changes can occur (Jammes et al., 1983).

It is of interest that patients who have difficulty being taken off mechanical ventilation and in whom the load on the respiratory muscle pump is excessive commonly adopt a pattern of rapid shallow breathing during unsuccessful weaning trials (Tobin et al., 1986). Such patterns of breathing reduce the PTI (below that predicted to result in muscle fatigue) (Milic-Emili, 1986) but at the expense of hypercapnia and weaning failure. These data suggest that the central nervous system reduces outgoing signals to avoid precipitating peripheral muscle fatigue.

In summary, it is argued that fatigue of the respiratory muscles may lead to hypercapnic respiratory failure, either as a result of muscle failure itself, or alteration in the strategy of breathing, or both (Roussos, 1982, 1984).

C. Factors Predisposing to Respiratory Muscle Fatigue

From Eq. (4) it is possible to draw conclusions regarding factors that predispose the inspiratory muscles to fatigue based on the premise that fatigue occurs when the load imposed on the respiratory muscles exceeds capacity and when the energy demands of the muscles exceed energy supply.

Energy Demands

Work of Breathing

When the work of breathing increases, or rather when the index of pressure × time (PTI) increases, the energy requirements increase and fatigue may occur.

Strength

The greater the fraction of maximum pressure developed by the inspiratory muscles, the greater the energy demands. This fraction can be increased either by increasing the pressure necessary to breathe (e.g., increased airway resistance) or by reducing the maximum force that the muscle can develop, as in diaphragmatic shortening

(Farkas and Roussos, 1984), hyperinflation (Roussos et al., 1979), and muscle myopathy, atrophy, prematurity, or neuromuscular disorders. Weakness may also be caused by metabolic and biochemical changes including sepsis, acidosis, hypercapnia, hypophosphatemia, and disorders of potassium and calcium metabo-lism. The effect of hyperinflation has been examined in normal subjects breathing at FRC plus half inspiratory capacity ($1/2$ IC); the critical pressure of the inspiratory muscles is decreased to about 25–35% of maximum (Fig. 16), and critical power is diminished to about 2.2 kg/min, compared to 50–70% and 6–8 kg/min, respectively, at FRC (Roussos et al., 1979).

Efficiency

For a given workload, the energy demands and oxygen cost of breathing increases as efficiency decreases. Differences in efficiency, as a result of experimental technique and the way different subjects use respiratory muscles to perform a given level of hyperventilation, as well as differences in respiratory rate and depth of breath affect the work of breathing. These are important factors that can explain the observed large differences in critical minute ventilation, which normal subjects can maintain indefinitely (Zocche et al., 1960; Shepard, 1967; Tenney and Reese, 1968; Freedman, 1970; Leith and Bradley, 1976). Resistive breathing is less efficient than hyperventilation, as pointed out by McGregor and Becklake (1961), who found that for a given external power, respiratory muscle efficiency decreased when breathing was done against resistance. In this situation, some inspiratory muscles may contract only to stabilize the chest wall, thus performing a quasi-isometric contraction (Macklem et al., 1978). This, of course, requires energy expenditure without the production of work. Consistent with this notion is the discrepancy between the values for critical power estimated by Roussos et al. (1979) during breathing through resistance (15–20 kcal/min) and those obtained by Tenney and Reese (1968) during hyperventilation (70/100 kcal/min).

Available Energy

Energy Supply

Energy supply is critically dependent on blood flow to muscle (Aubier et al., 1981b), which is itself determined by cardiac output and the ability of the muscle to increase blood flow parallel to increased work. The diaphragm has a greater capacity to increase blood flow than other skeletal muscles. However, it is likely that there is a limit to the amount that inspiratory muscle blood flow can increase. Such a limit is determined in part by the structure of muscle and the density of the vascular bed. However, it may also be determined by the intensity and duration of contraction. Skeletal muscle blood flow is impaired at high intensities of contraction (Barcroft and Milen, 1939; Humphreys and Lin, 1963). Thus, if the inspiratory muscles contract forcefully and do not relax during expiration, as occurs in asthma (Muller et al., 1980; Martin et al., 1980), the overall blood flow to the muscle may be less than required and fatigue will ensue.

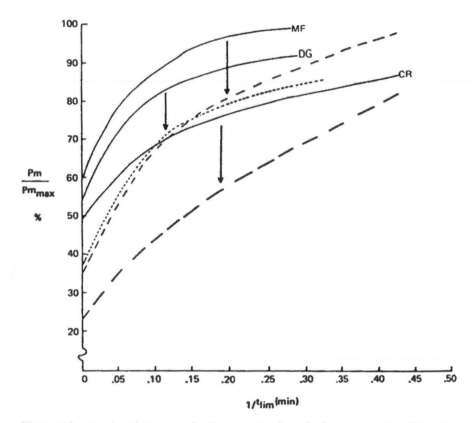

Figure 16 Relationship between Pm/Pm$_{max}$ and reciprocal of endurance time (1/t$_{lim}$) in three subjects at FRC (solid lines) and FRC + 1/2 IC (interrupted lines). In each subject intercept (Pm$_{crit}$) decreased at higher lung volume. (From Roussos et al., 1979.)

The oxygen supply to respiratory muscles is also dependent upon hemoglobin saturation and concentration (Jardim et al., 1981). Hypoxemia reduces the endurance time once W$_{crit}$ is exceeded, but it does not appear to influence W$_{crit}$ itself (Roussos and Macklem, 1977).

Other factors leading to fatigue can be predicted from experiments conducted on skeletal muscle and studies of whole body exercise. Substrate levels in the blood (glucose and free fatty acids) and the ability of the muscles to extract and utilize these sources of energy may potentially affect respiratory muscle performance.

Energy Stores

Poor nutritional status, catabolic states, or prolonged hyperventilation deplete glycogen and other energy stores, giving rise to respiratory muscle fatigue. In patients with acute respiratory failure, the concentrations of ATP and creatine phosphate in intercostal muscles are reduced (Gertz et al., 1977).

Although inspiratory muscle fatigue can be the result of an imbalance between energy supply and demand, there are undoubtedly cases, like with myasthenia gravis or partial curarization, in which failure of the muscle can be located at the neuromuscular junction and which are not apparently related to energetic imbalance. Similarly, with low-frequency fatigue, force generation at low stimulation frequencies can be dramatically and persistently reduced at a time when the metabolic composition of muscle is normal (Edwards et al., 1977a).

IV. Detection of Respiratory Muscle Fatigue

Muscle fatigue, in terms of failure of force generation, is best understood as a continuous process that starts whenever a muscle is subjected to an unsustainable load. Fatigue is therefore a normal physiological response to excessive load and is associated with a multitude of complex changes in muscle physiology that can affect all of the links in the chain of events from the central nervous system to the peripheral contractile machinery. Although fatigue is conveniently and conventionally defined in terms of force loss, other changes in physiological function can be useful indicators that the fatigue process is underway; indeed the notion that fatigue is a single endpoint (force loss) and all tests of fatigue should center on the detection of force loss is too narrow, from both a practical and an intellectual standpoint.

A. Measurement of Force (or Pressure)

Fatigue can be detected by techniques that directly measure the force of voluntary or electrically stimulated contractions or by measurements from which force is inferred (maneuvers such as VC). The measurement of force-frequency curves, as discussed previously, is a useful and specific technique for detecting peripheral fatigue. Measurement of the force-frequency curve of the diaphragm is made possible by stimulating the phrenic nerve and recording transdiaphragmatic pressure (Aubier et al., 1981a; Moxham et al., 1981a); the curve can easily be documented for the sternomastoid by stimulation of the muscle with surface electrodes (Moxham et al., 1980). Changes in the shape of the force-frequency curve provides information about the underlying mechanism of force loss. Loss of force at low frequencies indicates impairment of excitation-contraction coupling, whereas loss of force at high frequencies indicates impairment of neuromuscular junction transmission or membrane excitation.

Pressure-frequency relationships, obtained with unilateral phrenic stimulation, are complicated by uncontrolled movement and distortion of the contralateral hemidiaphragm. Bellemare et al. (1986) have shown that the pressure developed for any given frequency of stimulation is about 2.5 times greater during bilateral than during unilateral phrenic nerve stimulation, thus showing that the pressures developed by each side are not simply additive. Bilateral tetanic phrenic nerve stimulation is difficult, particularly at frequencies greater than 35 Hz, and likely to be of limited clinical use. However, partial pressure-frequency relationships can be constructed using paired stimuli and by varying the interval between the stimuli of each pair (Yan et al., 1993). This technique is simpler and better tolerated than tetanic stimulation and can provide information about high- and low-frequency fatigue of the diaphragm.

When normal subjects undertake treadmill exercise at 85–95% of maximum oxygen uptake to the point of exhaustion, twitch Pdi is reduced (Johnson et al., 1992). Twitch Pdi has also been shown to be reduced following maximum isocapnic voluntary ventilation for 2 min in normal subjects (Wragg et al., 1992). Data are therefore accumulating that, when pushed to the limit, the normal human diaphragm develops peripheral fatigue. The application of the twitch technique to patients with ventilatory failure is more difficult. For this purpose the more recent method of magnetic stimulation (Similowski et al., 1989) may have advantages.

A progressive decrease of maximum mouth pressure (PI_{max}) during an inspiratory task at a defined lung volume may provide some information regarding fatigue. However, under such conditions, there is always the possibility that inadequate effort may give false results. In this context the technique of twitch interpolation applied to the diaphragm is a powerful tool (Bellemare and Bigland-Ritchie, 1984, 1987).

B. Electromyographic Measurements

A reduction in the ratio of pressure generated to integrated EMG of the muscle (i.e., diaphragm Pdi/Edi) at constant length and geometry is a good index of muscle fatigue. Figure 9 (Aubier et al., 1981b) is an example of this index in keeping with earlier observations on other skeletal muscles by Lippold and coworkers (1960). The amplitude of the integrated electrical activity can also be used to monitor changes in the level of respiratory muscle activation. A close correspondence between the changes in the level of diaphragm activation, measured this way and by twitch interpolation, has been demonstrated by Bellemare and Bigland-Ritchie (1987) and by Hershenson and coworkers (1989).

The analysis of the EMG in its frequency domain delineates the power spectrum that shifts to lower frequencies with fatigue. This approach has been used for many years in other skeletal muscles (Lindstrom et al., 1977) and subsequently in the respiratory muscles (Gross et al., 1979). However, the underlying mechanism of the power spectral shift is not known. Among the factors thought to explain this shift is slowing of conduction velocity (Lindstrom et al., 1970). Thus, the spectral shift seen during fatigue could be explained by a progressive slowing of conduction velocity, which would in turn prolong the fiber action-potential wave form. It has been suggested (Mortimer et al., 1970) that slowing of conduction velocity may result from the accumulation of metabolites such as lactic acid. The accumulation of lactate is unlikely, in itself, to explain the EMG changes because patients with myophosphorylase deficiency, who do not produce lactic acid, have the same change in the EMG power spectrum with fatigue (Wiles et al., 1981). Supportive evidence for the conduction velocity theory is the fact that the measurement of conduction in single motor units of the biceps muscle, before and after contraction, has demonstrated a slowing of conduction velocity during fatigue (Broman, 1977). However, the findings of Bigland-Ritchie and coworkers (1981) indicate otherwise. They compared the relationship between the EMG power spectrum and nerve conduction velocity changes produced by fatigue and by cooling and found them to be different. They concluded that factors other than changes in the wave form of individual muscle fiber action potentials must contribute to the observed shift in the EMG power spectrum. However, their conduction velocity measurements included conduction over the nerve, which is greatly affected by cooling but not by fatigue, whereas the EMG power spectrum is not directly affected by nerve conduction. A good correspondence between the natural EMG power spectrum changes and the action potential wave form produced by supramaximal phrenic nerve stimulation has been found for the human diaphragm by Bellemare and Grassino (1982b). Phrenic stimulation offers a more direct method of evaluating changes in action potential propagation with fatigue that is not complicated by the potential effects of motor unit discharge rate or synchronization.

Further work is needed to elucidate the pathogenesis of the changes in the EMG power spectrum. Such studies will help us to understand the mechanism and site of fatigue. What is clear so far is that one cannot equate electromyographic indices of fatigue to contractile fatigue. It has been shown that changes in the EMG power spectrum are closely associated with high-frequency fatigue, although the spectrum remains normal in the presence of low-frequency fatigue (Moxham et al., 1982). Thus, it is possible that the EMG may help to detect fatigue due to a reduced frequency of central firing, neuromuscular junction failure, or failure of excitation of the sarcolemma, but it can give no information about excitation-contraction coupling failure or about the causes of failure of the contractile machinery (Fig. 17).

At the present time the value of the EMG for the detection of respiratory muscle fatigue is limited. Although the technique appeared to be a simple one when first applied to the respiratory muscles, experience has demonstrated that it is difficult to achieve useful information in this manner.

C. Respiratory Muscle Relaxation Rate

As a fatiguing contraction progresses, an early physiological event is the slowing of muscle relaxation rate (MRR), which has the important affect of facilitating a reduction in central firing frequency while maintaining plateau tension (Bigland-Ritchie et al., 1983). MRR is conventionally defined as the percentage loss of force or pressure in 10 ms. By recording respiratory pressures during a brief inspiratory effort and subsequent relaxation, MRR has been measured for the

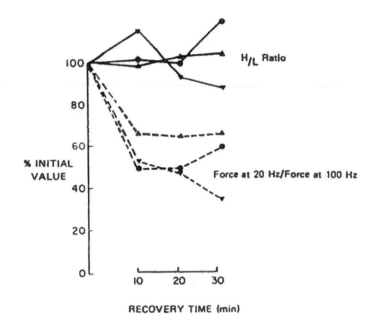

Figure 17   The force response to electrical stimulation at 20 Hz/force at 100 Hz following repeated submaximal voluntary contractions in the quadriceps (illustrating substantial low-frequency fatigue); EMG high/low ratio remains normal. (From Moxham et al., 1982.)

diaphragm in terms of transdiaphragmatic pressure and for the respiratory muscles as a whole by measuring mouth, nasopharyngeal, or esophageal pressures (Esau et al., 1983b; Levy et al., 1984; Koulouris et al., 1989; Mulvey et al., 1991b) (Fig. 10). The relaxation of muscle is an active energy-consuming process, and MRR is affected by temperature, thyroid status, the inherent speed of muscle, and fatigue. When skeletal muscle is subjected to an excessive load, there is an early slowing of MRR. Thus, MRR slows following exhaustive inspiratory resistive loading as well as maximum sustained ventilation. The MRR of the respiratory muscles is numerically similar to that of limb muscles and slows with exhaustive inspiratory loading in a similar way to loaded limb muscles. Furthermore, the recovery of MRR following exhaustive loading of the respiratory muscles is very similar to that for fatigued limb muscles. These observations suggest that respiratory muscle MRR, measured from respiratory pressures, reflects the relaxation rate of the respiratory muscles.

To date, although a number of studies have demonstrated slowing of MRR when the respiratory muscles are loaded in studies on normal subjects, there have been few investigations of MRR in patients. In a study of intubated patients on the intensive care unit, MRR has been measured from snifflike inspiratory maneuvers before and during weaning (Goldstone et al., 1994). Sequential measurements of

MRR demonstrated that in patients who weaned successfully, MRR remained unchanged, whereas in patients failing to wean, MRR slowed.

Although the measurement of MRR has many advantages when studying respiratory muscle fatigue, there are, in practice, many problems. The wide range of normal values for MRR makes it difficult to obtain useful information from a single measurement. Obtaining sequential measurements of MRR of sufficient quality is also a difficulty. As for limb muscles, the measurement of MRR during voluntary efforts, like a sniff, is dependent on the magnitude of the effort developed, presumably reflecting the recruitment of different motor unit types (Mulvey et al., 1991a). Theoretically some of these problems could be overcome by the measurement of the relaxation characteristics of twitch responses. However, the slowing of MRR, like the changes of the EMG power spectrum, is associated with high-intensity exercise and high-frequency fatigue (Esau et al., 1983a,b). As low-frequency fatigue is not associated with changes in relaxation rate (Jones, 1981), this type of fatigue cannot be detected with this single measurement (see also Yan et al., 1992).

D. Synergistic Behavior of Fatiguing Respiratory Muscles

A characteristic feature of fatiguing respiratory muscles is that each group of inspiratory muscles (diaphragm or intercostal/accessory) alternates its contribution to the breathing task (Roussos et al., 1979; Lopes et al., 1981). A typical example is shown in Figure 18, in which mouth pressure (Pm) and esophageal pressure (Pes) remain constant throughout the run, whereas transdiaphragmatic pressure (Pdi) and gastric pressure (Pga) vary, indicating changes in the strength of diaphragmatic contractions during a given fatiguing run. This alternation in the amplitude of Pdi may be interpreted as an indication of recruitment and derecruitment of the various groups of inspiratory muscles. A fall in abdominal pressure during inspiration to values lower than those obtained during relaxation at FRC indicates recruitment of intercostal/accessory muscles. An increase in abdominal pressure during inspiration greater than that occurring during an inspiration in which the diaphragm is the main muscle contracting signals recruitment of the abdominal muscles, which tends to preserve diaphragmatic length (Fig. 18, period C). When the abdominal pressure is maintained at its resting end-expiratory (FRC) value, the intercostal and accessory muscles are being recruited and the diaphragm shortens less (Fig. 18, period B). The alternation of the contributions of the diaphragm and intercostal/accessory muscles to the breathing task results predominantly in an outward motion of the abdomen or rib cage, respectively. This motion of parts of the chest wall is clearly demonstrated by the magnetometer tracings. However, the interpretation becomes difficult because the efforts of the subject far exceed the limits established by Konno and Mead (1967). Although deformation and artifacts complicate these tracings, their overall behavior is in accord with the pressure changes. The underlying physiological explanation of such alternation is unknown. Teleologically, however, the alternations may protect against the development of respiratory muscle fatigue

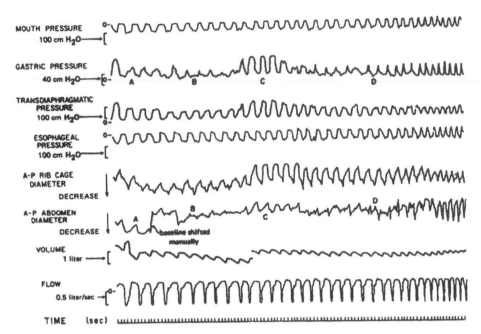

Figure 18 Recorded measurements of an experimental run at 75% of maximum mouth pressure (Pm_{max}). Except for transdiaphragmatic pressures (Pdi), all pressures were measured relative to atmospheric pressure. Swing in mouth pressure and esophageal pressure remained constant throughout run; those in gastric pressure (Pga) and Pdi varied. Increase in Pga during inspiration was associated with an increase of anteroposterior (AP) diameter of the abdomen (periods A and C); when Pga did not change, AP diameter of abdomen did not change either (period B); when Pga decreased, AP diameter also decreased (period D). (From Roussos et al., 1979.)

and thereby prolong endurance time. During periods when a smaller Pdi is developed, the diaphragm may recover from fatigue, whereas during periods when there are large positive abdominal pressure swings, the intercostal/accessory muscles are relatively relaxed and may undergo some recovery. This may postpone the eventual development of inspiratory muscle exhaustion.

References

Abbott, B. C. (1951). The heat production associated with the maintenance of a prolonged contraction and the extra heat produced during shortening. *J. Physiol.* (London), 112:438–445.

Agostoni, E., Thimm, F. F., and Fenn, W. O. (1959). Comparative features of breathing. *J. Appl. Physiol.*, 14:679–683.

Aldrich, T. K. (1987). Transmission failure of the rabbit diaphragm. *Respir. Physiol.*, 69:307–319.

Aubier, M., Murciano, D., Fournier, M., Milic-Emili, J., Pariente, R., and Derenne, J. P. (1980).

Central respiratory drive in patients with chronic obstructive lung disease in acute respiratory failure. *Am. Rev. Respir. Dis.*, 122:191–200.

Aubier, M., Farkas, G., De Troyer, A., Mozes, R., and Roussos, C. (1981a). Detection of diaphragmatic fatigue in man by phrenic stimulation. *J. Appl. Physiol.*, 50:538–544.

Aubier, M., Trippenbach, T., and Roussos, C. (1981b). Respiratory muscle fatigue during cardiogenic shock. *J. Appl. Physiol.*, 51:499–508.

Aubier, M., Viires, N., Syllie, G., Mozes, R., and Roussos, C. (1982). Respiratory muscles contribution to lactic acidosis. *Am. Rev. Respir. Dis.*, 126:648–652.

Balaban, R. S. (1990). Regulation of oxidative phosphorylation in the mammalian cell. *Am. J. Physiol.*, 258:C377–C389.

Barcroft, H., and Milen, J. L. E. (1939). The blood flow through muscle during sustained contraction. *J. Physiol.* (London), 97:17–31.

Bark, H., Supinski, G., Bundy, R., and Kelsen, S. (1988). Effect of hypoxia on diaphragm blood flow, oxygen uptake and contractility. *Am. Rev. Respir. Dis.*, 138:1535–1541.

Bazzy, A. R., and Donnelly, D. F. (1993). Diaphragmatic failure during loaded breathing: role of neuromuscular transmission. *J. Appl. Physiol.*, 74:1679–1683.

Bazzy, A. R., Akabas, S. R., Hays, A. P., and Haddad, G. G. (1988). Respiratory muscle response to load and glycogen content in type I and II fibers. *Exp. Neurol.*, 101:17–28.

Belanger, A. Y., and McComas, A. J. (1981). Extent of motor unit activation during effort. *J. Appl. Physiol.*, 51:1131–1135.

Bellemare, F., and Grassino, A. (1982a). Evaluation of the human diaphragm fatigue. *J. Appl. Physiol.*, 53:1196–1206.

Bellemare, F., and Grassino, A. (1982b). Effect of pressure and timing of contraction on human diaphragm fatigue. *J. Appl. Physiol.*, 53: 1190–1195.

Bellemare, F., Wight, D., Lavigne, C. M., and Grassino, A. (1983). Effect of tension and timing of contraction on the blood flow of the diaphragm. *J. Appl. Physiol.*, 54:1597–1606.

Bellemare, F., and Grassino, A. (1983). Force reserve of the diaphragm in patients with chronic obstructive pulmonary disease. *J. Appl. Physiol.*, 55:8–15.

Bellemare, F., Woods, J. J., Johansson, R., and Bigland-Ritchie, B. (1983). Motor unit discharge rates in maximal voluntary contractions of three human muscles. *J. Neurophysiol.*, 50:1380–1392.

Bellemare, F., and Bigland-Ritchie, B. (1984). Assessment of human diaphragm strength and activation using phrenic nerve stimulation. *Resp. Physiol.*, 58:263–277.

Bellemare, F., Bigland-Ritchie, B., and Woods, J. J. (1986). Contractile properties of the human diaphragm in vivo. *J. Appl. Physiol.*, 61:1153–1161.

Bellemare, F., and Bigland-Ritchie, B. (1987). Central components of diaphragmatic fatigue assessed by phrenic nerve stimulation. *J. Appl. Physiol.*, 62:1307–1316.

Bellemare, F., and Garzaniti, N. (1988). Failure of neuromuscular propagation during human maximal voluntary contractions. *J. Appl. Physiol.*, 64:1084–1093.

Bellemare, F. (1989). Respiratory muscle function. In *Textbook of Internal Medicine*. Vol. 2. Edited by W. N. Kelley. Philadelphia, J. B. Lippincott, p. 1843.

Bergstron, J., Hermansen, L., Hultman, E., and Saltin, B. (1967). Diet, muscle glycogen, and physical performance. *Acta Physiol. Scand.*, 71:140–150.

Bergstrom, J., Harris, R. C., Hultman, E., and Nordesjo, L. O. (1971). Energy rich phosphagen in dynamic and static work. *Adv. Exp. Med. Biol.*, 11:341–355.

Bigland-Ritchie, B., Jones, D. A., Hosking, G. P., and Edwards, R. H. T. (1978). Central and peripheral fatigue in sustained maximal voluntary contractions of human quadriceps muscle. *Clin. Sci. Mol. Med.*, 54:609–614.

Bigland-Ritchie, B., Jones, D. A., and Woods, J. J. (1979). Excitation frequency and muscle fatigue: electrical responses during human voluntary and stimulated contractions. *Exp. Neurol.*, 64:414–427.

Bigland-Ritchie, B. (1981). EMG and fatigue of human voluntary and stimulated contractions. In *Human Muscle Fatigue* (CIBA Foundation Symposium 82). Edited by R. Porter and J. Whelan. London: Pitman Medical, pp. 130–148.

Bigland-Ritchie, B., Donovan, E. F., and Roussos, C. (1981). Conduction velocity and EMG power spectrum changes in fatigue of sustained maximal efforts. *J. Appl. Physiol.*, 51:1300–1305.

Bigland-Ritchie, B., Johansson, R., Lippold, O. C. J., and Woods, J. J. (1983). Contractile speed and EMG changes during fatigue of sustained maximal voluntary contractions. *J. Neurophysiol.*, 50:313–324.

Bigland-Ritchie, B., Furbush, F., and Woods, J. J. (1986). Fatigue of intermittent, submaximal voluntary contractions: central and peripheral factors in different muscles. *J. Appl. Physiol.*, 61:421–429.

Bigland-Ritchie, B., Furbush, F., Gandevia, S. C., and Thomas, C. K. (1992a). Voluntary discharge frequencies of human motoneurons at different muscle lengths. *Muscle Nerve*, 15:130–138.

Bigland-Ritchie, B., Thomas, C. K., Rice, C. L., Howarth, J. V., and Woods, J. J. (1992b). Muscle temperature, contractile speed, and motoneuron firing rates during human voluntary contractions. *J. Appl. Physiol.*, 73:2457–2461.

Bongiovanni, L. G., and Hagbarth, K. E. (1990). Tonic vibration reflexes elicited during fatigue from maximal voluntary contractions in man. *J. Physiol.* (London), 423:1–14.

Broman, H. (1977). An investigation on the influence of a sustained contraction on the succession of action potentials from a single motor unit. *Electromyogr. Clin. Neurophysiol.*, 17:341–358.

Brown, G. L., and Burns, B. D. (1949). Fatigue and neuromuscular block in mammalian muscles. *Proc. R. Soc. Lond. (Biol)*, 136:182–195.

Buchthal, F., and Schmalbruch, H. (1970). Contraction times and fiber type in intact human muscles. *Acta Physiol. Scand.*, 79:435–452.

Burke, R. E., Levine, D. N., Zajac, F. E., Tsairis, P., and Engle, W. K. (1971). Mammalian motor units: physiological-histochemical correlation in three types of cat gastrocnemius. *Science*, 174:709–712.

Chance, B., Leigh, J. S., Jr., Clark, B. J., Maris, J., Kent, J., Nioka, S., and Smith, D. (1985). Control of oxidative metabolism and oxygen delivery in human skeletal muscle: a steady state analysis of the work/energy cost transfer function. *Proc. Natl. Acad. Sci.*, 82:8384–8388.

Citterio, G., Sironi, S., Piccoli, S., and Agostoni, E. (1983). Slow to fast shift in inspiratory muscle fibers during heat tachypnea. *Resp. Physiol.*, 52:259–274.

Close, R. E. (1972). The dynamic properties of mammalian skeletal muscles. *Physiol. Rev.*, 52:129–197.

Cohen, C., Zagelbaum, G., Gross, D., Roussos, C., and Macklem, P. T. (1982). Clinical manifestations of inspiratory muscle fatigue. *Am. J. Med.*, 73:308–316.

Collett, P. W., and Engel, L. A. (1986). Influence of lung volume on oxygen cost of resistive breathing. *J. Appl. Physiol.*, 61:16–24.

Comtois, A., Hu, F., and Grassino, A. (1991). Restriction of regional blood flow and diaphragm contractility. *J. Appl. Physiol.*, 70:2439–2447.

Crosfill, M. L., and Widdicombe, J. G. (1961). Physical characteristics of the chest and lungs and the work of breathing in different mammalian species. *J. Physiol.* (London), 158:1–14.

Davies, H. W., Haldane, J. S., and Priestly, J. G. (1919). The response to respiratory resistance. *J. Physiol.* (London), 53:60–69.

Davies, H. W., Brown, G. R., and Binger, C. A. L. (1925). The respiratory response to carbon dioxide. *J. Exp. Med.*, 41:37–52.

Dawson, M. J., Gardian, D. G., and Wilkie, D. R. (1978). Muscular fatigue investigated by phosphorus nuclear magnetic resonance. *Nature*, 274:861–866.

Desmedt, J. E., and Godaux, E. (1977). Ballistic contractions in man: characteristic recruitment pattern of single motor units of the tibialis anterior muscle. *J. Physiol.* (London), 264:673–693.

Dick, T. E., Kong, F. J., and Berger, A. J. (1987). Correlation of recruitment order with axonal conduction velocity for supraspinally driven diaphragmatic motor units. *J. Neurophysiol.*, 57:245–259.

Donaldson, S. K., Hermansen, L., and Bolles, L. (1978). Differential effects of H^+ on Ca^{2+}-activated force of skinned fibers from the soleus, cardiac and adductor magnus muscles of rabbits. *Pflügers Arch. Eur. J. Physiol.*, 376:55–65.

Dunn, F. T. (1955). The blockage of motor impulses in an asynchronized volley at the neuromuscular junction. *J. Cell Comp. Physiol.*, 46:348–350.

Edwards, R. H. T. (1978). Physiological analysis of skeletal muscle weakness and fatigue. *Clin. Sci. Mol. Med.*, 54:463–470.

Edwards, R. H. T., Hill, D. K., Jones, D. A., and Merton, P. A. (1977a). Fatigue of long duration in human skeletal muscle after exercise. *J. Physiol.* (London), 272:769–778.

Edwards, R. H. T., Young, A., Hosking, G. P., and Jones, D. A. (1977b). Human skeletal muscle function: description of tests and normal values. *Clin. Sci. Mol. Med.*, 52:283–290.

Edwards, R. H. T., Mills, K. R., and Newham, D. J. (1981). Greater low frequency fatigue produced by eccentric than concentric muscle contraction. *J. Physiol.* (London), 317:17.

Elliott, M. W., Mulvey, D. A., Moxham, J., Green, M., and Branthwaite, M. A. (1991). Domiciliary nocturnal nasal intermittent positive pressure ventilation in COPD: mechanisms underlying changes in arterial blood gas tensions. *Eur. Respir. J.*, 4:1044–1052.

Enoka, R. M., and Stuart, D. G. (1992). Neurobiology of muscle fatigue. *J. Appl. Physiol.*, 72:1631–1648.

Esau, S. A., Bellemare, F., Grassino, A., Permutt, S., Roussos, C., and Pardy, R. L. (1983a). Changes in relaxation rate with diaphragmatic fatigue in humans. *J. Appl. Physiol.*, 54:1353–1360.

Esau, S. A., Bye, P. T. P., and Pardy, R. L. (1983b). Changes in rate of relaxation of sniffs with diaphragmatic fatigue in humans. *J. Appl. Physiol.*, 55:731–735.

Fabiato, A., and Fabiato, F. (1978). Effects of pH on the myofilaments and the saracoplasmic reticulum of skinned cells from cardiac and skeletal muscles. *J. Physiol.* (London), 276:233–255.

Farkas, G., and Roussos, C. H. (1984). Acute diaphragmatic shortening: in vitro mechanics and fatigue. *Am. Rev. Respir. Dis.*, 130:434–438.

Faulkner, J. A., Jones, D. A., Roung, J. M., and Edwards, R. H. T. (1980). Dynamics of energetic process in human muscle. In *Exercise Bioenergetics and Gas Exchange*. Edited by P. Ceretelli and G. J. Whipp. New York, Elsevier-North Holland, pp. 81–90.

Fitts, R. H., and Holloszy, J. O. (1976). Lactate and contractile force in frog muscle during development of fatigue and recovery. *Am. J. Physiol.*, 231:430–433.

Freedman, S. (1970). Sustained maximum voluntary ventilation. *Respir. Physiol.*, 8:230–240.

Freedman, S., Cooke, N. T., and Moxham, J. (1983). Production of lactic acid by respiratory muscles. *Thorax*, 38:50–54.

Furguson, G. T., Irvin, C. G., and Cherniack, R. M. (1990). Effect of corticosteroids on diaphragm function and biochemistry in the rabbit. *Am. Rev. Respir. Dis.*, 141:156–163.

Gandevia, S. C., McKenzie, D. K., and Plassman, B. L. (1983). Endurance properties of respiratory and limb muscles. *Resp. Physiol.*, 53:47–61.

Gandevia, S. C., Macefield, G., Burke, D., and McKenzie, D. K. (1990). Voluntary activation of human motor axons in the absence of muscle afferent feedback. *Brain*, 113:1563–1581.

Garland, S. J., and McComas, A. J. (1990). Reflex inhibition of human soleus muscle during fatigue. *J. Physiol.* (London), 429:17–27.

Gauthier, A. P., Faltus, R. E., Macklem, P. T., and Bellemare, F. (1993). Effects of fatigue on the length-tetanic force relationship of the rat diaphragm. *J. Appl. Physiol.*, 74:326–332.

Gertz, I., Hedenstierna, G., Hellers, G., and Wahren, J. (1977). Muscle metabolism in patients with chronic obstructive lung disease and acute respiratory failure. *Clin. Sci. Mol. Med.*, 52:395–403.

Goldstone, J., Green, M., and Moxham, J. (1994). Maximum relaxation rate of the diaphragm during weaning from mechanical ventilation. *Thorax*, 49:54–60.

Graham, R., Jammes, Y., Delpierre, S., Grimaud, C., and Roussos, Ch. (1986). The effects of ischemia, lactic acid and hypertonic NaCl on phrenic afferent discharge during spontaneous diaphragmatic contraction. *Neurosci. Lett.*, 67(3):257–262.

Gribben, H. R., Gardiner, I. T., Heinz, C. J., Gibson, T. J., and Pride, N. B. (1983). The role of impaired inspiratory muscle function in limiting ventilatory response to CO_2 in chronic airflow obstruction. *Clin. Sci.*, 64:487–495.

Griggs, G. A., Findley, L. J., Suratt, P. M., Esau, S. A., Wilhoit, S. C., and Rochester, D. F. (1989). Prolonged relaxation rate of inspiratory muscles in patients with sleep apnea. *Am. Rev. Respir. Dis.*, 140:706–710.

Grimby, L., Hannertz, J., and Hedman, B. (1981). The fatigue and voluntary discharge properties of single motor units in man. *J. Physiol.* (London), 316:545–554.

Gross, D., Grassino, A., Ross, W. R. D., and Macklem, P. T. (1979). Electromyogram pattern of diaphragmatic fatigue. *J. Appl. Physiol.*, 46:1–7.

Gutierrez, G., Pohil, R. J., Andry, J. M., Strong, R., and Narayana, P. (1988a). Bioenergetics of rabbit skeletal muscle during hypoxemia and ischemia. *J. Appl. Physiol.*, 65:608–616.

Gutierrez, M., Beroiza, T., Contreras, G., Diaz, O., Cruz, E., Moreno, R., and Lisboa, C. (1988b). Weekly cuirass ventilation improves blood gases and inspiratory muscle strength in patients with chronic airflow limitation and hypercarbia. *Am. Rev. Respir. Dis.*, 138:617–623.

Hannerz, J., and Grimby, L. (1979). The afferent influence on the voluntary firing range of individual motor units in man. *Muscle Nerve*, 2:414–422.

Harris, R. C., Edwards, R. H. T., Hultman, E., Nordesjo, L. O., Nylind, B., and Sahlin, K. (1976). The time course of phosphorylcreatine resynthesis during recovery of the quadriceps muscle in man. *Pflygers Arch.*, 367:137–142.

Henneman, E., and Mendell, L. M. (1981). Functional organization of motor neuron pool and its inputs. In *Handbook of Physiology. The Nervous System. Motor Control*. Bethesda, Md., American Physiological Society, pp. 423–507.

Hershenson, M. B., Kikuchi, Y., and Loring, S. H. (1988). Relative strengths of the chest wall muscles. *J. Appl. Physiol.*, 65:852–862.

Hershenson, M. B., Kikuchi, Y., Tzelepis, G. E., and McCool, F. D. (1989). Preferential fatigue of the rib cage muscles during inspiratory resistive loaded ventilation. *J. Appl. Physiol.*, 66:750–754.

Hilaire, G., Gauthier, P., and Monteau, R. (1983). Central respiratory drive and recruitment order of phrenic and inspiratory laryngeal motoneurons. *Resp. Physiol.*, 51:341–359.

Hill, A. V. (1913). Heat production n prolonged contractions of an isolated frog's muscle. *J. Physiol.* (London), 47:305–324.

Hill, A. V., and Kupalov, P. (1929). Anaerobic and aerobic activity in isolated muscles. *Proc. R. Soc. Lond. [Biol.]*, 105:313.

Hultman, E., Bergstrom, J, and McLennan-Anderson, N. (1967). Breakdown and resynthesis of phosphoryl-creatine and adenosine triphosphate in connection with muscular work in man. *Scan. J. Clin. Lab. Invest.*, 19:56–66.

Hultman, E., Sjoholm, H., Sahlin, K., and Edstrom, L. (1981). Glycolytic and oxidative energy metabolism and contraction characteristics of intact human muscle. In *Human Muscle Fatigue: Physiological Mechanisms*. Edited by R. Porter and J. Whelan. London, Pitman, pp. 19–40.

Humphreys, P. S., and Lin, A. R. (1963). Blood flow through active and inactive muscle of the forearm during isolated hand grip contractions. *J. Physiol.* (London), 166:120–135.

Hussain, S. N., Magder, S., Chatillon, A., and Roussos, C. (1990). Chemical activation of thin fiber phrenic afferent:respiratory responses. *J. Appl. Physiol.*, 69:1002–1111.

Hussain, S. N. A., and Magder, S. (1991). Diaphragmatic intramuscular pressure in relation to tension, shortening and blood flow. *J. Appl. Physiol.*, 71:159–167.

Ikai, M., Yabe, K., and Ishii, K. (1967). Muskelkraft and muskulare Ermundung bei wilkurlicher Anspannung und elektrischer Reizung des Muskels. *Sportartz Sportmedizin*, 5:197–211.

Iscoe, S., Dankoff, J., Migicousky, R., and Polosa, C. (1976). Recruitment and discharge frequency of phrenic motor-neurons during inspiration. *Respir. Physiol.*, 26:113–128.

Jacobus, W. E. (1985). Respiratory control and the integration of heart high energy phosphate metabolism by mitochondrial creatine kinase. *Annu. Rev. Physiol.*, 47:707–725.

Jammes, Y., Bye, P. T. P., Pardy, R. L., and Roussos, C. (1983). Vagal feedback with expiratory threshold load under extracorporeal circulation. *J. Appl. Physiol.*, 55:316–322.

Jammes, Y., Buchler, B., Delpierre, S., Rasidakis, A., Grimaud, C., and Roussos, Ch. (1986). Phrenic afferents and their role in inspiratory control. *J. Appl. Physiol.*, 60(3):854–860.

Jardim, J., Farkas, G., Prefaut, C., Thomas, D., Macklem, P. T., and Roussos, C. (1981). The failing inspiratory muscles under normoxic and hypoxic conditions. Am. Rev. Respir. Dis., 124:274–279.

Jodkowski, J. S., Viana, F., Dick, T. E., and Berger, A. J. (1988). Repetitive firing properties of phrenic motoneurons in the cat. *J. Neurophysiol.*, 60:687–702.

Johnson, B. D., Babcock, M. A., Suman, O. E., and Dempsey, J. A. (1993). Exercise induced diaphragmatic fatigue in healthy humans. *J. Physiol.*, 460:385–405.

Jones, D. A. (1981). Muscle fatigue due to changes beyond the neuromuscular function. In *Human Muscle Fatigue: Physiological Mechanisms*. Edited by R. Porter and J. Whelan. London, Pitman Medical, pp. 178–190.

Jones, D. A., Bigland-Ritchie, B., and Edwards, R. H. T. (1979). Excitation frequency and muscle fatigue: mechanical responses during voluntary and stimulated contraction. Exp. Neurol., 64:401–413.

Jones, N. L., Sutton, J. R., Taylor, R., and Toews, C. J. (1979). Effect of pH on cardiorespiratory and metabolic response to exercise. *J. Appl. Physiol.*, 43:959–964.

Juan, G., Calverly, P., Talamo, C., Schnader, J., and Roussos, C. (1984). Effect of carbon dioxide on diaphragmatic function in human being. *N. Engl. J. Med.*, 310:874–879.

Juel, C., Bangsbo, J., Graham, T., and Saltin, B. (1990). Lactate and potassium fluxes from human skeletal muscles during and after intense, dynamic, knee extensor exercise. *Acta Physiol. Scand.*, 140:147–159.

Katz, A., and Hecht, H. (1969). The early "pump" failure and the ischemic heart. *Am. J. Med.*, 47:497–502.

Katz, L. A., Swain, J. A., Portman, M. A., and Balaban, R. S. (1989). Relation between phosphate metabolites and oxygen consumption of heart in vivo. *Am. J. Physiol.* 256:H265–H274.

Keens, T. G., Bryan, A. C., Levison, H., and Ianuzzo, C. D. (1978). Developmental pattern of muscle fibre types in human ventilatory muscles. J. Appl. Physiol., 44:909–913.

Kernell, D., and Monster, A. W. (1982). Motoneurone properties and motor fatigue. *Exp. Brain Res.*, 46:197–204.

Konno, K., and Mead, J. (1967). Measurements of the separate volume changes of rib cage and abdomen during breathing. *J. Appl. Physiol.*, 22:407–422.

Koulouris, N., Vianna, L. G., Mulvey, D. A., Green, M., and Moxham, J. (1989). Maximal relaxation rates of esophageal, nose, and mouth pressures during a sniff reflect inspiratory muscle fatigue. *Am. Rev. Respir. Dis.*, 139:1213–1217.

Krnjevic, K., and Miledi, R. (1959a). Failure of neuromuscular propagation in rats. *J. Physiol.* (London), 140:440–461.

Krnjevic, K., and Miledi, R. (1959b). Presynaptic failure of neuromuscular propagation in rats. *J. Physiol.* (London), 149:1–22.

Kugelberg, E., and Lindegren, B. (1969). Transmission and contraction fatigue of rat motor units in relation to succinate dehydrogenase activity of motor unit fibers. *J. Physiol.* (London), 288:285–300.

Kukulka, C. G., Moore, M. A., and Russel, A. G. (1986). Changes in human alpha motoneurone excitability during sustained maximum isometric contractions. *Neurosci. Lett.*, 68:327–333.

Kukulka, C. G., and Clamman, H. P. (1981). Comparison of the recruitment and discharge properties of motor units in human brachial biceps and adductor pollicis during isometric contractions. *Brain Res.*, 219:45–55.

Kushmerick, M. J., and Meyer, R. A. (1985). Chemical changes in rat leg muscle by phosphorus nuclear magnetic resonance. *Am. J. Physiol.* 248:C542–C549.

Lehman, C. F. (1851). Lehrbuch der physiologischen Chemie. 2nd ed. London, Cavendish Society.

Leith, D. E., and Bradley, M. (1976). Ventilatory muscle strength and endurance training. *J. Appl. Physiol.*, 41:508–516.

Levy, R. D., Esau, S. A., Bye, P. T. P., and Pardy, R. L. (1984). Relaxation rate of mouth pressure with sniffs at rest and with inspiratory muscle fatigue. *Am. Rev. Respir. Dis.*, 130:38–41.

Lieberman, D. A., Faulkner, J. A., Craig, A. B., and Maxwell, L. C. (1973). Performance and histochemical composition of guinea pig and human diaphragm. *J. Appl. Physiol.*, 34:233–237.

Lindstrom, L., Magnusson, R., and Petersen, I. (1970). Muscular fatigue and action potential conduction velocity changes studied with frequency analysis of EMG signal. *Electromyography*, 10:341–355.

Lindstrom, L., Kadefors, R., and Petersen, I. (1977). An electromyographic index for localised muscle fatigue. *J. Appl. Physiol.*, 43:750–754.

Lippold, O. C. J., Redfearn, J. W. T., and Vuco, J. (1960). The electromyography of fatigue. *Ergonomics*, 3:121–131.

Lockhat, D., Roussos, C., and Ianuzzo, C. D. (1988). Metabolite changes in the loaded hypoperfused and failing diaphragm. *J. Appl. Physiol.*, 65:1563–1571.

Lopes, J. M., Muller, N. L., Bryan, M. H., and Bryan, C. A. (1981). Synergistic behaviour of inspiratory muscles after diaphragmatic fatigue in newborn. *J. Appl. Physiol.*, 57:547–551.

Luttgau, H. C. (1965). The effect of metabolic inhibitors on the fatigue of the action potential in single muscle fibers. *J. Physiol.* (London), 178:45–67.

Macefield, G., Hagbarth, K. E., Gorman, R., Gandevia, S. C., and Burke, D. (1991). Decline in spindle support to a-motoneurones during sustained voluntary contractions. *J. Physiol.* (London), 440:497–512.

Macklem, P. T., Gross, D., Grassino, A., and Roussos, C. (1978). Partitioning of the inspiratory pressure swings between diaphragm and intercostal/accessory muscles. *J. Appl. Physiol.*, 44:200–208.

Manohar, M. (1990). Inspiratory and expiratory muscle perfusion in maximally exercised ponies. *J. Appl. Physiol.*, 68:544–548.

Manohar, M., and Hassan, A. S. (1991). Diaphragmatic energetics during prolonged exhaustive exercise. *Am. Rev. Respir. Dis.*, 144:415–418.

Marsden, C. D., Meadows, J. C., and Merton, P. A. (1971). Isolated single motor units in human muscle and their rates of discharge during maximum voluntary effort. *J. Physiol.* (London), 217:12P–13P.

Marsden, C. D., Meadows, J. C., and Merton, P. A. (1983). "Muscular wisdom" that minimizes fatigue during prolonged effort in man: peak rates of motoneuron discharge and slowing of discharge during fatigue. In *Motor Control Mechanisms in Health and Disease.* Edited by J. E. Desmedt. New York, Raven, pp. 169–211.

Martin, J., Powell, E., Shore, S., Emrich, J. J., and Engel, L. A. (1980). The role of respiratory muscles in the hyper-inflation of bronchial asthma. *Am. Rev. Respir. Dis.*, 121:441–447.

Mayock, D. E., Standdaert, T. A., Murphy, T. D., and Woodrum, D. A. (1991). Diaphragmatic force and substrate response to resistive loaded breathing in the piglet. *J. Appl. Physiol.*, 70:70–76.

McCool, F. D., McCann, D. R., Leith, D. E., and Hoppin, F. G., Jr. (1986). Pressure-flow effects on endurance of inspiratory muscles. *J. Appl. Physiol.*, 60:299–303.

McCool, F. D., Tzelepis, G. E., Leith, D. E., and Hoppin, F. C., Jr. (1989). Oxygen cost of breathing during fatiguing inspiratory resistive loads. *J. Appl. Physiol.*, 66:2045–2055.

McGregor, M., and Becklake, M. R. (1961). The relationship of oxygen cost of breathing to respiratory mechanical work and respiratory force. *J. Clin. Invest.*, 40:91–980.

McIlroy, M. D., Marshall, R., and Christie, R. V. (1954). The work of breathing in normal subjects. *Clin. Sci.*, 13:127–136.

McKenzie, D. K., and Gandevia, S. C. (1991). Recovery from fatigue of human diaphragm and limb muscles. *Resp. Physiol.*, 84:49–60.

McKenzie, D. K., Bigland-Ritchie, B., Gorman, R. B., and Gandevia, S. C. (1992). Central and peripheral fatigue of human diaphragm and limb muscles assessed by twitch interpolation. *J. Physiol.* (London), 454:643–656.

Mead, J. (1960). Control of respiratory frequency. *J. Appl. Physiol.*, 15:325–336.

Mense, S., and Stahnke, M. (1983). Responses in muscle afferent fibers of slow conduction velocity to contractions and ischemia in the cat. *J. Physiol.* (London), 342:383–397.

Merton, P. A. (1954). Voluntary strength and fatigue. *J. Physiol.* (London), 13:553–564.

Merton, P. A., Hill, D. K., and Morton, H. B. (1981). Indirect and direct stimulation of fatigued human muscle. In *Human Muscle Fatigue; Physiological Mechanisms.* Edited by R. Porter and J. Whelan. London, Pitman Medical, pp. 120–126.

Milic-Emili, J. (1986). Editorial: Is weaning an art or a science? *Am. Rev. Respir. Dis.*, 134:1107–1108.

Milic-Emili, J., and Petit, J. M. (1959). Il lavoro meccanicio della respirazione a varia frequenza respiratoria. *Arch. Sci. Biol.* (Bologna), 43:326–330.

Milner-Brown, H. S., Stein, R. B., and Yemm, R. (1973a). The orderly recruitment of human motor units during voluntary isometric contractions. *J. Physiol.* (London), 230:359–370.

Milner-Brown, H. S., Stein, R. B., and Yemm, R. (1973b). Changes in firing rate of human motor units during linearly changing voluntary contractions. *J. Physiol.* (London), 230:371–390.

Monod, H., and Scherrer, J. (1965). The work capacity of a synergic muscular group. *Ergonomics*, 8:329–337.

Mortimer, J. T., Magnusson, R., and Peterson, I. (1970). Conduction velocity in ischemic muscle: effect on EMG frequency spectrum. *Am. J. Physiol.*, 219:1324–1329.

Mosso, A. (1914). *Fatigue.* 3rd edition. Translated by M. Drummond. London, Allen and Urwin, p. 334.

Moulds, R. F. W., Young, A., Jones, D. A., and Edwards, R. H. T. (1977). A study of the contractility, biochemistry, and morphology of an isolated preparation of human skeletal muscles. *Clin. Sci. Mol. Med.*, 50:291–297.

Moxham, J., Wiles, C. M., Newham, D., and Edwards, R. H. T. (1980). Sternomastoid muscle function and fatigue in man. *Clin. Sci. Mol. Med.*, 59:463–468.

Moxham, J., Morris, A. J. R., Spiro, S. G., Edwards, R. H. T., and Green, M. (1981a). Contractile properties and fatigue of the diaphragm in man. *Thorax*, 36:164–168.

Moxham, J., Wiles, C. M., Newham, D., and Edwards, R. H. T. (1981b). Contractile function and fatigue. In *Human Muscle Fatigue: Physiological Mechanisms.* Edited by R. Porter and J. Whelan. London, Pitman Medical, pp. 197–205.

Moxham, J., Edwards, R. H. T., Aubier, M., De Troyer, A., Farkas, G., Macklem, P. T., and Roussos, C. (1982). Changes in the EMG power spectrum (high/low ratio) with force fatigue in man. *J. Appl. Physiol.*, 53:1094–1099.

Muller, N., Bryan, A. C., and Aamel, N. (1980). Tonic inspiratory activity as a cause of a hyperinflation in histamine induced asthma. *J. Appl. Physiol.*, 49:869.

Mulvey, D. A., Koulouris, N. G., Elliott, M. W., Moxham, J., and Green, M. (1991a). Maximal relaxation rate of inspiratory muscle can be effort dependent and reflect the activation of fast-twitch fibers. *Am. Rev. Respir. Dis.*, 144:803–806.

Mulvey, D. A., Koulouris, N. G., Elliott, M. W., Laroche, C. M., Moxham, J., and Green, M. (1991b). Inspiratory muscle relaxation rate after voluntary maximal isocapnic ventilation in humans. *J. Appl. Physiol.*, 70:2173–2180.

Nakamura, Y., and Schwartz, A. (1970). Possible control of intracellular calcium metabolism by (H+): sarcoplasmic reticulum of skeletal and cardiac muscle. *Biochem. Biophys. Res. Commun.*, 41:830–836.

Nassar-Gentina, V., Passonneau, J. V., Vergara, J. L., and Rapoport, S. I. (1975). Metabolic correlates of fatigue and of recovery from fatigue in single frog muscle fibers. *J. Gen. Physiol.*, 72:593–606.

Nava, S., Zanotti, E., Ambrosio, N., Fracchia, C., Scarabelli, C., and Rampula, C. (1992). Evidence of acute diaphragmatic fatigue in a "natural" condition. The diaphragm in labor. *Am. Rev. Respir. Dis.*, 146:1226–1230.

Nava, S., and Bellemare, F. (1989). Cardiovascular failure and apnea in shock. *J. Appl. Physiol.*, 66:184–189.

Needham, D. (1971). *Machina Carnia.* London, Cambridge University Press.

Newham, D. J., Mills, K. R., McPhail, G., and Edwards, R. H. T. (1982). Muscle damage in response to exercise. *Eur. J. Clin. Invest.*, 12:29.

NHLBI Workshop Respiratory Muscle Fatigue. (1990). Report of the Respiratory Muscle Fatigue Workshop Group. *Am. Rev. Respir. Dis.*, 142:474–480.

Nichols, D. G., Buck, J. R., Eleff, S. M., Shungu, D. C., Robotham, J. L., Koehler, R. C., and Traystman, R. J. (1993). Diaphragmatic fatigue assessed by 31P-magnetic resonance spectroscopy in vivo. *Am. J. Physiol.*, 264:C1111–1118.

Nordstrom, M. A., and Miles, T. S. (1991). Instability of motor unit firing rates during prolonged isometric contractions in human masseter. *Brain Res.*, 549:268–274.

Otis, A. B. (1954). The work of breathing. *Physiol. Rev.*, 34:449–458.

Person, R. S., and Kudina, L. B. (1972). Discharge frequency and discharge pattern of human motor units during voluntary contractions of muscle. *EEG Clin. Neurophysiol.*, 32:471–483.

Petrozzino, J. J., Scardella, A. T., Santiago, T. V., and Edelman, N. H. (1992). Dichloroacetate blocks endogenous opioid effects during inspiratory flow resistive loading. *J. Appl. Physiol.*, 72:590–596.

Reid, C. (1928). the mechanism of voluntary muscular fatigue. *Q.J. Exp. Psychol.*, 19:17–42.

Robertson, C. H., Jr., Pagel, M. A., and Johnson, R. L., Jr. (1977). The distribution of blood flow, oxygen consumption, and work output among the respiratory muscles during unobstructed hyperventilation. *J. Clin. Invest.*, 59:43–50.

Robertson, S., and Kerrick, W. (1976). The effect of pH on submaximal and maximal Ca^{++} activated tension in skinned frog skeletal fibers. *Biophys. J.*, 16:73A.

Roussos, C., and Macklem, P. T. (1977). Diaphragmatic fatigue in man. *J. Appl. Physiol.*, 43:189–197.

Roussos, C. (1979). Respiratory muscle fatigue in the hypercapnic patient. *Bull. Eur. Physiopathol. Respir.*, 15:117–123.

Roussos, C., Fixley, M., Gross, D., and Macklem, P. T. (1979. Fatigue of inspiratory muscles and their synergistic behavior. *J. Appl. Physiol.*, 46:897–904.

Roussos, C., and Aubier, M. (1981). Neural drive and electromechanical alterations in the fatiguing diaphragm. In *Human Muscle Fatigue: Physiological Mechanisms*. Edited by R. Porter and J. Whelan. London, Pitman Medical, pp. 213–233.

Roussos, C. (1982). The failing ventilatory pump. *Lung*, 160:59–84.

Roussos, C. (1984). Ventilatory muscle fatigue governs breathing frequency. *Clin. Respir. Physiol.*, 20:445–451.

Scardella, A. T., Parisi, R. A., Phair, D. K., Santiago, T. V., and Edelman, N. H. (1986). The role of endogenous opioids in the ventilatory response to acute flow-resistive loads. *Am. Rev. Respir. Dis.*, 133:26–31.

Scardella, A. T., Petrozzino, J. J., Mandel, M., Edelman, N. H., and Santiago, T. V. (1990). Endogenous opioids effects on abdominal muscle activity during inspiratory loading. *J. Appl. Physiol.*, 69:1104–1109.

Scardella, A. T., Santiago, T. V., and Edelman, N. H. (1989). Naloxone alters the early response to an inspiratory flow-resistive load. *J. Appl. Physiol.*, 67:1747–1753.

Shee, C. D., and Cameron, I. R. (1990). The effect of pH and hypoxia on function and intracellular pH of the rat diaphragm. *Resp. Physiol.*, 79:57–68.

Shepard, R. J. (1967). The maximum sustained voluntary ventilation in exercise. *Clin. Sci.*, 32:167–176.

Sieck, G. C., Fournier, M., and Blanco, C. E. (1991). Diaphragm fatigue resistance during postnatal development. *J. Appl. Physiol.*, 71:458–464.

Simolowski, T., Fleury, B., Launois, S., Cathala, H. P., Bouche P., and Derenne, J. P. (1989). Cervical magnetic stimulation: a painless method for bilateral phrenic nerve stimulation in conscious humans. *J. Appl. Physiol.*, 67:1311–1318.

Stephens, J. A., and Taylor, A. (1972). Fatigue of maintained voluntary muscle contraction in man. *J. Physiol.* (London), 220:1–18.

Supinski, G. S., Clary, S. J., Bark, H., and Kelsen, S. G. (1987). Effect of inspiratory muscle fatigue on perception of effort during loaded breathing. *J. Appl. Physiol.*, 62:300–307.

Supinski, G., Dimarco, A., Ketai, L., Hussein, F., and Altose, M. (1988). Reversibility of diaphragm fatigue by mechanical hyperperfusion. *Am. Rev. Respir. Dis.*, 138:604–609.

Supinski, G. S., DiMarco, A. F., Hussein, F., and Altose, M. D. (1989). Alterations in respiratory muscle activation in the ischemic fatigued diaphragm. *J. Appl. Physiol.*, 67:720–729.

Supinski, G. S., Dick, T., Stofan, D., and DiMarco, A. F. (1993). Effects of intraphrenic injection of potassium on diaphragm activation. *J. Appl. Physiol.*, 74:1186–1194.

Tenney, S. M., and Reese, R. E. (1968). The ability to sustain great breathing efforts. *Respir. Physiol.*, 5:187–201.

Thomas, C., Woods, J. J., and Bigland-Ritchie, B. (1989). Impulse propagation and muscle activation in long maximal voluntary contractions. *J. Appl. Physiol.*, 67:1835–1842.

Thomas, C. K., Bigland-Ritchie, B., and Johanson, R. S. (1991a). Force-frequency relationships of human thenar motor units. *J. Neurophysiol.*, 65:1509–1516.

Thomas, C. K., Johanson, R. S., and Bigland-Ritchie, B. (1991b). Attempts to physiologically classify human thenar motor units. *J. Neurophysiol.*, 65:1501–1508.

Tobin, M. J., Press, V., and Guenther, S. M. (1986). The pattern of breathing during successful and unsuccessful trials of weaning from mechanical ventilation. *Am. Rev. Respir. Dis.*, 134:1111–1118.

Tobin, M. J., Perez, W., Guenther, S. M., Lodato, R. F., and Dantzker, D. R. (1987). Does rib-cage abdominal paradox signify respiratory muscle fatigue? *J. Appl. Physiol.*, 63:851–860.

Tzelepis, G. E., McCool, F. D., Leith, D. E., and Hoppin, F. G., Jr. (1988). Increased lung volume impairs endurance of inspiratory muscles. *J. Appl. Physiol.*, 64:1796–1802.

Vianna, L. G., Koulouris, N., Lanigan, C., and Moxham, J. (1990). Effect of acute hypercapnia on limb muscle contractility in humans. *J. Appl. Physiol.*, 69(4):1486–1493.

Vigreux, B., Cnockaert, J. C., and Pertuzon, E. (1980). The effect of fatigue on the series elastic component of human muscle. *Eur. J. Appl. Physiol.*, 45:11–17.

Vollestad, N. K., Sejersted, O. M., Bahr, R., Woods, J. J., and Bigland-Ritchie, B. (1988). Motor drive and metabolic responses during repeated submaximal contractions in humans. *J. Appl. Physiol.*, 64:1421–1427.

Waller, A. D. (1891). The sense of effort: an objective study. *Brain*, 14:179–249.

Ward, M. E., Eidelman, D., Stubbing, D. G., Bellemare, F., and Macklem, P. T. (1988). Respiratory sensation and pattern of respiratory muscle activation during diaphragm fatigue. *J. Appl. Physiol.*, 65:2181–2189.

Westerblad, H., Lee, J. A., Lannergren, J., and Allen, D. G. (1991). Cellular mechanisms of fatigue in skeletal muscle. *J. Appl. Physiol.*, 261:C195–C209.

Wiles, C. M., Jones, D. A., and Edwards, R. H. T. (1981). Fatigue in human metabolic myopathy. In *Human Muscle Fatigue: Physiological Mechanisms*. Edited by R. Porter and J. Whelan. London, Pitman Medical, pp. 264–282.

Wilkie, D. (1981). Shortage of chemical fuel as a cause of fatigue. In *Human Muscle Fatigue: Physiological Mechanisms*. Edited by R. Porter and J. Whelan. London, Pitman Medical, pp. 102–114.

Wilson, S. H., Cooke, N. T., Moxham, J., and Spiro, S. G. (1984). Sternomastoid muscle function and fatigue in normal subjects and in patients with chronic obstructive pulmonary disease. *Am. Rev. Respir. Dis.*, 129:460–464.

Wragg, S., Aquilina, R., Moran, J., Hanmegerd, C., Green, M., and Moxham, J. (1992). Diaphragm fatigue following maximum ventilation in man. *Am. Rev. Respir. Dis.*, 145:A147 (abstract).

Yan, S., Similowski, T., Gauthier, A. P., Macklem, P. T., and Bellemare, F. (1992). Effect of fatigue on diaphragmatic at different lung volumes. *J. Appl. Physiol.*, 72:1064–1067.

Yan, S., Gauthier, A. P., Similowski, T., Faltus, R., Macklem, P. T., and Bellemare, F. (1993). Force-frequency relationships of in vivo human and in vitro rat diaphragm using paired stimuli. *Eur. Respir. J.*, 6:211–218.

Zocche, G. P., Fritts, H. W., and Cournard, A. (1960). Fraction of maximum breathing capacity available for prolonged hyperventilation. *J. Appl. Physiol.*, 15:1073–1074.

50

Inspiratory Pump Performance

A Pressure–Flow–Volume Framework

F. DENNIS McCOOL

Brown University Medical School
Providence
Memorial Hospital of Rhode Island
Pawtucket, Rhode Island

FREDERIC G. HOPPIN, Jr.

Brown University Medical School
Providence, Rhode Island

GEORGE E. TZELEPIS

Onassis Cardiosurgical Center
Athens, Greece

I. Introduction

The performance of the inspiratory pump can be characterized by the pressure, flow, and volume achieved, and these in turn depend on the force, velocity, and length of the inspiratory muscles (Rahn et al., 1946; Agostoni and Rahn, 1960; Agostoni and Fenn, 1960; Loring et al., 1985). The description of performance in terms of pressure, flow, and volume is analogous to that which has been applied so successfully over the past 30 years to the cardiac pump, leading to a better understanding of ventricular performance (Fry et al., 1964; Gault et al., 1968; Brutsaert and Sonnenblick, 1969; Strobeck and Sonnenblick, 1986) and to a number of routine invasive and noninvasive tests of cardiac performance. The situation in the respiratory system is different from the heart for several reasons. The inspiratory pump is comprised of a number of muscles that not only operate in concert with one another to sustain ventilation but are also used to perform nonrespiratory trunk tasks. These muscles vary in their operational lengths and the lung volume at which optimal tension is developed (Braun et al., 1982; Decramer and DeTroyer, 1984). The configuration of the respiratory system and the manner in which the muscles are coupled to the system profoundly impact on performance. Finally, the inspiratory pump depends on neural activation rather than pacemaker cells, and the degree of neural activation may vary among muscles and from breath to breath. Nonetheless, the classical force–velocity–length properties of skeletal muscle (Fenn and Marsh, 1935; Bahler et al., 1968) are readily apparent in pressure–flow–volume performance of the respiratory system as in the heart.

This chapter discusses how the pressure–flow–volume and force–velocity–length frameworks may be applied to the performance of the inspiratory pump, its energetics, its ability to sustain ventilation against a load, and how this approach may clarify some clinical issues.

II. Maximal Performance

Although the performance of the inspiratory pump may be characterized by three variables—pressure, flow, and volume—the focus historically has been largely on pairs of these variables.

Inspiratory pressure-volume relationships were first described during single maximal inspiratory efforts by Rahn et al. (1946). They attributed the difference between the pressure developed during muscular effort and that during relaxation condition to the muscles (P_{mus}). P_{mus} during maximal inspiratory efforts against an occluded airway ($P_{mus, max, stat}$) was greatest at volumes near the relaxation volume of the respiratory system (V_{relax}) and fell off at higher volumes (Fig. 1).

This effect of lung volume reflects in part the change of the mechanical advantage of the inspiratory muscles on the respiratory system (e.g., the decrease of the curvature of the diaphragm at high lung volumes) and in part the intrinsic force-length relationship of skeletal muscle, namely, that the tension developed by a muscle for a given level of activation is greatest at one length (l_o) and decreases at longer or shorter lengths. The greatest $P_{mus, max, stat}$ are seen at volumes close to

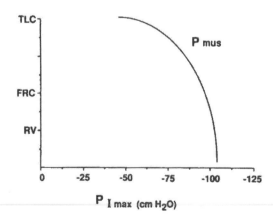

Figure 1 Pressure-volume relationships for the inspiratory muscles. The optimal volume for pressure generation is near FRC. (Adapted from Rahn et al., 1946.)

the relaxation volume of the respiratory system (V_{relax}) where diaphragm length is near its optimal for tension generation (l_o) and its configuration is most favorable (Kim et al., 1976; Road et al., 1986).

A similar relationship between volume and pressure has been shown for submaximal externally stimulated contractions of the diaphragm. Using transcutaneous stimulation of one phrenic nerve, Pengelly et al. (1971) demonstrated that the pressure generated by the human diaphragm (transdiaphragmatic pressure) decreases linearly with increasing lung volume. Smith and Bellemare (1987) extended these observations, using percutaneous twitch activation of the phrenic nerves. The decline in Pdi twitch amplitude with increasing lung volume was in close agreement with the in vitro force-length relationship of the diaphragm reported by others, suggesting that the diminished ability of the diaphragm to generate pressure at high lung volumes is due more to changes in length-tension properties of the diaphragm than to changes in mechanical advantage.

The above studies show that the effectiveness of the diaphragm as a pressure generator decreases with increasing lung volume. Less is known about the effect of increasing lung volume on the force-generating capacity of the rib cage muscles. In contrast to the diaphragm, which shortens by 30–40% (Braun et al., 1982; Newman et al., 1984), the parasternals in dogs only shorten by 7–8% over the inspiratory capacity range (Decramer and DeTroyer, 1984; Farkas et al., 1985). Furthermore, Brancatisano et al. (1993) found that the pressure generated by the rib cage muscles for a given degree of activation decreased at high lung volumes much more than would be expected just from changes in the length-tension properties of the muscle. These two observations suggest that, unlike the diaphragm, the ineffectiveness of the rib cage muscles in generating pressure at high lung volumes is predominantly due to changes in their mechanical advantage.

Inspiratory pressure-flow relationships were first described during single maximal inspiratory efforts by Agostoni and Fenn (1960). They showed that the inspiratory pressure recorded at a given lung volume decreases as inspiratory flow increases. This relationship is analogous to the force-velocity relationship described for isolated skeletal muscle (Wilke, 1950; Abbott and Wilke, 1953; Ritchie, 1954; Bahler et al., 1968), namely, for a given level of activation, the tension developed by a skeletal muscle decreases as the velocity of shortening increases.

Data for pressure-flow plots can be gathered by measuring esophageal pressure (Pes), inspiratory flow ($\dot{V}i$), and lung volume ($\dot{V}L$) during single maximal inspiratory efforts through varied external resistances. Values of Pes and $\dot{V}i$ are plotted at a given VL for each breath through the range of resistances (Fig. 2). As predicted by the force–velocity relationship, Pes and $\dot{V}i$ are negatively related (Agostoni and Fenn, 1960; Hyatt and Flath, 1966; McCool et al., 1990); $\dot{V}i$ is maximal when the inspiratory resistance is low such as during breaths with no external loads, and Pes is maximal when $\dot{V}i$ is zero, i.e., with complete airway occlusion. Topulos et al. (1987) extended these studies to pleiometric (lengthening) contractions and found, again as predicted from the force–velocity relationship of isolated skeletal muscle,

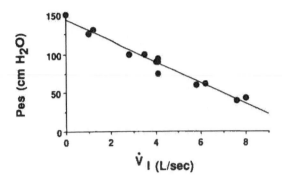

Figure 2 Inspiratory pressure-flow relationship. Analogous to the force-velocity relationship for muscle, maximal pressure (force) is achieved when external flow is zero. As inspiratory flow (velocity) increases, the pressure generated is less than maximal. (Adapted from Topulos et al., 1987.)

that the pressure generated is even greater when the muscle is being forcibly lengthened when it is activated. This phenomenon may be relevant to maneuvers designed to elicit maximal transdiaphragmatic pressure because subtle lengthening during voluntary maneuvers may increase measured pressure above truly static conditions (Gandevia and McKenzie, 1988).

Pressure is expected to relate directly to force and flow to velocity, however, the relationship of pressure to flow appears to be somewhat different from that of force to velocity. Although there is a modest degree of variation in the slopes of these relationships reported in different studies, the pressure–flow relationship is consistently reported to be linear, and this differs from the curvilinear force–velocity relationship reported for isolated muscle. The discrepancy may be illusory. In the respiratory system, even with no external loads, inspiration always has significant internal elastic and resistive properties. Thus the truly unloaded end of the force–velocity range has not been described in vitro. Indeed, the speed of shortening of the diaphragm during a maximal breathing capacity maneuver may be only half of the maximal unloaded speed of shortening of the truly unloaded diaphragm in vitro (Rochester, 1982). Another possible explanation is that the alinearity of the performance of the individual muscle groups contributing to the pressure–flow relationship is obscured as they act in concert to optimize performance.

The maximal inspiratory pressure–flow relationship may be altered transiently by fatiguing breathing tasks. Fatigue can be defined as a reversible decrease in performance and is quantifiable as depression of the pressure–flow curve. There has been some interest in the extent to which specific fatiguing tasks might have specific effects on the different ends of the maximal pressure–flow curve. Indeed, fatigue induced by high external resistance tasks appears to reduce maximal static pressure but not maximal flows (Fig. 3) (Bai et al., 1984; McCool et al., 1992). The explanation appears not to lie in the properties of the muscle itself; in isolated

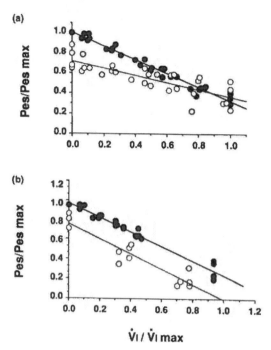

Figure 3 A composite of the inspiratory isovolume pressure–flow relationship during single maximal efforts for five subjects. (a) Control data (•); there is a greater reduction of pressure and a sparing of maximal inspiratory flow with fatigue induced by pressure loads (o). (b) Control data (•); there is a reduction of both pressure and flow with fatigue induced by hyperpnea (o). (Adapted from McCool et al., 1992.)

mammalian muscle, fatigue induced either by low force–high velocity contractions or by high force–low velocity contractions reduce both force and velocity (Seow and Stevens, 1988; Zhang and Kelsen, 1989). The explanation may instead lie in selective fatigue of the intrinsic muscles of the rib cage by high resistance tasks, sparing the diaphragm and thus sparing maximal inspiratory flow (Hershenson et al., 1989). In contrast, the fatigue induced by hyperpnea in normal subjects reduces both maximal static pressure and maximal inspiratory flow (McCool et al., 1992).

The maximal pressure–flow curve may also be altered by training. Here the effects appear to be specific to the type of training employed. In particular, the greatest increases in pressure occur following training with severe inspiratory resistive loads or with repetitive Mueller efforts, whereas the greatest increases in flow occur following training with hyperpnea or repetitive single maximal inspirations (Leith and Bradley, 1976; Tzelepis et al., 1992) (Fig. 4). These training-induced changes in the pressure–flow relationship also reflect known training-induced changes in muscle force–velocity relationships; isometric training specifically increases force, whereas

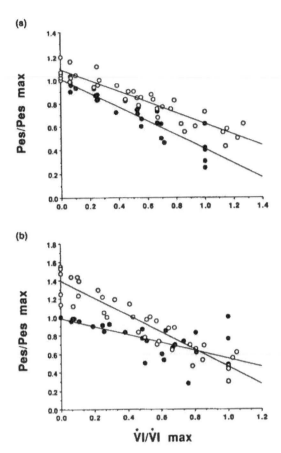

Figure 4 A composite of the inspiratory isovolume pressure–flow relationship for five subjects before (•) flow training (a) and pressure training (b). The greatest improvements in performance with both types of training (o) are in the area of the pressure–flow plane where the training occurs. (Adapted from Tzelepis et al., 1992.)

training with voluntary dynamic contractions increases maximum shortening velocity and not isometric force (Caiozzo et al., 1981; Coyle et al., 1981; Dachateau et al., 1984; Kanehisa and Miyashita, 1983). These varied effects of training may be relevant clinically when designing inspiratory muscle training protocols.

III. The Oxygen Cost of Breathing

At rest, the oxygen cost of breathing ($\dot{V}_{O_{2resp}}$) is only a small fraction (about 2%) of total body oxygen consumption. However, when the respiratory system is operating near its limits because of severe pressure (Roussos and Macklem, 1982) or flow loads (exercise hyperpnea) (Aaron et al., 1992), $\dot{V}_{O_2resp}$ increases substantially to values up to 1500 ml/min or approximately 10–15% of total body oxygen consumption.

Theoretical considerations predict that pressure and flow contribute independently to $\dot{V}_{O_2resp}$. During aerobic exercise, the oxygen consumed reflects the energetic costs of contraction. Mommaerts (1969) defined these costs in the equation:

$$DUt = W + ax + A + f(p,t) \qquad (1)$$

where DUt is the total energy cost of muscle contraction, W is the external work performed, ax is the heat associated with shortening (a is a constant with units of force and x is the distance by which the muscle shortens), A is the heat of activation, and f(p,t) is the heat related to the intensity and duration of external force maintained. Pressure and flow are major independent variables in this equation through force and velocity, respectively, W is the time integral of force times velocity, x is the time integral of velocity, and p is the force. Pressure and flow, then, should be major determinants of $\dot{V}_{O_2resp}$.

This prediction is borne out experimentally. Campbell et al. (1957) estimated the energy costs of breathing in humans by measuring total body $\dot{V}_{O_2}$ during resting tidal breathing and again when respiratory muscle activity was heightened by hyperpnea or resistive breathing loads. The increment in whole body oxygen consumption was then attributed to the respiratory muscles ($\dot{V}_{O_2resp}$). With this technique, inspiratory flow has been shown to affect $\dot{V}_{O_2resp}$ (Campbell et al., 1958; Bartlett et al., 1958; Milic-Emili, 1960; McGregor and Becklake, 1961; McKerrow and Otis, 1956). There are some differences in the reported oxygen cost of breathing for reasons that are not clear. However, there is general agreement that in healthy subjects, as inspiratory flow rates increase, $\dot{V}_{O_2resp}$ increases hyperbolically and the oxygen cost of breathing may be as great as 18 ml O_2 per liter of ventilation (Fig. 5). The differences among subjects within a series may be due to physiological variation among subjects, in particular to variations in patterns of respiratory muscle use.

Experimental observations also confirm that pressure has an independent effect on $\dot{V}_{O_2resp}$. Using direct measurements of $\dot{V}_{O_2resp}$ in dogs, Rochester and Bettini (1981) found a linear relation between the pressure-time product and oxygen consumption of the diaphragm. In humans, McGregor and Becklake (1961) first noted that inspiratory pressure was a reliable predictor of $\dot{V}_{O_2resp}$. Field et al. (1984) further demonstrated a strong correlation between the pressure-time product and $\dot{V}_{O_2resp}$ during resistive loaded breathing.

The product of pressure and flow is the work rate or power ($\dot{W} = \int P\dot{V}$). It represents a variable fraction of the total oxygen consumed (Rochester and Briscoe, 1979). For example, external work accounts for none of the metabolic costs during an isometric effort because no external work is performed. Measurements of power in healthy subjects have been found to correlate well with $\dot{V}_{O_2resp}$ during hyperpnea

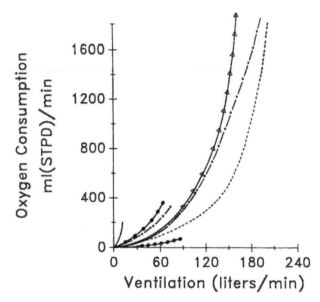

Figure 5 Results from several studies evaluating the oxygen cost of breathing at varying degrees of ventilation. As the minute ventilation increases, there is an increase in the oxygen cost of breathing. This relationship for patients with emphysema is depicted by the solid line. Note that the oxygen costs of breathing at any given level of ventilation is higher in these patients and that the maximal oxygen consumed is reduced when compared to normal subjects. (Adapted from Campbell et al., 1958.)

or breathing through minimal resistive loads (Collett et al., 1985) but have not been as tightly correlated with $\dot{V}_{O_{2resp}}$ as is the pressure-time product when measured during inspiratory resistive loading (Field et al., 1984). In this context, since less work is performed with severe pressure loads than with high ventilation loads, the pressure-time product may be more sensitive than power as a predictor of the energetic costs of muscle contraction.

Inspiratory muscle energetics have also been assessed by calculating the efficiency of breathing, i.e., the ratio of the work of breathing to the oxygen cost of breathing ($E_b = \Delta W / \Delta \dot{V}_{O_{2resp}}$). E_b has been calculated during inspiratory resistive loaded breathing (Field et al., 1984; Collett et al., 1985), hyperpnea (McCool et al., 1989), and breathing at varied lung volumes (Collett and Engel, 1986; McCool et al., 1989). The rather wide range of values for E_b among these studies is related in part to the inability to measure all components of work (e.g., elastic work of chest wall deformation). More importantly, however, it reflects systematic differences in the experimental design regarding inspiratory pressure, flow, and lung volume. Collett and Engel (1986) demonstrated that at high lung volumes, E_b was diminished by as much as 50% when subjects performed nonfatiguing inspiratory resistive breathing. McCool et al. (1989) extended their findings to fatiguing tasks performed over a wider range of flow rates and noted the E_b was also reduced during hyperpnea tasks performed at high lung volume. The reduction of efficiency at high lung volume may parallel similar changes in efficiency of skeletal muscle when activated at lengths less than l_0 (deHaan et al., 1986).

The reported effects of flow rate on efficiency are variable. Collett et al. (1985) found E_b to be nearly constant over a wide range of $\dot{V}I$ whereas Field et al. (1984) and McCool et al. (1989) noted that E_b varied with $\dot{V}I$. Differences between these studies may in part be related to studying fatiguing or nonfatiguing tasks. During fatiguing tasks, the efficiency of breathing is lower than for nonfatiguing tasks, probably due to the recruitment of other muscle groups that may not be as effective as the main inspiratory muscles. Furthermore, tasks performed through high external resistances may be less efficient than those performed at high flow rates. This may simply reflect the fact that the velocity of shortening in such tasks is less than the velocity at which peak efficiency of contraction occurs, i.e., about one third of the unloaded velocity (Baskin, 1965). Differences in the reported E_b among these studies may then be related to differences among fatiguing and nonfatiguing, resistive and hyperpnea loads.

IV. Inspiratory Muscle Endurance

A number of interactive factors determine the ability of the inspiratory pump to sustain its performance against loads (endurance). These include neural activation (Bellemare and Bigland-Ritchie, 1987), neural transmission across the neuromuscular junction (Aldrich et al., 1986), blood flow (Aubier et al., 1981), and impaired excitation-contraction coupling due to depletion of muscle energy stores or pH changes from lactic acid accumulation (Roussos and Macklem, 1982). The relationship between neural drive and fatigue has been reviewed in this book (i.e., central fatigue, transmission fatigue). This section focuses on factors that alter endurance of the inspiratory muscles themselves, in particular the effects of pressure, contraction time, flow, and lung volume. Finally, we discuss how these variables have been incorporated into indices for predicting inspiratory muscle endurance.

A. Pressure Effects

Inspiratory muscle endurance has been evaluated at the high-pressure pole of the pressure-flow relationship in experiments in which subjects breathed against high inspiratory resistive loads (Roussos and Macklem, 1977; Roussos et al., 1979, Bellemare and Grassino, 1982; McCool et al., 1986) (Fig. 6). Roussos and Macklem (1977) compared these pressure loads with the time that a breathing task could be sustained (T_{lim}) in normal subjects and found that the mean transdiaphragmatic pressure that could be sustained for prolonged periods was only 40% of its maximal

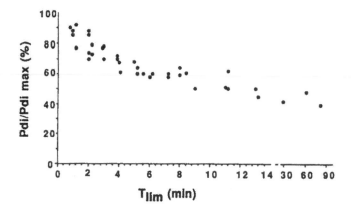

Figure 6 The relationship between mean transdiaphragmatic pressure developed per breath and the time an inspiratory resistive loaded breathing task can be sustained. The lower the ratio of Pdi to Pdi $_{max}$, the longer the task can be sustained. (Adapted from Roussos and Macklem, 1977.)

value (Pdi/Pdi $_{max}$ = 0.4). Pressure loads that required the muscles to generate greater forces led to earlier failure.

B. Contraction Time

Contraction time, uncontrolled in the study by Roussos and Macklem (1977), was subsequently evaluated by Bellemare and Grassino (1982). They found a systematic relationship between T_{lim} and the product of mean inspiratory pressure and duty cycle divided by maximal static Pdi (PTdi/Pdi $_{max}$). Breathing tasks characterized by PTdi/Pdi $_{max}$ of less than 0.15 could be sustained indefinitely, whereas those with PTdi/Pdi $_{max}$ of greater than 0.2 inevitably led to task failure.

C. Flow Effects

In the above studies the effects of inspiratory flow on endurance had not been evaluated. Indeed the findings of Roussos and Macklem (1977) and of Bellemare and Grassino (1982) were derived from studies performed over a wide range of inspiratory pressures but only a narrow range of inspiratory flow rates. By contrast, Tenney and Reese (1968) and Leith and Bradley (1976) evaluated inspiratory muscle endurance at the high flow pole of the pressure–flow relationship. In these experiments, during voluntary hyperpnea with eucapnia maintained by partial rebreathing or adding CO_2, T_{lim} decreased as the level of ventilation increased (Fig. 7). In general, a minute ventilation of less than 75% of the 12-s maximum breathing capacity (MBC) could be sustained indefinitely, whereas a greater ventilation load led to task failure.

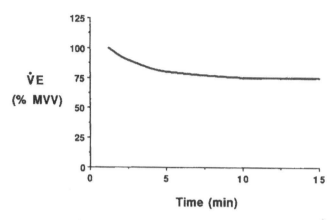

Figure 7 The relationship between ventilation expressed as a percent of the maximum voluntary ventilation and the time a hyperpnea breathing task can be sustained. As ventilation decreases to approximately 75% of the maximal voluntary ventilation, the hyperpnea can be sustained for at least 15 min. (Adapted from Leith and Bradley, 1976.)

D. Volume Effects

The effects of lung volume on inspiratory muscle endurance have also been described over the pressure-flow spectrum. Roussos et al. (1979) examined the effects of increased lung volume in the high-pressure range and showed that voluntary elevations in lung volume reduce the ability of normal subjects to breath against resistive loads. Tzelepis et al. (1988) extended their observations to include tasks at the intermediate and high-flow range. Again, increasing lung volume invariably decreased inspiratory muscle endurance. They attributed the diminished endurance to impairment of mechanical advantage or reduced muscle length. Although sustainable pressure is less, Clanton et al. (1993) showed that when expressed as a fraction of the maximal static pressure that can be achieved at the respective lung volumes, the sustainable pressures at high lung volumes are similar to those at lower lung volumes.

E. Interactions Among Factors

The above studies characterized inspiratory muscle endurance by utilizing tasks on the opposite ends of the pressure-flow spectrum. It seemed likely that these factors would interact in determining endurance. Indeed, the sustainable pressures at high flow rates were much lower in the study by Leith and Bradley (1976) than the sustainable pressures at low flow rates noted by Roussos and Macklem (1977). In order to explore such interactions and also to encompass the range of intermediate loads that might be imposed in exercise or disease, we evaluated endurance over a range of tasks from severe inspiratory resistive loads to unloaded hyperpnea (McCool et al., 1986) and found a linear tradeoff between the sustainable pressure-time product of esophageal pressure and inspiratory flow for tasks with a given T_{lim} (Fig. 8). This result is qualitatively similar to the pressure-flow behavior for single maximal efforts. The pressure-time product turned out to be a poor predictor of endurance when tested over the large range of flow rates studied, ranging from 0.31 for sustainable pressure-loaded tasks to 0.10 for sustainable flow-loaded tasks. Thus, a pressure-time product of less than 0.25 may be sustained indefinitely under the low flow circumstances studied by Bellemare and Grassino (1982) yet would lead to fatigue under the high-flow circumstances studied by Leith and Bradley (1976).

Clanton and coworkers (1993) also used the pressure–flow–volume framework to further evaluate the interrelationship of these variables on inspiratory muscle endurance. They found that, under varied conditions of pressure, flow, and volume, the pressure expressed as a fraction of the maximal pressure that the inspiratory pump can generate under the same conditions of pressure, flow, and volume ($P_{breath}/P_{dynamic\ max}$) can be used to predict endurance.

We postulated that the mechanism linking the effects of these variables might be a limiting rate of energy expenditure by the inspiratory muscles. This was supported by theoretical and experimental considerations (see above) that pressure and flow should contribute independently to energy consumption and by experimental results suggesting competition between pressure, flow, and duration of contraction in determining endurance. To test this hypothesis, we measured endurance (T_{lim}) and $\dot{V}_{O_{2resp}}$ in tasks with a wide range of pressures, flows, and volumes. We confirmed that $\dot{V}_{O_{2resp}}$, like T_{lim}, depended on pressure, flow, and volume. T_{lim}, moreover, was correlated with $\dot{V}_{O_{2resp}}$ and this relationship did not change with different combinations of pressure, flow, or volume (Fig. 9). There may be several mechanisms for the

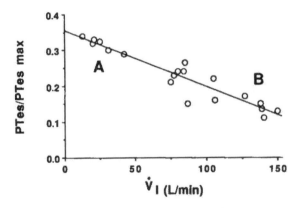

Figure 8 The tradeoff between pressure ($PTes/P_{max}$) and inspiratory flow ($\dot{V}_I$) for tasks that lead to fatigue in 8 min. Tasks labeled A are done through inspiratory resistive loads and are similar to those reported by Roussos and Macklem (1977). Tasks labeled B represent hyperpnea tasks and are similar to those reported by Leith and Bradley (1976). (Adapted from McCool et al., 1986.)

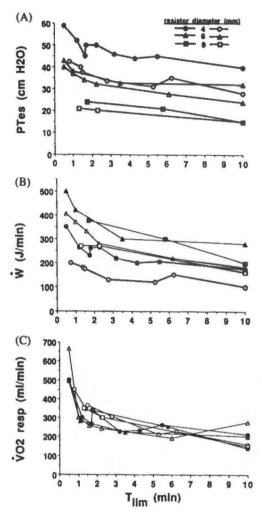

Figure 9 Relationship between T_{lim} and the esophageal pressure time product (A), work rate (B), and the oxygen cost of breathing (C) in one subject. In contrast to PTes and $\dot{W}$, there is no systematic variation of $\dot{V}_{O_{2resp}}$ with flow or lung volume at a given T_{lim}.

interactions between pressure, flow, and volume on $\dot{V}_{O_{2resp}}$ and endurance. The interaction of pressure and flow on energetics is presumably at the level of the sarcomere [Eq. (1)], whereas the interaction of lung volume may be through the gross mechanics of the system producing less pressure and flow for the same energy expenditure at high lung volumes. Whatever the mechanisms, the data are consistent with the notion that the endurance of the inspiratory muscles for a wide range of tasks depends on a limiting sustainable rate of energy consumption.

V. Clinical Relevance

Different diseases have rather distinct effects on the pressure–flow–volume capabilities of the inspiratory pump or on the pressure–flow–volume load presented to the inspiratory pump. Neuromuscular disorders (e.g., myasthenia, cachexia) primarily impair the pressure–flow capability of the pump. Thoracic deformity (e.g., kyphoscoliosis) may not reduce the pressure capability at FRC as much as it sharply constricts the volume axis of pump pressure–flow function. Flail chest and abnormal innervation of muscle groups (e.g., quadriplegia) lead to paradoxical movement of the chest wall, in effect impairing the flow capacity of the inspiratory pump. Restrictive diseases (e.g., pulmonary fibrosis, kyphoscoliosis, noncardiogenic pulmonary edema) impose pressure loads to ventilation. A different means of providing a pressure load may be seen in Parkinson's disease. Here, a pressure load is put on the agonist muscles of inspiration by activating antagonist muscles. In contrast, obstructive diseases generally impose a flow load through the increase of the V_D/V_T and a volume load by virtue of hyperinflation. In all these disorders, the ventilatory reserve (i.e., the extent to which sustainable performance exceeds ventilatory needs) is narrowed. The oxygen cost of breathing is likely increased in all disorders that impose pressure and flow loads and is documented to be increased and efficiency of breathing decreased in quadriplegia (Manning et al., 1992) and Parkinson's disease (Tzelepis et al., 1988) (Fig. 10). In Parkinson's disease this may be related to simultaneous activity of agonist and antagonist muscles and in quadriplegia to increased velocity of shortening of the diaphragm due to disordered

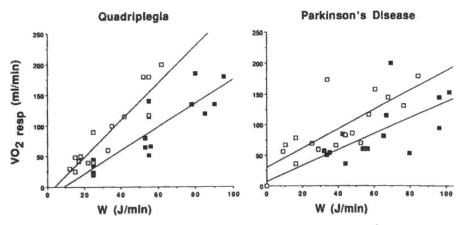

Figure 10   Relationship between oxygen cost of breathing ($\dot{V}_{O_{2resp}}$) and $\dot{W}_{tot}$ for normals (empty squares) and patients (filled squares) with quadriplegia or Parkinson's disease. Regression lines for the three groups are shown. The oxygen cost of breathing is higher in both patient groups when compared to normals. (Adapted from Tzelepis et al., 1988, and Manning et al., 1992.)

chest wall motion. It is likely that $\dot{V}_{O_{2resp}}$ and E_b are also reduced in restrictive diseases.

In view of the variety of pathological mechanisms, it should not be surprising that single indices of function have not been secure predictors of the ability to sustain ventilation when weaning from mechanical ventilation (Sahn and Lakshminar, 1973; Feeley and Hedley-White, 1975). Measurement of maximal inspiratory pressure (Black and Hyatt, 1969) addresses the capability of the inspiratory pump reasonably directly and is reduced by neuromuscular disorders or by hyperinflation as in acute asthma or excerbations of chronic obstructive pulmonary disease. It will not be very sensitive, however, to disorders affecting the pressure or flow load or flow capability of the inspiratory pump. Measurement of maximal flow has some appeal in theory, but in practice, it requires substantial patient cooperation and at best is not truly unloaded.

A less direct approach to assess weanability from mechanical ventilation is based on signs of distress in the breathing pattern, e.g., the ratio f/V_T (where f is frequency), essentially quantifying rapid shallow breathing (Tobin et al., 1986). A third approach has been to measure reserve directly comparing the pressure or flow load to the maximal pressure or flow capacity, the ratio $P_{breath}/P_{dynamic\ max}$ can be calculated as $(V_T/C_{rs})P_{dynamic\ max}$, where V_T is tidal volume and C_{rs} is the compliance of the respiratory system. Similarly, $\dot{V}_E/MVV$ can be calcalated where $\dot{V}_E$ is ventilation and MVV is maximal voluntary ventilation.

Combinations of such indices have been considered. Milic Emili (1986) derived the inspiratory effort quotient (IEQ), which consists of the elastic load to breathe (respiratory system compliance), breathing pattern (V_T and T_I/T_{TOT}), and the pressure reserve ($P_{I_{max}}$). Recently, Yang and Tobin (1991) calculated an index that also reflects the pressure load, breathing pattern, and pressure reserve in terms of respiratory system compliance, breathing frequency, and $P_{I_{max}}$, respectively. They found a positive predictive value of 0.71, which represented an improvement over measures of $P_{I_{max}}$ alone that had a positive predictive value of 0.59. Finally, Yang (1993) found that combining reserve ($P_I/P_{I_{max}}$) with an index of breathing pattern (f/V_T) provided the most accurate index of weanability yet with a sensitivity of 0.81 and a specificity of 0.93. These integrative indices represent improvements over single indices of pressure or flow demand and reserve. None tested have yet incorporated the full pressure-flow-volume assessment.

In summary, interpreting inspiratory pump performance in a pressure-flow-volume context clearly allows for a more complete description of performance than can be obtained by evaluating pairs of these variables alone. Furthermore, it facilitates comparisons with underlying mechanisms at the level of the sarcomere. These comparisons have already proved useful in understanding mechanisms of changes in pump performance that occur with changes in lung volume with fatigue or training and in disease. It may prove useful in providing a better framework to assess the ability of the pump to sustain required ventilation successfully.

References

Aaron, E. A., Seow, K. C., Johnson, B. D., and Dempsey, J. A. (1992). Oxygen cost of exercise hyperpnea: implications for performance. *J. Appl. Physiol.*, 72:1818–1825.

Abbott, B. C., and Wilkie, D. R. (1953). The relation between velocity of shortening and the tension-length curve of skeletal muscle. *J. Physiol.* (London), 120:214–223.

Agostoni, E., and Fenn, W. O. (1960). Velocity of muscle shortening as a limiting in respiratory airflow. *J. Appl. Physiol.*, 15:349–353.

Agostoni, E., and Rahn, H. (1960). Abdominal and thoracic pressures at different lung volumes. *J. Appl. Physiol.*, 15:1087–1092.

Aldrich, T. K., Shander, A., Chaudhry, I., and Nagashima, H. (1986). Fatigue of isolated rat diaphragm: Role of impaired neuromuscular transmission. *J. Appl. Physiol.*, 61:1077–1083.

Aubier, M., Trippenbach, T., and Roussos, C. (1981). Respiratory muscle fatigue during cardiogenic shock. *J. Appl. Physiol.*, 51:499–508.

Bahler, A. S., Fales, J. T., Zierler, K. L. (1968). The dynamic properties of mammalian skeletal muscle. *J. Gen. Physiol.*, 51:369–384.

Bai, T. R., Rabinovitch, B. J., and Pardy, R. L. (1984). Near-maximal voluntary hyperpnea and ventilatory muscle function. *J. Appl. Physiol.*, 57:1742–1748.

Bartlett, R. G., Jr., Brubach, H. F., Speecht, H. (1958). Oxygen cost of breathing. *J. Appl. Physiol.*, 12:413–424.

Baskin, R. J. (1965). The variation of muscle oxygen consumption with velocity of shortening. *J. Gen. Physiol.*, 49:9–15.

Bellemare, F., and Grassino, A. E. (1982). Effect of pressure and timing of contraction on human diaphragm fatigue. *J. Appl. Physiol.*, 53:1190–1195.

Black, L. F., and Hyatt, R. E. (1969). Maximal respiratory pressure: normal values and relationship to age and sex. *Am. Rev. Respir. Dis.*, 99:696–702.

Bradley, M. E., and Leith, D. E. (1978). Ventilatory muscle training and the oxygen cost of sustained hyperpnea. *J. Appl. Physiol.*, 45:885–892.

Brancatisano, A., Engel, L. E. and Loring, S. H. (1993). Lung volume and effectiveness of inspiratory muscles. *J. Appl. Physiol.*, 74:688–694.

Braun, N. M., Arora, N. S., and Rochester, D. F. (1982). Force-length relationship of the normal human diaphragm. *J. Appl. Physiol.*, 53:405–412.

Brutsaert, D. L., and Sonnenblick, E. H. (1969). Force-velocity-length-time relations of the contractile elements in heart muscle of the cat. *Circ. Res.*, 24:137–149.

Brutsaert, D. L., and Sonnenblick, E. H. (1974). Cardiac muscle mechanics in the evaluation of myocardial contractility and pump function: problems, concepts, and directions. *Prog. Cardiovasc. Dis.*, 16:337–361.

Caiozzo, V. J., Perrine, J. J., and Edgerton, V. R. (1981). Training induced adaptations of the in vivo force-velocity relationship of human muscle. *J. Appl. Physiol.*, 51:750–754.

Cala, S. J., Edyvean, J., Rynn, M. and Engel, L. A. (1992). O_2 cost of breathing; ventilatory vs pressure loads. *J. Appl. Physiol.*, 73:1720–1727.

Campbell, E. J. M., Westlake, E. K., Cherniack, R. M. (1957). Simple methods of estimating oxygen consumption and efficiency of the muscles of breathing. *J. Appl. Physiol.*, 11:303–308.

Campbell, E. J. M., Westlake, E. K., Cherniack, R. M. (1958). The oxygen consumption and efficiency of the respiratory muscles of young male subjects. *Clin. Sci.*, 18:55–64.

Clanton, T. L., Ameredes, B. T., Thomson, D. B., and Julian, M. W. (1990). Sustainable inspiratory pressures over varying flows, volumes, and duty cycles. *J. Appl. Physiol.*, 69:1875–1882.

Clanton, T. L., Hartman, E., and Julian, M. W. (1993). Preservation of sustainable inspiratory muscle pressure at increased end-expiratory lung volume. *Am. Rev. Resp. Dis.*, 147:385–391.

Collett, P. W., and Engel, L. A. (1986). Influence of lung volume on oxygen cost of resistive breathing. *J. Appl. Physiol.*, 61:16–24.

Collett, P. W., Perry, C., and Engel, L. A. (1985). Pressure-time product, flow, and oxygen cost of resistive breathing in humans. *J. Appl. Physiol.*, 58:1263–1272.

Coyle, E. F., Feiring, D. C., Rotkis, T. C., Cote, R. W., Roby, R. B., Lee, W., and Wilmore, J. H. (1981). Specificity of power improvements through slow and fast isokinetic training. *J. Appl. Physiol.*, 51:1437–1442.

Decramer, M., and DeTroyer, A. (1984). Respiratory changes in parasternal intercostal length. *J. Appl. Physiol.*, 57:1254–1260.

deHaan, A., deJong, J., van Doorn, J. E., Huijing, P. A., Woittiez, R. D., and Westra, H. G. (1986). Muscle economy of isometric contractions as a function of stimulation time and relative muscle length. *Pflugers Arch.*, 407:445–450.

Dodd, D. S., Collett, P. W., and Engel, L. A. (1988a). Influence of inspiratory flow rate and frequency on O2 cost of resistive breathing in humans. *J. Appl. Physiol.*, 65:760–766.

Dodd, D. S., Kelly, S., Collett, S. W., and Engel, L. A. (1988b). Pressure-time product, work rate, and endurance during resistive breathing in humans. *J. Appl. Physiol.*, 64:1397–1404.

Duchateau, J., and Hainut, K. (1984). Isometric or dynamic training: differential effects on mechanical properties of a human muscle. *J. Appl. Physiol.*, 56:296–301.

Farkas, G. A., Decramer, M., Rochester, D. F., and DeTroyer, A. (1985). Contractile properties of intercostal muscles and their functional significance. *J. Appl. Physiol.*, 59:528–535.

Feeley, T. W. and Hedley-White, J. (1975). Weaning from controlled ventilation and supplemental oxygen. *N. Engl. J. Med.*, 292:903–906.

Fenn, W. O., and Marsh, B. S. (1935). Muscular force at different speeds of shortening. *J. Physiol.*, 85:277–297.

Field, S., Sanci, S., and Grassino, A. (1984). Respiratory muscle oxygen consumption estimated by the diaphragm pressure-time index. *J. Appl. Physiol.*, 57:44–51.

Fry, D. L., Griggs, D. M., and Greenfield, J. C. (1964). Myocardial mechanics: Tension-velocity-length relationships in heart muscle. *Circ. Res.*, 14:73–85.

Gandevia, S. C., and McKenzie, D. K. (1988). Human diaphragmatic endurance during different maximal respiratory efforts. *J. Physiol.*, 395:625–638.

Gault, J. H., Ross, J., Jr., and Braunwald, E. (1968). Contractile state of the left ventricle in man. Instantaneous tension-velocity length relations in patients with and without disease of the left ventricular myocardium. *Circ. Res.*, 22:451–466.

Gordon, A. M., Huxley, A. F., and Julian, F. J. (1966). The variation in isometric tension with sarcomere length in vertebrate muscle fibers. *J. Physiol.* (London), 184:170–192.

Hershenson, M. B., Kikuchi, Y., Tzelepis, G. E., and McCool, F. D. (1989). Preferential fatigue of the rib cage muscles during inspiratory resistive loaded breathing. *J. Appl. Physiol.*, 66:750–754.

Hill, A. V. (1938). The heat of shortening and dynamic constants of muscle. *Proc. R. Soc. London Ser. B.*, 126:136–195.

Hill, A. V. (1964). The variation of total heat production in a twitch with velocity of shortening. *Proc. R. Soc. London Ser. B.*, 159:596–605.

Hyatt, R. E., and Flath, R. E. (1966). Relationship of airflow to pressure during maximal respiratory effort in man. *J. Appl. Physiol.*, 21:477–482.

Kanehisa, H., and Miyashita, M. (1983). Specificity of velocity in strength training. *Eur. J. Appl. Physiol.*, 52:104–106.

Kim, M., Druz, W. S., Dannon, J., Machnach, W., and Sharp, J. T. (1976). Mechanics of the canine diaphragm. *J. Appl. Physiol.*, 41:369–382.

Leith, D. E., and Bradley, M. (1976). Ventilatory muscle strength and endurance training. *J. Appl. Physiol.*, 41:508–516.

Loring, S. H., Mead, J., and Griscom, N. T. (1985). Dependence of diaphragmatic length on lung volume and thoracoabdominal configuration. *J. Appl. Physiol.*, 59:1961–1970.

Manning, A., McCool, F. D., Scharf, S. M., and Brown, R. (1992). Oxygen cost of resistive loaded breathing in quadriplegia. *J. Appl. Physiol.*, 73:825–831.

McCool, F. D., McCann, D. R., Leith, D. E., and Hoppin, F. G., Jr. (1986). Pressure-flow effects on endurance of inspiratory muscles. *J. Appl. Physiol.*, 60:299–303.

McCool, F. D., Tzelepis, G. E., Leith, D. E., and Hopping, F. G., Jr. (1989). Oxygen cost of breathing during fatiguing inspiratory resistive loads. *J. Appl. Physiol.*, 66:2045–2055.

McCool, F. D., Hershenson, M. B., Tzelepis, G. E., Kikuchi, Y., and Leith, D. E. (1992). Effects of fatigue on inspiratory muscle pressure-flow relationships. *J. Appl. Physiol.*, 73:36–43.

McGregor, M., and Becklake, M. R. (1961). The relationship of oxygen cost of breathing to respiratory mechanical work and respiratory force. *J. Clin. Invest.*, 40:971–980.

McKerrow, C. B., and Otis, A. B. (1956). Oxygen cost of hyperventilation. *J. Appl. Physiol.*, 9:375–379.

Milic-Emili, G., and Petit, J. M. (1960). Mechanical efficiency of breathing. *J. Appl. Physiol.*, 15:359–362.

Milic-Emili, J. (1986). Is weaning an art or a science? *Am. Rev. Respir. Dis.*, 134:1107–1108.

Mommaerts, W. F. (1969). Energetics of muscular contraction. *Physiol. Rev.*, 49:427–508.

Newman, S., Road, J., Bellemare, F., Clozel, J. P., Lavigne, C. M., and Grassino, A. (1984). Respiratory muscle length measured by sonomicrometry. *J. Appl. Physiol.*, 56:753–764.

Pengely, L. D., Anderson, A. M., and Milic-Emili, J. (1971). Mechanics of the diaphragm. *J. Appl. Physiol.*, 30:797–805.

Rahn, H., Otis, A. B., Chadwich, L. E., and Fenn, W. O. (1946). The pressure-volume diagram of the thorax and lung. *Am. J. Physiol.*, 146:161–178.

Ritchie, J. M. (1954). The relation between force and velocity of shortening in rat muscle. *J. Physiol.* (London), 123:633–639.

Road, J., Newman, S., Derene, J. P., Grassino, A. (1986). In vivo length-force relationship of canine diaphragm. *J. Appl. Physiol.*, 60:63–70.

Rochester, D. E., and Bettini, G. (1961). Diaphragmatic blood flow and energy expenditure in the dog. Effects of inspiratory airflow resistance and hyperpnea. *J. Clin. Invest.*, 40: 971–980.

Rochester, D. F., and Arora, N. S. (1983). Respiratory muscle failure. *Med. Clin. North Am.*, 67:573–597.

Rochester, D. F., and Briscoe, A. M. (1979). Metabolism of the working diaphragm. *Am. Rev. Respir. Dis.*, 119 (suppl):101–106.

Roussos, C., Fixley, M., Gross, D., et al. (1979). Fatigue of inspiratory muscles and their synergic behavior. *J. Appl. Physiol.*, 46:897–904.

Roussos, C., and Macklem, P. T. (1977). Diaphragmatic fatigue in man. *J. Appl. Physiol.*, 43:189–197.

Roussos, C., and Macklem, P. T. (1982). The respiratory muscles. *N. Engl. J. Med.*, 307:786–797.

Sahn, S. A., and Lakshminarayan, S. (1973). Bedside criteria for discontinuation of mechanical ventilation. *Chest*, 63:1003–1005.

Seow, C. Y., and Stephens, N. L. (1988). Fatigue of mouse diaphragm muscle in isometric and isotonic contractions. *J. Appl. Physiol.*, 64:2388–2393.

Smith, J., and Bellemare, F. (1987). Effects of lung volume on in vivo contraction characteristics of human diaphragm. *J. Appl. Physiol.*, 62:1893–1900.

Stainsby, W. M., and Barclay, J. K. (1976). Effect of initial length on relations between oxygen uptake and load in dog muscle. *Am. J. Physiol.*, 230:1008–1012.

Strobeck, J. E., and Sonnenblick, E. H. (1986). Myocardial contractile properties and ventricular performance. In *The Heart and Cardiovascular System*. Edited by H. A. Fozzard et al. New York, Raven Press, pp. 31–49.

Tenney, S. M., and Reese, R. E. (1958). The ability to sustain great breathing efforts. *Respir. Physiol.*, 5:187–201.

Tobin, M. J., Perez, W., Guenther, S. M., Semmes, B. J., Mador, M. J., Allen, S. J., Lodato, R. F., and Dantzker, D. R. (1986). The pattern of breathing during successful and unsuccessful trails of weaning from mechanical ventilation. *Am. Rev. Respir. Dis.*, 134:1111–1118.

Topulos, G. P., Reid, M. B., and Leith, D. E. (1987). Pleiometric activity of inspiratory muscles: maximal pressure-flow curves. *J. Appl. Physiol.*, 62:322–327.

Tzelepis, G. E., McCool, F. D., Friedman, J. H., and Hoppin, F. G., Jr. (1988a). Respiratory muscle dysfunction in Parkinson's disease. *Am. Rev. Resp. Dis.*, 138:266–271.

Tzelepis, G. E., McCool, F. D., Leith, D. E., and Hoppin, F. G., Jr. (1988b). Increased lung volume limits endurance of inspiratory muscles. *J. Appl. Physiol.*, 64:1796–1802.

Tzelepis, G. E., Vega, D., Patel, P., Fulambarker, A., and McCool, F. D. (1992). Pressure-flow specificity of inspiratory muscle training. *Am. Rev. Respir. Dis.*, 145:A151.

Wilkie, D. R. (1950). The relation between force and velocity in human muscle. *J. Physiol.* (London), 110:249–280.

Yang, K. L. (1993). Inspiratory pressure/maximal inspiratory pressure ratio: a predictive index of weaning outcome. *Intensive Care Med.*, 19:204–208.

Yang, K. L., and Tobin, M. J. (1991). A prospective study of indexes predicting the outcome of trials of weaning from mechanical ventilation. *N. Engl. J. Med.*, 324:1445–1450.

Zhang, R. A., and Kelsen, S. G. (1989). Effect of fatigue on diaphragmatic muscle shortening velocity and power output. *Am. Rev. Resp. Dis.*, 139:A167.

51

The Respiratory Muscles in Sepsis

JORGE BOCZKOWSKI

Institut National de la Santé et
de la Recherche Médicale
Faculté Xavier Bichat
Paris, France

MICHEL AUBIER

Université de Paris
Paris, France

I. Introduction

Sepsis remains an urgent medical problem, being an increasingly common cause of morbidity and mortality, particularly in elderly, immunocompromised, and critically ill patients. In fact, severe sepsis has been reported to be presently the most common cause of death in the noncoronary intensive care unit in the United States (Bone et al., 1992).

From the earliest observations of the sepsis phenomenon, it has been evident that respiratory failure is a major manifestation of this pathological condition. In fact, 25 years ago, Clowes and coworkers (1968) reported that "life-threatening respiratory insufficiency frequently accompanies extensive infections located in other parts of the body." From this moment to now, respiratory failure during sepsis has been traditionally related to secondary lung injury, defined by Petty and Ashbaug (1971) in the 1970s as the adult respiratory distress syndrome (ARDS). While not the sole cause of ARDS, sepsis remains the most common condition precipitating this catastrophic complication, which is associated, in septic patients, with mortality rates as high as 60–80% (Montgomery et al., 1985).

Recent experimental data suggest that ARDS is not the only cause of respiratory failure during sepsis. In fact, a large body of experimental evidence has become available in the last 5–10 years demonstrating failure of the respiratory muscles during sepsis. Since maintenance of ventilation depends on the ability of the respiratory muscles to generate force, dysfunction of these muscles during sepsis can lead to hypoventilation and respiratory failure, being thus life-threatening.

In this chapter, we will review first the effects of sepsis on respiratory muscle function and then the possible mechanisms involved in the genesis of this phenomenon.

II. Preliminary Considerations

Before describing the effects of sepsis on the respiratory muscles, two points must be stressed.

A. Definition of Sepsis

It is important to make clear the definition of sepsis to be used in this chapter. Until quite recently the general term "sepsis" was a source of considerable confusion in animal models and clinical studies because it referred to different conditions in different studies. In order to clarify this situation, a consensus definition of sepsis and its related conditions was recently proposed (Bone et al., 1992). From a clinical standpoint, sepsis can be defined as the systemic inflammatory response to infection manifested by two or more of the following conditions as the result of infection: (1) temperature $>38°C$ or $<36°C$; (2) heart rate >90 beats per minute; (3) respiratory rate > 20 breaths/min or $Pa_{CO_2} < 32$ mm Hg; and white blood cell count $>12,000/cu$ mm, $<4000/cu$ mm, or $>10\%$ immature forms. Sepsis and its sequelae represent a continuum of clinical and physiopathological severity. In this context, "septic shock" is defined as sepsis-induced hypotension, persisting despite adequate fluid resuscitation, along with the presence of hypoperfusion abnormalities and organ dysfunction (Bone et al., 1992).

These definitions were established in order to be utilized in clinical practice. Since in this chapter we will describe almost exclusively animal studies, we will adapt the definitions cited above to the experimental setting. For the purpose of this review, we will follow Wichterman and associates (1980) for whom "sepsis" refers to an infectious episode wherein an animal is toxic (febrile, weak, anorexic, lethargic, etc.) because of invasive infection and "septic shock" refers to the effects of sepsis leading to circulatory collapse. In consequence, we will consider septic shock as a subset of the septic condition, and we will utilize almost exclusively the term "sepsis" to refer to both situations unless specified.

B. Methodological Considerations

It must be noted that all of the studies regarding the effects of sepsis on respiratory muscles have been performed in animals, and no clinical research has confirmed experimental data. The reason for this situation probably lies in the complexity of the septic condition and in its association with other pathological entities that may impair respiratory muscle function by themselves, e.g., hypocalcemia (Aubier et al., 1985), metabolic acidosis (Howell et al., 1985), and undernutrition (Dureuil et al., 1989). Animal models of sepsis, from which data describing the effects of sepsis on the respiratory muscles have originated, are not generally comparable in the stage of clinical sepsis they purport to represent. The host response to a focus of infection describes a spectrum of physiopathological abnormalities that are not precisely reproduced by any of the different animal models of sepsis currently available. Consequently, from a clinical point of view, available data concerning the effects of sepsis on respiratory muscles must be interpreted with caution.

III. Effects of Sepsis on Respiratory Muscle Function

Physiopathology of organ dysfunction during sepsis is a complex and multifactorial process. For this reason presentation of data describing the effects of sepsis on respiratory muscle function can be performed in several ways, depending on which physiopathological variable is considered to be prominent. We choose a schematic and rather simplistic "time-related" presentation because it seems that different physiopathological aspects of muscle dysfunction are prominent at different periods after the beginning of the septic process.

A. Immediate Effects of Sepsis on Respiratory Muscle Function

Hussain and associates (1985b) first described the immediate effects of sepsis on respiratory muscle function by evaluating in spontaneously breathing dogs the effects of intravenous administration of a lethal dose of *E. coli* endotoxin on diaphragmatic strength and electrical activity. They also measured phrenic nerve output as an index of respiratory center activity. Endotoxin is a lipoprotein-carbohydrate complex found in the cell wall of all gram-negative bacteria (Raetz et al., 1991), which is currently used in experimental studies of sepsis physiopathology as a model of gram-negative infection.

This experimental model of sepsis was characterized hemodynamically by a rapid fall in cardiac output and blood pressure amounting to 40% of preinoculation values, with very little change until the death of the animals, which occurred 150–270 min after injection. Phrenic nerve output and diaphragmatic electrical activity increased during the first hour of the experiment. This was accompanied by a parallel increase in muscular strength, mean inspiratory flow rate, and minute ventilation. After this period, diaphragmatic strength decreased in spite of the fact that phrenic nerve output and diaphragmatic electrical activity continued to rise (Fig. 1). This failure of the diaphragm as a pressure generator despite increased central inspiratory neural drive, and muscle excitation revealed occurrence of diaphragmatic fatigue. As a consequence, minute ventilation decreased and CO_2 rose. Finally, as

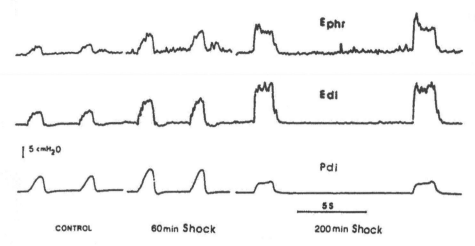

Figure 1 Representative tracing of one dog during endotoxic shock showing changes in integrated phrenic neurogram (E_{phr}) (top), integrated diaphragmatic electromyogram (E_{di}) (middle), and transdiaphragmatic pressure (P_{di}) (bottom). Left, during control; middle, 60 minutes after onset of endotoxic shock; right, 200 minutes after onset of endotoxic shock and prior to death of animal. (From Hussain et al., 1985b.)

the muscle approached exhaustion, frequency of breathing decreased followed by central apnea. Cardiac arrest occurred within 1–2 min as the P_{O_2} decreased.

This study shows unequivocally that respiratory failure is the precipitating factor leading to death in this experimental model of septic shock. The underlying mechanism responsible for respiratory failure is fatigue of the respiratory muscles due to impairment of the contraction process in the face of increasing muscle excitation.

Occurrence of respiratory muscle dysfunction precociously after intravenous inoculation of *E. coli* endotoxin was also reported by our laboratory (Leon et al., 1992). We evaluated diaphragmatic strength and electrical activity by measuring, during bilateral phrenic stimulation in rats, transdiaphragmatic pressure (P_{di}) and muscle electromyogram, respectively. In contrast with the study of Hussain and colleagues (1985b), diaphragmatic function was evaluated in mechanically venti-lated animals, a procedure that places the respiratory muscles at rest (Rochester et al., 1977). This fact has interesting physiopathological implications since fatigue is thought to occur as the result of an imbalance between muscular energy supply and energy demands (Roussos et al., 1982). As a consequence, one can expect that placing the respiratory muscles at rest could preserve muscle contractile function during the earlier stages of sepsis by reducing muscle energy demands.

As in a study by Hussain and coworkers (1985b), intravenous inoculation of endotoxin resulted in a marked decrease in blood pressure, which amounted to 70% of preinoculation values at the end of the experience. Diaphragmatic strength decreased significantly within 1 h of endotoxin inoculation. This decrease was restricted to the P_{di} generated at high frequencies of phrenic nerve stimulation (50 and 100 Hz) and was accompanied by a parallel reduction in the electrical activity of the diaphragm. Twitch and low-frequency P_{di} as well as muscle relaxation rate remained unchanged. This finding suggests that the reduction in diaphragmatic strength for high-frequency stimulations could be related to an impairment of the neuromuscular transmission. Finally, endurance capacity of the diaphragm was curtailed in septic animals: p_{di} at the end of a continuous stimulation at 10 Hz during a 30-s period amounted to 75% of the initial value, whereas it remained unchanged in control animals.

The results of this study show like the work of Hussain and associates (1985b), that respiratory muscle function is impaired early after the onset of the septic process. This impairment exists even if the respiratory muscles are placed at rest, a condition that reduces muscle energy demands. However, in contrast with the Hussain et al. study, the decrease in diaphragmatic strength appears to be related to an impairment in neuromuscular transmission, whereas no change in diaphragmatic contractility was noted: twitch P_{di} amplitude and relaxation remaining unchanged. Furthermore, we found in septic animals a decrease in diaphragmatic resting membrane potential. This phenomenon, which was reported in critically ill patients with various diseases (Cunningham et al., 1971) and in septic animal models (Illner et al., 1981), could impair action potential generation (Sperelakis et al., 1985) resulting in failure of neuromuscular transmission due to a postsynaptic membrane depolarization as well as an impaired propagation of electrical excitation along diaphragmatic fibers. The reason(s) for the discrepancy between our results and those of Hussain and coworkers (1985b) is unclear. It could be related to differences in animal species and/or in the experimental protocols, particularly in the methodological assessment of diaphragmatic function and neuromuscular transmission.

A major common aspect of the two studies cited above is that blood pressure was significantly reduced in septic animals. It is well known that blood pressure is a major determinant of muscle metabolic substrate delivery and contractile function. In fact, the results of Hussain and coworkers (1985b) are very close to those reported by Aubier and associates (1981) in nonseptic hypotensive spontaneously breathing dogs. This phenomenon raises the question of the role of hypotension in the physiopathology of the immediate effects of sepsis on respiratory muscle function.

Murphy and colleagues (1992a) evaluated this point in 4-week-old piglets. These authors investigated in spontaneously breathing animals the effects on diaphragmatic strength of a continuous group B streptococcus infusion at a level that caused a decrease in cardiac output but that avoided hypotension. Diaphragmatic strength was evaluated by measuring P_{di} generated during bilateral phrenic stimulation. The main result of this study was that P_{di} remained unchanged in septic animals over a 4-h experimental period (Fig. 2). However, another study from the same laboratory (Murphy et al., 1992b) showed that increasing the dose of streptococcus inoculum, while avoiding significant hypotension, resulted in a

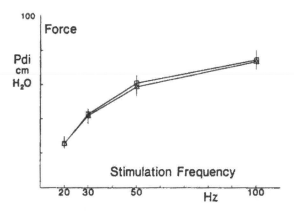

Figure 2 Relationship between frequency of stimulation and transdiaphragmatic pressure (P_{di}) before and after 4 h of group B streptococcus inoculation in piglets. No change was observed in the P_{di} frequency curves over 4 h of group B streptococcus infusion. (From Murphy et al., 1992a.)

transitory but significant decrease in diaphragmatic strength. Hurtado and coworkers (1992) investigated the role of hypotension in peripheral muscle dysfunction during sepsis. These authors evaluated the effects of a similar level of septic and nonseptic hypotension on peripheral muscle metabolism and strength generation in rabbits. Blood pressure decreased by approximately 22% of baseline values in both groups of animals. By the end of the experiment (180 min after onset of hypotension) hindlimb force was significantly reduced in septic animals for all frequencies of stimulation. However, a similar reduction was observed in nonseptic animals. Collectively, these studies suggest that hypotension contributes to the genesis of the immediate effects of sepsis on respiratory and peripheral muscle function.

B. Late Effects of Sepsis on Respiratory Muscle Function

Once the first reports on the immediate effects of sepsis on respiratory muscle function were published, investigators began to be interested by the consequences of septic processes lasting several days. Using an in vivo rat model, we evaluated the modifications of diaphragmatic function 3 days after *Streptococcus pneumoniae* injection (Boczkowski et al., 1988) and 2 days after inoculation of *E. coli* endotoxin (Boczkowski et al., 1990; Van Surell et al., 1992). Both inoculations were performed subcutaneously, and both models of sepsis were nonlethal, with no changes in blood pressure, serum electrolytes, and acid-base status. Inoculated animals developed fever, were anorexic, and lost body weight. Since undernutrition impairs respiratory muscle function (Dureuil et al., 1989), septic animals were compared with pair-fed controls. The results of these studies were similar: 2 or 3 days of experimental sepsis in rats impaired diaphragmatic function without affecting muscle mass and histological aspect. Contractile force in response to phrenic stimulation was reduced without concomitant decrease in the electrical activity of the muscle. Muscle relaxation rate was prolonged, and the diaphragms of septic animals fatigued rapidly in response to a stimulation regimen that was without effect on diaphragms of control animals (Fig. 3).

Similar results were reported by Shindoh and associates (1992) in *E. coli* endotoxin–inoculated hamsters. These authors evaluated diaphragmatic force generation and fatigability after 2 days of sublethal *E. coli* endotoxin intraperitoneal administration. Muscular contractility was evaluated in vitro during direct muscle stimulation. Diaphragmatic force was reduced for all frequencies of muscle stimulation. This was accompanied by a slight increase in muscle relaxation and by an increased muscular fatigability.

The deleterious effects of 2–3 days of sepsis on muscular function are not limited to the respiratory muscles. Ruff and Secrist (1984) have shown utilizing an in vitro preparation that in rats the strength of the limb muscles soleus and extensor digitorium longus was reduced after 3 days of pneumococcal sepsis. In this study, limb muscle mass decreased significantly. When limb muscle tension was corrected for muscle mass, it was still reduced, indicating contractile impairment out of proportion to muscle wasting.

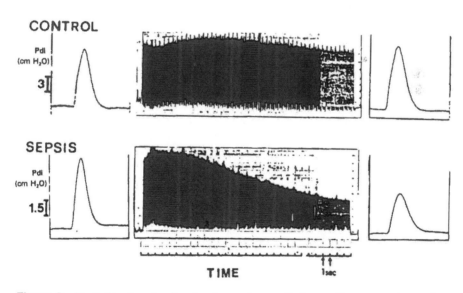

Figure 3   Typical tracing showing the changes in transdiaphragmatic pressure (P_{di}) during a continuous 30-s electrical stimulation of the phrenic nerves at 10 Hz in a control and a *Streptococcus pneumoniae* septic animal. Before and after the 30-s stimulation period, P_{di} for single twitch stimulation is also shown. A marked decrease in twitch P_{di} can be observed after the stimulation period in the septic animal, whereas no change was noted in the control. (From Boczkowski et al., 1988.)

C. Chronic Effects of Sepsis on Respiratory Muscle Function

Finally, Drew and colleagues (1988) examined the effects of a chronic infection lasting several weeks, visceral leishmaniasis, on the function of the diaphragm and the peripheral muscles soleus and plantaris. Muscular function was assessed in vitro. Infected animals (intracardiac inoculation of *Leishmania donovani* amastigotes) were maintained for 7–12 weeks until advanced disease characterized by anorexia, weight loss, and weakness was evident. To distinguish between effects of reduced caloric intake and infection per se, the authors studied healthy control animals and noninfected animals subjected to caloric restriction. Body weight and the mass of the diaphragm, soleus, and plantaris were reduced in septic animals. Absolute contractile force of the diaphragm and soleus muscles was moderately reduced, and only to the extent that muscle mass was decreased. Force normalized to muscle mass or cross-sectional area was not impaired. In contrast, the force of the plantaris, a fast twitch muscle, was severely reduced even after correcting for loss of muscle mass. The effects of leishmaniasis on the diaphragm and soleus muscles were not different from those of semistarvation with equivalent weight loss, but this model of sepsis produced a much greater loss in plantaris force than occurred with semistarvation.

IV. Mechanisms of Respiratory Muscle Dysfunction During Sepsis

The underlying mechanisms of respiratory muscle dysfunction during the early phase and after several days of sepsis are certainly different. Indeed, energetic impairment appears to be a major physiopathological determinant of the early dysfunction. This hypothesis is supported by the fact that early respiratory muscle dysfunction is closely related to the presence of hypotension, which can lead to a decreased muscle blood flow (Hussain et al., 1988), and thus, a reduced muscle metabolic subtracts delivery. By contrast, the late respiratory muscle dysfunction is clearly independent of hypotension. Indeed, muscle metabolic alterations during sepsis are complex and long-lasting, and it is possible that metabolic alterations are involved in the genesis of muscular dysfunction not only in the short but also in the long term. In this connection, it is interesting to note that metabolic alterations are triggered by mediators released as a part of the host response to the infectious aggression. We will discuss, therefore, the mechanisms involved in respiratory muscle dysfunction during sepsis by considering first the energetic aspect and, second, the muscular metabolic and functional alterations linked to the release of inflammatory mediators.

A. Energetics

From a general point of view respiratory muscle dysfunction is thought to occur when blood supply of energetic substrates to the muscle is not sufficient to meet the muscle's metabolic needs (Supinski, 1986). The efficiency of energy substrate uptake by these muscles mainly depends upon the total blood flow that reaches them, the conditions of perfusion of the microvascular network, and the ability of muscle cells to utilize metabolic substrate. Sepsis can alter all of these processes. In addition, sepsis induces long-lasting and complex alterations in muscular carbohydrate and protein metabolism. In the following section, we will analyze each of these points.

Respiratory Muscle Blood Flow During Sepsis

Like other skeletal muscles, the working respiratory muscles (especially the diaphragm) respond to increase energy requirements in part by an increase in muscle blood flow and in part by increasing extraction of oxygen from blood perfusing these muscles (Robertson et al., 1977; Reid et al., 1983; Hussain et al., 1988). Intramuscular determinants of muscle blood flow include factors such as regional, neural, and humoral control of the circulation, the anatomical arrangement of the vasculature within a given muscle, and the strength and duration of muscle contraction (Supinski, 1986). External determinants of muscle blood flow include hemodynamic variables such as mean arterial pressure and cardiac output. Under some circumstances, these variables assume paramount importance in determining muscle blood flow; however, the most important determinant of respiratory muscle blood flow is their level of activity (Supinski, 1986).

Sepsis is characterized hemodynamically by an initial hyperdynamic phase, whose hallmarks are an increased cardiac output, a decreased total peripheral resistance, and a normal or near-normal arterial blood pressure (Bone, 1991). As the infectious aggression continues and overwhelms the various host defense systems, cardiac function worsens, peripheral resistance rises, and blood pressure falls. Systemic hemodynamic changes are accompanied by a generalized blood flow maldistribution among the different organs, including the skeletal muscles. Some studies showed an increase in blood flow to the peripheral muscles (Wright et al., 1971; O'Donnell et al., 1974), however, the great majority of authors reported that, independently of the systemic hemodynamic state, blood flow to the peripheral skeletal muscles is reduced during sepsis (Wyler et al., 1969, 1970; Ferguson et al., 1978; Romanosky et al., 1981; Bond, 1983; Lang et al., 1984; Van Lambakgen et al., 1984; Hussain et al., 1985a; Fish et al., 1986; Jepson et al., 1987; Breslow et al., 1987). These results have been observed in resting muscles, which have low oxygen requirements. By contrast, few data are available in the current literature concerning the effect of sepsis in active contracting peripheral muscles. Romanosky and coworkers (1981) showed that increased hindlimb activity by electrical stimulation in septic dogs induced an increase in blood flow as compared to the resting state. However, blood flow through stimulated muscle in septic animals increased somewhat less than in controls, a difference that could be attributed to the low arterial pressure observed in these septic animals. Since these authors did not perform measurements in an hypotensive nonseptic group, it is not possible to know if in sepsis the well-established relationship between muscle oxygen consumption and blood flow in active muscles is preserved or not.

Blood flow to the respiratory muscles was also involved in the interorgan maldistribution of cardiac output during sepsis. However, as observed in peripheral muscles, this phenomenon was modulated by the degree of contractile activity. Indeed, either immediately or after the beginning of the septic process or somewhat later, if the diaphragm is at rest, its blood flow decreases (Hussain and Roussos, 1985a), whereas if it contracts, blood flow can be unchanged (Lang et al., 1984) or increased (Ferguson et al., 1978; Hussain and Roussos, 1985a). This late difference in the amount of diaphragmatic blood flow might be related itself to a different degree of contractile activity between the cited studies. Indeed, diaphragmatic blood flow was unchanged during 4 days of sustained nonhypotensive sepsis (Lang et al., 1984), an experimental model that can be considered as equivalent to the models utilized to describe the late effects of sepsis on respiratory muscle function. By contrast, blood flow increased during 3–4 h of lethal septic shock in dogs (Hussain and Roussos, 1985a) and in guinea pigs (Ferguson et al., 1978). An increase in minute ventilation and in the work of breathing could be more important in severe septic shock than in sustained nonhypotensive sepsis. This can lead to a more important diaphragmatic contractile activity, energy requirements and hence blood flow in the former than in the latter situation.

The increase in respiratory muscle blood flow during septic shock can reach dramatic levels. Hussain and Roussos (1985a) showed in spontaneously breathing dogs that 60 min after a lethal dose of *E. coli* endotoxin blood flow to the respiratory muscles increased significantly whether expressed in terms of percentage of the cardiac output or in absolute values. In fact, in spite of a reduction in blood pressure or in cardiac output of about 60–70% of baseline, 8.8% of the cardiac output was received by the respiratory muscles in comparison to 1.9% in animals in which the muscles were placed at rest by mechanical ventilation (Fig. 4). The large share of the cardiac output taken up by the respiratory muscles in spontaneously breathing animals resulted in reduced blood flow to the brain, the gastrointestinal tract, and other skeletal muscles as compared with mechanically ventilated animals with a similar reduction in cardiac output (Hussain and Roussos, 1985a) (Fig. 5). It is predictable that in this state, the function of the vital organs other than the respiratory muscles will be compromised. For example, the average value of cerebral blood flow for the spontaneously breathing animals in the Hussain and Roussos study (1985a) dropped to the level of ischemia sufficient to induce cerebral metabolic dysfunction (Raymond et al., 1976).

Certainly the values for diaphragmatic blood flow observed during septic shock by Hussain and Roussos (1985a) are much lower than the reported maximum in normotensive dogs. Indeed, whereas the diaphragm seems capable of receiving up to 360 ml/100 g/min in normotensive dogs during inspiratory resistive load (Robertson, et al., 1977), it received only 50 ml/100 g/min in hypotensive septic

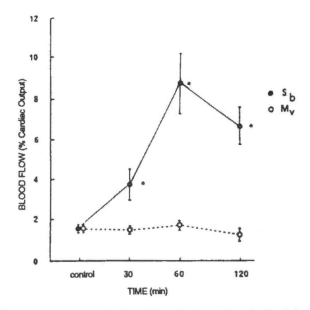

Figure 4 Total respiratory muscle blood flow during endotoxic shock in spontaneously breathing (SB) dogs (filled circles) and mechanically ventilated (MV) dogs (open circles). At any time during shock, fractional distribution of cardiac output to the respiratory muscles was higher in SB group ($p < 0.05$) compared with MV group. (From Hussain and Roussos, 1985a.)

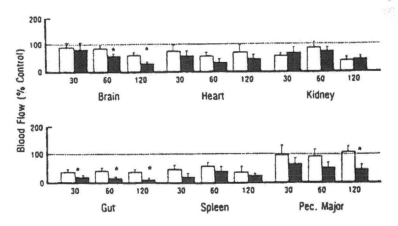

Figure 5 Mean blood flow to various organs at control (C), 30, 60, and 120 minutes of endotoxic shock in spontaneously breathing (SB) dogs (filled squares) and mechanically ventilated (MV) dogs (open squares). In MV group, blood flow of brain, gut, and pectoralis major was significantly increased (*$p < 0.05$) compared with SB group. (From Hussain and Roussos, 1985a.)

animals. This difference could be related to the low cardiac output and blood pressure of septic animals. However, the increase in blood flow in septic animals was greater for any given energy demand of the diaphragm, as judged by the relationship between pressure-time index (PTI) and diaphragmatic blood flow. PTI is well correlated with diaphragm V_{O_2} (Rochester et al., 1976; Robertson et al., 1977) and blood flow (Rochester and Bettini, 1976; Hussain et al., 1988). Although the slope of the relationship between diaphragmatic blood flow and PTI varies considerably between different studies, in conditions similar to those of septic animals in the Hussain and Roussos study it was roughly linear (Magder et al., 1985). Thus, since in septic animals PTI increased twofold, one might expect a twofold increase in diaphragmatic blood flow and not the sixfold increment observed. The reason for this finding is not clear. It may reflect a specific effect of sepsis resulting in a greater degree of diaphragmatic vasodilatation and hence greater blood flow for a given level of PTI as compared to a nonseptic situation.

Considerable evidence suggests that sepsis decreases vascular reactivity and vasomotor tone in peripheral skeletal muscle vessels as well as in other vascular territories (see Sibbald et al., 1991 for review). This hyporreactivity is the result of an impairment of vasoconstriction and of an enhancement of vasodilatation. The diminished vascular contractility caused by sepsis might be mainly due to alterations of the common contractile mechanism beyond the membrane receptors. On the other hand, enhancement of vasodilatation could be related to activation of the L-arginine:nitric oxide pathway through an endothelium-independent mechanism (Julou-Schaeffer et al., 1990).

Hyporreactivity of the respiratory muscle vasculature may explain the disproportionate increase of diaphragmatic blood flow with respect to the level of PTI in septic dogs (Hussain and Roussos, 1985a). However, no direct data are available to confirm or reject this hypothesis. We investigated recently the effects of *E. coli* endotoxin administration on the microcirculation of the resting rat diaphragm by in vivo videomicroscopy (Boczkowski et al., 1992). The protocol of endotoxin administration we utilized induced a significant fall in blood pressure throughout the experimental period (60 min). The endotoxic rats exhibited progressive and highly significant reductions in diameters of the largest arterioles studied contrasting with less impressive modifications of the smaller arterioles (Fig. 6). These constrictions may explain the reduction of blood flow in the resting diaphragm during experimental sepsis reported by Hussain and Roussos (1985a). The changes in arteriolar diameter with endotoxin injection could be explained by the decline in arterial pressure observed in these animals and not due to endotoxin itself. To test this possibility, we studied a group of animals in which blood pressure was matched to that of the endotoxic group by a graded hemorrhage. In this group we observed a constriction of large vessels similar to that observed in septic animals, suggesting that arteriolar constriction of the resting diaphragm during endotoxemia could be due to hypotension. It is interesting to note that, for the same level of hypotension, a tendency to a less important constriction in arterioles of septic than of nonseptic

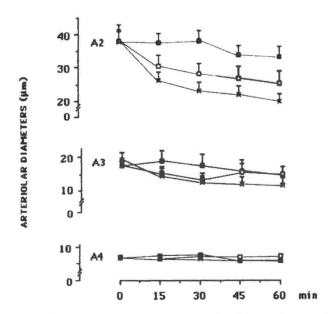

Figure 6 Comparison of second (A2), third (A3), and fourth (A4) order arteriolar diameters in control (group C, plain squares), endotoxic (group E, empty squares), and endotoxic (group H, asteriks) hypotensive-matched animals at baseline (0 min) and at 15, 30, 45, and 60 min after beginning of the experimental protocol. The SEMs for A4 were too small to be shown on the graph. The time-dependent changes in A2 diameters were not significantly different in groups E and H, while both these groups were significantly different from group C ($p <$ 0.05 in both cases). For A3 and A4 arterioles, no significant changes in diameter were found. (From Boczkowski et al., 1992.)

animals was observed. Although this tendency was not statistically significant, it suggests that a degree of arteriolar hyporeactivity to hypotensive constrictor stimuli possibly occurred in the diaphragm of septic animals.

Finally, the question arises if the amount of diaphragmatic vasodilatation during sepsis is the maximum that the muscle could reach for the level of blood pressure. Hussain and Roussos (1985a) compared the values of muscle blood flow in septic animals with the maximum theoretical values this parameter could reach as estimated by Reid and Johnson's mathematical model (Reid and Johnson, 1983). This comparison showed that the calculated blood flow should be 20% higher than they observed. By contrast, in nonseptic shock (cardiac tamponade) this limitation was not observed (Viires et al., 1983). Therefore it is possible to conclude that, although blood flow was significantly increased during sepsis and even greater than expected for the PTI they observed, a septic-induced limitation to the maximal blood flow was operational. This limitation could be situated at the microcirculatory level, as will be discussed later.

O₂ Extraction by the Respiratory Muscles During Sepsis

As stated above, the oxygen requirements of the respiratory muscles are met not only by increasing blood flow but also by increasing extraction of oxygen from blood perfusing the muscles. The maximum capacity to extract O_2 is a function of the metabolic profile of the muscle fibers and of the capillary density. It has been demonstrated in normoxic animals that the arteriovenous O_2 difference across the diaphragm can increase from 6.4 ml/dl during quiet breathing to values as high as 18–19 ml/dl during breathing against high inspiratory resistance (Rochester and Bettini, 1976; Reid and Johnson, 1983), a value that corresponds to 80–95% extraction of the delivered oxygen.

Sepsis is characterized by severe alterations in systemic O_2 metabolism. It has been shown in humans and in animal models that a severe defect exists in the physiological mechanisms that enables tissues to increase their O_2 extraction ratio as O_2 delivery is lowered. However, in contrast with the whole body, it is difficult to assess the importance of such O_2 extraction defect in skeletal muscle. In fact, although some studies showed that O_2 extraction by resting skeletal muscle was depressed during sepsis (Harken et al., 1975; Bredle et al., 1989; Hurtado et al., 1992), this depression was slight, less important than the whole body defect, and transitory. In addition, other authors demonstrated that O_2 extraction was unaltered (Samsel et al., 1988) or increased (Romanosky et al., 1981). Conversely, experimental data showed a similar increase in muscular O_2 extraction during submaximal muscular contraction in septic and in control animals (Romanosky et al., 1981). Collectively, these studies suggest that O_2 extraction capacity by resting or submaximally contracting skeletal muscle is not severely impaired during sepsis. However, we do not know if extraction capacity is limited or not during maximal contractile activity or, in other words, if sepsis impairs skeletal muscle capacity to extract O_2 under maximal demand.

Oxygen extraction by the respiratory muscles during sepsis was measured by Hussain and coworkers (1986) in spontaneously breathing animals. In contrast with peripheral muscles, no data are available concerning resting muscles. These authors showed that diaphragmatic O_2 extraction increased significantly in spontaneously breathing animals during hypotensive sepsis as compared to controls. This extraction was more important than in the peripheral skeletal muscle gastrocnemius but was similar to that observed in hypotensive nonseptic animals breathing spontaneously with similar levels of energy requirement, as judged by the PTI (Hussain et al., 1988). However, since, as we stated before, a limitation in diaphragmatic blood flow was observed in sepsis but not in hypotensive nonseptic animals, it appears that sepsis could impair O_2 extraction by the diaphragm under maximal demand. In fact, when data from Hussain and associates (1988) are compared with data from other studies, it appears that minimal phrenic venous O_2 content was much higher in septic dogs than in nonseptic dogs during resistive loading breathing (Rochester and Bettini, 1976; Robertson et al., 1977). Thus, as observed in peripheral muscles, it seems that a defect in O_2 extraction by the respiratory muscles exists during sepsis. The mechanism of this impairment is not clear. It could be related to deleterious effects of sepsis on muscular oxidative capacity and/or on the microcirculation.

Few authors have evaluated the effects of sepsis on oxidative potential of skeletal muscle (Tavakoli et al., 1982; Friman et al., 1984). A decrease in muscle oxidative capacity of varying degrees depending on the experimental conditions has been reported. By contrast, divergent results have been reported by the studies investigating the effects of sepsis on muscle microcirculation. Siegel and coworkers (1967) postulated occurrence of precapillary arteriovenous shunting during sepsis, but direct evidence of this phenomenon is lacking. Baker (1982) demonstrated in the mesenteric circulation of septic hypotensive cats an impairment in red blood cell transit across microcirculatory pathways that was not present in hypotensive nonseptic animals. Such impairment could limit the diffusion of O_2 from the blood to the surrounding tissue cells. By contrast, other authors postulated that microcirculatory heterogeneity does not increase in skeletal muscle during sepsis when evaluated by measurement of tissue P_{O_2} (Gutierrez et al., 1991; Hurtado et al., 1992). In order to study the effects of sepsis on respiratory muscles capillary perfusion, we measured in vivo the number of diaphragmatic capillaries perfused with red blood cells during hypotensive sepsis in rats (Boczkowski et al., 1992). We found a marked alteration in diaphragmatic capillary perfusion pattern in septic animals since the number of nonperfused capillaries was multiplied by a factor of 4 as compared to the baseline values (Fig. 7). This finding cannot be related to the low arterial pressure observed in

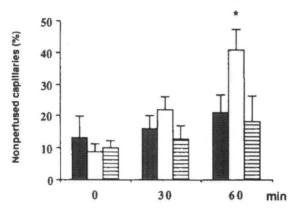

Figure 7 Percentage of nonperfused capillaries per optical field at baseline (0 min), 30, and 60 min in control (group C, black columns), endotoxic (group E, white columns), and endotoxic (group H, hatched columns) hypotensive-matched animals. After 60 min the percentage of nonperfused capillaries was found to be significantly different among the three groups. This percentage was significantly higher in group E than in groups C and H (*$p <$ 0.05 in both cases) and was not different between groups C and H. (From Boczkowski et al., 1992.)

this condition, since the percentage of nonperfused capillaries did not increase in hypotensive nonseptic controls. The impaired capillary perfusion could be due to capillary obstruction by granulocytes (Bagge et al., 1982; Harlan, 1985) and/or due to endothelial cells swelling (Harlan, 1985). Regardless of the mechanism(s) by which endotoxemia altered diaphragmatic capillary perfusion, this finding of a large functional capillary derecruitment may have important functional implications concerning metabolic subtracts exchanges and O_2 extraction capacity by diaphragmatic myofibrils and capillary washout of metabolic toxic products.

Lactate Production by the Respiratory Muscles During Sepsis

The reduced O_2 extraction by the respiratory muscles during sepsis was accompanied by an increase in muscle lactate concentration (Hussain et al., 1986) and by a decrease in glycogen concentration (Hussain et al., 1986; Leon et al., 1992). Although these findings suggest a shift from aerobic to anaerobic metabolism, and thus support the conclusion that blood flow and O_2 extraction were limited during sepsis, other factors could contribute to this increase in lactic acid concentration. Indeed, Hussain and coworkers (1986) found that the diaphragm of septic animals produced lactate at higher levels of phrenic venous P_{O_2} than reported in nonseptic conditions (Robertson et al., 1977). In addition, Hurtado and associates (1992) showed lactic acidosis during hypotensive sepsis in rabbits as compared to nonseptic hypotensive controls in spite of similar peripheral muscle tissue P_{O_2} and adenine nucleotides and phosphocreatine concentrations in these two groups of animals. Interestingly, similar findings were reported by Chaudry and coworkers (1979) in peripheral muscle of nonhypotensive peritonitic rats. These data suggest a direct effect of sepsis on muscular energetic metabolism leading to increased lactate production.

From a metabolic point of view, the septic episode has been described as an acquired disease of intermediary metabolism (Siegel, 1981). In particular, alterations in carbohydrate metabolism have been implicated as playing an important role in the development and outcome of the septic process. During sepsis, skeletal muscle presents an impairment in energetic metabolism characterized by a resistance to the action of insulin, which makes it unable to increase oxidation of glucose in response to insulin stimulation (Beisel, 1984). This leads to an increased production of lactate even in absence of tissue hypoxia (Beisel, 1984). Although these abnormalities may be related to the endocrine distrubances occurring during sepsis, they may be the result of a direct effect of the septic process. In fact, Vary and colleagues (1986) demonstrated in peripheral muscle of septic rats a decrease in the concentration of the active form of the enzyme pyruvate dehydrogenase, which is one of the major determinants of glucose oxidation in vivo. This reduction occurred in spite of unchanged concentration of muscle adenine nucleotides.

Alterations in Muscular Protein Metabolism During Sepsis

The alterations in muscular oxidative and carbohydrate metabolism reported previously are only a part of the host metabolic response to sepsis. In fact, this is an exceedingly complex phenomenon during which every metabolic pathway can become involved. A very striking feature is that generalized infectious disease are catabolic forms of illness, marked by weight loss and a decrease in muscle mass and strength (Beisel, 1984).

Numerous authors reported during sepsis an increase in net skeletal muscle protein degradation mainly related to an accelerated protein breakdown (see Hasselgren et al., 1988 for review). Muscular and particularly contractile proteins appear to serve as a stored reserve of "labile" nitrogen, which can be tapped during periods of infection. After their release from the contractile proteins, some of the branched amino acids are used by the muscles as a direct source of energy, whereas other amino acids are taken up by other tissues, especially the liver, where they are used for protein (acute-phase reactants, antibodies) synthesis. A limitation in the supply of metabolic fuel to muscle tissue is an important factor conditioning the increase in muscle protein degradation. Indeed, muscle is insulin resistant and unable to increase its utilization of glucose in response to insulin stimulation, while simultaneously blood free fatty acids and ketones are below those of normal fasting individuals (Ryan, 1976). The key fuels for muscle are therefore available to it in limited supply during sepsis, and it is possible that the observed increase in the oxidation of branched-chain amino acids may be necessary to supply the energy needs of the tissue. Proteolysis could be at least partly due to increased cathepsin B activity (Ruff and Secrist, 1984).

By contrast with the numerous biochemical studies of skeletal muscle metabolic alterations during sepsis, very few authors have investigated the functional repercussions of increased protein breakdown. As stated above, Ruff and Secrist (1984) reported in a rat model of 3 days' *Streptococcus pneumoniae* sepsis that twitch and tetanic tensions generated by limb muscles were reduced after correction for muscle mass, indicating contractile impairment out of proportion to muscle wasting. This was accompanied by an increase in the activity of muscular cathepsin B, an enzyme involved in protein degradation (Hummel et al., 1988). Both these phenomena were prevented when the animals were treated with leupeptin, a cathepsin B inhibitor, suggesting the role of muscular proteolysis in the decreased muscular contractility.

To our knowledge, no study directly investigated protein metabolism alterations in the respiratory muscles during sepsis. Indirect information about this phenomenon can be obtained by analyzing previous data obtained in rats after 2–3 days' sepsis (Boczkowski et al., 1988). In those studies, we found that diaphragmatic mass was not significantly affected, whereas peripheral muscle mass decreased significantly. Peripheral muscle atrophy was probably related to an increase in the net breakdown of muscular proteins, as demonstrated by other authors. Therefore, the discrepancy in muscular mass changes between peripheral and diaphragmatic muscles may have been related to differences in their muscular protein breakdown rates. This could be related to the different activity patterns of these muscles, as demonstrated in other catabolic situations such as trauma (Tischler et al., 1983), the most active muscle, the diaphragm, being less susceptible to septic wastage than the less active peripheral muscles. An impairment in diaphragmatic contractility was observed in septic animals, and this occurred in spite of a conserved muscle mass, arising doubts about the functional significance of protein breakdown in diaphragmatic function. However, we cannot definitively rule out such physiopathological elements until direct experimental evidence is available.

B. Mediators

For many years it has been recognized that the septic process is the result of extensive triggering of the body defense mechanisms by invading microorganisms and their products. These defense mechanisms include the release of cytokines into the circulation, activation of neutrophils and monocytes, and activation of plasma protein cascade systems such as the complement system, the intrinsic (contact system) and extrinsic pathways of coagulation, and the fibrinolytic system. In addition, these inflammatory mediators can act on target cells by the intermediary of locally produced molecules such as prostaglandins. In the literature there is now abundant evidence that, to some extent, all of these inflammatory mediator systems become activated during sepsis. It is now becoming apparent that numerous metabolic and circulatory changes observed during sepsis are initiated by these mediators; however, their interrelationships as well as their precise role in sepsis are poorly understood. The same applies to their role in the physiopathology of muscular dysfunction. Recent studies showed evidence that respiratory muscle dysfunction during sepsis can be ascribed to the actions of endogenously produced mediators, such as prostaglandins, and secretory products of activated neutrophils and monocytes such as toxic metabolites of oxygen and cytokines. In this section we will review these studies and discuss the mechanism(s) of action of each mediator.

Prostaglandins

Several lines of evidence suggest that prostaglandins are involved in the physiopathology of sepsis (see Fletcher, 1983, and Metz et al., 1990, for review). Prostaglandin (PG) production is increased after endotoxin inoculation in several species. Elevated levels of $PGF_{2\alpha}$ have been demonstrated in patients with clinical sepsis. A correlation exists between decreased levels of prostaglandins induced by prostaglandin synthesis inhibitors such as indomethacin or fatty acid deficiency and improved hemodynamics and survival in experimental septic shock. These data have implicated prostaglandins as mediators of physiopathological changes of sepsis, though their mechanisms of action have not yet been established.

Several studies indicate that prostaglandins play a role in the development of peripheral skeletal muscle dysfunction during septic states (Ruff and Secrist, 1984). Indeed, elevated PGE_2 levels have been found in peripheral muscles of septic animals (Turinsky et al., 1985; Hasselgren et al., 1985), and pharmacological inhibition of prostaglandins synthesis has been shown to protect septic animals from peripheral skeletal muscle impairment (Ruff and Secrist, 1984).

We evaluated the effects on prostaglandin synthesis inhibition by indomethacin on diaphragmatic dysfunction during sepsis, utilizing an in vivo rat model (Boczkowski et al., 1990). Sepsis was induced by a 2-day sublethal *E. coli* endotoxin administration, as described in the section referring to the long-term effects of sepsis on the respiratory muscles. This study showed that indomethacin significantly prevented the reduction of diaphragmatic strength found in septic animals. In addition, this agent prevented peripheral muscle atrophy. To our knowledge, this is the only work concerning the role of prostaglandins in respiratory muscle dysfunction during sepsis.

Improving the energetic metabolism of the respiratory muscles, which is altered during sepsis as stated before, could explain at least in part the preventive effects of indomethacin. Indeed, several studies have shown that indomethacin and other prostaglandin synthesis inhibitors attenuated hypotension and prolonged survival in experimental septic shock models (Feuerstein et al., 1981; Fletcher, 1982; Jacobs et al., 1982). In addition, it has been demonstrated in the rat cremaster muscle that prostaglandins are involved in microcirculatory alterations after live *E. coli* inoculation (Cryer et al., 1990).

Another metabolic disturbance that could be prevented by indomethacin is an increase in muscle protein breakdown. Indeed, skeletal muscle protein breakdown is accelerated following in vivo intraarterial infusion of PGE_2 in rats (Pressler et al., 1985) and after in vitro addition of PGE_2 to incubated normal rat muscles (Rodemann et al., 1982; Goldberg et al., 1988). These findings suggest that the prevention of peripheral muscle atrophy we found in septic animals treated with indomethacin was probably related to prevention of increased protein degradation. In addition, Ruff and Secrist (1984) reported that indomethacin not only prevented wasting but also improved contractility of peripheral muscles in septic rats. These findings support the hypothesis that prostaglandins impair skeletal muscle function during sepsis by increasing contractile protein breakdown. However, as stated above, the role of increased protein breakdown in respiratory muscle contractile impairment during sepsis is not clearly determined.

Toxic Metabolites of Oxygen

Highly toxic metabolites of oxygen are generated normally by aerobic metabolism in most cells, and this generation is often greatly increased in pathological conditions. When this oxidant flux exceeds the capability of the multiple endogenous antioxidant mechanisms, tissue injury ensues mainly as a consequence of peroxidation of polyunsaturated fatty acids (Marx, 1987). During experimental sepsis, products of lipid peroxidation such as malondialdehyde accumulate in many organs such as lungs, liver, and brain (Takeda et al., 1986), providing indirect evidence of tissue damage by oxidant stress. These data are in line with other studies suggesting that reactive oxygen metabolites are involved in the pathophysiology of sepsis (McKechnie et al., 1986; Morgan et al., 1988). Thus, it is conceivable that reactive oxygen metabolites may also be implicated in the respiratory muscle impairment observed during sepsis.

Recent studies have examined in vitro and in vivo the involvement of reactive oxygen metabolites on diaphragmatic strength and fatigability during sepsis (Supinski et al., 1990; Shindoh et al., 1992; Van Surell et al., 1992). These studies were performed in hamsters and in rats, evaluating the immediate (3 h) and long-term (2 days) effects of *E. coli* endotoxin inoculation with and without concomitant administration of toxic oxygen metabolite scavengers. In two of these studies (Shindoh et al., 1992; Van Surell et al., 1992) malondialdehyde concentration in the diaphragm was measured. It must be noted that, in contrast with data concerning prostaglandins, no study is available regarding the role of oxygen metabolites on peripheral skeletal muscle dysfunction during sepsis. The results of these studies are concordant: administration of scavengers largely ablated the effects of endotoxin inoculation on the diaphragm, with muscles of animals given endotoxin and the scavenger generating similar strength as controls and substantially more than animals given endotoxin alone (Fig. 8). Scavengers also improved diaphragmatic fatigability. Malondialdehyde content was elevated in diaphragmatic samples taken from endotoxin inoculated animals when compared to controls; this elevation was not present when endotoxin animals received oxygen metabolite scavengers (Fig. 9).

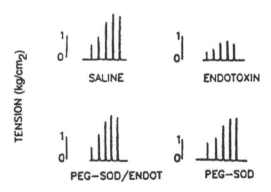

Figure 8 Force-frequency curves (1, 10, 20, 50, 100 Hz) from individual saline-treated control (upper left), and endotoxin-treated (upper right), endotoxin/PEG-SOD-treated (lower left), and PEG-SOD-treated (lower right) animals. The diaphragm of the endotoxin-treated animal generated lower tensions for a given stimulus frequency than the tensions produced by the diaphragm from control animal. PEG-SOD administration significantly blunted the effect of endotoxin on the diaphragm force-frequency relationship, with the animal given both PEG-SOD and endotoxin having a force-frequency curve similar to that elicited in the control animal. (From Shindoh et al., 1992.)

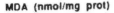

MDA (nmol/mg prot)

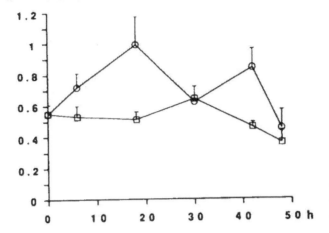

MDA (nmol/mg prot)

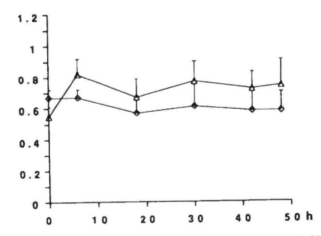

Figure 9 Diaphragmatic malondialdehyde (MDA) content before and 6, 18, 30, 42, and 48 h after the first endotoxin or saline inoculation in control (C, open triangles) and endotoxemic (E, open circles) animals (top), and in control plus *N*-acetylcysteine (C-NAC, filled triangles), and endotoxemic plus *N*-acetylcysteine (E-NAC, filled circles) animals (bottom). Diaphragmatic MDA content was significantly higher in E as compared to C animals at 18 and 42 h ($p < 0.05$, respectively). No significant difference was observed in E-NAC as compared to C and to C-NAC animals. (From Van Surell et al., 1992.)

As stated before, malondialdehyde is one of the final products of membrane lipid peroxidation (Reilly et al., 1991), a process that alters membrane ionic permeability and function (Maridonneau et al., 1983). Since skeletal muscle membranes are involved in excitation-contraction coupling, the rise in diaphragmatic malondialdehyde observed in septic animals suggests that lipid peroxidation of cell membranes could be involved in the reduced diaphragmatic strength and endurance observed in these animals. Lipid peroxidation results from the attack of reactive oxygen metabolites on phospholipids of the biomembrane (McCord, 1985; Demling et al., 1989). Consequently, the increased diaphragmatic malondialdehyde in septic animals suggests that diaphragmatic dysfunction could be related to muscle oxidant injury during endotoxemia. Furthermore, the finding that scavengers prevented both the increase in diaphragmatic malondialdehyde content and muscle dysfunction observed in septic animals supports the hypothesis that these findings are oxidant induced and probably cause-effect related.

Reactive oxygen metabolites can impair respiratory muscle function in several ways. They can limit metabolic supply to the muscles. Indeed, it has been shown that oxygen scavengers can improve cardiac output in experimental models of sepsis (McKechnie et al., 1986). In addition, recent data suggest that reactive oxygen metabolites are involved in the genesis of microcirculatory alterations during sepsis, such as an increase in microvascular leakage of macromolecules (Matsuda et al., 1991) and arteriolar hyporreactivity (Gryglewski et al., 1986). Furthermore, these molecules can increase proteins sensitivity to degradation (Fliegel et al., 1984), thus theoretically favoring proteolysis during sepsis. Finally, in vitro studies have shown that reactive oxygen metabolites can produce loss of mitochondrial, sarcoplasmic reticulum, and endoplasmic reticulum integrity in skeletal muscle (Davies et al., 1982), shortening of the action potential, changes in tension, and depletion of high-energy phosphates in cardiac muscle (Goldhaber et al., 1989).

Cytokines and Other Monocyte Inflammatory Mediators

A class of mediators that has attracted the most recent attention in the pathogenesis of sepsis are the protein mediators called cytokines. This class of mediators includes tumor necrosis factor (TNF) and proteins from the interleukin (IL), interferon, and macrophage-stimulating factor families. They are typically small proteins that are released by a wide variety of cell sources, including macrophages, lymphocytes, and fibroblasts, in response to injurious stimuli such as endotoxin and bacterial exotoxins. There is now compelling evidence that cytokines belonging to the interleukin family (IL-1, IL-6, IL-8) and TNF are major elements in the pathophysiology of sepsis.

Several lines of evidence allow one to think that cytokines, mainly TNF and IL-1, could mediate skeletal muscle dysfunction during sepsis. TNF induced changes in skeletal muscle membrane potential similar to those observed in peripheral and respiratory muscles during sepsis (Tracey et al., 1986). Furthermore, these cytokines can impair muscle metabolic substrate delivery by acting at the organ blood flow level. Indeed, TNF and IL-1 can induce vascular hyporeactivity similar to that observed during sepsis. This has been demonstrated in nonmuscular (Beasley et al., 1989) and in muscular vessels (Vicaut et al., 1991). Finally, it has been demonstrated in vivo that inoculations of TNF and IL-1 induce a cachectic state with muscular wastage (Fong et al., 1989) and increased skeletal muscular protein degradation (Flores et al., 1989).

In spite of the body of evidence indicating that TNF and IL-1 could impair skeletal muscle function, no study has investigated this question in the locomotor muscles. By contrast, several laboratories have evaluated the effects of TNF on respiratory muscle function. In vitro studies showed that TNF at a concentration of 50–400 ng/ml did not impair diaphragmatic force generation in rats (Diaz et al., 1991), whereas a concentration of 10 μg/ml of the cytokine elicited a significant decrease in force for all the frequencies of stimulation in hamsters (Wilcox et al., 1992a). A similar decrease was observed when diaphragmatic strips were incubated 1 h in endotoxin-stimulated monocyte supernatant medium, which contained 146 ng/ml of TNF [a concentration that alone did not impair diaphragmatic contractility (Diaz et al., 1991)] and 30,000 U/ml of Il-1 (Wilcox et al., 1992b) (Fig. 10). This suggests a synergistic effect of a combination of TNF and IL-1 on diaphragmatic contractility. Furthermore, in vivo TNF induced a significant decrease in diaphragmatic force in dogs beginning 4 h after administration (Wakai et al., 1991). Although in the latter study cardiac output tended to decrease after TNF administration, it was maintained within normal values by fluid administration. However, no information about blood pressure was provided. Collectively, these studies suggest that TNF induces a decrease in diaphragmatic force generation.

Interaction Between Different Mediators

Many relationships have been shown between the various mediators discussed above. Reactive oxygen metabolites are generated as byproducts during prostaglandin synthesis (Samuelsson et al., 1978), and administration of ibuprofen, a prostaglandin synthesis inhibitor, prevents oxidant lung injury and in vitro lipid peroxidation after phosgene inhalation (Kennedy et al., 1990). In addition, administration of catalase, an antioxidant enzyme, prevents thromboxane synthesis after endotoxin administration in sheep (Seekamp et al., 1988), and dimethyl sulfoxide, a reactive oxygen metabolites scavenger, inhibits prostacyclin production by endothelial cells incubated in vitro with endotoxin. Furthermore, prostaglandins are involved in the genesis of cremaster arteriolar vasodilatation (Vicaut et al., 1991), and diaphragmatic impaired contractility (Wilcox and Bressler, 1992a) induced by TNF administration.

V. Conclusion and Perspectives

The reviewed studies clearly demonstrate that sepsis impairs the function of the respiratory muscles. This impairment is observed soon after the beginning of the

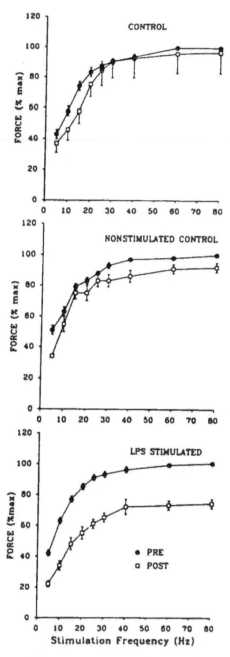

Figure 10 Comparison of force frequency response before and after incubation in Krebs solution (upper panel), nonstimulated (NS) monocyte supernatant (middle panel), and lipopolysaccharide-stimulated monocyte supernatant (lower panel). Force is expressed as a percentage of maximal preincubation tetanus. Preincubation values are represented by closed symbols, and postincubation values are represented by open symbols. There is a decline in force postincubation at all stimulation frequencies for the lipopolysaccharide-stimulated group ($p < 0.05$) with no significant difference in the control and NS groups. (From Wilcox et al., 1992b.)

septic process, and it may still be present after several weeks, depending on the duration of the infectious aggression. However, several differences arise between time-related results concerning the role of hypotension, the site of muscle failure, and the importance of undernutrition.

The early dysfunction is strongly related to the hypotension that can be present in this condition. In contrast, the more delayed effects (days to weeks) appear to be independent from hemodynamic alterations, probably being related to physio-pathological processes that need some time to develop.

Respiratory muscle impairment occurring some time after the beginning of the septic process is probably located at the muscle contractile machinery level since muscular strength is reduced when the muscles are directly stimulated in vitro. However, neurotransmission failure is also postulated to occur immediately after the beginning of the septic process.

Finally, chronic effects of sepsis on the diaphragm are not different from those of semistarvation with equivalent weight loss. These results differs from those observed after 2–3 days of sepsis in which diaphragmatic dysfunction occurred independently of the nutritional status of the septic animals.

Changes in respiratory energetic metabolism during sepsis may partly explain the observed decline of the contractile function in this situation. Blood flow to the respiratory muscles was decreased if the muscles were at rest and was unchanged or increased if they contracted. This increase could reach dramatic proportions, depriving the rest of the body of adequate energy supply. However, despite the conservation or increase in blood flow, spontaneously breathing animals showed respiratory muscle contractile dysfunction.

Lactate concentration was increased in the respiratory muscles of septic animals. This phenomenon could be related to an impaired aerobic metabolism of these muscles, as suggested by the reported limitations in O_2 extraction. However, a direct metabolic effect of the septic process on muscle lactate metabolism might also be considered. Whatever the mechanism of the increased muscular lactate concentration, this phenomenon has important implications concerning the physio-pathology of respiratory muscles dysfunction during sepsis. Indeed, an association between the accumulation of lactate and impairment of the skeletal muscle ability to perform work has been demonstrated (Tesch et al., 1978). This has been attributed to the resultant decrease in intracellular pH, which has been shown to inhibit excitation-contraction coupling (Metzger et al., 1987). It must be noted that the majority of studies describing blood flow to and O_2 extraction and lactate production by the respiratory muscles concerned the early period of sepsis. Whether the described changes are still present some time after the beginning of the septic process, their importance in the genesis of the impaired contractility observed in this situation is not clear. Other metabolic alterations such as protein breakdown are prominent later on in the evolution of the septic process. This phenomenon is probably involved in the genesis of the impaired contractile function of peripheral skeletal muscles observed later (2–3 days) in the evolution of the septic process.

By contrast, indirect evidence raises doubts about the occurrence of such phenomena in the respiratory muscles. Since direct experimental data are lacking, this subject clearly deserves further investigation.

Respiratory muscle dysfunction during sepsis appears to be related to the action of mediators such as prostaglandins, oxygen-reactive metabolites, and TNF acting alone or in concert. This is a new and rapidly growing field of research, and the exact mechanisms by which prostaglandins, oxygen-reactive metabolites, and TNF impair muscular function remain to be elucidated as do the roles of other inflammatory molecules.

From an integrated point of view, it is possible to postulate that sepsis impairs respiratory muscle function by acting at two levels. The first is an impairment at different steps of the chain of muscular energetic supply: blood flow and metabolic substrate extraction and utilization. The second is a direct impairment of the contractile process. These effects of sepsis are probably the result of the action of inflammatory mediators.

Clearly, sepsis is a exceedingly complex phenomenon and much more work must be done to have a clear comprehension of its effects on the respiratory muscles as well as to assess the clinical impact of this impairment.

References

Aubier, M., Trippenbach, T., and Roussos, C. (1981). Respiratory muscle failure during cardiogenic shock. *J. Appl. Physiol.*, 51:499–508.

Aubier, M., Viires, N., Piquet, J., Murciano, D., Blanchet, F., Marty, C., Gherardi, R., and Pariente, R. (1985). Effects of hypocalcemia on diaphragmatic strength generation. *J. Appl. Physiol.*, 58:2054–2061.

Bagge, U., and Braide, M. (1982). Leukocyte plugging of capillaries in vivo. In *White Blood Cells: Morphology and Rheology as Related to Function*. Edited by U. Bagge, G. V. R. Born, and P. Gaehtgens. The Hague, Martinus Nijhoff Publishers, pp. 89–98.

Baker, C. (1982). Arteriolar to venular red cell and plasma dispersion in hemorrhage and endotoxin-shocked cats. *Adv. in Shock Res.*, 8:35–51.

Beasley, D., Cohen, R., and Levinsky, N. (1989). Interleukin-1 inhibits contraction of vascular smooth muscle. *J. Clin. Invest.*, 83:331–335.

Beisel, W. (1984). Metabolic effects of infection. *Prog. Food Nutr. Sci.*, 8:43–75.

Boczkowski, J., Dureuil, B., Branger, C., Pavlovic, D., Murciano, D., Pariente, R., and Aubier, M. (1988). Effects of sepsis on diaphragmatic function in rats. *Am. Rev. Respir. Dis.*, 138:260–265.

Boczkowski, J., Dureuil, B., Pariente, R., and Aubier, M. (1990). Preventive effects of indomethacin on diaphragmatic contractile alterations in endotoxemic rats. *Am. Rev. Respir. Dis.*, 142:193–198.

Boczkowski, J., Vicaut, E., and Aubier, M. (1992). In vivo effects of Escherichia coli endotoxemia on diaphragmatic microcirculation in rats. *J. Appl. Physiol.*, 72:2219–2224.

Bond, R. (1983). Peripheral vascular adrenergic depression during hypotension induced by *E. coli* endotoxin. *Adv. Shock Res.*, 9:157–169.

Bone, R. (1991). Gram-negative sepsis. Background, clinical features, and intervention. *Chest*, 100:802–808.

Bone, R., Balk, R., Cerra, F., Dellinger, R., Fein, A., Knaus, W., Schein, R., and Sibbald, W.

(1992). Definitions for sepsis and organ failure and guidelines for the use of innovative therapies in sepsis. *Chest*, 101:1644–1655.

Bredle, D., Samsel, R., Schumacker, P., and Cain, S. (1989). Critical O_2 delivery to skeletal muscle at high and low P_{O_2} in endotoxemic dogs. *J. Appl. Physiol.*, 66:2553–2558.

Breslow, M., Miller, C., Parker, S., Walman, A., and Traystman, R. (1987). Effect of vasopresors on organ blood flow during endotoxin shock in pigs. *Am. J. Physiol.*, 252(21): H291–H300.

Chaudry, I., Wichterman, K., and Baue, A. (1979). Effect of sepsis on tissue adenine nucleotide levels. *Surgery*, 85:205–211.

Clowes, G., Zuschneid, W., Turner, M., Blackburn, G., Rubin, J., Toala, P., and Green, G. (1968). Observations of the pathogenesis of the pneumonitis associated with severe infections in other parts of the body. *Ann. Surg.*, 167:63–69.

Cryer, H., Garrison, R., Harris, P., Greenwald, B., and Alsip, N. (1990). Prostaglandins mediate skeletal muscle arteriole dilation in hyperdynamic bacteremia. *Am. J. Physiol.* 259:H728–H734.

Cunningham, J., Carter, N., Rector, F., and Seldin, D. (1971). Resting transmembrane potential difference of skeletal muscle in normal subjects and severely ill patients. *J. Clin. Invest.*, 50:49–59.

Davies, J. A., Quintanilha, A. T., Brooks, G. A., and Packer, L. (1982). Free radicals and tissue damage produced by exercise. *Biochem. Biophys. Res. Comm.*, 107:1198–1205.

Demling, R., and Lalonde, C. (1989). Relationship between lung injury and lung lipid peroxidation caused by recurrent endotoxemia. *Am. Rev. Respir. Dis.*, 139:1118–1124.

Diaz, P., Julian, M., and Clanton, T. (1991). Endotoxin and tumor necrosis factor do not directly affect in vitro diaphragm force production and fatigability (abstract). *Am. Rev. Respir. Dis.*, 143:A561.

Drew, J., Farkas, G., Pearson, R., and Rochester, D. (1988). Effects of a chronic wasting infection on skeletal muscle size and contractile properties. *J. Appl. Physiol.*, 64:460–465.

Dureuil, B., Viires, N., Veber, B., Pavlovic, D., Pariente, R., Desmonts, J. M., and Aubier, M. (1989). Acute diaphragmatic changes induced by starvation in rats. *Am. J. Clin. Nutr.*, 49:738–744.

Ferguson, J., Spitzer, J., and Miler, H. (1978). Effects of endotoxin on regional blood flow in the unanesthetized guinea pig. *J. Surg. Res.*, 25:236–243.

Feuerstein, G., Dimicco, J., Ramu, A., and Kopin, I. (1981). Effect of indomethacin on the blood pressure and plasma catecholamine responses to acute endotoxaemia. *J. Pharm. Pharmacol.*, 33:576–579.

Fish, R., Lang, C., and Spitzer, J. (1986). Regional blood flow during continuous low-dose endotoxin infusion. *Circ. Shock*, 18:267–275.

Fletcher, J. (1982). The role of prostaglandins in sepsis. *Scand. J. Infect. Dis.*, 31(suppl):55–60.

Fletcher, J. (1983). Prostaglandin synthetase inhibitors in endotoxin or septic shock. A review. *Adv. Shock Res.*, 10:9–14.

Fliegel, S., Lee, E., McCoy, J., Johnson, K., and Varani, J. (1984). Protein degradation following treatment with hydrogen peroxide. *Am. J. Pathol.*, 115:418–425.

Flores, E., Bistrian, B., Pomposelli, J., Dinarello, C., Blackburn, G., and Istfan, N. (1989). Infusion of tumor necrosis factor/cachectin promotes muscle catabolism in the rat. *J. Clin. Invest.*, 83:1614–1622.

Fong, Y., Moldawer, L., Marano, M., Wei, H., Barber, A., Manogue, K., Tracey, K., Kuo, G., Fischman, D., Cerami, T., and Lowry, S. (1989). Cachectin/TNF or IL-1 alpha induces cachexia with redistribution of body proteins. *Am. J. Physiol.*, 256:R659–R665.

Friman, G., Ilback, N., and Beisel, W. (1984). Effects of *Streptococcus pneumoniae*, *Salmonella typhimurium*, and *Francisella tularensis* infections on oxidative, glycolitic and lysosomal enzyme activity in red and white skeletal muscle in the rat. *Scand. J. Infect. Dis.*, 16:111–119.

Golberg, A., Kettelhut, I., Furuno, K., Fagan, J., and Baracos, V. (1988). Activation of protein breakdown and prostaglandin E_2 production in rat skeletal muscle in fever is signaled by a macrophage product distinct from interleukin 1 or other known monokines. *J. Clin. Invest.* 81:1378–1383.

Goldhaber, J. I., Ji, S., Lamp, S. T., and Weiss, J. N. (1989). Effects of exogenous free radicals on electromechanical function and metabolism in isolated rabbit and guinea pig ventricle. *J. Clin. Invest.*, 83:1800–1809.

Gryglewski, R., Palmer, R., and Moncada, S. (1986). Superoxide anion is involved in the breakdown of endothelium-derived relaxing factor. *Nature*, 320:454–456.

Gutierrez, G., Lund, N., and Palizas, F. (1991). Rabbit skeletal muscle P_{O_2} during hypodynamic sepsis. *Chest*, 99:224–229.

Harken, A., Woods, M., and Wright, C. (1975). Influence of endotoxin on tissue respiration and oxygen dissociation in an isolated canine hindlimb. *Ann. Surg.*, 41:704–709.

Harlan, J. (1985). Leukocyte-endothelial interaction. *Blood*, 65:513–525.

Hasselgren, P., Talamini, M., Lafrance, R., James, J., Peters, J., and Fisher, J. (1985). Effect of indomethacin on proteolysis in septic muscle. *Ann. Surg.*, 202:557–562.

Hasselgren, P., Pedersen, P., Sax, H., Warner, B., and Fisher, J. (1988). Current concepts of protein turnover and amoni acid transport in liver and skeletal muscle during sepsis. *Arch. Surg.*, 123:982–999.

Howell, S., Fitzgerald, R. S., and Roussos, C. (1985). Effects of uncompensated and compensated metabolic acidosis on canine diaphragm. *J. Appl. Physiol.*, 59:1376–1382.

Hummel, R., James, J., Warner, B., Hasselgren, P. and Fischer, J. (1988). Evidence that cathepsin B contributes to skeletal muscle protein breakdown during sepsis. *Arch. Surg.*, 123:221–224.

Hurtado, F., Gutierrez, A., Silva, N., Fernandez, E., Khan, A., and Gutierrez, G. (1992). Role of tissue hypoxia as the mechanism of lactic acidosis during *E. coli* endotoxemia. *J. Appl. Physiol.*, 72:1895–1901.

Hussain, S., and Roussos, C. (1985a). Distribution of respiratory muscle and organ blood flow during endotoxic shock in dogs. *J. Appl. Physiol.*, 59:1802–1808.

Hussain, S., Simkus, G., and Roussos, C. (1985b). Respiratory muscle fatigue: a cause of ventilatory muscle failure in septic shock. *J. Appl. Physiol.*, 58:2033–2040.

Hussain, S., Graham, R., Rutledge, F., and Roussos, C. (1986). Respiratory muscle energetics during endotoxic shock in dogs. *J. Appl. Physiol.*, 60:486–493.

Hussain, S., Roussos, C., and Magder, S. (1988). Autoregulation of diaphragmatic blood flow in dogs. *J. Appl. Physiol.*, 64:329–36.

Illner, H., and Shires, G. (1981). Membrane defect and energy status of rabbit skeletal muscle cells in sepsis and septic shock. *Arch. Surg.*, 116:1302–1305.

Jacobs, E., Soulsby, M., and Bone, R. (1982). Ibuprofen in canine endotoxic shock. *J. Clin. Invest.*, 70:536–541.

Jepson, M. M., Cox, M., Bates, P. C., Rothwell, N. J., Stock, M. J., Cady, E. B., and Millward, D. J. (1987). Regional blood flow and skeletal muscle energy status in endotoxemic rats. *Am. J. Physiol.*, 252:E581–587.

Julou-Schaeffer, G., Gray, G., Fleming, I., Schott, C., Parrat, J., and Stoclet, J. (1990). Loss of vascular responsiveness induced by endotoxin involves L-arginine pathway. *Am. J. Physiol.*, 259:H1038–H1043.

Kennedy, T., Rao, N., Noah, W., Michael, J., Jafri, M., Gurtner, G., and Hoidal, J. (1990). Ibuprofen prevents oxidant lung injury and in vitro lipid peroxidation by chelating iron. *J. Clin. Invest.*, 86:1565–1573.

Lang, C., Bagby, G., Ferguson, J., and Spitzer, J. (1984). Cardiac output and redistribution of organ blood flow in hypermetabolic sepsis. *Am. J. Physiol.*, 246:R331–R337.

Leon, A., Boczkowski, J., Dureuil, B., Desmonts, J., and Aubier, M. (1992). Effects of endotoxic shock on diaphragmatic function in mechanically ventilated rats. *J. Appl. Physiol.*, 72:1466–1472.

Magder, S., Lockhat, D., Luo, B., and Roussos, C. (1985). Respiratory muscle and organ blood flow with elastic loading and shock. *J. Appl. Physiol.*, 58:1148–1156.

Maridonneau, I., Braquet, P., and Garay, R. P. (1983). Na^+ and K^+ transport damage induced by oxygen free radicals in human red cell membranes. *J. Biol. Chem.*, 258:3107–3113.

Marx, J. (1987). Oxygen free radicals linked to many diseases. *Science*, 235:529–531.

Matsuda, T., Eccleston, C., Rubinstein, I., Rennard, S., and Joyner, W. (1991). Antioxidants attenuate endotoxin-induced microvascular leakage of macromolecules in vivo. *J. Appl. Physiol.*, 70:1483–1489.

McCord, J. M. (1985). Oxygen free radicals in postischemic tissue injury. *N. Engl. J. Med.*, 312:159–163.

McKechnie, K., Furman, B., and Parratt, J. (1986). Modification by oxygen free radical scavengers of the metabolic and cardiovascular effects of endotoxin infusion in conscious rats. *Circ. Shock*, 19:429–439.

Metz, C., and Sheagren, J. (1990). Ibuprofen in animal models of septic shock. *J. Crit. Care*, 5:206–211.

Metzger, J., and Fitts, R. (1987). Role of intracellular pH in muscle fatigue. *J. Appl. Physiol.*, 62:1392–1397.

Montgomery, A., Stager, M., Carrico, C., and Hudson, L. (1985). Causes of mortality in patients with the adult respiratory distress syndrome. *Am. Rev. Respir. Dis.*, 132:485–489.

Morgan, R., Manning, P., Coran, A., Drongowski, R., Till, G., Ward, P., and Oldham, K. (1988). Oxygen free radical activity during live *E. coli* septic shock in the dog. *Circ. Shock*, 25:319–323.

Murphy, T., Mayock, D., Standaert, T., Gibson, R., and Woodrum, D. (1992a). Group B streptococcus has no effect on piglet diaphragmatic force generation. *Am. Rev. Respir. Dis.*, 145:471–475.

Murphy, T., Standaert, T., Gibson, R., Mayock, D., and Woodrum, D. (1992b). Group B streptococcal (GBS) shock impairs diaphragmatic contractility in the piglet (abstract). *Am. Rev. Respir. Dis.*, 145:A560.

O'Donnell, T., Clowes, G., Blackburn, G., and Ryan, N. (1974). Relationship of hindlimb energy fuel metabolism to the circulatory responses in severe sepsis. *J. Surg. Res.*, 16:112–123.

Petty, T., and Ashbaugh, D. (1971). The adult respiratory distress syndrome—clinical features, factors influencing prognosis and principles of management. *Chest*, 70:233–239.

Pressler, V., Fagan, J., Scott, T., McMillen, A., and Wilmore, D. (1985). Intra-arterial infusion of PG E_2 produces increased skeletal muscle protein degradation in rats. *Surg. Forum*, 37:52–53.

Raetz, C., Ulevitch, R., Wright, S., Sibley, C., Ding, A., and Nathan, C. (1991). Gram-negative endotoxin: an extraordinary lipid with profound effects on eukaryotic signal transduction. *FASEB J.*, 5:2652–2660.

Raymond, R., and Emerson, T. (1976). Cerebral metabolism during endotoxin shock (abstract). *Fed. Proc.*, 35:794.

Reid, M., and Johnson, R. (1983). Efficiency, maximal blood flow and aerobic work capacity of canine diaphragm. *J. Appl. Physiol.*, 54:763–772.

Reilly, P. M., Schiller, H. J., and Bulkley, G. B. (1991). Pharmacologic approach to tissue injury mediated by free radicals and other reactive oxygen metabolites. *Am. J. Surg.*, 161:488–503.

Robertson, C., Foster, G., and Johnson, R. J. (1977). The relationship of respiratory failure to the oxygen consumption of, lactate production by, and distribution of blood flow among respiratory muscles during increasing respiratory resistance. *J. Clin. Invest.*, 59:31–42.

Rochester, D., and Bettini, G. (1976). Diaphragmatic blood flow and energy expenditure in the dog. Effects of inspiratory airflow resistance and hypercapnia. *J. Clin. Invest.*, 57:661–672.

Rochester, D., Braun, N., and Laine, S. (1977). Diaphragmatic energy expenditure in chronic respiratory failure: the effect of assisted ventilation with body respirators. *Am. J. Med.*, 63:223–232.

Rodemann, H., and Goldberg, A. (1982). Arachidonic acid, prostaglandin E_2 and F_2 influences rates of protein turnover in skeletal and cardiac muscle. *J. Biol. Chem.*, 257:1632–1638.

Romanosky, A., McGuinness, O., Bagby, G., and Spitzer, J. (1981). Increased muscle oxygen consumption during electrical stimulation following endotoxin administration. *Adv. Shock Res.*, 6:121–129.

Roussos, C., and Macklem, P. (1982). The respiratory muscles. *N. Engl. J. Med.*, 307:786–797.

Ruff, R. L., and Secrist, D. (1984). Inhibitors of prostaglandin synthesis or cathepsin B prevent muscle wasting due to sepsis in the rat. *J. Clin. Invest.*, 73:1483–1486.

Ryan, N. (1976). Metabolic adaptations for energy production during trauma and sepsis. *Surg. Clin. North Am.*, 56:1073–1090.

Samsel, R., Nelson, D., Sanders, W., Wood, L., and Schumacker, P. (1988). Effect of endotoxin on systemic and skeletal muscle O_2 extraction. *J. Appl. Physiol.*, 65:1377–1382.

Samuelsson, B., Goldyne, M., Granström, E., Hamberg, M., Hammarström, S., and Malmstem, C. (1978). Prostaglandins and thromboxanes. *Ann. Rev. Biochem.*, 47:997–1029.

Seekamp, A., Lalonde, C., Zhu, D., and Demling, R. (1988). Catalase prevents prostanoid release and lung lipid peroxidation after endotoxemia in sheep. *J. Appl. Physiol.*, 65:1210–1216.

Shindoh, C., Dimarco, A., Nethery, D., and Supinski, G. (1992). Effect of PEG-superoxide dismutase on the diaphragmatic response to endotoxin. *Am. Rev. Respir. Dis.*, 145:1350–1354.

Sibbald, W., Fox, G., and Martin, C. (1991). Abnormalities of vascular reactivity in the sepsis syndrome. *Chest*, 100:155s–159s.

Siegel, J., Greespan, M., and Del Guercio, L. (1967). Abnormal vascular tone, defective oxygen transport and myocardial failure in human sepstic shock. *Ann. Surg.*, 165:504–517.

Siegel, J. (1981). Relations between circulatory and metabolic changes in sepsis. *Ann. Rev. Med.*, 32:175–194.

Sperelakis, N., and Fabiato, A. (1985). Electrophysiology and excitation-contraction coupling in skeletal muscle. In *The Thorax*. Edited by C. Roussos and P. T. Macklem. New York, Marcel Dekker, pp. 45–67.

Supinski, G. (1986). Control of respiratory muscle blood flow. *Am. Rev. Respir. Dis.*, 134:1078–1079.

Supinski, G., Shindoh, C., Netherly, A., and Dimarco, A. (1990). Effect of SOD on the diaphragmatic response to endotoxin (abstract). *FASEB J.*, 4:A949.

Takeda, K., Shimada, Y., Okada, T., Amano, M., Sakai, T., and Yoshiya, I. (1986). Lipid peroxidation in experimental septic rats. *Crit. Care Med.*, 14:719–723.

Tavakoli, H., and Mela, L. (1982). Alteratons of mithocondrial metabolism and protein concentration in subacute septicemia. *Infect. Immun.*, 38:536–541.

Tesch, P., Sjodin, B., Thorstensson, A., and Karlsson, J. (1978). Muscle fatigue and its relation to lactate accumulation and LDH activity in man. *Acta Physiol. Scand.*, 103:413–420.

Tischler, M., and Fagan, J. (1983). Response to trauma of protein, amino acid and carbohydrate metabolism in injured and uninjured rat skeletal muscles. *Metabolism*, 32:853–867.

Tracey, K., Lowry, S., Beutler, B., Cerami, A., Albert, J., and Shires, G. (1986). Cachectin/Tumor necrosis factor mediates changes of skeletal muscle plasma membrane potential. *J. Exp. Med.*, 164:1368–1373.

Turinsky, J., and Loegering, D. (1985). Prostaglandin E_2 and muscle protein turnover in *Pseudomonas aeruginosa* sepsis. *Biochem. Biophys. Acta*, 840:137–140.

Van Lambakgen, A., Bronsveld, W., Van Den Bos, G., and Thijs, K. (1984). Distribution of cardiac output, oxygen cosumption, and lactate production in canine endotoxin shock. *Cardiovasc. Res.*, 18:195–201.

Van Surell, C., Boczkowski, J., Pasquier, C., Du, Y., Franzini, E., and Aubier, M. (1992). Effects of N-acetylcysteine on diaphragmatic function and malondialdehyde content in *E. coli* endotoxemic rats. *Am. Rev. Respir. Dis.*, 146:730–734.

Vary, T., Siegel, J., Nakatani, T., Sato, T., and Aoyama, H. (1986). Effect of sepsis on activity of pyruvate dehydrogenase complex in skeletal muscle and liver. *Am. J. Physiol.*, 250:E634–E640.

Vicaut, E., Hou, X., Payen, D., Bousseau, A., and Tedgui, A. (1991). Acute effects of tumor necrosis factor on the microcirculation of rat cremaster muscle. *J. Clin. Invest.*, 87:1537–1540.

Viires, N., Syllie, G., Aubier, M., Rassidiakis, A., and Roussos, C. (1983). Regional blood flow distribution in dog during induced hypotension and low cardiac output. *J. Clin. Invest.*, 72:935–947.

Wakai, Y., Wilcox, P., Cooper, J., Walley, K., and Road, J. (1991). The effect of tumor necrosis factor α TNF α) on diaphragmatic contractility in anesthetized dogs (abstract). *Am. Rev. Respir. Dis.*, 143:A560.

Wilcox, P., and Bressler, B. (1992a). Effects of tumor necrosis factor α on in vitro hamster diaphragm contractility (abstract). *Am. Rev. Respir. Dis.*, 145:A457.

Wilcox, P., Osborne, S., and Bressler, B. (1992b). Monocyte inflammatory mediators impair in vitro hamster diaphragm contractility. *Am. Rev. Respir. Dis.*, 146:462–466.

Witcherman, K., Bave, A., and Chaudry, J. (1980). Sepsis and septic shock. A review of laboratory models and a proposal. *J. Surg. Res.*, 189–201.

Wright, C., Duff, J., McLean, A. and McLean, L. (1971). Regional capillary blood flow and oxygen uptake in severe sepsis. *Surg. Gynecol. Obstet.*, 132:637–644.

Wyler, F., Forsyth, R., Nies, A., Neuze, J., and Melmon, K. (1969). Endotoxin-induced regional circulatory changes in the unanesthetized monkey. *Circ. Res.*, 24:777–786.

Wyler, F., Neutze, J., and Rudolph, A. (1970). Effects of endotoxin on distribution of cardiac output in unanesthetized rabbits. *Am. J. Physiol.*, 219:246–251.

52

Gravity

MARC ESTENNE

Erasme University Hospital
Brussels, Belgium

LUDWIG A. ENGEL

Westmead Hospital
Sydney, Australia

MANUEL PAIVA

Université Libre de Bruxelles
Brussels, Belgium

I. Introduction

The normal respiratory system is exquisitely sensitive to gravity, which causes regional differences in intrapleural pressure, alveolar size, ventilation and perfusion, gas exchange, and parenchymal stresses within the lungs (West, 1977, 1991; Engel, 1991) and determines the configuration of the relaxed chest wall (Agostoni and Mead, 1964). Despite this susceptibility, there have been relatively few experimental observations on the respiratory function under conditions of microgravity. In part this is due to the difficulty in creating gravity-free environments. Also, weightlessness affects many organs in the body and the resultant functional disturbances are generally more important than in the case of the lung. In fact, ventilatory function during space flights has appeared to be adequately maintained, and no major respiratory problems have been identified so far.

Many ground-based studies have assessed the effect of microgravity on the respiratory system using extrapolations from hypergravity experiments or supposed analogs of weightlessness such as water immersion and changes in the orientation of the gravitational field with respect to the body between the upright ($+1$ Gz) and supine ($+1$ Gx) or head-down ($-$ Gz) postures. None of these indirect approaches, however, creates true gravity-free conditions because residual hydrostatic pressure gradients are always present. These conditions can only be produced during space flights or aboard high-powered jet aircraft flying through a Keplerian arc (Fig. 1). During such flights the aircraft is first pitched up to a 45° nose-high altitude, which increases head-to-foot acceleration to ~+1.8 Gz. Then the nose is lowered to abolish wing lift, and engine thrust is reduced to balance drag (producing near 0 Gz). A ballistic parabolic flight profile results and is maintained until the aircraft nose is 45° below the horizon; this allows 0 Gz to be sustained for 20–25 s. A +1.8 Gz pullout lasting for ~20 s brings the aircraft back to steady horizontal flight at 1 Gz and the whole cycle can be repeated. Because many parabolas may be performed during a single flight, this approach offers the advantage of multiple measurements and reproducibility testing. In addition, because measurements may be obtained at 1 and 0 Gz within less than 1 min, they should not be influenced by factors other than gravity itself. However, observations during parabolic flights are by necessity limited to the brief period immediately following entry into the weightless state and therefore no information is obtainable about less rapid and/or adaptative physiological changes. Furthermore, the short period of hypergravity preceding the period of weightlessness may potentially influence the measurements.

In contrast, during space flight, time constraints limit the number of repeated measurements, and variables other than gravity may play a role. Nevertheless, manned space flights offer the only opportunity to study human adaptation to prolonged exposure to microgravity. Until recently, studies of lung function during space flight had been limited to isolated measurements of vital capacity among U.S. and Soviet crew members. In 1991 and 1993, however, extensive measurements of

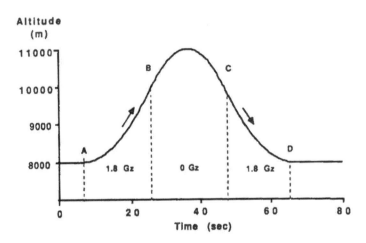

Figure 1   Maneuver profile during a parabola. (A) From a horizontal flight path at ~8,000 m, aircraft commences a pull-up with an acceleration of 1.7–2.0 Gz. (B) Engine thrust is reduced, and aircraft begins a free-falling parabolic trajectory and a period of microgravity. (C) Pull-out from dive path with an acceleration of 1.7–2.0 Gz. (D) Return to horizontal flight at Gz. (From Estenne et al., 1992.)

cardiopulmonary function were performed on Spacelab Life Sciences-1 (SLS-1) and D-2 missions, which were the first Spacelab flights primarily dedicated to life sciences (West, 1992).

In this chapter, we will summarize and discuss data obtained during direct exposure to weightlessness and report some results from hypergravity experiments. In the first section, we describe the impact on the cardiorespiratory system of the redistribution of blood volume and extracellular fluid due to changes in hydrostatic pressure gradient. Then we discuss the effects of changing Gz on lung and chest wall mechanics. The last section describes changes in ventilation and perfusion distribution. The bulk of microgravity data have been obtained during parabolic flights at the very onset of weightlessness. The Spacelab flights scheduled in the coming years will hopefully provide more information on the cardiorespiratory adaptations to prolonged weightlessness.

II. Redistribution of Blood Volume and Extracellular Fluid

A. Increase in Central Blood Volume

Redistribution of blood volume and extracellular fluid due to removal of the hydrostatic pressure gradient is a major response to weightlessness. Its importance to the cardiorespiratory system is the expected rise in intrathoracic blood volume and consequent alterations in pulmonary diffusing capacity and cardiac output. Studies of leg volumes by multiple girth measurements in Skylab IV and subsequent shuttle flights have shown reductions of 1.5–2.0 liters (Thornton et al., 1987), and astronauts commonly experience a sensation of fullness in the head, stuffy nose, nasal voice, and burning eyes (Johnston and Dietlein, 1977; Thornton et al., 1977). In addition, jugular veins of subjects submitted to 0 Gz appear to be distended (Levy and Talbot, 1983), and photographs taken during orbital flights frequently show evidence of facial edema with periorbital swelling. These observations suggest that the headward shift of blood produced by gravitational unloading may be substantial.

From studies using postural changes from upright to supine, head-out immersion, head-down tilt bedrest, and inflation of fracture splints or anti-G-suit around the limbs, it has been estimated that the increase in central blood volume produced by these various experimental conditions is between 200 and 700 ml (Sjöstrand, 1951, 1952; Weissler et al., 1957; Arborelius et al., 1972; Blomqvist and Stone, 1983; Chadha et al., 1983; Kimball et al., 1986) and that it results in a 6–12 torr rise in central venous pressure (Echt et al., 1974; Norsk et al., 1987). An increase in this pressure has also been reported in an orbiting macaque monkey (Meehan, 1971) and immediately after entry into weightlessness during parabolic flights (Norsk et al., 1987). On the other hand, Kirsch et al. (1984) documented a decrease in central venous pressure estimated from antecubital vein measurements 22 h after launch in four Spacelab-1 astronauts. This unexpected finding has been recently confirmed by direct measurements of central venous pressure, which was continuously recorded from 5 h before launch until 9 h into the flight in one crew member of the SLS-1 mission (Buckey et al., 1993). Central venous pressure increased during launching because of a threefold increase in acceleration but then decreased in weightlessness below preflight values. This observation, which was not predicted by ground-based models, might be related to the absence of any pressure within tissues in microgravity. This could alter compliance throughout the cardiovascular system so that the same blood volume is contained at a lower pressure.

Redistribution of blood volume to the thorax in weightlessness has been qualitatively demonstrated by a reduction in thoracic impedance (Lathers et al., 1989). However, using simultaneous measurements of thoracoabdominal and lung volumes, Paiva et al. (1989) were unable to detect a significant increase in thoracic blood volume after entry into weightlessness during parabolic flights. They considered it unlikely that a blood volume shift in excess of ~200 ml could have been missed, which suggests that the increase in central blood volume during short periods of microgravity may be smaller than that induced by postural changes, head-out immersion, or inflation of anti-G-suit at 1 Gz.

During prolonged exposure to weightlessness, a variety of neurohumoral factors rapidly come into play, resulting in contraction of circulating blood volume (Bungo and Johnson, 1983; Guy and Prisk, 1989). This response is in part responsible for the 2–3 kg weight loss that has been found in Skylab crewmembers (Thornton et al., 1977; Thornton and Ord, 1977) and more recently in Spacelab astronauts (Bungo et al., 1987). A qualitatively similar response is seen during bedrest, head-down tilt, and water immersion (Blomqvist and Stone, 1983). In addition, the usual prelaunch position (supine with legs elevated) for up to 4 h before space flights induces some fluid redistribution even before weightlessness is experienced, which probably accelerates these compensatory changes (Lathers et al., 1989; Mukai et al., 1991). Among other factors, contraction of circulating blood volume contributes to the development of orthostatic intolerance upon return to 1 Gz after space flight. Postflight faintness on standing is common, and lower body negative pressure (LBNP) typically produces more disturbances postflight than preflight (Blomqvist and Stone, 1983).

B. Effect on Pulmonary Diffusing Capacity and Its Subdivisions

Comprehensive measurements of pulmonary diffusing capacity (D_L), pulmonary capillary blood volume (V_c), and membrane diffusing capacity (D_m) have been obtained in four subjects exposed to 9 days of microgravity during the SLS-1 mission (Prisk et al., 1993). Measurements were performed pre- and postflight in the standing and supine postures, and in-flight after approximately 24 h of exposure to microgravity and on days 4 and 9. The results can be summarized as follows. Microgravity produced increases in D_L, V_c, and D_m which, on average, were ~28%

greater than the control preflight standing values (Fig. 2). All variables remained unchanged for the duration of the flight and immediately returned to control levels postflight. The changes in V_c with microgravity were quantitatively similar to those seen on transition from standing to supine; in contrast, whereas such postural changes have no significant effect on D_m, microgravity caused it to rise substantially. To the extent that V_c and D_m are the two components of D_L, one can thus understand why the increase in D_L observed at 0 Gz was almost twice as great as that elicited by the standing-to-supine transition (Fig. 2).

The large increase in D_m during microgravity compared to the supine posture suggests that there is considerably more surface available for gas exchange. This is because hydrostatic differences in vascular pressures are completely abolished at 0 Gz. As a result the increase in V_c due to removal of blood pooling in the periphery is associated with an uniform capillary filling and hence a large increase in the surface area of the blood-gas barrier (Prisk et al., 1993). In contrast, such extensive capillary recruitment does not occur, or does so only to a limited extent, on transition from standing to supine because capillaries are not fully recruited in the upper regions of the lung where vascular pressures remain relatively low.

The rise in diffusing capacity in weightlessness is thus directly related to an

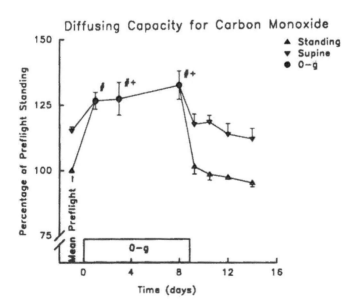

Figure 2 Means of individually normalized data obtained from four crew members, preflight and postflight in the standing and supine position, and in-flight during the SLS-1 mission. Error bars, ±SE. Data that differ significantly from the standing pre- and postflight values ($^{#}p < 0.05$) and from the supine pre- and postflight values ($^{+}p < 0.05$) are marked. (From Prisk et al., 1993.)

increase and a more uniform distribution of capillary blood volume throughout the lung. These changes were maintained for the whole duration of the SLS-1 mission despite large reductions in plasma volume and therefore presumably also in circulating blood volume (Prisk et al., 1993). This suggests that contraction of blood volume occurred primarily in the systemic veins, which contain approximately 70% of total blood volume (Blomqvist and Stone, 1983).

C. Effect on Cardiac Function

Estimates of cardiac function derived from measurements of thoracic impedance indicate that both cardiac index and stroke volume increased during short periods of weightlessness, whereas heart rate decreased (Lathers et al., 1989; Mukai et al., 1991). These changes have been attributed to the headward shift of blood volume, which directly increases cardiac filling pressures and reduces heart rate by stimulation of cardiovascular receptors. In-flight echocardiograms obtained during space flights have also shown a trend toward early increases in left ventricular end-diastolic and stroke volumes, but these changes were small in magnitude and were not maintained for more than 1–4 days after launch (Pourcelot et al., 1983; Charles and Lathers, 1991).

Using rebreathing techniques, Prisk et al. (1993) measured stroke volume and pulmonary capillary blood flow—which reflects cardiac output—at various time intervals before, during, and after the SLS-1 mission. Cardiac output rose to preflight supine levels after 24 h of exposure to microgravity but decreased thereafter and remained intermediate to preflight standing and supine values. However, taken as a whole, in-flight cardiac output was elevated compared to preflight standing (Fig. 3). Similarly, stroke volume was elevated on mission days 2 and 4 to approximately supine preflight levels, and then gradually decreased. Altogether these data indicate that redistribution of blood volume in microgravity produces an initial increase in cardiac output and stroke volume in much the same way as water immersion or going from upright to supine does (Blomqvist and Stone, 1983). Both changes tend to lessen within a few days of exposure to weightlessness, but the time required for a complete adaptation is unknown as yet.

In opposition to microgravity, increasing gravitational stresses accentuates orthostatic fluid shifts from the thorax to the legs, and hence reduces end-diastolic ventricular volume, stroke volume, and cardiac output. Conversely, heart rate increases in an almost linear fashion with increasing Gz (Blomqvist and Stone, 1983; Boutellier et al., 1985; Arieli et al., 1986).

III. Lung and Chest Wall Mechanics

A. Lung and Chest Wall Volumes at End-Expiration

Gravity exerts a major influence on lung and chest wall volumes at end-expiration. In an early analysis, Agostoni and Mead (1964) predicted that functional residual

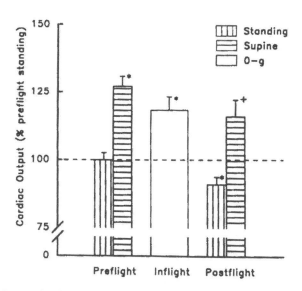

Figure 3 Means of individually normalized data obtained from four crew members, preflight and postflight in the standing and supine position, and in-flight during the SLS-1 mission. In-flight data are an average over 9 days of the flight. Error bars, SE. Data that differ significantly from the preflight standing value (*$p < 0.05$) and from the preflight supine value ($^+p < 0.05$) are marked. (From Prisk et al., 1993.)

capacity (FRC) in the weightless state should be intermediate between those found in the upright and in the supine postures, i.e., it should decrease by about 10% ongoing from 1 to 0 Gz. However, early measurements of FRC in parabolic flights have been inconclusive (von Baumgarten et al., 1980; Wetzig, 1986; Wetzig and von Baumgarten, 1987), and chest radiographs made at FRC in five seated normal subjects after 10 s of microgravity showed no significant differences between 1 and 0 Gz, although the lung tended to become somewhat shorter and wider (Michels et al., 1979). On the other hand, more recent studies by several groups of investigators have consistently demonstrated a 200- to 500-ml decrease in FRC during short periods of microgravity (Fig. 4); as expected, there was a concomitant rise in end-expiratory esophageal pressure (Paiva et al., 1989; Prisk et al., 1990; Edyvean et al., 1991; Kays et al., 1993). Similarly, repeated measurements performed on four astronauts during the SLS-1 mission have shown that although pre- and postflight FRC values were not different, the in-flight FRC was on average 15% (520 ml) lower than the preflight standing FRC. This decrease was sustained throughout the 9-day mission (Elliott et al., 1994). These data thus provide unequivocal evidence that both short and prolonged exposure to microgravity produce a substantial reduction in FRC. This reduction may be potentially due to blood volume shifts into the thorax and mechanical factors.

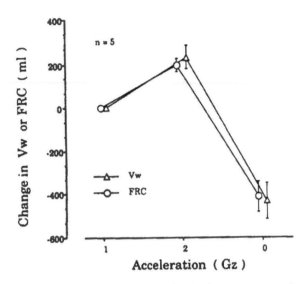

Figure 4 Changes in end-expiratory thoracoabdominal volume (Vw) or functional residual capacity (FRC) as a function of acceleration (Gz) in the sequence observed during parabolic flight paths in five normal seated subjects. Error bars, ±SE. (From Paiva et al., 1989.)

Blood Volume Shifts

All other things being equal, changes in blood volume within the thoracoabdominal cavity are expected to cause reciprocal changes in chest wall and lung volumes (Agostoni and Mead, 1964), in much the same way as a pleural effusion (Estenne et al., 1983; Gilmartin et al., 1985) or a pneumothorax (Heaf and Prime, 1954) does. The distribution of the volume changes between the chest wall and the lung depends primarily on the relative compliances of these two structures, i.e., the more compliant the lung relative to the chest wall, the greater the decrease in lung volume and the smaller the increase in chest wall volume, and vice versa. Studies in normal humans using inflation of fracture splints (Kimball et al., 1986) or inflation of a 1-liter balloon in the stomach (Gilroy et al., 1985), as well as studies of induced pleural effusions in upright dogs (Krell and Rodarte, 1985), have shown that in these various experimental conditions the supplementary volume added to the respiratory system is primarily accommodated by the chest wall. The increase in chest wall volume was in general twice as great as the decrease in lung volume, indicating a relatively effective protection of intrathoracic gas volume.

The distribution of the increased blood volume between the lung and the chest wall in weightlessness is unknown. Although this increase is expected to minimize the decrease in thoracoabdominal volume while amplifying the decrease in lung volume, Paiva et al. (1989) were unable to find a difference between the reduction in thoracoabdominal volume and that in FRC after entry into weightlessness during parabolic flights (Fig. 4). As already stressed, this suggests that blood volume shifts are relatively small in magnitude during short periods of microgravity. In addition, if two thirds of the volume change are accommodated by the chest wall, as reported in the above-mentioned studies, then blood volume shifts at 0 Gz should only have a minor effect on FRC. Its reduction in microgravity would thus be due primarily, if not exclusively, to mechanical factors.

Mechanical Factors

Using a respiratory inductance plethysmograph, Paiva et al. (1989) and Edyvean et al. (1991) found that the decrease in FRC in microgravity was primarily due to a decrease in the volume of the abdominal compartment of the chest wall (Fig. 5). They observed that changes in end-expiratory abdominal volume followed closely changes in Gz and were remarkably reproducible during each parabolic maneuver. A change from the upright to the supine posture (1 Gz to 1 Gx) and immersion of seated subjects to the xiphoid process are also associated with an inward displacement of the anterior abdominal wall, a cranial displacement of the diaphragm, and a fall in FRC (Agostoni and Mead, 1964; Agostoni et al., 1966; Prefaut et al., 1976). In microgravity these changes occur because the weight of the abdominal contents is removed.

Whereas changes in end-expiratory abdominal volume during parabolic flights proved to be very consistent, changes in end-expiratory rib cage volume were more

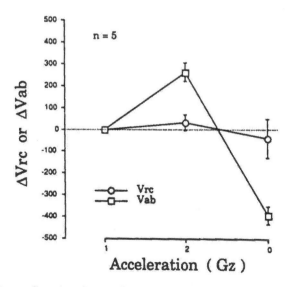

Figure 5   Changes in end-expiratory rib cage (ΔVrc) and abdominal (ΔVab) volumes as a function of acceleration (Gz) in the sequence observed during parabolic flight paths in five normal seated subjects. Error bars, $\pm$SE. (From Paiva et al., 1989.)

variable. This volume did not change at 0 Gz compared to 1 Gz in one study (Fig. 5) (Paiva et al., 1989), but it was found to increase at 0 Gz in a subsequent study by the same group of investigators (Edyvean et al., 1991). In part, this variability may be due to the fact that removal of gravitational stresses does not affect all rib cage dimensions uniformly. Using pairs of magnetometers to measure changes in rib cage dimensions in five normal seated subjects during parabolic flights, Estenne et al. (1992) found that microgravity was associated with a consistent motion of the sternum in the cranial direction and an increase in the anteroposterior diameter of the lower rib cage (measured at the level of the 5th intercostal space). In contrast, there was a systematic decrease in the transverse diameter of the lower rib cage, which therefore adopted a more circular shape in weightlessness (Fig. 6).

The increase in rib cage anteroposterior diameter at 0 Gz was anticipated. In the upright posture at 1 Gz, gravitational loading of the abdomen produces a hydrostatic gradient of pressure that lengthens and stretches passively the ventral abdominal wall. Because the abdominal muscles insert on the sternum and the lower ribs, this passive tension is applied to the lower rib cage and acts to pull it downward. By removing the weight of the abdominal contents, transition to weightlessness removes the tension in the abdominal wall, and transabdominal pressure becomes nearly zero (Fig. 7) (Edyvean et al., 1991). As a result, the sternum and the ribs move upward and the ventral rib cage expands. A similar change is observed during immersion of seated subjects from hips to lower sternum (Reid et al., 1986). It is more difficult to understand why the transverse diameter of the lower rib cage did

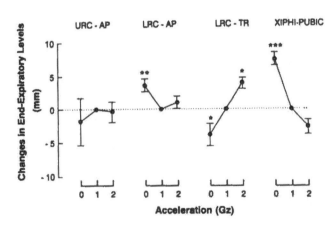

Figure 6 Average changes in rib cage dimensions at end expiration relative to 1 Gz in five normal seated subjects during parabolic flights. URC-AP, upper rib cage anteroposterior diameter; LRC-AP, lower rib cage anteroposterior diameter; LRC-TR, lower rib cage transverse diameter. Error bars, ±SE. Each point represents mean of five subjects except for URC-AP diameter, for which mean of four subjects is shown. $*p < 0.05$; $**p < 0.025$; $***p < 0.01$ vs. 1 Gz. (From Estenne et al., 1992.)

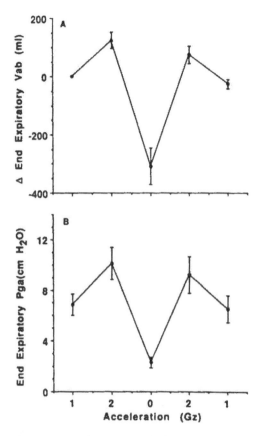

Figure 7   Changes in (A) end-expiratory abdominal volume (ΔVab) and (B) end-expiratory gastric pressure (Pga) as a function of acceleration (Gz) in the sequence observed during parabolic flight paths in five normal seated subjects. Error bars, $\pm$SE. (From Edyvean et al., 1991.)

not similarly increase at 0 Gz. The more likely explanation is that this dimension is primarily driven by transabdominal pressure. To the extent that the transverse diameter was measured in the abdomen-apposed portion of the rib cage (Estenne et al., 1992), its dimension at end-expiration should be primarily influenced by transabdominal rather than transthoracic pressure. The observation that the former consistently decreased ongoing from 1 to 0 Gz (Edyvean et al., 1991) might thus account for the response of the transverse diameter. The much smaller length of diaphragm apposed to the ventral as compared to the lateral aspects of the rib cage (Estenne and De Troyer, 1985; Whitelaw, 1987; Paiva et al., 1992; Gauthier et al., 1993) presumably explains why the fall in transabdominal pressure did not act to decrease the anteroposterior diameter.

Despite the greater facility for studying the effects of increased acceleration, experimental studies of the effect of hypergravity on FRC have provided conflicting results. Although Glaister (1970) observed a descent of the diaphragm dome at 3 Gz, suggesting an increased abdominal volume, Grassino et al. (1978) did not find any consistent change in end-expiratory abdominal cross-section or FRC between 1 and 3 Gz. Similarly, Boutellier et al. (1985) and Arieli et al. (1986) found no change in FRC with a threefold increase in head-to-foot acceleration. On the other hand, three studies during parabolic flights showed a increase in FRC during the 1.8 Gz period preceding the onset of weightlessness (Fig. 4) (Paiva et al., 1989; Edyvean et al., 1991; Kays et al., 1993). In addition, one of these studies (Kays et al., 1993) and a study recently performed in a human centrifuge (Estenne et al., 1995) reported that changes in FRC were associated with decreases in end-expiratory esophageal pressure.

These discrepant results may be due to at least two factors. First, measurements of FRC were obtained using different techniques. For example, Grassino et al. (1978) inferred changes in FRC from measurements of vital capacity and inspiratory capacity, Boutellier et al. (1985) and Arieli et al. (1986) used a rebreathing technique and Kays et al. (1993) used a body plethysmograph. Second, it is well known that the distension of the ventral abdominal wall that occurs ongoing from supine to upright elicits tonic contraction of the abdominal muscles (De Troyer, 1983). This response, which opposes the increase in abdominal volume and the descent of diaphragm dome, may also be elicited in response to hypergravity and hence may minimize or even prevent the increase in FRC that would otherwise occur. Therefore, depending on the level of abdominal muscle activity, increasing gravitational stresses may have different effects on abdominal volume and FRC (Estenne et al., 1995).

B. Static Lung Volumes

During early measurements in parabolic flights, several investigators found no consistent changes in vital capacity (VC) between 1 and 0 Gz in seated normal subjects (Foley and Tomashefski, 1969; Michels and West, 1978). Similarly, chest radiographs taken at residual volume (RV) and total lung capacity (TLC) after 10 s of microgravity showed no significant effect of weightlessness (Michels et al., 1979). On the other hand, Paiva et al. (1989) noted an 8% decrease in slow expiratory VC at 0 Gz in four subjects seated in an aircraft flying parabolic trajectories. A somewhat lower but significant decrease in forced expiratory VC was also recently found during weightlessness in seven of nine subjects who performed a large number of forced expiratory maneuvers during parabolic flights (Guy et al., 1991). When present, the decrease in VC was entirely accounted for by a reduction in TLC since there was no change (Paiva et al., 1989) or even a slight decrease (Kays et al., 1993) in residual volume at 0 Gz relative to 1 Gz.

The first measurements of VC during prolonged exposure to weightlessness were obtained during the last 2 weeks of the Skylab III mission in 1973 and at various intervals throughout the 84-day Skylab IV mission in 1973–74. Of the six astronauts studied, four showed a decrease in in-flight VC approaching 10% of the preflight control value (Sawin et al., 1976). Although this change has been attributed in part to the low barometric pressure inside the spacecraft (equivalent to 27,000-ft altitude), recent measurements performed in Spacelab where ambient pressure was 759 mm Hg have shown that VC was reduced by about 5% (~200 ml) on flight day 2 compared to the standing 1 Gz preflight value (Elliott et al., 1994; Guy et al., 1994). This reduction, however, was no longer present on subsequent flight days (Fig. 8).

Altogether these data indicate that gravitational unloading produces a very slight and transient reduction in VC. Although smaller in magnitude, this change is qualitatively similar to that elicited in normal subjects by water immersion to the neck (Hong et al., 1969; Prefaut et al., 1976; Elliott et al., 1989), simultaneous inflation of an abdominal bladder and of antishock trousers to lower limbs (Regnard et al., 1990), and postural changes such as head-down tilt and changing from upright

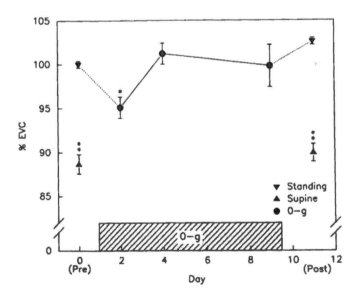

Figure 8 Means of individually normalized expired vital capacity (EVC) obtained from four crewmembers during the SLS-1 mission. Means from all the preflight sessions are pooled and displayed at day 0. Error bars, ±SE. Data that differ significantly from the standing control value are marked: $*p < 0.05$; $**p < 0.001$. The postflight data shown, obtained from three crew members, was compared to the preflight data on these three subjects. (From Guy et al., 1994.)

to supine (Agostoni and Mead, 1964). The reduction in VC (and TLC) seen in these various experimental conditions as well as in weightlessness is likely to be due, at least in part, to blood volume shifts to the thorax.

In contrast to weightlessness, increases in gravitational stresses up to 3 Gz do not produce consistent changes in VC (Foley and Tomashefski, 1969; Grassino et al., 1978; Pyszczynski et al., 1985; Guy et al., 1991).

C. Forced Expiratory Volumes and Flows

Studies during parabolic flights have shown that short periods of weightlessness generally produce a slight decrease in forced expiratory volume in one sec (FEV_1), FEV_1/VC ratio, and maximum expiratory flow rates (Foley and Tomashefski, 1969; Guy et al., 1991). In addition, in their study of maximum expiratory flow-volume (MEFV) curves, Guy et al. (1991) found that flow rates were higher at large lung volumes and smaller at low lung volumes at 0 Gz compared to 1 Gz. These alterations, however, were small in magnitude and were not present in all subjects. Qualitatively similar changes in the descending limb of the MEFV curve have been reported during head-out immersion (Prefaut et al., 1976; Elliott et al., 1989) and in the supine as opposed to the upright posture (Castille et al., 1982; Guy et al., 1991). They have been attributed to alterations in lung recoil pressure due to vascular engorgement (Prefaut et al., 1976) and subsequent changes in local airway stresses that alter location and motion of airway choke points during forced expiration. Similar mechanisms might account for the observations made in microgravity.

D. Pattern of Breathing

Although early observations during parabolic flights suggested that breathing frequency may increase in microgravity without concomitant changes in tidal volume (von Baumgarten et al., 1980), more recent studies have shown that 20-s periods of weightlessness produce only small and inconsistent changes in tidal volume, breathing frequency, mean inspiratory flow rate, and inspiratory duty cycle (Fig. 9) (Paiva et al., 1989; Edyvean et al., 1991; Kays et al., 1993). This is consistent with the effects of posture and head-out immersion, which do not alter the temporal pattern of breathing at rest (Burki, 1977; Reid et al., 1986). In contrast, prolonged exposure to microgravity may well have a different effect. Recent measurements performed during the SLS-1 mission have shown a 15% reduction in tidal volume accompanied by an increase in breathing frequency in-flight compared to preflight (Elliot et al., 1994). Measurements performed by Prisk et al. (1993) in the same mission provided evidence that this change was not due to increases in interstitial lung fluid and stimulation of J receptors, which may result in rapid shallow breathing. The explanation for the different effect of short and prolonged exposure to microgravity remains therefore to be determined.

Separate measurements of rib cage and abdominal volume indicate that the

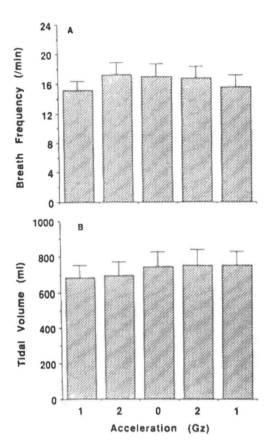

Figure 9 Breathing frequency (A) and tidal volume (B) as a function of Gz during parabolic maneuvers. Each value represents mean of five normal seated subjects. Error bars, SE. (From Edyvean et al., 1991.)

relative contribution of the two chest wall compartments to tidal volume is markedly altered by changes in Gz. In two successive studies, Paiva et al. (1989) and Edyvean et al. (1991) found that in seated normal subjects, the contribution of the abdomen increased from 0.33–0.39 to 0.51–0.57 ongoing from 1 Gz to 0 Gz (Fig. 10). The value found in microgravity is intermediate between that found in the upright and in the supine posture (Sharp et al., 1975; Druz and Sharp, 1981). The greater contribution of the abdomen to tidal volume at 0 Gz is due to increased abdominal compliance, which results from removal of tension in the ventral abdominal wall (Fig. 11). On transition to weightlessness, abdominal compliance increased on average ~60% relative to 1 Gz in the five subjects studied by Edyvean et al. (1991). Abdominal compliance also increases ongoing from upright to supine (Agostoni and

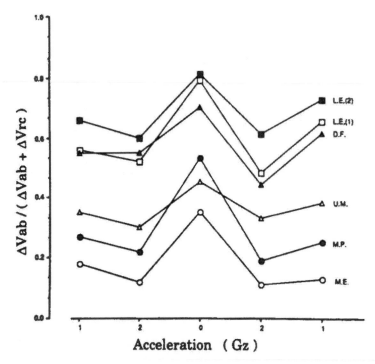

Figure 10 Abdominal contribution to tidal breathing [ΔVab/(ΔVab + ΔVrc)] at different levels of acceleration (Gz) in five normal seated subjects. Data represent average values based on measurements during 4–10 parabolas. Results on LE are shown separately for flights 1 and 2, respectively. (From Paiva et al., 1989.)

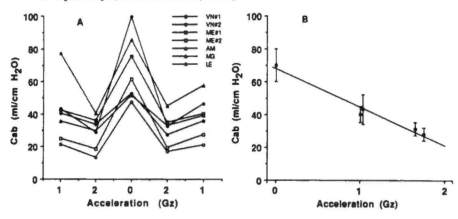

Figure 11 (A) Abdominal compliance (Cab) as a function of Gz during parabolic maneuvers in five normal seated subjects, two of whom were studied in duplicate on different flights. Each symbol is mean of 5–8 parabolas. (B) Cab vs. Gz. Symbols represent mean of five subjects. Error bars, ±SE. (From Edyvean et al., 1991.)

Mead, 1964; Konno and Mead, 1968; Estenne et al., 1985). Conversely, it decreased by ~35% ongoing from 1 to 1.8 Gz (Edyvean et al., 1991).

The increased abdominal contribution to tidal volume at 0 Gz was accompanied by a reciprocal decrease in rib cage contribution. Measurements with magnetometers have shown that this results from a reduced tidal expansion of both upper and lower portions of the rib cage along the anteroposterior diameter (Fig. 12) (Estenne et al., 1992). The smaller expansion of the lower rib cage may be explained by the increased abdominal compliance, which reduces the insertional and appositional components of the expanding action of the diaphragm (De Troyer, 1991). This mechanism, however, cannot account for the reduced tidal expansion of the upper rib cage because the expanding forces produced by diaphragm contraction do not apply, or apply only to a limited extent, to the upper portion of the cage (Estenne and De Troyer, 1985). This alteration is likely to be related to derecruitment of the scalene muscles at 0 Gz. Direct electromyographic recordings from these muscles, which inflate the upper portion of the rib cage during quiet inspiration at 1 Gz (De Troyer and Estenne, 1984; Estenne and De Troyer, 1985), have shown a consistent decrease in phasic inspiratory activity in weightlessness (Estenne et al., 1992). This adjustment may be part of the reflex referred to as operational length compensation (Green et al., 1978). When the operating length of the diaphragm increases, as it presumably does in microgravity, the inspiratory activation of all inspiratory muscles is reduced in order to keep tidal volume constant. This mechanism has been demonstrated during postural changes from upright to supine (Druz and Sharp, 1981) and during hip-to-xiphoid immersion (Reid et al., 1986).

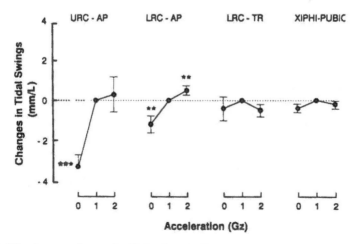

Figure 12 Average changes in tidal swings in rib cage dimensions relative to 1 Gz in five normal seated subjects during parabolic flights. Same abbreviations as in Figure 6. Each point represents mean of five subjects except for URC-AP diameter, LRC-AP diameter at 2 Gz, and LRC-TR diameter at 2 Gz, for which means of four subjects are shown. Error bars, ±SE. **$p < 0.025$, ***$p < 0.01$ vs. 1 Gz. (From Estenne et al., 1992.)

IV. Ventilation and Perfusion Distribution

It is well documented that gravity is responsible for topographical differences in pulmonary blood flow, ventilation, and gas exchange (West, 1977). In the upright posture, blood flow decreases from the lung base up to the apex, where it reaches very low values. Similarly, because the lung distorts under its own weight, the alveoli at the base of the lung are relatively compressed compared with the apical alveoli (regional TLC/RV ratios increase from apex to base), and because poorly expanded alveoli are more compliant, ventilation increases down the upright lung. These apico-basal gradients increase as gravitational forces increase (Bryan et al., 1966) and retain their orientation along the gravitational vector as posture is changed (Kaneko et al., 1966). In addition to the direct effect of gravity, however, nongravitational mechanisms also produce inhomogeneities of ventilation and perfusion. Microgravity experiments offer the best approach to evaluate the relative role played by these gravitational and nongravitational factors. In this section, we summarize experimental data on the distribution of pulmonary ventilation and perfusion obtained at 0 Gz during paraboic flights (Michel and West, 1978) and during the SLS-1 mission (Guy et al., 1994).

A. Ventilation

Ventilation inequality was measured by performing VC single-breath nitrogen (N_2) washouts during which a 150-ml bolus of 79% argon (Ar) and 21% oxygen was inhaled at residual volume followed by a maximal inspiration of pure oxygen. When performed at 1 Gz, the concentrations of N_2 and Ar first increase rapidly in the expired air and then rise much more slowly over most of the VC. This slowly ascending portion of the washout curve is referred to as the alveolar plateau (Phase III) and may be characterized by its slope and by the amplitude of the superimposed oscillations of expired gas concentrations related to the heartbeat (cardiogenic oscillations). The alveolar plateau ends at a point where there is a sudden increase in expired gas concentrations. This terminal rise (Phase IV) may be described by its height and volume, i.e., the volume from the end of Phase III to end expiration. For the sake of clarity, we will first discuss the effects of microgravity on cardiogenic oscillations and Phase IV and then analyze the changes in Phase III.

Cardiogenic Oscillations and Phase IV

Nitrogen and Ar oscillations decreased significantly in microgravity to about 44% and 24% of the control preflight standing values, respectively. Similarly, N_2 Phase IV height and volume decreased to 18% and 43% of control at 0 Gz. In contrast, Ar Phase IV height decreased to only 40% of control and Ar Phase IV volume did not change in microgravity. In addition, the presence of Ar Phase IV never became questionable at 0 Gz (Figs. 13, 14).

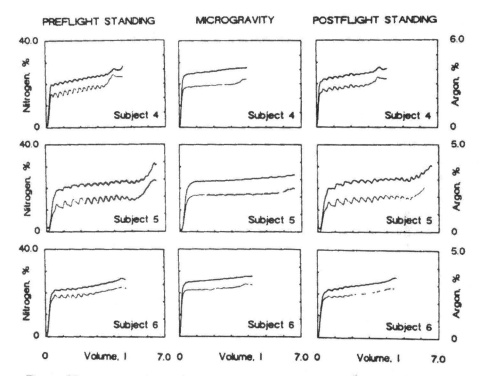

Figure 13 Representative tracings from three crew members obtained in the standing position preflight, postflight, and in-flight during the SLS-1 mission. (From Guy et al., 1994.)

The terminal rise in N_2 and Ar concentrations that is seen at 1 Gz is generally thought to be caused by basal airway closure and thus cessation of flow from units that have low N_2 concentrations because of their large TLC/RV ratios and low Ar concentrations resulting from their closure in early inspiration when the Ar bolus is inhaled. The magnitude of cardiogenic oscillations also primarily reflects TLC/RV expansion differences, but it is independent of sequential lung-emptying between different lung regions (Engel, 1986). The observation that both height and volume of N_2 Phase IV and the size of cardiogenic oscillations were substantially reduced in microgravity thus indicates that TLC/RV ratios became much more uniform throughout the lung in weightless conditions.

However, the persistence of detectable N_2 and Ar terminal rises at 0 Gz as well as the unchanged Ar phase IV volume demonstrate that airway closure still occurs in the absence of gravity. Although the mechanisms responsible for airway closure in weightlessness are unknown, Engel et al. (1975) and, more recently, Crawford et al. (1989) have shown that some airways may be closed while others remain open within small regions of the lung at 1 Gz. Such intraregional

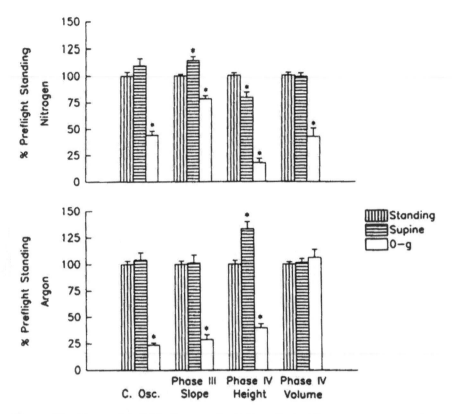

Figure 14 Means of individually normalized data obtained from seven crewmembers, preflight in the standing and supine position, and in-flight during the SLS-1 mission. Preflight standing controls are 100% by definition. Error bars, SE. Data that differ significantly from the standing control value are marked (*$p < 0.05$). C. Osc., cardiac oscillations. (From Guy et al., 1994.)

inhomogeneity of airway closure may also be present in microgravity, the site of airway closure being then widely dispersed throughout the lung rather than confined to the lung base.

Phase III

During exposure to a prolonged period of microgravity the slope of Phase III for N_2 was reduced by 22% relative to the preflight standing value (Figs. 13, 14). In contrast, no significant effect was observed during parabolic flights, but the results showed considerable intersubject variability. Early work on the distribution of ventilation has suggested that the slope of the alveolar plateau for N_2 is largely gravity dependent, i.e., the sloping of phase III would be due to the fact that apical lung units with low TLC/RV ratios and large N_2 concentration contribute progressively greater proportions of their initial volume during the course of expiration (Anthonisen et al., 1970). However, the observation that the N_2 slope was only slightly reduced at 0 Gz despite much more uniform TLC/RV ratios argues against this hypothesis. In contrast, it suggests, in agreement with recent studies (Engel et al., 1986; Paiva and Engel, 1987, 1989), that most of the N_2 slope may be due to diffusion-dependent mechanisms emanating from small lung regions (corresponding roughly to a single acinus).

On the other hand, the more uniform TLC/RV ratios in weightlessness produced a marked reduction in Ar slope, which decreased to 29–39% of the standing 1 Gz control value during both short and prolonged (Figs. 13, 14) exposure to microgravity. The greater sensitivity of the Ar slope to apico-basal gradients of regional lung expansion may be accounted for by the fact that when a bolus of Ar is inhaled at the start of inspiration, it is exclusively distributed to nonclosed airways, which in 1 Gz conditions results in large apico-basal gradients of gas concentration.

Summary

Altogether these data indicate that topographical differences in lung expansion and ventilation are substantially reduced in weightlessness. However, the maintenance of alveolar plateaus with positive slopes, cardiogenic oscillations, and terminal rises at 0 Gz provides unequivocal evidence for considerable nongravitational ventilatory inhomogeneity in the normal human lung.

B. Perfusion

Radiographs of seated subjects showed consistent differences in lung density and vascular markings between 1 and 0 Gz (Michels et al., 1979). In both posteroanterior and lateral views, lung density was greater at 0 Gz than at 1 Gz in the upper lung fields relative to the lower lung fields. Similarly, the upper lung field vascular shadows were larger in microgravity. Distribution of pulmonary blood flow has been assessed more directly during parabolic flights (Michel and West, 1978) and during the SLS-1 mission (G. K. Prisk, personal communication) by measuring expired P_{O_2} and P_{CO_2} during a constant-flow VC exhalation. Immediately before that, the subjects hyperventilated for several seconds and then held their breath at TLC for ~15 s. The rationale for the method was that during breath-holding regional gas exchange would be determined by blood flow, and the amplitude of the cardiogenic oscillations during the subsequent exhalation should reflect topographical differences in blood flow per unit lung volume. In microgravity, the height of Phase IV was almost abolished, thus providing strong evidence that large-scale hydrostatically generated topographical inequalities of blood flow were grossly reduced under weightless conditions. The cardiogenic oscillations were also almost eliminated during short periods of microgravity, but they persisted at 60% of the standing preflight value during the SLS-1 mission. The latter finding suggests that perfusion inhomogeneities in areas of the lung that are relatively close to each other may persist in weightlessness.

Increased acceleration has been shown to exaggerate the normal regional differences in perfusion, i.e., at high Gz levels blood flow is confined at the base of the lung (Bryan et al., 1965; Michel and West, 1978). Because at the same time ventilation is confined to the upper regions due to basal airway closure, gas exchange is greatly impaired (Glaister, 1970; Nunneley, 1976).

Acknowledgment

This work was supported in part by Contract PAI 21 with the Ministère de la Politique Scientifique.

References

Agostoni, E., and Mead, J. (1964). Statics of the respiratory system. In *Handbook of Physiology. Respiration*. Vol. I. Edited by W. O. Fenn and H. Rahn. Washington, D.C., American Physiological Society, pp. 387–409.

Agostoni, E., Gurtner, G., Torri, G., and Rahn, H. (1966). Respiratory mechanics during submersion and negative pressure breathing. *J. Appl. Physiol.*, 21:251–258.

Anthonisen, N. R., Robertson, P. C., and Roos, W. R. D. (1970). Gravity-dependent sequential emptying of lung regions. *J. Appl. Physiol.*, 28:589–595.

Arborelius, M., Balldin, U. I., Lilja, B., and Lundgren, C. E. G. (1972). Hemodynamic changes in man during immersion with the head above water. *Aerosp. Med.*, 43:592–598.

Arieli, R., Boutellier, U., and Farhi, L. E. (1986). Effect of water immersion on cardiopulmonary physiology at high gravity (+ Gz). *J. Appl. Physiol.*, 61:1686–1692.

Blomqvist, C. G., and Stone, H. L. (1983). Cardiovascular adjustments to gravitational stress. In *Handbook of Physiology. The Cardiovascular System.*, Vol. III. Edited by J. T. Shepherd and F. M. Abboud. Washington, D.C., Amercan Physiological Society, pp. 1025–1063.

Boutellier, U., Arieli, R., and Farhi, L. E. (1985). Ventilation and CO_2 response during + Gz acceleration. *Resp. Physiol.*, 62:141–151.

Bryan, A. C., Macnamara, W. D., Simpson, J., and Wagner, H. N. (1965). Effect of acceleration on the distribution of pulmonary blood flow. *J. Appl. Physiol.*, 20:1129–1132.

Bryan, A. C., Milic-Emili, J., and Pengelly, D. (1966). Effect of gravity on the distribution of pulmonary ventilation. *J. Appl. Physiol.*, 21:778–784.

Buckey, J. C., Gaffney, F. A., Lane, L. D., Levine, B. D., Watenpaugh, D. E., and Blomqvist, C. G. (1993). Central venous pressure in space. *N. Engl. J. Med.*, 328:1853–1854.

Bungo, M. W., and Johnson, P. C., Jr. (1983). Cardiovascular examinations and observations of deconditioning during the space shuttle orbital flight test program. *Aviat. Space Environ. Med.*, 54:1001–1004.

Bungo, M. W., Goldwater, D. J., Popp, R. L., and Sandler, H. (1987). Echocardiographic evaluation of space shuttle crewmembers. *J. Appl. Physiol.*, 62:278–283.

Burki, N. K. (1977). The effects of changes in functional residual capacity with posture on mouth occlusion pressure and ventilatory pattern. *Am. Rev. Respir. Dis.*, 116:895–900.

Castille, R., Mead, J., Jackson, A., Wohl, M. E., and Stokes, D. (1982). Effects of posture on flow-volume curve configuration in normal humans. *J. Appl. Physiol.*, 53:1175–1183.

Chadha, T. S., Lopez, F., Jenouri, G., Birch, S., and Sackner, M. A. (1983). Effects of partial anti-G suit inflation on thoracic volume and breathing pattern. *Aviat. Space Environ. Med.,* 54:324–327.

Charles, J. B., and Lathers, C. M. (1991). Cardiovascular adaptation to spaceflight. *J. Clin. Pharmacol.,* 31:1010–1023.

Crawford, A. B. H., Cotton, D. J., Paiva, M., and Engel, L. A. (1989). Effect of airway closure on ventilation distribution. *J. Appl. Physiol.,* 66:2511–2515.

De Troyer, A. (1983). Mechanical role of the abdominal muscles in relation to posture. *Respir. Physiol.,* 53:341–353.

De Troyer, A., and Estenne, M. (1984). Coordination between rib cage muscles and diaphragm during quiet breathing in humans. *J. Appl. Physiol.,* 57:899–906.

De Troyer, A. (1991). Respiratory muscles. In *The Lung. Scientific Foundations.* Vol. I. Edited by R. G. Crystal and J. B. West. New York, Raven Press, pp. 869–883.

Druz, W. S., and Sharp, J. T. (1981). Activity of respiratory muscles in upright and recumbent humans. *J. Appl. Physiol.,* 51:1552–1561.

Echt, M., Lange, L., and Gauer, O. H. (1974). Changes in peripheral venous tone and central transmural venous pressure during immersion in a thermoneutral bath. *Pflügers Arch.,* 352:211–217.

Edyvean, J., Estenne, M., Paiva, M., and Engel, L. A. (1991). Lung and chest wall mechanics in microgravity. *J. Appl. Physiol.,* 71:1956–1966.

Elliott, A. R., Prisk, G. K., and Guy, H. J. B. (1989). Effect of immersion on flow-volume curve configuration (abst). *FASEB J.,* 3:6240.

Elliott, A. R., Prisk, G. K., and Guy, H. J. B., and West, J. B. (1994). Lung volumes during sustained microgravity on Spacelab SLS-1. *J. Appl. Physiol.,* 77:2005–2014.

Engel, L. A., Grassino, A., and Anthonisen, N. R. (1975). Demonstration of airway closure in man. *J. Appl. Physiol.,* 38:1117–1125.

Engel, L. A. (1986). The dynamic distribution of gas flow. In *Handbook of Physiology. The Respiratory System.* Vol. III. Edited by J. Mead and P. T. Macklem. Washington, D.C., American Physiolical Society, pp. 575–593.

Engel, L. A. (1991). Effect of microgravity on the respiratory system. *J. Appl. Physiol.,* 70:1907–1911.

Estenne, M., Yernault, J. C., and De Troyer, A. (1983). The mechanism of relief of dyspnea after thoracocentesis in patients with large pleural effusions. *Am. J. Med.,* 74:813–819.

Estenne, M., and De Troyer, A. (1985). Relationship between respiratory muscle EMG and rib cage motion in tetraplegia. *Am. Rev. Respir. Dis.,* 132:53–59.

Estenne, M., Yernault, J. C., and De Troyer, A. (1985). Rib cage and diaphragm—abdomen compliance in humans: effects of age and posture. *J. Appl. Physiol.,* 59:1842–1848.

Estenne, M., Gorini, M., Van Muylem, A., Ninane, V., and Paiva, M. (1992). Rib cage shape and motion in microgravity. *J. Appl. Physiol.,* 73:946–954.

Estenne, M., Van Muylem, A., Kinnear W., Gorini, M., Ninane, V., Engel, L. A., and Paiva, M. (1995). Effects of increased & Gz on chest wall mechanics in humans. *J. Appl. Physiol.* (in press).

Foley, M. F., and Tomashefski, J. F. (1969). Pulmonary function during zero-gravity maneuvers. *Aerosp. Med.,* 40:655–657.

Gauthier, A., Verbanck, S., Estenne, M., Segebarth, C., Macklem, P. T., and Paiva, M. (1994). Three-dimensional reconstruction of the in vivo human diaphragm shape at different lung volumes. *J. Appl. Physiol.,* 76:405–506.

Gilmartin, J. J., Wright, A. J., and Gibson, J. J. (1985). Effects of pneumothorax or pleural effusion on pulmonary function. *Thorax,* 40:60–65.

Gilroy, R. J., Jr, Lavietes, M. H., Loring, S. H., Mangura, B. T., and Mead, J. (1985). Respiratory mechanical aspects of abdominal distension. *J. Appl. Physiol.,* 58:1997–2003.

Glaister, D. H. (1970). Ventilation and mechanics of breathing. In *The Effects of Gravity and Acceleration on the Lung.* Edited by D. H. Glaister. Slough, England: Technivision Services, pp. 19–36.

Grassino, A. E., Fokert, L., and Anthonisen, N. R. (1978). Configuration of the chest wall during increased gravitational stress in erect humans. *Respir. Physiol.*, 33:271–278.

Green, M., Mead, J., and Sears, T. A. (1978). Muscle activity during chest wall restriction and positive pressure breathing in man. *Respir. Physiol.*, 35:283–300.

Guy, H. J. B., and Prisk, G. K. (1989). Heart-lung interactions in aerospace medicine. In *Heart-Lung Interactions in Health and Disease*. Vol. 42. Edited by S. M. Sharf and S. S. Cassidy. New York, Marcel Dekker, pp. 519–563.

Guy, H. J. B., Prisk, G. K., Elliott, A. R., and West, J. B. (1991). Maximum expiratory flow-volume curves during short periods of microgravity. *J. Appl. Physiol.*, 70:2587–2596.

Guy, H. J. B., Prisk, G. K., Elliott, A. R., Deutschman, III, R. A., and West, J. B. (1994). Inequality of pulmonary ventilation during sustained microgravity as determined by single-breath washouts. *J. Appl. Physiol.*, 76:1719–1729.

Heaf, P. J. D., and Prime, F. J. (1954). Mechanical aspects of artificial pneumothorax. *Lancet*, ii:468–470.

Hong, S. K., Cerretelli, P., Cruz, J. C., and Rahn, H. (1969). Mechanics of respiration during submersion in water. *J. Appl. Physiol.*, 27:535–538.

Johnston, R. S., Dietlein, L. F., eds. (1977). *Proceedings of the Skylab Life Science Symposium*. Washington, D.C., National Aeronautics and Space Administration.

Kaneko, K., Milic-Emili, J., Dolovich, M. B., Dawson, A., and Bates, D. V. (1966). Regional distribution of ventilation and perfusion as a function of body position. *J. Appl. Physiol.*, 21:767–777.

Kays, C., Choukroun, M. L., Techoueyres, P., Varenne, P., and Vaida, P. (1993). Lung mechanics during parabolic flights (abstr.) *Fifth European Symposium on Life Sciences Research in Space*, pp. RES-0-03.

Kimball, W. R., Kelly, K. B., and Mead, J. (1986). Thoracoabdominal blood volume change and its effect on lung and chest wall volumes. *J. Appl. Physiol.*, 61:953–959.

Kirsch, K. A., Röcker, L., Gauer, O. H., Krause, R., Leach, C., Wicke, H. J., and Landry, R. (1984). Venous pressure in man during weightlessness. *Science* (Wash.), 225:218–219.

Konno, K., and Mead, J. (1968). Static volume-pressure characteristics of the rib cage and abdomen. *J. Appl. Physiol.*, 24:544–548.

Krell, W. S., and Rodarte, J. R. (1985). Effects of acute pleural effusion on respiratory system mechanics in dogs. *J. Appl. Physiol.*, 59:1458–1463.

Lathers, C. M., Charles, J. B., Elton, K. F., Holt, T. A., Mukai, C., Bennett, B. S., and Bungo, M. W. (1989). Acute hemodynamic responses to weightlessness in humans. *J. Clin. Pharmacol.*, 29:615–627.

Levy, M. N., and Talbot, J. M. (1983). Cardiovascular deconditioning of space flight. *Physiologist*, 26:297–303.

Meehan, J. P. (1971). Biosatellite 3: a physiological interpretation. *Life Sci. Space Res.*, 9:83–98.

Michels, D. B., and West, J. B. (1978). Distribution of pulmonary ventilation and perfusion during short periods of weightlessness. *J. Appl. Physiol.*, 45:987–998.

Michels, D. B., Friedman, P. J., and West, J. B. (1979). Radiographic comparison of human lung shape during normal gravity and weightlessness. *J. Appl. Physiol.*, 47:851–857.

Mukai, C. N., Lathers, C. M., Charles, J. B., Bennett, B. S., Igarashi, M., and Patel, S. (1991). Acute hemodynamic responses to weightlessness during parabolic flight. *J. Clin. Pharmacol.*, 31:993–1000.

Norsk, P., Foldager, N., Bonde-Petersen, F., Elmann-Larsen, B., Johansen, T. S. (1987). Central venous pressure in humans during short periods of weightlessness. *J. Appl. Physiol.*, 63:2433–2437.

Nunneley, S. A. (1976). Gas exchange in man during combined + Gz acceleration and exercise. *J. Appl. Physiol.*, 40:491–495.

Paiva, M., and Engel, L. A. (1987). Theoretical studies of gas mixing and ventilation distribution in the lung. *Physiol. Rev.*, 67:750–796.

Paiva, M., and Engel, L. A. (1989). Gas mixing in the lung periphery. In *Respiratory Physiology*. Vol. 40. Edited by H. K. Chang and M. Paiva. New York, Marcel Dekker, pp. 245–276.

Paiva, M., Estenne, M., and Engel, L. A. (1989). Lung volumes, chest wall configuration, and pattern of breathing in microgravity. *J. Appl. Physiol.*, 67:1542–1550.

Paiva, M., Verbanck, S., Estenne, M., Poncelet, B., Segebarth, C., and Macklem, P. T. (1992). Mechanical implications of in vivo human diaphragm shape. *J. Appl. Physiol.*, 72:1407–1412.

Pourcelot, L., Pottier, J. M., Patat, F., Arbeille, P., Kotovskaya, A., Genin, A., Savilov, A., Bistrov, A., Golovkina, O., Bost, R., Simon, P., and Guell, A. (1983). Cardiovascular exploration in microgravity. French-Soviet Flight Aboard Salyut VII Flight. *Proc. Int. Astronaut. Fed. Budapest*, pp. 92–105.

Prefaut, C., Lupi-H, E., and Anthonisen, N. R. (1976). Human lung mechanics during water immersion. *J. Appl. Physiol.*, 40:320–333.

Prisk, G. K., Elliott, A. R., Guy, H. J. B., and West, J. B. (1990). Lung volumes and esophageal pressures during short periods of microgravity and hypergravity (abstr) *Physiologist*, 33:A83.

Prisk, G. K., Guy, H. J. B., Elliott, A. R., Deutschmann, III, R. A., and West, J. B. (1993). Pulmonary diffusing capacity, capillary blood volume, and cardiac output during sustained microgravity. *J. Appl. Physiol.*, 75:15–26.

Pyszczynski, D., Mink, S. N., and Anthonisen, N. R. (1985). Increased gravitational stress does not alter maximum expiratory flow. *J. Appl. Physiol.*, 59:28–33.

Regnard, J., Baudrillard, P., Salah, B., Xuan, T. D., Cabanes, L., and Lockhart, A. (1990). Inflation of antishock trousers increases bronchial response to metacholine in healthy subjects. *J. Appl. Physiol.*, 68:1528–1533.

Reid, M. B., Loring, S. H., Banzett, R. B., and Mead, J. (1986). Passive mechanics of upright human chest wall during immersion from hips to neck. *J. Appl. Physiol.*, 60:1561–1570.

Sawin, C. F., Nicogossian, A. E., Rummel, J. A., and Michel, E. L. (1976). Pulmonary function evaluation during the Skylab and Appollo-Soyouz missions. *Aviat. Space Environ. Med.*, 47:168–172.

Sharp, J. T., Goldberg, N. B., Druz, W. S., and Danon, J. (1975). Relative contribution of rib cage and abdomen to breathing in normal subjects. *J. Appl. Physiol.*, 39:608–618.

Sjöstrand, T. (1951). Determination of changes in the intrathoracic blood volume in man. *Acta Physiol. Scand.*, 22:114–128.

Sjöstrand, T. (1952). The regulation of blood distribution in man. *Acta Physiol. Scand.*, 26:312–327.

Thornton, W. E., and Ord, J. (1977). Physiological mass measurements in Skylab. In *Biomedical Results from Skylab*. Edited by R. S. Johnston and L. F. Dietlein. Washington, D.C., National Aeronautics and Space Administration, SP-377.

Thornton, W. E., Hoffler, G. W., and Rummel, J. A. (1977). Anthropometric changes and fluid shifts. In *Biomedical Results from Skylab*. Edited by R. S. Johnston and L. F. Dietlein. Washington, D.C., National Aeronautics and Space Administration, SP-377.

Thornton, W. E., Moore, T. P., and Pool, S. L. (1987). Fluid shifts in weightlessness. *Aviat. Space Environ. Med.*, 58:86–90.

von Baumgarten, R. J., Baldrighi, G., Vogel, H., and Thumler, R. (1980). Physiological response to hyper- and hypogravity during rollercoaster flight. *Aviat. Space Environ. Med.*, 51:145–154.

Weissler, A. M., Leonard, J. J., and Warren, J. V. (1957). Effects of posture and atropine on cardiac output. *J. Clin. Invest.*, 36:1656–1662.

West, J. B., ed. (1977). *Regional Differences in the Lung*. New York, Academic Press.

West, J. B. (1991). Space. In *The Lung. Scientific Foundations*. Vol. 2. Edited by R. G. Crystal and J. B. West. New York, Raven Press, pp. 2133–2141.

West, J. B. (1992). Life in space. *J. Appl. Physiol.*, 72:1623–1630.

Wetzig, J. (1986). Respiration measurements in the weightlessness of parabolic flight. In *ESTEC Working Paper 1457*. Edited by D. L. Frimout, A. Gonfalone, and V. Pletser. Noordwijk.

Wetzig, J., and von Baumgarten, R. (1987). Respiratory parameters aboard an aircraft performing parabolic flights. In *Proceedings of the Third European Symposium on Life Sciences Research in Space* (ESA SP-271; 47–50).

Whitelaw, W. A. (1987). Shape and size of human diaphragm in vivo. *J. Appl. Physiol.*, 62:180–186.

53

Chest Wall Mechanics in the Newborn

SANDRA J. ENGLAND

UMDNJ-Robert Wood Johnson
  Medical School
New Brunswick, New Jersey

CLAUDE GAULTIER

Hôpital Antoine Beclere
Paris, France

A. CHARLES BRYAN

Hospital for Sick Children
Toronto, Ontario, Canada

I. Introduction

The thorax has a profound effect on lung mechanics in infancy. The chest wall is highly compliant. Agostoni (1959) has pointed out that at birth this is a substantial advantage, as it maintains the lung close to residual volume (RV), thus reducing the volume of intrapulmonary fluid, and facilitates the compression of the thorax through the birth canal. The problem is that when the fluid is resorbed, the lung may remain close to RV. Furthermore, the chest wall is so compliant that in the preterm infant with even mild respiratory distress, it looks like a "flail chest." The extent of paradoxical inward movement of the rib cage during inspiration has, in fact, been exploited as a simple method of detecting lung disease (Allen et al., 1990; Sivan et al., 1990). Thus the diaphragm dissipates a substantial fraction of its power sucking in ribs rather than fresh air. The mechanisms capable of stabilizing the thorax appear to be switched off in rapid eye movement (REM) sleep, which is the infant's predominant behavioral state. Histochemically, the diaphragm appears poorly equipped to deal with high work-loads. Despite all this, under normal conditions the thorax works well enough, but with any departure from normality, such as prematurity or quite trivial lung disease, the thorax becomes a problem.

II. Structural Changes in the Rib Cage

At birth, the ribs are mainly cartilage and extend almost at right angles from the vertebral column, resulting in a more circular rib cage than in the adult (Fig. 1) (Takahashi and Atsumi, 1955; Openshaw et al., 1984; Devlieger et al., 1991). This mechanical arrangement seems inefficient. In the adult, the volume of the rib cage can be increased by raising the ribs, which increases the contained volume by both the bucket-handle and pump-handle effects (Jordanoglou, 1970). In the infant, the ribs are already "raised" (Fig. 2), and this may be one of the reasons that motion of the rib cage contributes so little to tidal volume. This orientation of the ribs does not change substantially until the infant assumes the upright posture, which alters the forces acting on the rib cage. The direct action of gravity on the ribs and the action of the trunk muscles inserted into them causes a caudad inclination of the ribs. This leads to a relative lengthening of the thoracic cavity, and it loses its circular cross section (Howatt and Demuth, 1965). Assuming the upright posture also changes the effect of the abdominal contents on the thorax. In the supine position, the abdominal contents apply a positive pressure to the diaphragm, reducing lung volume, particularly in the dependent region. In the upright position, the abdominal contents apply a negative pressure to the diaphragm, increasing lung volume. However, in infants, since the abdominal hydrostatic column is small, these changes are likely to be quite minimal. Concurrently with the changes in rib position, there is a progressive mineralization of the ribs. These changes in shape and structure have major importance in "stiffening" the rib cage.

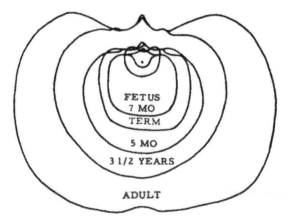

Figure 1   Changes in the shape of the thoracic cross section with age.

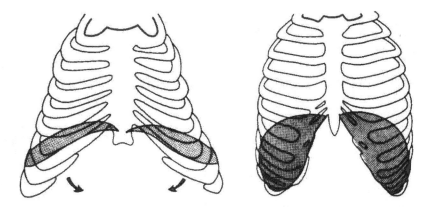

Figure 2 Comparison of the infant and adult rib cage and diaphragm. In the infant the diaphragm is much less curved and has a small area of apposition. (From Devlieger et al., 1991.)

III. Passive Compliance of the Chest Wall

In newborn animals and humans, chest wall compliance (Cw) is high (Agostoni, 1959; Avery and Cook, 1961; Richards and Blackman, 1961; Nightingale and Richards, 1965; Reynolds and Esten, 1966; Fisher and Mortola, 1980; Gerhardt and Bancalari, 1980; Davis et al., 1988). The measurement of passive Cw in human infants presents some formidable technical challenges. It is therefore not surprising that reported values of Cw with growth are scanty and inconsistent. A major point of discussion has been the validity of esophageal pressure measurements in infants with chest wall distortion (LeSouef et al., 1983) due to respiratory disease or prematurity and in intubated infants (Heaf et al., 1983; Thomson et al., 1983). However, some investigators have found that a valid pressure can be determined even in the presence of severe lung disease (Gerhardt et al., 1987; Davis et al., 1988).

Gerhardt and Bancalari (1980) reported a Cw of 6.4 ml/cm H_2O/kg body weight in premature infants under 32 weeks gestational age, decreasing to 4.2 ml/cm H_2O/kg in term infants. Davis et al. (1988) reported lower values (2.4–3.8 ml/cm H_2O/kg) in preterm infants of 31–34 weeks gestational age studied during relaxed expiration during the first 3 weeks of life. Reynolds and Etstan (1966), in much older infants (mean age 41 days), reported a Cw of 6 ml/cm H_2O/kg, similar to Gerhardt and Bancalari's data in premature infants. Rasanen et al. (1991) found a much stiffer chest wall in infants less than 1 year of age after open heart surgery. This may reflect the sternotomy but it was also clearly an effect of lung volume as there were large increases in compliance as the lungs were inflated, with a distinct inflection point around 5 cm H_2O.

Part of the problem may be methodological, but part is certainly due to difficulties in normalizing for growth. Mead (1979) has pointed out how difficult this is and has suggested that lung weight might be the best (but here unobtainable) normalizing factor. Normalizing by body weight in infants is potentially highly misleading. A 32-week gestational age infant is about half the body weight of a term infant, primarily due to the almost total absence of adipose tissue in the preterm infant (Widdowson, 1968).

Although in animals Cw decreases rapidly with growth (Agostoni, 1959; Avery and Cook, 1961), this does not appear to be the case in humans, as there is no major change in Cw in the first 6 months of life (Richards and Blackman, 1961). Sharp et al. (1970) measured the total respiratory compliance of children between the ages of 5 and 16. They showed a progressive fall in total compliance, which they attributed to changes in Cw. The uncertainties about the way in which Cw changes with age are unfortunate. Chest wall compliance has a major influence on both the maintenance of lung volume and stabilization of ventilation.

IV. Functional Residual Capacity

Functional residual capacity (FRC) is defined as the static passive balance of forces between the lung and the chest wall. In the adult, this establishes an FRC that is about 50% of the total lung capacity (TLC) in the upright position and about 40% of TLC in the supine position (Fig. 3). In the infant, the outward recoil of the chest wall is very small (Fagan, 1977). Consequently, the static passive balance of forces would dictate an FRC of about 10% of TLC. Such a small FRC seems incompatible with stability of the terminal airways or adequate gas exchange. From the measured FRC in infants (Nelson et al., 1963; Gaultier et al., 1979) and anatomical estimates of TLC (Fagan, 1977), the dynamic FRC/TLC ratio appears to be about 40%, that

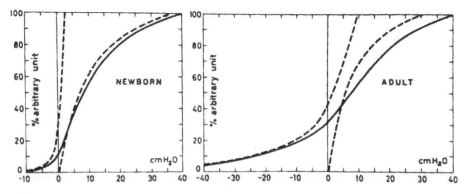

Figure 3 Comparison of compliance of the lung and chest wall in newborn and adult animals, illustrating the very low passively determined FRC in the newborn.

is, similar to that in the supine adult. Thus, the dynamic end-expiratory lung volume (EELV) appears to be substantially higher than the passively determined FRC.

The most obvious evidence for this is that during an apnea the end-expiratory volume generally falls to a substantially lower level, presumably the passively determined FRC, than that of preceding breaths (Fig. 4). It has also been shown that in infants, in contrast to the adult, expiration is terminated at substantial flow rates, suggesting an active interruption of relaxed expiration (Fig. 5) (LeSouef et al., 1983; Kosch and Stark, 1984). Kosch and Stark (1984) estimated, by linear extrapolation of the expired flow-volume curve to zero flow, that the dynamic end-expiratory volume is about 14 ml above the relaxation volume. This appears to be a common phenomenon in small mammals whose chest wall is highly compliant. Vinegar et al. (1979) argued that the end-expiratory volume was determined by the interplay between expiratory time (T_E) and the expiratory time constant. Thus the shorter the T_E and the longer the time constant, the greater the volume "trapped" at end-expiration. The end-expiratory volume in infants is variable depending on a balance between T_E and several mechanisms that lengthen the time

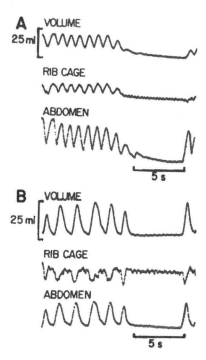

Figure 4 Volume and rib cage and abdominal magnetometer signals (upward deflection coincides with increasing diameter) during breathing and an unobstructed apnea in non-REM (A) and REM (B) sleep. End-expiratory lung volume falls substantially during apnea in non-REM sleep, but not during REM sleep. (Adapted from Stark et al., 1987.)

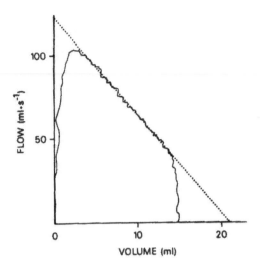

Figure 5 Flow-volume curve of an infant during passive expiration depicting the abrupt onset of inspiratory flow before passive end-expiratory volume is reached.

constant. The age at which EELV is no longer dynamically elevated above passive FRC is not known. Colin et al. (1989), based on the shape of expiratory flow-volume curves, estimate that the transition occurs at about 12 months of age.

In the lamb (Harding et al., 1978) and the dog pup (England et al., 1985) the adductor muscles of the larynx are active during expiration, increasing airflow resistance and acting as a brake on airflow in wakefulness and non-REM sleep. The time constant is substantially increased by this adduction of the vocal cords (England and Stogryn, 1986). The evidence for this expiratory airflow braking in human infants is rather indirect (Kosch et al., 1988) but very persuasive. Fisher et al. (1982) have shown that glottic closure appears to be a very important mechanism for establishing lung volume in the immediate postnatal period. Muller et al. (1979b) have suggested that tonic activity in both the diaphragm and intercostal muscles hold the lung at a higher active end-expiratory volume in the awake and non-REM sleep states. Kosch et al. (1988) have shown substantial braking of expiratory airflow in human infants during breaths with tonic expiratory activation of the diaphragm (Fig. 6).

The effect of sleep state on the end-expiratory volume is still highly controversial. Henderson-Smart and Read (1979) demonstrated a large (30%) fall in EELV during REM sleep by body plethysmography in full-term infants. This was supported by indirect measurements of changes in EELV with change in state by Lopes et al. (1981) and a very rigorous study by Stark et al. (1987). However, repeated studies using direct helium dilution measurements of EELV (Moriette et al., 1983; Walti et al., 1986; Beardsmore et al., 1989; Stokes et al., 1989) have

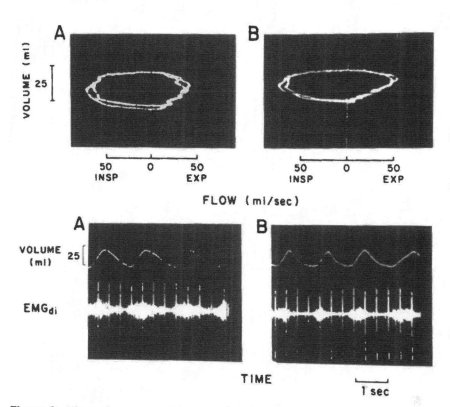

Figure 6 Flow-volume curves (upper panel) and time-based volume and diaphragmatic electromyogram (EMG$_{di}$) (lower panel) for breaths during non-REM (A) and REM (B) sleep in a week-old infant. During non-REM sleep, postinspiratory diaphragmatic activity occurs coincident with low peak inspiratory flow and convex shape of the volume-time trace, indicating expiratory airflow braking. During REM sleep, diaphragmatic activity is absent during expiration and peak inspiratory flow is higher falling linearly to zero at end-expiration. (Adapted from Stark et al., 1987.)

failed to find any significant changes in EELV with state change. In these papers more rigid electrophysiological criteria of state were used. In the study by Walti et al. (1986) small but significant decreases in EELV were observed in REM sleep, but only when there was gross paradoxical chest wall motion during inspiration.

It is difficult to resolve these conflicting sets of observations. However, logically the EELV should fall in REM sleep. It is well documented that expiratory airflow braking mechanisms are disabled in REM sleep. Both Lopes et al. (1981) and Stark et al. (1987) have clearly shown that postinspiratory diaphragmatic activity is reduced in REM. Animal studies have demonstrated a substantial reduction of laryngeal adduction during expiration in REM sleep (Harding et al., 1979; England et al., 1985). Further, flows during quiet sleep in human infants show clear evidence of expiratory braking, whereas during REM sleep the flow volume curves appear to be passive with no evidence of braking (Fig 6.) (Stark et al., 1987). Thus the expiratory time constant is shorter in REM, and a number of studies (Haddad et al., 1979; Hathorn, 1979; Stark et al., 1987) have shown that T_E is longer in REM. Both of these factors would result in lung volume falling close to the passively determined FRC at end-expiration. The lengthening of T_E is difficult to explain. However, a study by Fedorko et al. (1988) showed that vagal reflexes were crucial in determining expiratory time in the newborn, and Phillipson (1978) has shown that the Hering Breuer reflex was disabled in REM sleep, which could explain the lengthened expiratory time in infants during REM.

Thus there is evidence for a long T_E and a short time constant in the infant during REM sleep, both factors of which should decrease the "trapped" volume and result in a lower EELV. The fall in oxygenation that accompanies REM sleep has been attributed to a lowered EELV in this state (Martin et al., 1979). Despite this logic, the fact remains that very carefully performed studies using helium dilution have failed to demonstrate a fall in EELV during REM sleep.

V. Ventilation

In the adult, roughly half of the total impedance of the respiratory system is in the chest wall; thus, about half of the force generated by the respiratory muscles is dissipated in moving the chest wall rather than inflating the lung. From this point of view, the highly compliant chest wall of the infant would appear to be an advantage, but in fact this is the problem. The lung is driven by two generators in the chest wall: the caudal surface of the lung is driven by the diaphragm and the remaining surface by the rib cage. These two generators oppose one another (Goldman et al., 1976, 1978; Grassino et al., 1978). The inspiratory action of each generator lowers the pleural pressure, and if only one is active, the other will move paradoxically. Thus, if the diaphragm is paralyzed, inspiration by the intercostals will suck the diaphragm cephalad.

The more common situation occurs when the intercostal muscles are inhibited, when shortening of the diaphragm will cause paradox of the rib cage. The magnitude of this paradoxical motion depends on the relative compliances of the lung and chest wall, since the diaphragm acts on these two in parallel and divides its displacement accordingly. The ratio of the passive compliance of the chest wall to the passive compliance of the lung in the preterm infants is about 6:1 (Gerhardt and Bancalari, 1980). Thus, theoretically it is much easier to move the chest wall than it is the lung, and ventilation would become impossible. However, passive properties imply total relaxation of any muscle or structure that might influence pressure development. During inspiration the system is not totally relaxed, and the relevant number is the active or effective compliance of the system.

Several attempts have been made to measure the active compliance of infants (Adler et al., 1976; Boychuk et al., 1977). Gerhardt and Bancalari (1980) and Mortola et al. (1982), using entirely different methodologies, concluded that the effective compliance of full-term babies was about 2.5 ml/cm H_2O, substantially lower than their estimates of passive compliance. However, Gerhardt and Bancalari (1980) were unable to show any difference between the active and passive compliance of very premature infants. The problem probably lies in the method of measurement, which assumes that the respiratory system will expand along its relaxation configuration. Any distortion of the rib cage will substantially decrease the effective compliance but will not be included in the standard methods of measurement. Heldt and McIlroy (1987) showed that with marked distortion in preterm infants that the effective compliance increased about 10-fold. Several factors combine to stiffen the system. Since the intercostal muscles and the diaphragm have force/length characteristics, they will reduce the compliance of the chest wall progressively as their force of contraction increases. A further stabilizing factor is that the lower rib cage and the portion of the diaphragm opposed to it form part of the abdominal wall. The diaphragm acts on the rib cage directly through its insertions and indirectly by increasing abdominal pressure. These forces tend to elevate and evert the lower rib cage. However, this mechanical coupling is much more effective in the upright than in the supine position, and babies in most Western societies are usually kept in the prone or supine position. Furthermore, for the diaphragmatic action on the rib cage to be effective in changing lung volume, actions applied to the lower rib cage must be transmitted to the upper rib cage, and this transmission depends on rib cage compliance. If the rib cage is very compliant, motion of the lower ribs is not transmitted, and there is paradoxical breathing, that is, splaying of the lower rib cage and sternal retraction. This is particularly obvious in REM sleep, when phasic activity of the intercostal muscles is depressed, which allows independent motion of the ribs (Fig. 7). Finally, distortion of the rib cage itself from the relaxation configuration is probably a critical factor in increasing the active compliance of the chest wall.

In the very premature infant, in whom REM sleep is the predominant behavioral state (Dreyfus-Brisac, 1968, 1970) and whose ribs are very compliant, paradoxical breathing is almost constant (Davi et al., 1979). As the infant matures, paradoxical breathing is more clearly confined to episodes of REM sleep, but even in non-REM sleep there is very little outward motion of the rib cage during inspiration despite phasic inspiratory activity of the intercostals (Fig. 7). The extent of paradoxical movement of the rib cage during REM decreases progressively with maturation (Gaultier et al., 1987) but is present even in older children (Tabachnik et al., 1981) and adults (Tusiewicz et al., 1977).

VI. Respiratory Muscles

With growth, there is a progressive increase in the bulk of the muscles of respiration. There are also important changes in the fiber composition, fiber size, oxidative capacity, and contraction characteristics of the diaphragm (see Sieck and Fournier,

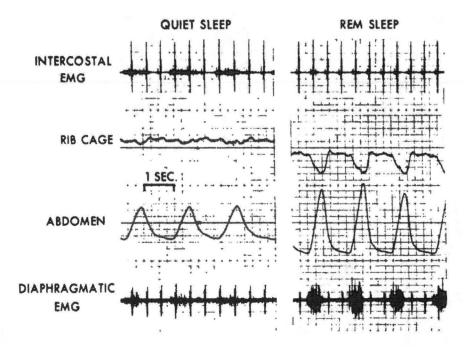

Figure 7 Surface intercostal and diaphragmatic EMG and motion of rib cage and abdomen (magnetometer) in an infant in NREM (quiet) and REM sleep. Note the almost complete suppression of the intercostal EMG and the marked increase in the diaphragmatic EMG. Also note the paradoxical motion of the rib cage and increase in abdominal motion in REM.

1991, for a comprehensive review of this topic). Coincident with these changes in muscle bulk and composition, there is a progressive increase in the maximum inspiratory and expiratory pressures with substantial differences between the sexes at all ages (Cook et al., 1964; Gaultier and Zinman, 1983). Yet the maximum pressures exerted by children are surprisingly high compared to adults, much higher than other indices of muscle strength. This is probably related to the small radius of curvature of the rib cage, diaphragm, and abdomen, which by the Laplace relationship will convert small tensions into relatively high pressures. Esophageal pressures of up to –70 cm H_2O have been recorded in infants during the first breath (Karlberg and Koch, 1962). Pressures in excess of –60 cm H_2O have been reported in anesthetized children just prior to extubation (Malsch, 1978), and inspiratory and expiratory pressures of about 120 cm H_2O have been recorded during crying in normal infants and toddlers (Shardonofsky et al., 1989).

A. Diaphragm Fiber Type, Size, and Oxidative Capacity

In the preterm infant, the diaphragm is composed of less than 10% type I fibers (slow-twitch) (Keens et al., 1978), and low percentages of type I fibers have been found in neonatal animals of various species with a high percentage of type II fibers, particularly type IIc (Maxwell et al., 1983; Lesouef et al., 1988; Sieck et al., 1991). The subtypes of type II fibers (fast-twitch) also change postnatally, with the proportion of type IIa increasing, then decreasing, type IIb increasing, and type IIc decreasing. Mean cross-sectional area of all fiber types increases postnatally (Sieck et al., 1991).

The total oxidative capacity of the diaphragm, defined as succinyl dehydrogenase (SDH) activity, is low at birth (Sieck and Fournier, 1991). Type I fibers are commonly defined as high and type II fibers as low oxidative, suggesting that this difference between the oxidative capacities of neonatal and adult diaphragms reflects the paucity of type I fibers in the neonate. However, the distinct differences in SDH activities between type I and II fibers found in the adult are not detectable in the diaphragm during the early postnatal period.

B. Contractile Properties

Twitch contraction and half-relaxation times of the diaphragm are longer in neonates than in adults (Sieck et al., 1991; Sieck and Fournier, 1991). Slow muscle contraction and relaxation are also reflected in the low frequency required for elicitation of tetanic contraction and the leftward shift of the force-frequency curve relative to the adult diaphragm. Developing muscle fibers express neonatal isoforms of myosin heavy chains (Kelly, 1983; Reiser et al., 1985) correlating with slow cross-bridge cycling. Also the sarcoplasmic reticulum is less extensive in neonatal muscle fibers (Belacastro, 1987), a property that could result in slow release and reuptake of calcium during contractions.

VII. Respiratory Muscle Fatigue

The fatiguability of the neonatal respiratory muscles in relation to the adult remains a controversial issue. The paucity of fatigue-resistant type I fibers, high proportion of fatigue-susceptible type IIc fibers, and low oxidative capacity of the neonatal diaphragm suggest that muscle should be relatively prone to fatigue. However, a number of in vitro studies of the neonatal diaphragm (Maxwell et al., 1983; Sieck and Fournier, 1991; Sieck et al., 1991) have shown exactly the opposite, that the muscle is inherently fatigue resistant despite its histochemical properties.

In contrast, Muller et al. (1979a,c) showed that an increase in the low-frequency and decrease in the high-frequency power in the surface diaphragmatic EMG in preterm infants during periods of marked chest wall distortion were invariably associated with increasing end-tidal CO_2. Such changes in the power spectrum of an EMG precede the loss of force in a muscle developing high-frequency fatigue (Bigland-Ritchie et al., 1981). In rabbits in which the diaphragm was stimulated via the phrenic nerve to contract against an occluded airway, fatigue, defined as loss of airway pressure over time with each diaphragmatic contraction, occurred more quickly in neonatal than adult animals (LeSouef et al., 1988). In contrast, Sieck et al. (1991) performed in situ stimulations of the cat diaphragm, albeit with the muscle free of its normal attachments, and found neonatal animals to be relatively fatigue resistant.

There are several possible explanations for the discrepancies cited above. The diaphragmatic fatigue seen in the premature infant and in the neonatal rabbit as studied by LeSouef et al. (1988) might be of central rather than peripheral origin. Fatigue in vivo might also reflect failure at the neuromuscular junction rather than fatigue of the muscle fibers (Sieck and Fournier, 1991). Also the high fatiguability in the neonate when diaphragmatic contractions occur against the inherent mechanical properties of the respiratory system and at the muscle length existant in vivo reflect the ability of this muscle to maintain ventilation. In contrast, in the in vitro and in situ animal studies cited above, the diaphragm was separated from its attachments, contracted without lung inflation, and its length adjusted to result in maximal tension development.

As has been repeatedly stressed in this chapter, the highly compliant chest wall makes the respiratory pump intrinsically inefficient. This problem is compounded during REM sleep, which markedly depresses the intercostal muscles. In consequence, the diaphragm dissipates a large fraction of its force in distorting the rib cage rather than effecting volume exchange. Further, infants use their abdominal muscles to optimize diaphragmatic length, and this abdominal muscle activity is inhibited in REM sleep (Praud et al., 1991). To maintain alveolar ventilation in REM sleep, there is a substantial increase in the activation of the diaphragm, as measured by surface EMG, and in shortening of the diaphragm, as measured by abdominal excursion (Muller et al., 1979a) (Fig. 7). This results in an increased diaphragmatic work of breathing (Guslits et al., 1987). The respiratory rate is high, sharply limiting the adult option of increasing expiratory time to give the diaphragm a rest. Furthermore, acidosis and hypoxia, both of which increase the fatiguability of muscle, are not uncommon in the sick premature infant. All of these factors increase the potential for diaphragmatic fatigue to occur in the infant.

References

Adler, S. A., Thach, B. T., and Franz, J. D. (1976). Maturational change of effective elastance in the first 10 days of life. *J. Appl. Physiol.*, 40:539–542.

Agostoni, E. (1959). Volume-pressure relationships to the thorax and lung in the newborn. *J. Appl. Physiol.*, 14:909–913.

Allen, J. L., Wolfson, M. R., McDowell, K., and Shaffer, T. H. (1990). Thoracoabdominal asynchrony in infants with airflow obstruction. *Am. Rev. Respir. Dis.*, 141:337–342.

Avery, M. E., and Cook, C. D. (1961). Volume-pressure relationships of lungs and thorax in fetal, neonatal, and adult goats. *J. Appl. Physiol.*, 16:1034–1038.

Beardsmore, C. S., MacFadyen, U. M., Moosavi, S. S., Wimpress, S. P., Thompson, J., and Simpson, H. (1989). Measurement of lung volumes during active and quiet sleep in infants. *Ped. Pulmonol.*, 7:71–77.

Belacastro, A. N. (1987). Myofibril and sarcoplasmic reticulum changes during muscle development: activity vs inactivity. *Int. J. Biochem.*, 19:945–948.

Bigland-Ritchie, B., Donovan, E. F., and Roussos, Ch. (1981). Conduction velocity and EMG power spectrum changes in fatigue of sustained maximal efforts. *J. Appl. Physiol.*, 51:1300–1305.

Boychuk, R. B., Seshia, M. M. K., and Rigatto, H. (1977). The effect of gestational age on the effective elastance of the respiratory system in neonates. *Pediatr. Res.*, 11:791–793.

Colin, A. A., Wohl, M. E., Mead, J., Ratken, A., Glass, G., and Stark, A. R. (1989). Transition from dynamically maintained to relaxed end-expiratory volume in human infants. *J. Appl. Physiol.*, 67(5):2107–2111.

Cook, C. D., Mead, J., and Ozales, M. M. (1964). Static volume-pressure characteristics of the respiratory system during maximum effort. *J. Appl. Physiol.*, 19:1016–1022.

Davi, M., Sankaran, K., MacCallum, M., Cates, D., and Rigatto, H. (1979). Effect of sleep state on chest distortion and on the ventilatory response to CO_2 in neonates. *Pediatr. Res.*, 13:982–986.

Davis, G. M., Coates, A. L., Papageorgiou, A., and Bureau, M. A. (1988). Direct measurement of static chest wall compliance in animal and human neonates. *J. Appl. Physiol.*, 65:1093–1098.

Devlieger, H., Daniels, H., Marchal, G., Moerman, Ph., Casaer, P., and Eggermont, E. (1991). The diaphragm of the newborn infant: anatomical and ultrasonographic studies. *J. Develop. Physiol.*, 16:321–329.

Dreyfus-Brisac, C. (1968). Sleep ontogenesis in early human prematurity from 24–27 weeks of conceptional age. *Dev. Psychobiol.*, 1:162–169.

Dreyfus-Brisac, C. (1970). Ontogenesis of sleep in human prematures after 32 weeks of conceptual age. *Dev. Psychobiol.*, 3:91–121.

England, S. J., Kent, G., and Stogryn, H. A. F. (1985). Laryngeal muscle and diaphragm activities in conscious dog pups. *Respir. Physiol.*, 60:95–108.

England, S. J., and Stogryn, H. A. F. (1986). Influence of the upper airway on breathing pattern and expiratory time constant in dog pups. *Respir. Physiol.*, 66:181–192.

Fagan, D. G. (1977). Shape changes in V-P loops for children's lungs related to growth. *Thorax*, 32:198–202.

Fedorko, L., Kelly, N., and England, S. J. (1988). Importance of vagal afferents in determining ventilation in newborn rats. *J. Appl. Physiol.*, 65(3):1033–1039.

Fisher, J. T., and Mortola, J. P. (1980). Statics of the respiratory system in newborn animals. *Respir. Physiol.*, 41:155–172.

Fisher, J. T., Mortola, J. P., Smith, J. B., Fox, G. S., and Weeks, S. (1982). Respiration in newborns: Development of the control of breathing. *Am. Rev. Respir. Dis.*, 56:650–657.

Gaultier, Cl., Boule, M. Allaire, Y., Clement, A., and Girard, F. (1979). Growth of lung volumes during the first three years of life. *Bull. Eur. Physiopathol. Respir.*, 15:1103–1116.

Gaultier, C., and Zinman, R. (1983). Maximal static pressures in healthy children. *Respir. Physiol.*, 51:45–61.

Gaultier, C., Praud, J. P., Canet, E., Delaperche, M. F., and D'Allest, A. M. (1987). Paradoxical inward rib cage motion during rapid eye movement sleep in infants and young children. *J. Dev. Physiol.*, 9:391–397.

Gerhardt, T., and Bancalari, E. (1980). Chest wall compliance in full term and premature infants. *Acta Paediatri. Scand.*, 69:359–364.

Gerhardt, T., Hehre, D., Feller, R., Reifenberg, L., and Bancalari, E. (1987). Serial determination of pulmonary function in infants with chronic lung disease. *J. Pediatr.*, 110:448–456.

Goldman, M. D., Grimby, G., and Mead, J. K. (1976). Mechanical work of breathing derived from rib cage and abdominal V-P partitioning. *J. Appl. Physiol.*, 41:752–763.

Goldman, M. D., Grassino, A., Mead, J., and Sears, T. A. (1978). Mechanics of the human diaphragm during voluntary contractions: dynamics. *J. Appl. Physiol.*, 44:840–848.

Grassino, A., Goldman, M. D., Mead, J., and Sears, T. A. (1978). Mechanics of the human diaphragm during voluntary contraction: statics. *J. Appl. Physiol.*, 44:829–839.

Guslits, B., Gaston, S., Bryan, M. H., England, S. J., and Bryan, A. C. (1987). Diaphragmatic work of breathing in premature human infants. *J. Appl. Physiol.*, 62(4):1410–1415.

Haddad, G., Epstein, R., Epstein, M., Leistner, H., Marino, P., Mellins, R. (1979). Maturation of ventilation and ventilatory pattern in normal sleeping infants. *J. Appl. Physiol.*, 46:998–1002.

Harding, R., Johnson, P., and McClelland, M. E. (1979). The expiratory role of the role of the larynx during development and the influence of behavioral state. In *Central Nervous Control Mechanisms of Breathing*. Edited by C. Von Euler and H. Lagercrantz. Oxford, Pergamon Press, pp. 353–359.

Hathorn, M. (1979). The rate and depth of breathing in newborn infants in different sleep states. *J. Physiol. (London)*, 243:110–113.

Heaf, D., Turner, H., Stocks, K., and Helms, P. (1983). The accuracy of esophageal pressure measurements in convalescent and sick intubated infants. *Pediatr. Pulmonol.*, 2:5–8.

Heldt, G. P., and McIlroy, M. B. (1987). Distortion of chest wall and work of diaphragm in preterm infants. *J. Appl. Physiol.*, 62(1):164–169.

Henderson-Smart, D. J., and Read, D. J. C. (1979). Reduced lung volume during behavioral active sleep in the newborn. *J. Appl. Physiol.*, 46:1081–1085.

Howatt, W. F., and Demuth, G. R. (1965). Configuration of the chest wall. *Pediatrics*, 25:177–184.

Jordanoglou, J. (1970). Vector analysis of rib movement. *Respir. Physiol.*, 10:109–120.

Karlberg, P., and Koch, G. (1962). Respiratory studies in newborn infants. *Acta. Paediatr. Scand.* 105 (suppl):439–448.

Keens, T. G., Bryan, A. C., Levison, H., and Ianuzzo, C. D. (1978). Developmental pattern of muscle fiber types in human ventilatory muscle. *J. Appl. Physiol.*, 44:909–913.

Kelly, A. M. (1983). Emergence of muscle specialization. In *Handbook of Physiology*. Sec 10. Skeletal Muscle. Edited by L. D. Peachey and R. H. Adrian. Bethesda, MD, American Physiological Society, pp. 507–537.

Kosch, P. C., and Stark, A. R. (1984). Dynamic maintenance of end-expiratory lung volume in full-term infants. *J. Appl. Physiol. Respirat. Environ. Exercise Physiol.*, 57(4):1126–1133.

Kosch, P. C., Hutchison, A. A., Wozniak, J. A., Carlo, W. A., and Stark, A. R. (1988). Posterior cricoarytenoid and diaphragm activities during tidal breathing in neonates. *J. Appl. Physiol.*, 64(5):1968–1978.

LeSouef, P. N., Lopes, J. M., England, S. J., Bryan, M. H., and Bryan, A. C. (1983). Influence of chest wall distortion on esophageal pressure. *J. Appl. Physiol.*, 55:353–358.

LeSouef, P. N., England, S. J., Stogryn, H. A. F., and Bryan, A. C. (1988). Comparison of diaphragmatic fatigue in newborn and older rabbits. *J. Appl. Physiol.*, 65:1040–1044.

Lopes, J., Muller, N. L., Bryan, M. H. and Bryan, A. C. (1981). Importance of inspiratory muscle tone in the maintenance of the functional residual capacity in the newborn. *J. Appl. Physiol.*, 51:830–834.

Malsch, E. (1978). Maximal inspiratory force in infants and children. *S. Afr. Med. J.*, 71:842–849.

Martin, R. J., Okkern, A., and Rubin, D. (1979). Arterial oxygen tension during active and quiet sleep. *J. Pediatr.*, 94:271–274.

Maxwell, L. C., McCarter, J. M., Keuhl, T. J., and Robotham, J. L. (1983). Development of histochemical and functional properties of baboon respiratory muscles. *J. Appl. Physiol.*, 54:551–561.

Mead, J. (1979). The problems in interpreting common tests of pulmonary function. In *The Lung in the Transition Between Health and Disease*. Edited by P. T. Macklem and S. Permutt. New York, Marcel Dekker, pp. 43–52.

Moriette, G., Chaussain, M., Radvanyi-Bouvet, M. F., Walti, H., Pajot, N., and Relier, J. P. (1983). Functional residual capacity and sleep states in the premature infant. *Biol. Neonate*, 43:125–133.

Mortola, J. P., Fisher, J. T., Smith, B., Fox, G., and Weeks, S. (1982). Dynamics of breathing in infants. *J. Appl. Physiol.*, 52:1209–1215.

Muller, N. L., Gulston, G., Cade, D., Whitton, J., Froese, A. B., Bryan, M. H., and Bryan, A. C. (1979a). Diaphragmatic muscle fatigue in the newborn. *J. Appl. Physiol.*, 46(6):688–695.

Muller, N. L., Volgyesi, G., Becker, L., Bryan, M. H., and Bryan, A. C. (1979b). Diaphragmatic muscle tone. *J. Appl. Physiol.*, 47:279–284.

Muller, N. L., Volgyesi, G., Bryan, M. H., and Bryan, A. C. (1979c). The consequence of diaphragmatic muscle fatigue in the newborn infant. *J. Pediatr.*, 95:793–797.

Nelson, N., Prod'ham, L., Cherry, R., Pipsitz, P., and Smith, C. (1963). Pulmonary function in the newborn infant. *J. Clin. Invest.*, 42:1850–1857.

Nightingale, D. A., and Richards, C. C. (1965). Volume-pressure relationship of the respiration system of curarized infants. *Anesthesiology*, 26:710–714.

Openshaw, P., Edwards, S., and Helms, P. (1984). Changes in rib cage geometry during childhood. *Thorax*, 39:624–627.

Phillipson, E. A. (1978). Respiratory adaptation in sleep. *Ann. Rev. Respir. Dis.*, 40:133–156.

Praud, J. P., Egreteau, L., Benlabed, M., Curzi-Dascalova, L., Nedelcoux, H., and Gaultier, C. (1991). Abdominal muscle activity during CO_2 rebreathing in sleeping neonates. *J. Appl. Physiol.*, 70:1344–1350.

Rasanen, J., Peltola, K., and Leijala, M. (1991). Lung mechanics and airway pressure transmission in infants after open heart surgery. *Eur. J. Cardio-Thorac Surg.*, 5:253–257.

Reiser, P. J., Moss, R. L., Giulian, G. G., and Greaser, M. L. (1985). Shortening velocity and myosin heavy chains of developing rabbit muscle fibers. *J. Biol. Chem.*, 260:14403–14405.

Reynolds, R. N., and Etstan, B. E. (1966). Mechanics of respiration in apneic anesthetized infants. *Anesthesiology*, 27:13–19.

Richards, C. C., and Blackman, L. (1961). Lung and chest wall compliance in apneic paralyzed infants. *J. Clin. Invest.*, 40:273–278.

Shardonofsky, F. R., Perez-Chada, D., Carmuega, E., and Milic-Emili, J. (1989). Airway pressures during crying in healthy infants. *Pediatr. Pulmonol.*, 6:14–18.

Sharp, M., Druz, W., Balgot, R., Bandelin, V., and Damon, J. (1970). Total respiratory compliance in infants and children. *J. Appl. Physiol.*, 2:775–779.

Sieck, G. C., and Fournier, M. (1991). Developmental aspects of diaphragm muscle cells, structural and functional organization. In *Developmental Neurobiology of Breathing*. Edited by Haddad and Farber. Marcel Dekker, New York, pp. 375–428.

Sieck, G. C., Fournier, M., and Blanco, C. E. (1991). Diaphragm muscle fatigue resistance during postnatal development. *J. Appl. Physiol.*, 71(2):458–464.

Sivan, Y., Deakers, T. W., and Newth, C. J. L. (1990). Thoraco abdominal asynchrony in acute airway obstruction in small children. *Am. Rev. Respir. Dis.*, 142:540–544.

Stark, A. R., Cohlan, B. A., Waggener, T. B., Frantz, I. D., and Kosch, P. C. (1987). Regulation of end-expiratory lung volume during sleep in premature infants. *J. Appl. Physiol.*, 62(3):1117–1123.

Stokes, G. M., Milner, A. D., Newball, E. A., Smith, N. J., Dunn, C., and Wilson, A. J. (1989). Do lung volumes change with sleep state in the neonate? *Eur. J. Pediatr.*, 148:360–364.

Tabachnik, E., Muller, N. L., Bryan, A. C., and Levison, H. (1981). Changes in ventilation and chest wall mechanics during sleep in normal adolescents. *J. Appl. Physiol.*, 51:557–564.

Takahashi, E., and Atsumi, H. (1955). Age differences in thoracic form as indicated by the Thoracic Index. *Human Biol.*, 27:65–74.

Thomson, A., Elliott, J., and Silverman, M. (1983). Pulmonary compliance in sick low birthweight infants. How reliable is the measurement of esophageal pressure? *Arch. Dis. Child.*, 58:891–896.

Tusiewicz, K., Moldofsky, H., Bryan, A. C., and Bryan, M. H. (1977). Mechanics of the rib cage and diaphragm during sleep. *J. Appl. Physiol.*, 42:600–602.

Vinegar, A., Sinnet, E. E., and Leith, D. E. (1979). Dynamic mechanisms determine functional residual capacity in mice *Musculus*. *J. Appl. Physiol.*, 46:867–871.

Walti, H., Moriette, G., Radvanyi-Bouvet, M. F., Chaussain, M., Morel-Kahn, F., Pajot, N., and Relier, J. P. (1986). Influence of breathing pattern on functional residual capacity in sleeping newborn infants. *J. Develop. Physiol.*, 8:167–172.

Widdowson, E. M. (1968). Growth and composition of the fetus and newborn. In *Biology and Gestation*. Vol 2. The Fetus and Neonate. Edited by N. S. Assali. New York, Academic Press, pp. 1–49.

54

Respiration During Diving

YVES JAMMES

Institut Jean Roche
Marseille, France

CHARIS ROUSSOS

National and Kapodistrian University
 of Athens Medical School
Athens, Greece
McGill University
Montreal, Quebec, Canada

I. Historical Aspects

One of the most exciting human dreams has been the exploration and conquest of the underwater world. However, for centuries, underwater excursions have been limited to depths of a few meters. A compilation of the processes used by divers of old, including rigid diving bells, hypothetical respiratory apparatus, and breath-hold diving, may be found in *De Re Militari* by Vegece (sixteenth century). A large number of physiological problems associated with the investigation of the underwater environment take place during breath-hold diving. Until the experiments with barometric pressure by Pascal (*L'équilibre des Liqueurs*, 1648), the consequences of elevated ambient pressure on an immersed individual, principally on chest wall mechanics, were totally ignored. Based on the knowledge of the necessity to equilibrate pressure between the inspired air and the medium surrounding the chest, several inventors proposed models for diving helmets connected via an umbilicus to a pump delivering compressed air (Fréminet, 1774; Klingert, 1797; Siebe, 1819).

 A new step in the conquest of the underwater environment was made when the diver became autonomous, i.e., independent of a source of pressurized air at sea level. This was achieved in 1860 by B. Rouquayrol and A. Denayrouze, who built and marketed the first autonomous diving suit, consisting of a self-carried compressed air tank, which delivered the inspired gas at pressure equilibrated to that of the ambient water. However, due to the heaviness of the diving suit, the divers were very limited, and true autonomous diving was only realized in 1933 by Y. Le Prieur and then more successfully in 1943 by E. Gagnan and J. Y. Cousteau. The narcotic effects exerted by high partial pressure of nitrogen (N_2) combined with the increased density of inspired air and elevated pressure limited the maximal depth to 30–40 meters of sea water (msw). The necessity of using other dilutant gases of low density, such as helium (He) and, more recently, hydrogen (H_2), associated or not with N_2, has necessitated modification of the composition of the inspired gas mixture with depth and also warming of the inspired gas and the diving suit. This limits the autonomy of deep sea divers, who must use a tube to deliver gases and fluids, but allows excursional diving at a depth reaching 500 msw as well as experimental human diving in pressure chambers at 71 atmospheres absolute (ATA) (700 msw).

The present study focuses on the consequences of diving—including breath-hold diving—on the thorax. This includes the effects of elevated pressure on the chest wall and pulmonary mechanics as well as on the heart and hemodynamics. In addition, specific problems of deep sea diving, in particular, enhanced respiratory heat loss and the influences of the high-pressure nervous syndrome on respiratory control, will also be discussed.

All aspects of pulmonary and chest wall dysfunctions under hyperbaric conditions have been extensively commented upon in a recent general review (Jammes et al., 1992).

II. Breath-Hold Diving

During apnea in the course of a dive, the major problem is tissue tolerance of hypoxia. Various adaptations exist in diving animals, including mammals (e.g., seals, dolphins, whales), birds, and reptiles, some of whom reach depths of 600 msw (the Weddell seal, *Leptonychotes weddelli*) or even 1500 msw (the whale *Physeter catodon*) (Hui, 1975), the apneic duration being 1 h or more. In some human divers who have reached depths of 65 msw (Craig, 1968) or more (110–118 msw), the duration of apnea was limited to 110–130 s (Ferrigno et al., 1991). Ventilatory arrest is responsible for progressive asphyxia caused by physical work (swimming), which increases oxygen consumption and CO_2 production. The P_{O_2}-P_{CO_2} diagram in Figure 1 shows the changes in the alveolar gas composition during apnea that is maintained at sea level or during a dive combining apnea and swimming. In both cases the composition of the alveolar gas tends to reach the mixed venous blood, but during diving two phenomena delay this event. First, the muscular work induces a leftward shift in the position of the mixed venous point. Second, the intrathoracic pressure increases with the ambient hydrostatic pressure (the increase in ambient pressure is one ATA, i.e., one bar, for each 10 m depth

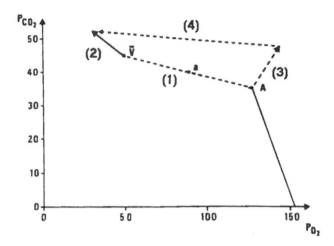

Figure 1 Theoretical changes in alveolar gas composition (A), arterial (a) and mixed venous blood (v) during apnea performed at sea level in a resting (1) or exercising (2) subject or during a breath-hold dive (3) associated with swimming (4).

in sea water and each 10.4 m in fresh water). According to the Boyle-Mariotte law, this results in a proportional increase in the partial pressures of alveolar gases.

In a recent study, Qvist et al. (1993) confirmed compression hyperoxia ($Pa_{O_2} = 141$ torr) and hypercapnia ($Pa_{CO_2} = 47$ torr) in Korean female divers who dove to a fixed depth of 4–5 m. When a breath-hold diver returns from a dive, the reverse phenomenon occurs: PA_{O_2} decreases and the alveolar-to-arterial P_{O_2} gradient may be inversed, resulting in increased arterial hypoxemia. In humans, arterial P_{O_2} was 54 torr at the end of a 2-min dive at 10 m (Hill, 1973), whereas in the harbor seal (*Phoca vitulina*), Pa_{O_2} was only 10 torr after a 23-min dive (Kerem and Elsner, 1973). Usually, human divers hyperventilate before they dive in order to enhance the oxygen stores in the arterial blood and to prolong apneic duration. In this case, the breath-hold time may increase to 90–130 s during a dive at 10 msw (Hill, 1973). However, due to prolonged apneic duration, the final PA_{O_2} value is lowered (only 37 torr in the study by Hill). Hypercapnia has been inconsistently observed at the end of 2- to 3-min breath-hold dives in humans; this results mostly from the high CO_2 diffusibility in extra- and intracellular fluids and also initial hypocapnia induced by the hyperventilation before the dive. However, in the harbor seal, Pa_{CO_2} reaches 100 torr after a 23-min dive (Kerem and Elsner, 1973) and metabolic acidosis also occurs within a period of a few minutes after the dive, as measured in the Weddell seal (Kooyman et al., 1981). These differences between human divers and diving mammals (also birds or reptiles) result from the high oxygen stores, the reduction of cellular O_2 consumption, and the tolerance to acidosis in the latter (Dejours, 1975; Leith, 1989); thus, in the seal *Cystophora cristata* total O_2 stores are 2.3 mmol/kg compared to 0.9 mmol/kg in humans. This results from higher hemoglobin and myoglobin concentrations and storage of oxygenated blood in the arterial networks. Enhanced O_2 stores are associated with a marked reduction in cellular oxygen consumption, assessed by the progressive decrease in arteriovenous O_2 concentration throughout the dive, measured in seals, ducks, and alligators (Andersen, 1969). In such hypoxia-tolerant animals, the cellular adaptations essentially correspond to an arrest in oxidative metabolism and glycolytic activation (Hochachka, 1989). This phenomenon is particularly marked in some organs, such as the liver and kidneys, and also in the limb muscles, where the blood supply falls markedly during diving (Behrisch and Elsner, 1984). Reduced blood supply to peripheral tissues results from the reflex bradycardia, which reaches 50% of baseline heart frequency (f_H) in humans (Irving, 1963) and only 10% of control f_H in the seal; the diving bradycardia is associated with reduced strength of cardiac contraction in diving mammals and birds (Ferrante and Opdyke, 1963) and humans (Gross et al., 1976), and also vasoconstriction in the limb muscles, the skin, the kidneys, and the digestive tract, with the redistribution of blood towards the heart, lungs, and brain (Zapol et al., 1979). Bradycardia and peripheral vasospasm result from reflex mechanisms initiated by the stimulation of cold receptors in the nose and the face, pulmonary stretch receptors, and also arterial baroreceptors (Song et al., 1969). However, continuous exposure of the face to cold water abolished the cardiac response to diving (Sterba and Lundgren, 1988), probably by a cold adaptation of facial thermoreceptors. The degree of bradycardia and peripheral vasospasm during breath-hold immersion decreases when the intrathoracic pressure increases (Song et al., 1969); this may be attributed to the activation of the pulmonary vagal stretch receptors and also the reduced activity of arterial baroreceptors in the aortic arch due to decreased transmural pressure. These reflex responses are enhanced when apnea is performed under high ambient pressure (Smith and Hong, 1977) (see below). Cardiac arrhythmia is never observed in diving animals despite the fact that their heart rates decrease drastically. In contrast, in humans many ECG irregularities, such as supraventricular and ventricular premature complexes, have been recorded coincidently with the lowest heart rates (Ferrigno et al., 1991); this presumably reflects increased vagal tone, but hypoxemia is also known to make the myocardium irritable.

The combination of the different reflex influences seems to determine the breath-hold time. Hypoxemia stimulates the arterial chemoreceptors and reflexly activates the respiratory centers, eliciting the breaking point of apnea. On the other hand, sustained lung hyperinflation induces inhibitory reflexes due to the activation of the pulmonary vagal stretch receptors and also, probably, chest wall and diaphragmatic receptors, their sensory paths prolonging the breath-hold duration. The existence of these opposite reflex influences in the determination of the breaking point of apnea has been demonstrated by the significant prolongation of the breath-hold time by a deep inspiration of an hypoxic gas mixture at the end of an apnea performed at sea level (Grimaud et al., 1968).

Chest wall compression by the elevated hydrostatic pressure is marked in some animals that dive 600–1000 msw (61–101 ATA). This phenomenon is less pronounced in humans despite the fact that some breath-hold divers have reached a depth of 100 msw. In humans, the compressibility of the thorax is low, and two factors combine to determine the reduction in alveolar gas volume (Craig, 1968):

1. the ratio between the residual volume (RV) and the total lung capacity (TLC): theoretical considerations tend to fix the limits of human breath-hold diving at the maximal depth of 40 msw, which corresponds to the minimal value of the RV/TLC ratio (0.20). However, some divers have reached greater depths, for example 65 msw, at which a further 0.6-liter decrease in intrathoracic gas volume was measured.
2. A blood volume shift from peripheral tissues towards the thoracic cavity: this allows the maintainence of pressure equalization, because the shift in blood volume roughly corresponds to the lung volume reduction.

The latter phenomenon is enhanced in most diving mammals, where the thoracic retia mirabilia may contain a very large volume of blood. In these animals the high value of the chest wall compliance thoracic squeeze, and their airways, armored by cartilage rings, do not close and trap gas in the lungs (Leith, 1989).

III. Breathing During Diving

There must be a measure of agreement between the pressure of the breathing source and the hydrostatic pressure on the diver's chest. Thus, any discrepancy between the breathing gas delivery pressure and the hydrostatic pressure on the chest causes positive or negative pressure breathing.

A. Biophysical Consequences of Dense-Gas Breathing

Due to the constant value of the pressure × volume product measured at constant temperature in perfect gases, the density (ρ) of a gas mixture increases linearly with the absolute pressure, expressed in ATA (Fig. 2). Then the density of compressed room air measured at 11 ATA (100 msw) is multiplied by around 10. Due to the molecular interactions within the inspired gas mixture, the increase in gas density with elevated ambient pressure must be corrected by a factor of $+2.4$ to -3.0%, depending on the nature of the dilutant gas (N_2, He, or H_2). As shown in Figure 2, the use of dilutant gases of low density, as He or H_2 (Table 1), allows a marked reduction in the slope of the density versus ambient pressure relationship. Nevertheless, at 46 ATA (450 msw), the depth maintained for 12 days during the experimental human dive ENTEX XI (Marine Nationale Française), the density of the He-O_2 and He-N_2-O_2 gas mixtures successively breathed by the subjects was 8.7 and 11 g/liter, respectively. The gas density is the major factor in the Reynolds number, which determines the magnitude of turbulent airflow stream. Its enhancement under hyperbaric condition constitutes the main reason for the limitation of

Gas density, g·L⁻¹

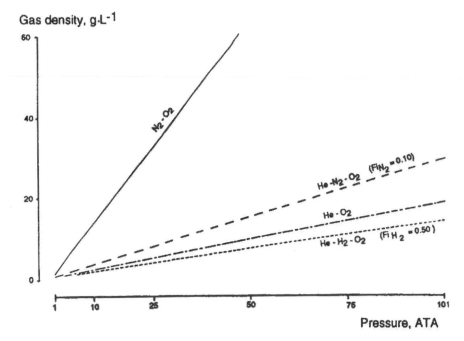

Figure 2 Changes in density of inspired gas mixtures containing oxygen (O_2) plus nitrogen (N_2), helium (He), and/or hydrogen (H_2) with the elevated ambient pressure. In all cases the inspired P_{O_2} has been fixed to around 300 mm Hg, as during human deep diving.

the pulmonary mechanics at depth. Other physical parameters allow one to characterize a breathing mixture. This mostly depends on the choice of the dilutant gases, because the inspired fractional concentration of oxygen is always low during deep dives ($\leq 1\%$) in order to maintain the inspired P_{O_2} value below 300 mm Hg. This avoids reaching the oxygen toxicity threshold. Also, this relatively high PI_{O_2} facilitates respiratory gas exchanges, which may be altered under hyperbaric conditions (see later). The dynamic viscosity (μ) plays a determinant role in the

Table 1 Physical Characteristics of Dilutant Gases Constituting the Inspired Mixtures Breathed under Hyperbaric Conditions

	Density, ρ g/L	Dynamic viscosity, μ poise (10^{-5})	Specific heat, Cp Kcal/K°/kg	Thermal conductivity, K Cal.s.m/K°(10^{-3})
Nitrogen (N_2)	1.19	16.58	0.25	5.73
Helium (He)	0.17	18.64	1.24	34.07
Hydrogen (H_2)	0.09	8.40	3.42	40.21

resistances that oppose the laminar gas flow. The value of μ slightly increases (+5%) under 51 ATA. This may accentuate the discrepancies between gas mixtures containing N_2 and/or He, the value of μ for the latter already being higher at sea level (Table 1). A lung function test used for the evaluation of peripheral airway obstruction is based on this physical difference between He and N_2. The eventual consequences of increased resistance in the small airways in subjects breathing helium for several days or months during saturation dives have never been studied. Other physical parameters, as the specific heat (Cp) and thermal conductivity (K), determine the thermal exchanges through the respiratory apparatus. They do not change significantly under hyperbaric conditions. However, baseline Cp values for He and H_2 are 5 and 14 times higher than that for N_2, and the K coefficient of these low-density gases is 6 and 7 times higher than for N_2, respectively. Actually, the combined effects of elevated gas density with ambient pressure and the relatively high Cp and K values of gas mixtures containing He and/for H_2 severely increase the respiratory heat losses, namely, the convective heat loss ($\dot{H}c = \dot{V}_E \cdot \rho \cdot Cp(T^\circ_E - T^\circ_I)$). The convective respiratory heat loss has been measured at 25 ATA in He-O_2 (Jammes et al., 1988), 45 ATA in He-N_2-O_2 (Burnet et al., 1990), and recently 30 ATA with gas mixtures containing hydrogen (Burnet et al., 1992b). Therefore, due to these physical factors, the heat loss required to increase the temperature of one degree in a He-O_2 gas mixture ($\Delta\dot{H}c/\Delta T^\circ_I$) is multiplied by 20 at 11 ATA and by 59 at 31 ATA compared to 1 ATA (Fig. 3). This effect is accentuated when H_2 is used as a dilutant gas (Burnet et al., 1992b).

B. Limitation of Lung Mechanics

Air Flow Limitation

Numerous human studies conducted in subjects inhaling different gas mixtures containing N_2, He, Neon (Ne), or sulfur hexafluoride (SF_6), at normal or elevated ambient pressure, have clearly demonstrated that the maximal mechanical performances of the ventilatory system (the maximal voluntary ventilation, the forced expiratory volume measured at 1 s, and the peak expiratory flow rate) decrease as the square root of the increased gas density (reviewed by Spaur et al., 1977). This is mostly due to enhanced turbulent airflow in the large airways, because instantaneous flow rates, measured at 50% and 25% of the vital capacity, do not vary with the elevated pressure (Broussolle et al., 1976). The extrathoracic trachea is not shielded from the environmental pressure by pleural pressure; it has been shown that the transmural pressures that can occur during a dive at 300 msw (31 ATA) are high enough to cause dynamic compression of the cervical trachea during forced inspiratory maneuvers (Flook and Fraser, 1989). Thus, the diver's capacity for performing work is limited by the respiratory system. The more significant observations are that airway resistances increase with elevated pressure in the inspired gas even during eupneic ventilation. This has been demonstrated using a body plethysmograph (Varène et al.,

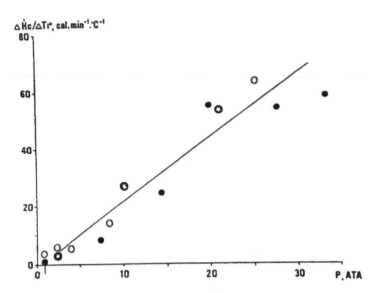

Figure 3 The convective respiratory heat loss ($\Delta\dot{H}c$), normalized to the decrease in inspired temperature ($\Delta TI°$) during a cold test, increases in proportion to the pressure of inspired gas mixture: room air at sea level and He-O_2 under pressure. (Adapted from Hoke et al., 1976, and Jammes et al., 1988.)

1967) and airflow interruptive method (Clarke et al., 1982)—these two methods measuring the sole resistance of the central airways—and also from the recording of transpulmonary pressure with an esophageal balloon (Jammes et al., 1988; Burnet et al., 1990). This reveals that the total lung resistance (R_L) increases linearly with the density of the breathing mixture (Fig. 4). For example, at 46 ATA (gas density = 11 g/liter) the R_L value is multiplied by 3.5 in resting individuals (Burnet et al., 1990). Consequently, the work of breathing (W) increases in proportion to the elevated pressure of the inspired gas mixture as shown by our group during 12 days of diving at 46 ATA (Lenoir et al., 1990), the value of W measured during eupnea is multiplied by around 3 at this depth (Fig. 5). The diaphragm seems to support most of this incremental work, indeed the electromyographic recordings of chest wall and abdominal muscles do not reveal any spontaneous rhythmic activities (Lenoir et al., 1990). When subjects perform a physical performance and, thus, hyperventilate, the work of breathing obviously increases in proportion to the value of minute ventilation ($\dot{V}_E$). However, as demonstrated by Vorosmarti et al. (1975), any increase in the flow resistance due to dense-gas breathing (range of densities: 1–15 g/liter) markedly enhances the slope of the W vs. $\dot{V}_E$ curvilinear relationship: thus, for a moderate hyperventilation ($\dot{V}_E$ = 40 liters/min), the resting value of W is multiplied by 5 when the gas density is 10 g/liter, compared to a corresponding 20% increase measured in the same individual breathing room air at sea level (density: 1 g/liter) (Fig. 5).

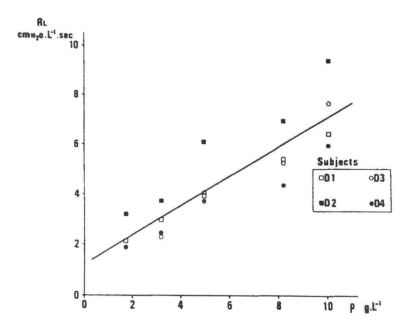

Figure 4 During eupneic ventilation, total lung resistance (R_L) increases linearly with the gas density in human subjects breathing a He-N_2-O_2 mixture at pressure up to 46 ATA. (From Burnet et al., 1990.)

Three other factors may accentuate the alterations in lung mechanics under hyperbaric conditions: (1) the occurrence of hyperbaric tremor recorded in skeletal muscles and in the diaphragm, (2) increased diaphragmatic tonic activity demonstrated under very high ambient pressure (these two phenomena will be commented on later), and (3) a reflex bronchospasm, sometimes associated with mucus hypersecretion, produced by an insufficient warming of the inspired gas mixture.

Cold-Induced Bronchospasm

As commented above, the respiratory heat loss severely increases during deep diving. This makes it necessary to warm the inspired gas and the ambient gas mixture in the diving chamber, the thermal comfort being obtained at an ambient temperature of 30°C at 19 ATA (180 msw) (Webb, 1970). The use of hydrogen as a dilutant gas requires enhanced warming of the inspired gas. Dyspnea and excessive upper respiratory tract secretions have been reported in divers breathing a cold (1°C) He-O_2 mixture at 27 ATA (Hoke et al., 1976). The measurement of lung resistance (R_L) has allowed us to demonstrate that the inhalation of relatively fresh He-O_2 or He-N_2-O_2 gas mixtures (7–8°C) at pressures up to 8 ATA enhanced the R_L value, and this effect is proportional to the elevated pressure

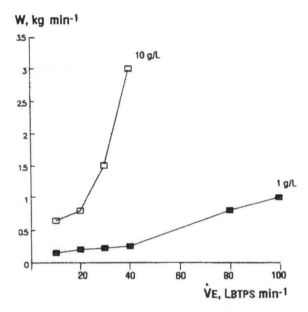

Figure 5 Dense-gas breathing (density = 10 g/liter) markedly increases the mean slope of the relationship between the work of breathing (W) and minute ventilation ($\dot{V}_E$), compared to that measured at sea level (density: 1 g/liter). (Adapted from Vorosmarti et al., 1975, and Lenoir et al., 1990.)

(Jammes et al., 1988; Burnet et al., 1990). The mean increase in R_L measured in divers breathing an insufficiently warmed gas mixture at a depth at 450 msw was around 50% of control R_L value (warm gas), but the response may be twice as high in some individuals (Jammes et al., 1988). However, the same subjects did not present any change in R_L value when they breathed room air at the same temperature at sea level. On the basis of animal studies (Jammes et al., 1983a, 1986) and of some experiments on healthy humans (Heaton et al., 1983), the airway response to the inhalation of cold gas has been attributed to a vagal reflex resulting from the stimulation of thermosensitive units in the larynx and the upper trachea. The participation of thermosensory pathways to the respiratory control system is reinforced by the observation of the perception of an unpleasant sensation of cold or very cold inspired gas in the upper airways when the divers inhaled a cold He-O_2 mixture at 25 ATA, whereas they could not detect the same temperature variations at lesser depths (Jammes et al., 1988). In any case, the airway response to cold was found to correlate directly to the magnitude of the respiratory heat loss and not to the absolute value of the inspired temperature (Burnet et al., 1990). This corroborates electrophysiological studies in cats that have shown that the thermoreceptors in the upper airways act as sensors of the thermal flux through the airway wall (Jammes et al., 1987).

C. Alterations in Respiratory Gas Exchanges

The elevated ambient pressure, with the associated increase in gas density, combined to the specific physical properties of the different inspired gases in the breathing mixture, may theoretically alter the respiratory gas exchanges by convection and/or diffusion. Indeed, the airflow stream limitation in the central airways may enhance the distribution inequalities within the alveolar spaces. Moreover, the transport of respiratory gases by diffusion through the peripheral airways and the alveoli may be modified by the use of dilutant gases other than nitrogen. In fact, as shown in Table 2, the binary diffusion coefficients of O_2 or CO_2 in He or H_2 are higher than that measured in N_2 (room air) at the same ambient pressure. Paganelli (1987) has shown that the binary coefficient of respiratory gases in He or N_2 decreases with the elevated ambient pressure. However, the quantity of gas transported by diffusion depends on the product of the capacitance of the gas phase (the same for all gases at a given temperature) multiplied by the D coefficient and the partial pressure difference, the latter being proportional to the ambient pressure (P). In consequence, as calculated by Paganelli (1987), the DP product for He-O_2 does not vary with pressure up to 90 ATA. The theoretical considerations of the diffusion limitation under hyperbaric conditions also take into account the diffusion time throughout each breathing cycle. Thus, a mathematical model proposed by Lanphier and Camporesi (1982) suggests that at 51 ATA, diffusion limitation may occur when the respiratory frequency is higher than 9 min^{-1} (diffusion time inferior to 7 s), a circumstance often reproduced during quiet breathing in humans. However, none of these mathematical models take into account that the inspired P_{O_2} value is in the range of 220–300 mm Hg during experimental and also off-shore dives, and not 150 mm Hg as when subjects breath room air at sea level.

   Human observations and animal studies reveal some modifications in respiratory gas exchange under hyperbaric conditions. In resting goats studied at 20 ATA of

Table 2 Diffusion Coefficients of Dilutant Gases (Primary D) Constituting the Inspired Gas Mixture Used Under Hyperbaric Conditions and Values of Binary Diffusion Coefficients of Respiratory Gases in the Corresponding Dilutant Gas

	Primary D coefficient (cm^2/s)	Binary D coefficient	
		Oxygen	Carbon dioxide
N_2	0.22	0.23	0.17
He	1.69	0.78	0.63
H_2	1.50	0.83	0.66

Values measured at 1 ATA.
Source: L'Air liquide, 1976.

a He-O_2 mixture, Chouteau and coworkers (reviewed by Chouteau, 1971) have reported clinical and EEG signs of acute hypoxemia when the inspired P_{O_2} was 150 mm Hg: these manifestations disappeared after P_{IO_2} was elevated. A polarographic O_2 electrode introduced into the abdominal aorta has confirmed that Pa_{O_2} falls (to around 75 torr) at 21 ATA in anesthetized rabbits (Chouteau, 1971). However, these observations were not corroborated in resting humans breathing dense-gas mixtures containing Ne or SF_6 at normal or elevated pressure (Saltzman et al., 1971; Wood et al., 1976; Giry et al., 1987). Then the convection requirement for oxygen ($\dot{V}_E/\dot{V}_{O_2}$) remains constant at pressure up to 36 ATA (density: 9 g/liter). Moreover, sea level animal studies have even demonstrated that the alveolar-to-arterial P_{O2} difference decreases with the elevated density of the breathing mixture (Worth et al., 1976). The CO_2 transport at rest is unchanged or slightly modified under hyperbaric conditions. Thus, in 18 human volunteers, studied under ambient pressure varying from 1 to 66 ATA, no correlation was found between the end-tidal P_{CO_2} value (PET_{CO_2}) and the gas density (maximal value: 20 g/liter) (Dwyer et al., 1977; Gelfand et al., 1983; Giry et al., 1987). However, transcutaneous measurement of P_{CO_2} in anesthetized rats, ventilated at constant minute volume under 42 ATA, has revealed a significant but moderate increase (1.5–3.0 mm Hg) in this variable, independent on any alveolar hypoventilation of central origin (Furset et al., 1987). During incremental exercise performed under hyperbaric condition, Fagraeus et al. (1973) have not evidenced change in the $\dot{V}_E$ vs. $\dot{V}_{O_2}$ relationship at a work rate inferior to 50% of the maximal $\dot{V}_{O_2}$. At higher work rates the results are contradictory. A reduction in the aerobic power is observed and seems to depend on the experimental circumstances. Indeed, in immersed individuals at 43.4 ATA (a condition closer to that of commercial deep diving), reduced aerobic power was reported by Dwyer et al. (1977), whereas in dry hyperbaric experiments, Fragraeus et al. (1973) and Anthonisen et al. (1976) did not observe this phenomenon. When a diver is immersed upright and breathes a gas mixture from a mouth-held demand regulator or even gas from a diving chamber, the mean hydrostatic pressure acting on the thorax exceeds the gas delivery pressure. This is physically analogous to negative-pressure breathing, a circumstance responsible for elevated total respiratory static work as well as the flow-resistive pulmonary work due to increased airway resistance (Taylor and Morrison, 1990). This may explain the observations by Dwyer et al. (1977). In addition, at exercise levels superior to the anaerobic threshold, the $\dot{V}_E/\dot{V}_{O_2}$ ratio decreases at depth, whereas this ratio normally increases at sea level. The most striking fact is the phenomenon of "CO_2 retention" commonly observed in humans exercising under high pressure, the magnitude of hypercapnia being proportional to the minute ventilation (see the review by Lanphier and Camporesi, 1982, and also Taylor and Morrison, 1990). Such inadequate respiratory response to exertion may be compared to that measured in patients with severe chronic obstructive pulmonary disease (COPD), who often exhibit a rise in arterial P_{CO_2} during exercise (Jones, 1988). Although this pattern of response was classically attributed to a combination of an increase in the work of breathing and reduced central responsiveness to CO_2, the latter phenomenon has not been confirmed (see the review by Rebuck and

Slutsky, 1986). Thus, the decreased ventilatory response to CO_2-driven breathing in COPD patients seems to be more a consequence of a failure of the ventilatory pump to overcome the mechanical load than the result of any decrease in the neural drive. As reported already, the work of breathing increases greatly when healthy subjects hyperventilate during the inhalation of a high-density gas mixture. Moreover, further modifications in respiratory function occur with dense-gas breathing. As shown in Figure 6, the combination of dense-gas breathing plus exercise hyperventilation markedly increases the physiological deadspace (Salzano et al., 1984), and the alveolar gas distribution is inversed in such circumstances (Wood et al., 1976). Both phenomena may be responsible for the occurrence of CO_2 retention in working divers. In addition, neurological factors may also depress the chemoreflex drive of breathing when normal individuals remain under high gas pressures. Thus, when divers exercise at the same work rate and elevated ambient pressure, PET_{CO_2} is significantly higher if the inspired gas mixture contains hydrogen (Giry, 1990), a dilutant gas that has the lowest density but a narcotic power much higher than helium.

In summary, the aforementioned data obtained at simulated depths clearly show that respiratory gas exchange is not altered in resting individuals, but some limitations in oxygen inflow and CO_2 outflow occur during the hyperventilation associated with physical exercise.

D. Adaptative and Nonadaptative Ventilatory Responses

Breathing high-density gas mixtures constitutes a condition of resistive internal ventilatory loading. The same experimental circumstance is difficult to reproduce

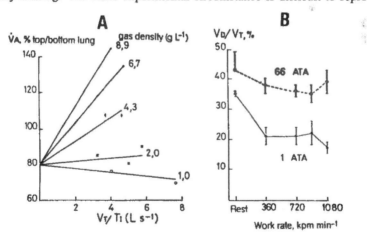

Figure 6 (A) Dense-gas breathing combined with hyperventilation (increased mean inspiratory flow rate, V_T/T_I) severely enlarges the relative alveolar ventilation measured in the lung top and, thus, the deadspace effect in upright individuals. (From Wood and Bryan, 1971.) (B) This results in a global increase in the physiological deadspace in subjects exercising under high pressure (66 ATA), compared to the V_D/V_T ratio measured at the same work load at sea level (From Salzano et al., 1984.)

at sea level in individuals, because dense-gas breathing and drug-induced broncho-spasm (internal load) and even the addition of resistors to the respiratory system (external load) are always limited in duration. In addition, the elevated hydrostatic pressure and/or the high partial pressures of the dilutant gases may exert various influences on the central nervous system, including respiratory control: the excitatory effects are classically attributed to the hydrostatic pressure changes, whereas the dilutant gases exert an anesthetic influence; the maximal effect is observed with nitrogen and the minimal with helium (Rostain et al., 1987).

Minute Ventilation and Breathing Pattern

In resting individuals $\dot{V}_E$ increases in proportion to the density of the breathing mixture, whatever the nature of the dilutant gas, including N_2, He, H_2, Ne, or SF_6 (Fig. 7); this statistical linear relationship derives from data reported in 33 healthy subjects by Saltzman et al. (1971), Wood et al. (1976), Dwyer et al. (1977), Giry et al. (1987), and Lenoir et al. (1990). Concomitantly, the respiratory frequency slows down and, thus, the tidal volume increases. These observations are confirmed in conscious cats compressed at 101 ATA in He-O_2 or He-N_2-O_2 (Burnet and Naraki, 1988; Burnet et al., 1992a). In contrast, in anesthetized animals breathing a dense-gas

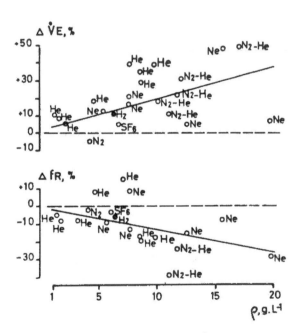

Figure 7 Percentage changes in minute ventilation ($\dot{V}_E$) and respiratory frequency (f) measured in human subjects during the quiet breathing of different gas mixtures at normal or elevated ambient pressure (maximal depth: 650 msw or 66 ATA). (From Saltzman et al., 1971, Wood et al., 1976, Dwyer et al., 1977, Giry et al., 1987, and Lenoir et al., 1990.)

mixture (SF_6 plus O_2) at sea level, we measured hypoventilation, characterized by bradypnea with no change in tidal breath (Barrière et al., 1993): this response disappeared after bivagotomy. Thus, the hyperventilation reported in awake individuals (humans and animals) during dives is attributed to the general excitatory influence exerted by hydrostatic pressure changes, which is accentuated during periods of compression (Linnarson and Hesser, 1978; Gelfand et al., 1980, 1983). The biochemical properties of dilutant gases may play also a role. Indeed, in cats the hyperventilation measured at 101 ATA is higher with the He-O_2 than with a He-N_2-O_2 gas mixture (Burnet and Naraki, 1988). The diving bradypnea may correspond to a reflex adaptative response, which opposes the elevated impedance of the respiratory system due to increased gas density, but the accompanying enhanced amplitude of the tidal breath must accentuate the increase in respiratory muscle work. The sole positive element is the observation that the duty cycle (inspiratory period above total cycle time) does not change, even at pressures up to 46 ATA (Lenoir et al., 1990). This may delay the occurence of diaphragmatic fatigue, a phenomenon believed to occur during deep diving (see below).

Chemoreflex Drive of Breathing

Several human studies conducted under high ambient pressure as well as sea level observations performed in subjects breathing dense-gas mixtures have shown that the respiratory sensitivity to hypercapnia, mostly evaluated by the rebreathing method, decreases in proportion to the inspired gas density (see results and also review by Gelfand et al., 1980). A similar reduction of the response to hypoxia has not been reported (Doell et al., 1983). Thus, these particular circumstances seem to affect the central chemosensitivity and not the arterial chemoreflex drive for breathing. Several explanations for the reduced central CO_2 sensitivity under high pressure may be proposed. The high-pressure nervous syndrome cannot be involved, because this phenomenon occurs in subjects breathing dense-gas mixture at normal or slightly elevated ambient pressures (Gelfand et al., 1980). The narcotic properties of dense gases may be partly responsible for this phenomenon. Also, central interactions between the different respiratory afferents, activated under the condition of severe ventilatory loading, may also explain the reduced CO_2 sensitivity. Indeed, animal studies at normal ambient pressure have already shown that the enhanced sensory pathway from respiratory muscles, contracting against a high and prolonged expiratory threshold load, markedly depresses the response to hypercapnia (Jammes et al., 1983b). Whatever the mechanism of the reduced chemosensitivity to CO_2 under hyperbaric conditions or with dense-gas breathing at sea level, this phenomenon may also explain that hypercapnia often develops in response to exercise during experimental diving.

Recruitment of Respiratory Muscles

Electromyographic recordings of the spontaneous diaphragmatic activity in human volunteers compressed at pressure up to 46 ATA (gas density: 8–11 g/liter) (Lenoir et al., 1990) and in cats studied up to 101 ATA (gas density: 25 g/liter) (Burnet et al., 1992a) have revealed a marked recruitment of diaphragmatic motor units in parallel to the increased amplitude of tidal breaths. This is associated with changes in the EMG power spectrum, characterized by reduced centroid frequency corresponding to decreased ratio in a high/low band of EMG frequencies. These EMG changes persisted, with no accentuation, during 12 days at 46 ATA (Fig. 8) or 3 days at 101 ATA (Fig. 9). They are not proportional to the elevated pressure, as was shown in cats where the decrease in centroïd frequency was already maximal at 31 ATA. Simultaneous EMG recordings of abdominal and intercostal muscles and also nonrespiratory muscles (trapezius and deltoid muscles in cats, adductor pollicis in humans) have demonstrated that the changes in the EMG power spectrum were not found in the skeletal muscles or in the abdominal muscles, which did not participate to the resting ventilation at depth (Lenoir et al., 1990; Derrien et al., 1990; Burnet et al., 1992a). However, the leftward shift in EMG spectrum was present in intercostal muscles, which rhythmically contracted under high pressure (Burnet et al., 1992a). Thus, the EMG power changes are closely associated with the increased respiratory muscle work due to severe and prolonged ventilatory

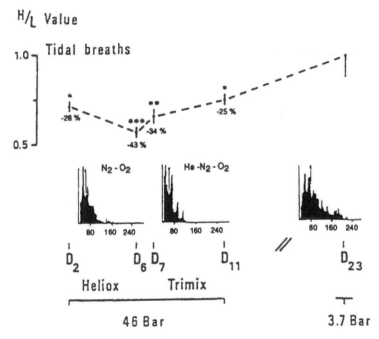

Figure 8 Compared to control condition near sea level (3.7 ATA), changes in diaphragmatic EMG spectrum are present during quiet ventilation in four human volunteers during a 12-day sojourn at 46 ATA. This results in both reduced ratio of high to low bands of EMG frequencies (H/L) and a leftward shift in power spectrum. (Adapted from Lenoir et al., 1990.)

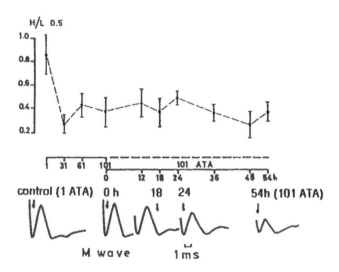

Figure 9 The same changes in diaphragmatic EMG spectrum are measured in conscious cats compressed until 101 ATA with the He-N$_2$-O$_2$ mixture. In this species, the mass action potential (diaphragmatic M wave) in response to a direct muscle stimulation is markedly modified from the 18th to 24th hour of stay at maximal pressure. (From Burnet et al., 1992.)

loading with dense-gas breathing. Normobaric studies have clearly demonstrated that the mechanical failure of an exercising skeletal or respiratory muscle is preceded by an increase in the low-frequency component of the EMG of that muscle (Gross et al., 1979). It is thus attractive to attribute the EMG changes observed at depth to the neuromuscular signs of respiratory muscle fatigue. Recent sea level studies strongly suggest that the leftward shift in EMG spectrum mostly results from a rate-limiting factor, regulating the neural discharge rate, which is determined by a sensory feedback from the activation of nerve endings in muscles contracting at a high strength (Bigland-Ritchie and Woods, 1984; Jammes and Balzamo, 1992). Thus, these EMG power changes reflect more the variations in the recruitment strategy of motor units than the slowing of action potential conduction velocity in muscle fibers, as was initially suggested by Lindström et al. (1970). However, at pressures up to 101 ATA the analysis of the diaphragmatic EMG response to direct muscle stimulation reveals a marked prolonged duration of the mass action potentials (Burnet et al., 1992a). This may be attributed to a slowing of the time course of muscular electrogenesis under high pressure because this phenomenon also occurs in an isolated phrenic-to-diaphragm preparation (Kendig and Cohen, 1976).

In addition to the changes in the recruitment strategy of diphragmatic and also intercostal motor units hyperbaric animal studies at pressures up to 91 ATA (gas density around 20 g/liter) have also shown a marked increase in the tonic diaphragmatic activity (Imbert et al., 1981) (Fig. 10). This phenomenon is similar

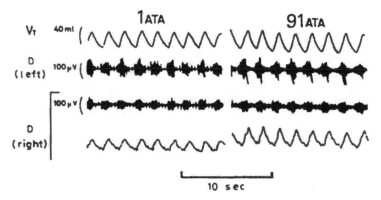

Figure 10   Tonic EMG activity in the diaphragm occurs in conscious cats exposed to very high He-O$_2$ pressure (91 ATA), as assessed by elevated baseline integrated diaphragmatic EMG (bottom trace).

to that observed during acute bronchospasm (Muller et al., 1980); its mechanism involves the participation of pulmonary vagal afferents, strongly stimulated under the circumstances of drug-induced bronchospasm (Badier et al., 1990). It may be hypothesized that the same reflex pathways are elicited during the condition of severe internal resistive loading produced by dense-gas breathing.

The peripheral manifestations of the high-pressure nervous syndrome, mostly represented by the hyperbaric tremor, may also modify the efficiency of the chest wall muscles and the diaphragm. Indeed, in humans (Lenoir et al., 1990) hyperbaric tremor at 11–14 Hz is recorded in all skeletal muscle groups, as well as the diaphragm and other respiratory muscles studied.

IV.   Cardiovascular Function Under High Pressure

The cardiovascular consequences of breathing high-density gas mixtures have been mostly focused on the changes in heart rate and systemic blood pressure. A bradycardia is often reported under a hyperbaric environment in humans (Kerem and Salzano, 1974; Wilson et al., 1977) and animals (Shida and Lin., 1981; Stuhr et al., 1990) and also in an isolated heart exposed to high pressure (Doubt and Hogan 1978; Gennser and Ornhagen, 1989). On the other hand, inconsistent cardiac responses have been reported in humans (Bühlman et al., 1970; Joulia et al., 1992), showing no change in heart rate or even increased cardiac frequency. Human studies involving the hyperbaric He-O$_2$ environment have shown that the eventual changes in heart rate were independent of the pressure level and the density for deep dives (Flynn et al., 1972; Joulia et al., 1992). Moreover, bradycardia was not detected when in vivo or in vitro studies were performed under normoxic conditions at ambient pressure up to 71 ATA (Hordness and Tyssebotn, 1985). Limited information is available concerning ECG variations during compression and prolonged residence under high pressure. Abberrent cardiac rhythms ranging from coupled extrasystoles to conduction blocks have sometimes been observed during human saturation dives in air (Wilson et al., 1977) or He-O_2 (Argeles et al., 1977) and also during hyperbaric experiments on isolated myocardial strips (Doubt and Evans, 1982). Tall peak T waves were reported by Wilson et al. (1977) during a 7-h human dive at 7 ATA of compressed air with normal oxygen pressure (175 mm Hg). Our observations of divers participating in a 73-day saturation dive at 25.5 ATA by COMEX (Hydra IX) (gas mixtures containing He and/or H_2) and of conscious dogs compressed to 91 ATA in a He-N_2-O_2 mixture (Joulia et al., 1992) showed that the T-wave amplitude increases in proportion to the gas density, whatever the composition of the inspired gas mixture. These T-wave changes cannot be explained by the positional changes in QRS or T vectors. No satisfactory explanation of these T-wave changes has yet been proposed. More detailed reports on cardiovascular changes at pressure are fragmentary. The use of different techniques to measure the cardiac output in humans or animals may explain the opposite changes in this variable reported at depth. Measurements of cardiac output and regional blood flow distribution in rats using radioactive labeled microspheres (Aanderud et al., 1985) and in dogs with chronically implanted Doppler flow meters (Barthelemy, 1990) at pressure up to 71 ATA (rats) or 91 ATA (dogs) have not shown significant changes in aortic blood flow, but they reveal reduced perfusion to the kidneys, surrenals, skeletal muscles, and brain. In dogs the changes in regional blood flow have been compared in two circumstances that favor (He-O_2) or attenuate (He-N_2-O_2 mixture) the excitatory effects of elevated pressure on the central nervous system (Barthélemy, 1990); thus, the decrease in limb muscle, mesenteric, or carotid blood flow observed at pressure superior to 61 ATA in animals breathing the He-O_2 mixture is weak or absent even at higher pressure with the ternary mixture containing nitrogen. The excitatory effects of high helium pressure on the nervous system and perhaps also the sympathetic motor control to blood vessels may be responsible for the reduced organ perfusion under high ambient pressure. Baroreceptor reflexes have been studied in humans at 46 ATA using a noninvasive technique (Bowser-Riley, 1990). A neck collar device allowed the application of positive or negative pressure to the carotid sinus baroreceptor sensitivity to the ensuing changes in heart rate were assessed. The reflex heart rate response to applied positive pressure to the carotid sinus, which reduces the transmural pressure, is accentuated at depth, whereas the baroreflex response to increased transmural sinus pressure (negative pressure) is depressed. This leads to the conclusion that elevated hydrostatic pressure exerted on the surrounding tissues may modify the gain of the sinusal baroreflex arch. Similar observations were reported by Barthélemy et al. (1993), who found that the increase in blood pressure in response to the Vasalva maneuver (decreased transmural pressure in the thoracic aorta) is accentuated at 26 ATA, whereas the magnitude of reverse blood pressure changes accompanying a maximal inspiratory effort (Müller maneuver) that increases the transmural aortic pressure is not modified. However, in no case does the systemic blood pressure significantly vary during human deep diving.

Actually, it seems that the hyperbaric environment modifies the cardiovascular function through the elevated hydrostatic pressure or the changes in intrathoracic pressure with dense-gas breathing. However, it cannot be ignored that the high pressure of dilutant gases may also influence the nervous control of the vasomotor tone.

V. Pulmonary Function of Deep Divers

The main question for a chest physician is, what are the consequences of the repetitive exposure to high pressure of gases on the pulmonary function of commercial and military divers? The answer may be based on the comparison between lung function tests performed in a population of professional divers and standardized normal values and also on longitudinal studies in the same individuals repetitively exposed to high pressure.

A. Lung Function of Professional Divers

The results obtained with 897 deep divers are collected in Table 3. The predictive value of these observations is limited by variation of the individual diving experience, which ranges from 1 to 17 years, and also by the maximal depth. However, for the 36 divers examined by our team (groups 3 and 6) and by the laboratory of the Marine Nationale (CERB) (groups 4 and 5), the experience of diving is homogeneous (6–15 years), and all of them have worked at 16–46 ATA. All these observations concern commercial or military divers, some of who have also participated in experimental dry dives in a pressure chamber (groups 3, 4, 5, and 6). This horizonal statistical study does not reveal any significant modification in lung volumes, maximal forced expiratory capacity, or diffusing capacity of these divers compared to the normal values measured in sedentary male individuals of the same age and height.

B. Short-Term Consequences of a Deep Dive

Pre- and postdive lung function tests were performed in our laboratory on a group of 13 professional divers participating in an "off-shore" dive at 300 msw in the North Sea (total time of dive: 18 days; breathing mixture: He-O_2). Postdive measurements were performed within 8 days of surfacing. Then, only the expiratory flow rates measured at small lung volume and the diffusing capacity for carbon monoxide (breath-hold diffusion test), adjusted for hemoglobin changes, were significantly reduced: the midexpiratory time increased from 74 ± 5 ms (predive) to 82 ± 3 ms (postdive) and the DL_{CO}/V_A value decreased from 5.3 ± 0.4 to 4.6

Table 3 Pulmonary Function of Professional Divers

	Number of divers	Diving experience (y)	Maximal depth (msw)	Age (y)	VC (% of normal)	TLC (% of normal)	FEV$_{1.0}$/FVC (%)	DLCO/VA (%)	Ref.
Group 1	26	2–14	?	32 ± 5	84	118	67 ± 4	112	
Group 2	858	?	15–300	30 ± 5	111	?	82 ± 6	?	
Group 3 ENTEX X	3	6–11	250	34 ± 9	100	94	80 ± 9	?	
Group 4 HYDRAV	6	>5	300–450	34 ± 3	111	?	73 ± 6	?	
Group 5 ENTEX XI	4	8–15	450	34 ± 6	122	?	77 ± 5	?	
Group 6	23	9–12	150	34 ± 9	114	100	78 ± 12	98	

± 0.6 ml/min/torr/liter after the dive. These abnormalities were not found when the subjects were examined again 2 months after surfacing. The same observations of postdive reduction in the diffusing capacity after a 18-day simulated saturation dive at 33 ATA (320 msw) with P_{IO_2} around 400 mm Hg were reported by Suzuki et al. (1991). These changes were still observed 13 days after surfacing, but they disappeared 48 days later. The authors have attributed the transient decrease in DL_{CO}/V_A to the pulmonary oxygen toxicity caused by long-term exposure to oxygen close to 0.5 ATA. Indeed, decreased diffusing capacity no longer occurred after a saturation dive at the same pressure but with a lower P_{IO_2} (310 mm Hg). Examination of the three divers who participated in the 71 ATA Hydra 10 COMEX experiment has also shown a reduction in maximal strength of the inspiratory muscles (PI_{max}), which recovered control values progressively within 2 months of decompression. These data must be confirmed, but they suggest that severe and prolonged ventilatory loading during the dive may alter diaphragmatic function.

C. Longitudinal Studies of Lung Function of Professional Divers

Davey et al. (1984) examined during a period of 5 years 255 divers, each of whom reached the depth of 300 msw several times. The annual reduction in the forced vital capacity (FVC) and the forced expired flow rates at small lung volumes, but not the FEV $_{1.0}$/FVC ratio, was positively correlated with the maximal depth reached during the same period of time. Thus, repetitive exposure to high-pressure gases (most often the He-O_2 mixture) seems to induce a weak but nonnegligible limitation of the pulmonary function, mostly evidenced at the periphery of the airway tract. Several factors may be responsible for such progressive chronic obstructive pulmonary disease: the elevated airway pressure resulting from the combined effects of increased resistances opposing airflow plus enhanced respiratory muscle work and perhaps also the bronchorrhea and the associated bronchospasm in response to the cooling of airway mucosa. Indeed, if the conditioning of inspired temperature in the range of 30–33°C is easy during experimental dives in a pressure chamber, the maintenance of this relatively high temperature value in the helmet of deep divers maneuvering in a cold water environment is much more difficult despite the relative efficiency of thermal exchanger devices used during "off-shore" operations.

VI. Conclusion

Diving exposes the respiratory apparatus to very extreme conditions, which force the respiratory gas exchanger and also the ventilatory pump to work near their limits. Except for the obvious ergonomic interest to concisely determine human tolerance to breath-hold diving and hyperbaric exposure, experimental studies performed in pressure chambers reproduce very interesting conditions of prolonged ventilatory loading difficult or even impossible to generate in sea-level experiments. The physiological measurements made during the survey of human volunteers during deep dives may serve to provide better knowledge of the mechanical consequences of dense-gas breathing on respiratory muscle mechanics and the cardiovascular system.

References

Aanderud, L., Onarheim, J., and Tyssebotn, I. (1985). Effects of 71 ATA He-O_2 on organ blood flow in the rat. *J. Appl. Physiol.*, 59:1369–1375.

Air Liquide. (1976). *Encyclopédie des Gaz.* Amsterdam, Elsevier.

Andersen, H. T. (1969). *The Biology of Marine Animals.* New York, Academic Press.

Anthonisen, N. R., Utz, G., Kryger, M. H., and Urbanette, J. S. (1976). Exercise tolerance at 4 and 6 ATA. *Undersea Biomed. Res.*, 3:95–102.

Argeles, H. J., Freezor, M. D., and Saltzman, H. A. (1977). Human vector electrocardiographic responses at increased pressure to 1000 msw. *Undersea Biomed. Res.*, 4:A30.

Badier, M., Jammes, Y., Romero-Colomer, P., and Lemerre, C. (1989). Tonic activity in inspiratory muscles and phrenic motoneurones by stimulation of vagal afferents. *J. Appl. Physiol.*, 66:1613–1619.

Barrière, J. R., Delpierre, S., DelVolgo, M. J., and Jammes, Y. (1993). Comparisons among external resistive loading, drug-induced bronchospasm and dense-gas breathing in cats: roles of vagal and spinal afferents. *Lung*, 171:125–136.

Barthélemy, P. (1990). La distribution des débits circulatoires régionaux sous haute pression. *Arch. Intern. Physiol. Biochem.*, 98:A389–A392.

Barthélemy, P., Joulia, F., Burnet, H., and Jammes, Y. (1993). Etude de la fonction cardiovasculaire chez l'homme au cours de plongées expérimentales à 26 ATA (mélange hélium-azote-oxygène). *Arch. Intern. Physiol. Biochem.*, 101:341–345.

Behrisch, H. W., and Elsner, R. (1984). Enzymatic adaptations to asphyxia in the harbour seal and dog. *Respir. Physiol.*, 55:239–254.

Bigland-Ritchie, B., and Woods, J. J. (1984). Changes in muscle contractile properties and neural control during human muscular fatigue. *Muscle Nerve*, 7:691–699.

Bowser-Riley, F. (1990). Cardiovascular function and vasomotor reflexes during deep diving. *Arch. Intern. Physiol. Biochem.*, 98:A385–A388.

Broussolle, B., Chouteau, J., and Hyacinthe R. (1976). Respiratory function during a simulated saturation dive to 51 ATA with a helium-oxygen mixture. In *Underwater Physiology V.* Edited by C. J. Lambert. Bethesda, Md., FASEB, pp. 79–89.

Bühlman, A. A., Matthys, H., Overrath, G., Bennett, P. B., Elliott, D. H., and Gray, S. P. (1970). Saturation exposures at 31 ATA in ann oxygen-helium atmosphere with excursions to 36 ATA. *Aerospace Med.*, 41:394–403.

Burnet, H., and Naraki, N. (1988). Ventilatory failure in cats during prolonged exposure to very high pressure. *Undersea Biomed. Res.*, 15:19–30.

Burnet, H., Lucciano, M., and Jammes, Y. (1990). Respiratory effects of cold gas breathing in humans under hyperbaric environment. *Respir. Physiol.*, 81:413–424.

Burnet, H., Lenoir, P., and Jammes, Y. (1992a). Changes in respiratory muscle activity in conscious cats during experimental dives at 101 ATA. *J. Appl. Physiol.*, 73:465–472.

Burnet, H., Raynaud-Gobert, M., Lucciano, M., and Jammes, Y. (1992b). Relationships between inspired and expired gas temperature under hyperbaric environment. *Respir. Physiol.*, 90:377–386.

Chouteau, J. (1971). Respiratory gas exchanges in animals during exposure to extreme ambient pressure. In *Underwater Physiology IV.* Edited by C. J. Lambertsen. New York, Academic Press, pp. 395–398.

Clarke, J. R., Jaeger, M. J., Zumrick, J. L., O'Bryan, R., and Spaur, W. H. (1982). Respiratory resistance from 1 to 46 ATA measured with the interrupter technique. *J. Appl. Physiol.*, 52:549–555.

Craig, A. B. (1968). Depth limits of breath-hold diving (an example of Fennology). *Respir. Physiol.*, 5:14–22.

Crosbie, W. A., Reed, J. W., and Clarke, M. C. (1979). Functional characteristics of the large lungs found in commercial divers. *J. Appl. Physiol.*, 46:633–645.

Davey, T. S., Cotes, J. E., Reed, J. W. (1984). Relationships of ventilatory capacity to hyperbaric exposure in divers. *J. Appl. Physiol.*, 56:1655–1658.

Dejours, P. (1975). *Principles of Comparative Respiratory Physiology*. New York, Elsevier.

Derrien, I., Lenoir, P., and Jammes, Y. (1990). Etude comparative des muscles diaphragme et adducteur du pouce lors de contractions statiques fatigantes à 25 ATA (Entex XVI); *Arch. Intern. Physiol. Biochem.*, 98:A424.

Doell, D., Zutter, M., Anthonisen, N. R. (1973). Ventilatory response to hypercapnia and hypoxia at 1 and 4 ATA. *Respir. Physiol.*, 18:338–346.

Doubt, T. J., and Evans, D. E. (1982). Hyperbaric exposures alter cardiac excitation-contraction coupling. *Undersea Biomed. Res.*, 9:131–145.

Doubt, T. J., and Hogan, P. M. (1978). Effects of hydrostatic pressure on conduction and excitability in rabbit atria. *J. Appl. Physiol.*, 45:24–32.

Dwyer, J., Saltzman, H. A., and O'Bryan, R. (1977). Maximal physical work capacity of man at 43.4 ATA. *Undersea Biomed. Res.*, 4:359–372.

Fagraeus, L., Karlsson, J., Linnarsson, D., and Saltin, B. (1973). Oxygen uptake during maximal work at lowered and raised ambient pressure. *Acta Physiol. Scand.*, 87:411–421.

Ferrante, F. L., and Opdyke, D. F. (1969). Mammalian ventricular function during submersion asphyxia. *J. Appl. Physiol.*, 26:561–570.

Ferrigno, M., Grassi, B., Ferretti, G., Costa, M., Marconi, C., Cerretelli, P., and Lundgren, C. (1991). Electrocardiogram during deep breath hold dives by elite divers. *Undersea Biomed. Res.*, 18:81–91.

Flook, V., and Fraser, I. M. (1989). Inspiratory flow limitation in divers. *Undersea Biomed. Res.*, 16:305–311.

Flynn, E. T., Berghage, T. E., and Coil, E. F. (1972). Influence of increased ambient pressure and gas density on cardiac rates in man. *Naval Exp. Diving Unir Rep.*, 4:1–22.

Furset, K., Aanderud, L., Segedal, K., and Tyssebotn, I. (1987). Transcutaneous measurement of P_{CO_2} at high ambient pressure (41 bar). *Undersea Biomed. Res.*, 14:51–62.

Gelfand, R., Lambertsen, C. J., and Peterson, R. E. (1980). Human respiratory control at high ambient pressures and inspired gas densities. *J. Appl. Physiol.*, 48:528–539.

Gelfand, R., Lambertsen, C. J., Strauss, R., Clark, J. M., and Puglia, C. D. (1983). Human respiration at rest in rapid compression and high pressures and gas densities. *J. Appl. Physiol.*, 54:290–303.

Gennser, M., and Ornhagen, H. C. (1989). Effects of hydrostatic pressure, H_2, He and N_2 on beating frequency of rat atria. *Undersea Biomed. Res.*, 16:153–164.

Giry, P. (1990). Les échanges gazeux respiratoires en milieu hyperbare. *Arch. Intern. Physiol. Biochem.*, 98:A357–A360.

Giry, P., Battesti, A., Burnet, H., Jouen, P., Rua, P., and Hyacinthe, R. (1987). Mesures de physiologie respiratoire pratiquées au cours de la plongée Hydra V. In *Hydra V Final Report*. Edited by Comex.

Giry, P., Cosson, P., Bouaicha, A., Marnet, Ph., and Battesti, A. (1988). Respiratory measurements during the Entex XI dive (450 msw). In *Entex XI Final Report*. edited by Ministere de la Defense, DRET 861025.

Grimaud, C., Vanuxem, P., Fondarai, J., and Coutant, P. (1968). Le point de rupture de l'apnée volontaire. *C. R. Soc. Biol.*, 162:1542–1546.

Gross, D., Grassino, A., Ross, W. R. D., and Macklem, P. T. (1979). Electromyogram pattern of diaphragmatic fatigue. *J. Appl. Physiol.*, 46:1–7.

Gross, P. M., Terjung, R. L., and Lohman, T. G. (1976). Left ventricular performance in man during breath-holding and simulated diving. *Undersea Biomed. Res.*, 3:351–360.

Heaton, R. W., Henderson, A. F., Gray, B. J., and Costello, J. F. (1983). The bronchial response to cold air challenge: evidence for different mechanisms in normal and asthmatic subjects. *Thorax*, 38:506–511.

Hill, P. (1973). Hyperventilation, breath-holding and alveolar oxygen tensions at the breaking point. *Respir. Physiol.*, 19:201–209.

Hochachka, P. W. (1989). Molecular mechanisms of defense against oxygen lack. *Undersea Biomed. Res.*, 16:375–380.

Hoke, B., Jackson, D. L., Alexander, J. M., and Flynn, E. T. (1976). Respiratory heat loss and pulmonary function during cold gas breathing at high pressures. In *Underwater Physiology V*. Edited by C. J. Lambertsen. Bethesda, Md., FASEB, pp. 725–740.

Hordness, C., and Tyssebotn, I. (1985). Effect of high ambient pressure and oxygen tension on organ blood flow in conscious trained rats. *Undersea Biomed. Res.*, 12:115–128.

Hui, C. A. (1975). Thoracic collapse as affected by the retia thoratica in the dolphin. *Respir. Physiol.*, 25:63–70.

Imbert, G., Jammes, Y., Naraki, N., Duflot, J. C., and Grimaud, C. (1981). Ventilation, pattern of breathing and activity of respiratory muscles in awake cats during oxygen-helium simulated dives (1000 msw). In *Underwater Physiology VII*. Edited by A. J. Bachrach and M. M. Matzen. Bethesda, Md., Undersea Medical Society, pp. 273–282.

Irving, L. (1963). Bradycardia in human divers. *J. Appl. Physiol.*, 18:489–491.

Isabey, D. (1990). Mélanges de haute densité et mécanique ventilatoire. *Arch. Intern. Physiol. Biochem.*, 98:A361–A364.

Jammes, Y., Barthélemy, P., and Delpierre, S. (1983a). Respiratory effects of cold air breathing in anesthetized cats. *Respir. Physiol.*, 54:41–54.

Jammes, Y., Bye, P. T. P., Pardy, R. L., Katsardis, C., Esau, S., and Roussos, (1983b). Expiratory threshold load under extracorporeal circulation: effects of vagal afferents. *J. Appl. Physiol.*, 55:307–315.

Jammes, Y., Barthélemy, P., Fornaris, M., and Grimaud C. (1986b). Cold-induced bronchospasm in normal and sensitized rabbits. *Respir. Physiol.*, 63:347–360.

Jammes, Y., Nail, B., Mei, N., and Grimaud, C. (1987). Laryngeal afferents activated by phenyldiguanide and their response to cold air or helium-oxygen. *Respir. Physiol.*, 67:379–389.

Jammes, Y., Burnet, H., Cosson, P., and Lucciano, M. (1988). Bronchomotor response to cold air or helium-oxygen at normal and high ambient pressures. *Undersea Biomed. Res.*, 15:179–192.

Jammes, Y., and Balzamo, E. (1992). Changes in afferent and efferent phrenic activities with electrically-induced diaphragmatic fatigue. *J. Appl. Physiol.*, 73:894–902.

Jammes, Y., Broussolle, B., Giry, P., and Hyacinthe, P. (1992). Physiologie respiratoire et plongée. In *Physiologie et Médecine de la Plongée*. Edited by B. Broussolle. Poitiers, Ellipses, pp. 121–154.

Jones, N. L. *Clinical Exercise Testing*. Philadelphia, W. B. Saunders.

Joulia, F., Barthélemy, P., Guerrero, F., and Jammes, Y. (1992). T wave changes in humans and dogs during experimental dives. *J. Appl. Physiol.*, 73:1708–1712.

Kendig, J. J., and Cohen, E. N. (1976). Neuromuscular function at hyperbaric pressures: pressure-anesthetic interactions. *Am. J. Physiol.*, 230:1244–1249.

Kerem, D., and Elsner, R. (1973). Cerebral tolerance to asphyxial hypoxia in the harbor seal. *Respir. Physiol.*, 19:188–200.

Kerem, D., and Salzano, J. (1974). Effect of high ambient pressure on human apneic bradycardia. *J. Appl. Physiol.*, 37:108–111.

Kooyman, G. L., Castellini, M. A., and Davis, R. W. (1981). Physiology of diving in marine animals. *Ann. Rev. Physiol.*, 43:343–356.

L'Air liquide. In *Encyclopédie des Gaz*. Amsterdam, Elsevier.

Lanphier, E. H., and Camporesi, E. (1982). Respiration and exercise. In *The Physiology and Medicine of Diving*. Edited by P. B. Bennett and D. H. Elliott. San Pedro, Cal., Best Publishing Company, pp. 99–156.

Leith, D. E. (1989). Adaptations to deep breath hold diving: respiratory and circulatory mechanisms. *Undersea Biomed. Res.*, 16:345–353.

Lenoir, P., Jammes, Y., Giry, P., Rostain, J. C., Burnet, H., Tomei, C., and Roussos, C. (1990). Electromyographic study of respiratory muscles during human diving at 46 ATA. *Undersea Biomed. Res.*, 17:121–137.

Lindström, L., Magnusson, R., and Petersen, I. (1970). Muscular fatigue and action potential conduction velocity changes studied with frequency analysis of EMG signals. *Electromyography*, 4:341–356.

Linnarson, D., and Hesser, C. M. (1978). Dissociated ventilatory and central respiratory responses to CO_2 at raised N_2 pressure. *J. Appl. Physiol.*, 45:758–761.

Muller, N., Bryan, A. C., and Zamel, N. (1980). Tonic inspiratory muscle activity as a cause of hyperinflation in histamine-induced asthma. *J. Appl. Physiol.*, 49:869–874.

Paganelli, C. V. (1987). Gas-phase diffusion of O_2 in helium and nitrogen under pressure. In *Underwater Physiology IX*. Bethesda, Md., Undersea and Hyperbaric Medical Society, pp. 439–446.

Qvist, J., Hurford, W. E., Park, S., Radermacher, P., Falke, K. J., Ahn, D. W., Guyton, G. P., Stanek, K. S., Hong, S. K., Weber, R. E., and Zapol, W. M. (1993). Arterial blood gas tensions during breath-hold diving in the Korean ama. *J. Appl. Physiol.*, 75:285–293.

Rebuck, A. S., and Slutsky, A. S. (1986). Control of breathing in diseases of the respiratory tract and lungs. In *Handbook of Physiology*, section 3: *The Respiratory System*. Vol. II. Part 2. Edited by A. P. Fishman. Bethesda, American Physiological Society, pp. 771–791.

Rostain, J. C., Lemaire, C., and Naquet, R. (1987). Deep diving: neurological problems. In *Comparative Physiology of Environmental Adaptations*. Vol. 2. Edited by P. Dejours. Basel, Karger, pp. 38–47.

Salzano, J. V., Camporesi, E. M., Stolp, B. W., and Moon, R. E. (1984). Physiological response to exercise at 47 and 66 ATA. *J. Appl. Physiol.*, 57:1055–1068.

Saltzman, H. A., Salzano, J. V., Blenkarn, G. O., and Kylstra, J. A. (1971). Effects of pressure on ventilation and gas exchange in man. *J. Appl. Physiol.*, 30:443–449.

Shida, K. K., and Lin, Y. C. (1981). Contribution of environmental factors in development of hyperbaric bradycardia. *J. Appl. Physiol.*, 50:731–735.

Smith, R. M., and Hong, S. K. (1977). Heart rate response to breath holding at 18.6 ATA. *Respir. Physiol.*, 30:69–79.

Song, S. H., Lee, W. K., Chung, Y. A., and Hong, S. K. (1969). Mechanism of apneic bradycardia in man. *J. Appl. Physiol.*, 27:323–327.

Spaur, W. H., Raymond, L. W., Knott, M. M., Crothers, J. C., Braithwaite, W. R., Thalmann, E. D., and Uddin, D. F. (1977). Dyspnea in divers at 49.5 ATA: mechanical, not chemical in origin. *Undersea Biomed. Res.*, 4:183–198.

Sterba, J. A., and Lundgren, C. E. G. (1988). Breath-hold duration in man and the diving response induced by face immersion. *Undersea Biomed. Res.*, 15:361–375.

Stuhr, L. E. B., Ask, J. A., and Tyssebotn, I. (1990). Cardiovascular changes in anesthetized rats during exposure to 30 bar. *Undersea Biomed. Res.*, 17:383–393.

Suzuki, S., Ikeda, T., and Hashimoto, A. (1991). Decrease in the single-breath diffusing capacity after saturation dives. *Undersea Biomed. Res.*, 18:103–109.

Taylor, N. A. S., and Morrison, J. B. (1990). Effects of breathing-gas pressure on pulmonary function and work capacity during immersion. *Undersea Biomed. Res.*, 17:413–428.

Varène, P., Timbal, J., and Jacquemin, C. (1967). Effect of different ambient pressures on airway resistance. *J. Appl. Physiol.*, 22:699–706.

Vorosmarti, J., Bradley, M. E., and Anthonisen, N. R. (1975). The effects of increased gas density on pulmonary mechanics. *Undersea Biomed. Res.*, 2:1–10.

Webb, P. (1970). Body heat loss in undersea gaseous environments. *Aerosp. Med.*, 41:1282–1288.

Wilson, J. M., Klighfield, P. D., Adams, G. M., Harvey, C., and Schaeffer, K. E. (1977). Human ECG changes during prolonged hyperbaric exposures breathing N_2-O_2 mixtures. *J. Appl. Physiol.*, 42:614–623.

Wood, L. D. H., and Bryan, A. C. (1971). Mechanical limitations of exercise ventilation at increased ambient pressure. In *Underwater Physiology IV*. Edited by C. J. Lambertsen. New York, Academic Press, pp. 307–316.

Wood, L. D. H., Bryan, A. C., Bau, S. K., Weng, T. R., and Levison, H. (1976). Effects of increased gas density on pulmonary gas exchange in man. *J. Appl. Physiol.*, 41:206–210.

Worth, H., Takahashi, H., Willmer, H., and Piiper, J. (1976). Pulmonary gas exchange in dogs ventilated with mixtures of oxygen with various inert gases. *Respir. Physiol.*, 28:1–15.

Zapol, W., Liggins, G. C., Schneider, R. C., Qvist, J., Snider, M. T., Creasy, R. K., and Hochachka, P. W. (1979). Regional blood flow during simulated diving in the conscious Weddell seal. *J. Appl. Physiol.*, 47:968–973.

55

Influence of Anesthesia on the Thorax

DAVID O. WARNER and KAI REHDER

Mayo Clinic
Rochester, Minnesota

I. Introduction

It has long been appreciated that anesthetic drugs alter chest wall function. For example, in 1858 John Snow observed that during chloroform anesthesia breathing was "sometimes performed only by the diaphragm whilst the intercostal muscles are paralyzed." Indeed, observations of the pattern of breathing were employed for many years as a clinically useful guide to the proper administration of anesthesia. More recently, anesthetic effects on chest wall function have attracted attention as a possible explanation for the impairment of pulmonary gas exchange observed during anesthesia. Also, anesthetic-induced changes in respiratory muscle activity may be useful to deduce the function of these muscles.

Before discussing the effects of anesthesia on the thorax, two difficulties must be acknowledged. First, many relevant variables (e.g., the shape and motion of the diaphragm) are difficult to measure, so that even basic descriptive information is often limited. Second, there is no suitable animal model. The chest wall of quadrupeds differs fundamentally from that of humans in both form and function. For example, during quiet breathing in dogs, phasic activity is prominent in muscles with expiratory actions (De Troyer et al., 1989). This activity may be responsible for a significant portion of the tidal volume (Krayer et al., 1988; Warner et al., 1989). In contrast, awake humans in the supine position have little or no active expiratory muscle activity during quiet breathing (Druz and Sharp, 1981; De Troyer et al., 1987). Drug-induced muscle paralysis and mechanical ventilation may increase the functional residual capacity (FRC) in dogs by eliminating active expiration (Hubmayr et al., 1987; Warner et al., 1989), in marked distinction to human subjects, in whom FRC is reduced after anesthesia with pharmacological paralysis (Rehder and Marsh, 1986). Because of these differences between quadrupeds and humans, this chapter will focus on data obtained in human subjects.

This chapter begins by reviewing current concepts of how anesthesia with spontaneous breathing (referred to as "anesthesia") and anesthesia with drug-induced paralysis and mechanical ventilation (referred to as "anesthesia-paralysis") influence chest wall function. The potential impact of these changes on pulmonary mechanics, intrapulmonary inspired gas distribution, and pulmonary gas exchange will then be examined.

II. Anesthesia and Functional Residual Capacity

In the majority of recumbent human subjects, the induction of general anesthesia reduces FRC (Fig. 1) (Rehder and Marsh, 1986). This decrease occurs rapidly after induction (Howell and Peckett, 1957; Bergman, 1982), does not appear to change with time (Don et al., 1972; Westbrook et al., 1973, Hewlett, 1974), and is not

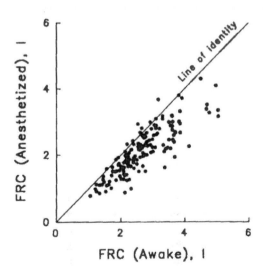

Figure 1 Comparative measurements of FRC ($n = 157$) between awake and anesthetized states for recumbent subjects (Don et al., 1970, 1972; Westbrook et al., 1973; Hewlett et al., 1974; Rehder et al., 1972, 1974, 1977; Juno et al., 1978; Hedenstierna et al., 1981; Bickler et al., 1987; Krayer et al., 1987). Mean FRC awake is 2.69 ± 0.07 (SE) liters whereas mean FRC anesthetized or anesthetized-paralyzed is 2.15 ± 0.06 liters.

affected by inspired oxygen concentration (Don et al., 1970; Hewlett et al., 1974). During barbiturate/narcotic anesthesia, muscular paralysis does not further decrease FRC (Westbrook et al., 1973). FRC does not fall if anesthesia is induced in the sitting position (Rehder et al., 1972). Most anesthetic drugs, including thiopental, methoxyflurane, halothane, and isoflurane, decrease FRC; however, FRC is not affected by ketamine anesthesia (Shulman et al., 1985; Mankikian et al., 1986). The mechanisms causing the decrease in FRC remain unclear. Current hypotheses focus on a loss of tonic activity in chest wall muscles (both rib cage and diaphragm) and changes in the volume of blood in the thoracoabdominal cavity. Increases in lung elastic recoil caused by anesthesia may also contribute to decreased FRC and will be discussed in a following section.

Some studies suggest that both inspiratory rib cage muscles and the diaphragm possess tonic activities that contribute to normal chest wall recoil (Muller et al., 1979; De Troyer et al., 1980; Druz and Sharp, 1981; Drummond, 1987). However, in most studies this tone is minimal in the supine position (Tusiewicz et al., 1977; Druz and Sharp, 1981), and its presence in the diaphragm is controversial (Druz and Sharp, 1981; Krayer et al., 1987). Nevertheless, if such tone existed, it would be abolished by anesthesia and paralysis, altering chest wall shape; some anesthetic drugs may also reduce this tone during spontaneous breathing (Drummond, 1987).

Several studies have documented changes in chest wall shape with induction of anesthesia, but the descriptions differ. Froese and Bryan (1974) examined the diaphragmatic silhouette with fluoroscopy in two subjects and found that induction of anesthesia caused a cephalad shift of the end-expiratory position of the dependent regions of the diaphragm; paralysis did not further change end-expiratory diaphragmatic position (Fig. 2). Shifts in the nondependent regions of the diaphragm were inconsistent in these two subjects. Hedenstierna et al. (1985) deduced a cephalad shift of the diaphragm from CT scans taken before and after induction of anesthesia/paralysis. However, both of these studies were limited by the inability to image the entire diaphragm, forcing the investigators to infer diaphragmatic position from either a silhouette (Froese and Bryan, 1974) or a single CT slice (Hedenstierna et al., 1985). In contrast to these two studies, three studies using high-speed three-dimensional CT scanning to image the entire diaphragm have found no consistent net cephalad shift in end-expiratory diaphragmatic position with induction of anesthesia or anesthesia/paralysis in subjects lying supine (Krayer et al., 1987; Krayer et al., 1989; Warner et al., unpublished observations); similar results have been obtained using ultrasound to image the diaphragm (Drummond et al., 1986). However, all the latter studies did note a consistent change in diaphragmatic shape, as dependent diaphragmatic regions tended to shift cephalad and nondependent regions tended to shift caudad (Fig. 2). We conclude that the contribution of the diaphragm to reductions in FRC caused by anesthesia may be smaller than originally thought.

Phasic electrical expiratory activity develops in abdominal muscles during

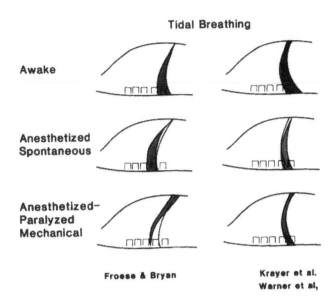

Figure 2 Diagrammatic representation of diaphragm motion in subjects lying supine, measured using fluoroscopy (left panel) (modified from Froese and Bryan, 1974) or three-dimensional CT scans (right panel) (modified from Krayer et al., 1989; Warner et al., unpublished observations) are shown. Solid line in each panel indicates the end-expiratory position in the awake state. Stippled area depicts motion of diaphragm during active inspiration (spontaneous) or passive inflation (paralyzed). (From Froese and Bryan, 1974.)

halothane anesthesia in subjects lying supine (Freund et al., 1964; Kaul et al., 1973). This activity may contribute to the reduction in FRC, but such activity is not necessary for a decreased FRC (Westbrook et al., 1973).

The shape of the rib cage also is changed by anesthesia. Anesthesia-paralysis decreases the external anteroposterior diameter and increases the lateral diameter of the thorax and abdomen (Fig. 3) (Vellody et al., 1978). Although some initial studies suggested otherwise (Jones et al., 1979; Hedenstierna et al., 1981), it is now apparent that the internal rib cage cross-sectional area consistently decreases with the anesthesia-paralysis (Hedenstierna et al., 1985; Krayer et al., 1987), so that the volume bounded by the inner surface of the rib cage above the diaphragm decreases by approximately 0.2 liter. This reduction in overall volume is accomplished by nonuniform changes in internal chest wall dimensions that exhibit considerable intersubject variability (Krayer et al., 1987).

Increases in intrathoracic blood volume can decrease FRC (Kimball et al., 1985). Krayer et al. (1987) estimated intrathoracic tissue volume as the difference between total thoracic volume measured during apnea with a three-dimensional CT scanner and thoracic gas volume measured by N_2 washout immediately following

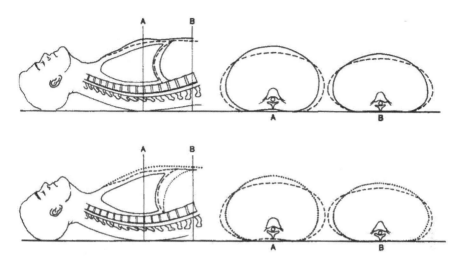

Figure 3 (Upper panel) Diagrammatic representation of chest wall shape during the awake (————) and anesthetized-paralyzed (- - - - -) states in a subject lying supine. Transverse sections of the thorax (A) and abdomen (B) are shown. Anesthesia-paralysis decreases the anteroposterior diameters and increases the lateral diameters. (Lower panel) With anesthesia-paralysis, mechanical inflation of the lung from FRC (- - - - -) to end-inspiration (. . . . .) increases anteroposterior diameters and decreases lateral diameters.

scanning. They assumed that changes in this tissue volume would reflect shifts of blood in or out of the thorax. Anesthesia-paralysis decreased total thoracic volume less than thoracic gas volume, suggesting an increase in intrathoracic tissue volume (mean increase of approximately 0.3 liter), although there was considerable intersubject variability. Similar results were obtained in an early study by Hedenstierna et al. (Hedenstierna et al., 1981), using measurements of external dimensions to estimate total thoracic volume. However, in a later study (Hedenstierna et al., 1985) these investigators measured central blood volume by a thermal-dilution technique and found that anesthesia-paralysis *decreased* this variable by 0.3 liter. In addition to differences in measurement techniques, these later measurements of Hedenstierna et al. were made during intermittent positive pressure ventilation, which may decrease intrathoracic blood volume (Warner et al., 1989). Nevertheless, it is apparent that changes in intrathoracic blood volume caused by anesthesia could be of sufficient magnitude to affect FRC.

   One feature common to all studies of factors affecting FRC during anesthesia is marked intersubject variability. Thus, it is unlikely that any single factor consistently dominates; the magnitude of effect in any patient depends on an interaction of several factors. This variability also may reflect the technical difficulties of measuring such factors as diaphragmatic position and intrathoracic blood volume.

III. Anesthesia and Chest Wall Motion

In addition to effects on the end-expiratory position of the chest wall, as reflected by changes in FRC, anesthesia also has significant effects on the pattern of chest wall motion.

A. Spontaneous Breathing

During spontaneous breathing, chest wall motion is determined by the balance between force applied by the respiratory muscles and the passive impedances of the chest wall structures.

The effects of anesthetics on chest wall motion depend on the anesthetic agent. During quiet breathing in subjects lying supine, the relative contribution of the rib cage to tidal volume as measured by external thoracic dimensions is decreased by halothane anesthesia (Fig. 4) (Tusiewicz et al., 1977; Jones et al., 1979). This attenuation of rib cage motion also affects the chest wall response to CO_2 rebreathing, such that there is little increase in rib cage motion as minute ventilation increases (Tusiewicz et al., 1977). At high minute ventilation, paradoxic motion of the rib cage during early inspiration may occur. These changes in motion are accompanied by a decrease in the normal phasic inspiratory electrical activity of parasternal intercostal muscles (Tusiewicz et al., 1977); this decrease in activity may contribute to decreased rib cage motion. In addition, phasic expiratory activity in the abdominal muscles during halothane anesthesia (Freund et al., 1964; Kaul et al., 1973) may affect chest wall motion. However, because the different abdominal

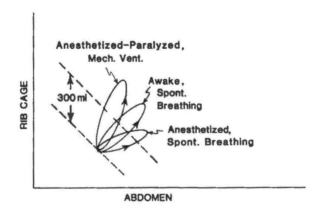

Figure 4 Diagrammatic representation of rib cage and abdomen-diaphragm contributions to tidal volume in three states: awake, anesthetized with spontaneous breathing, and anesthetized-paralyzed. Compared with the awake state, the relative rib cage contribution decreases during anesthesia with spontaneous breathing and increases with anesthesia-paralysis.

muscles have different effects on the rib cage (Mier et al., 1985) and because it is not known which abdominal muscles are recruited during halothane anesthesia, the possible affects of this activity on rib cage motion are uncertain.

In contrast to halothane, intravenous anesthetics either have no effect [methohexital (Bickler et al., 1987)] or actually increase [ketamine (Mankikian et al., 1986)] the rib cage contribution to tidal volume. One may speculate that these agents have less effect on intercostal muscle activity, especially as both these agents have been reported not to affect FRC (Shulman et al., 1985; Mankikian et al., 1986; Bickler et al., 1987).

During eupnea, the pattern of diaphragmatic motion in subjects anesthetized with halothane resembles that observed in awake recumbent subjects, i.e., the relative motion of the dependent regions of the diaphragm is greater than that of the nondependent regions (Fig. 2) (Froese and Bryan, 1974; Warner et al., unpublished observations). This pattern is also present in the lateral decubitus position.

B. Anesthesia-Paralysis and Mechanical Ventilation

During mechanical ventilation, the motion of the chest wall is produced by a relatively uniform increase in alveolar pressure, so that motion is determined by the regional impedances of the relaxed respiratory system.

The relative contribution of the rib cage to tidal volume increases with mechanical ventilation in the supine position (Fig. 4) (Grimby et al., 1975; Vellody et al., 1978). The anteroposterior diameters of both the rib cage and abdomen increase during a tidal breath, while the lateral diameters decrease, in contrast to the more uniform expansion observed during spontaneous breathing (Fig. 3) (Vellody et al., 1978).

The pattern of diaphragmatic motion during mechanical ventilation has been examined in two studies. Froese and Bryan (1974) examined the diaphragmatic silhouette in three supine subjects and found a predominate motion of the nondependent regions of the diaphragm during tidal volumes matched to those present during spontaneous breathing (4.6–6.3 ml/kg) and a more uniform, pistonlike diaphragm motion during larger tidal volumes (14.5–25.9 ml/kg) (Fig. 2). Similar results were obtained in a lateral decubitus position. A uniform motion is expected if the vertical gradients of pleural and abdominal pressures remain constant with lung inflation and the diaphragm behaves as an isotropic membrane with sufficient passive tension to prevent shape distortion. Krayer et al. (1989) also matched tidal volumes during mechanical ventilation to those present during spontaneous breathing (approximately 11.5 ml/kg) and measured diaphragmatic motion using high-speed three-dimensional CT scanning. With subjects in the supine position, the pattern of motion was pistonlike (Fig. 2). In contrast, in prone subjects motion was greatest in nondependent regions. This latter finding is not as expected for a uniform increase in transdiaphragmatic pressure across an isotropic membrane and suggests that the distribution of passive tension in the diaphragm may not be uniform (as expected from its anatomical properties), that motion depends on thoracoabdominal coupling of the diaphragm, that abdominal or pleural pressures are not described by simple linear pressure gradients, or other possibilities.

IV. Anesthesia and Pressure-Volume Relationships

As would be expected from these effects on the chest wall, anesthesia changes the relationships between applied pressures and volumes of the lung and chest wall. In general, the elastic recoil of the total respiratory system increases with induction of anesthesia (Westbrook et al., 1973; Rehder et al., 1974), so that a greater inflation pressure is required to maintain a given lung volume. This increase is not affected by the depth of anesthesia or the addition of paralysis to anesthesia (Rehder et al., 1974), is not progressive with time, and cannot be prevented by repeated inflations of the lungs to high airway pressures (Westbrook et al., 1973).

The static compliance of the respiratory system is also decreased by anesthesia in most studies. The primary source of decreased static compliance appears to be the lung (Westbrook et al., 1973). Static chest wall compliance appears to be little affected over most of the range of lung volumes; at low lung volumes chest wall recoil may be decreased, although it is technically difficult to estimate pleural pressures at low lung volumes in subjects lying supine (Westbrook et al., 1973). The mechanism(s) leading to decreased static lung compliance during anesthesia are unclear. Anesthesia could have a *primary* action on the lung by stimulating smooth muscle or other contractile elements in the airways or lung parenchyma, by causing airway closure or atelectasis, by changing surfactant function, or several other possibilities. However, studies to date do not strongly support any of these mechanisms as a primary cause of decreased static lung compliance. Alterations in static lung compliance could also be *secondary* to changes in chest wall function, especially as lung elastic properties are quite dependent on the conditions of lung ventilation. Conditions where ventilation occurs at low lung volumes, such as produced by external strapping of the chest wall, are associated with a decrease in lung compliance (Scheidt et al., 1981). Changes in surfactant properties have been advanced to explain this decrease (Young et al., 1970). Thus, the primary effect of anesthesia may be to change the shape and motion chest wall, leading to secondary changes in static lung compliance; however, direct effects of anesthesia on the lung are possible.

V. Anesthesia, Ventilation Distribution, and Gas Exchange

The lung must conform in shape to the surrounding chest wall. Thus, nonuniform deformations in chest wall shape, such as those caused by anesthesia, must distort the underlying lung and may therefore affect regional ventilation (Hoppin and Hildebrandt, 1977). Mechanisms such as the slippage of lung lobes, mechanical interdependence of lung parenchyma, and collateral ventilation defend against major perturbations in regional ventilation (Hubmayr et al., 1987), and consequently changes in pulmonary gas exchange. Thus, it is difficult to make simple predictions of changes in inspired pulmonary gas distribution based on observations of chest wall motion, as the following studies demonstrate.

Inspired pulmonary gas distribution is not uniform in awake, spontaneously breathing subjects, with ventilation per unit lung volume greater in dependent lung regions in all body positions (Rehder et al., 1972, 1977, 1978) (Fig. 5). The effect of anesthesia-paralysis on inspired pulmonary gas distribution depends on body position. In subjects in either the supine or lateral decubitus position, ventilation/unit lung volume becomes more uniform, in seated subjects it becomes less uniform, and in prone subjects it is unchanged. These alterations in regional ventilation caused by anesthesia-paralysis can be related to changes in diaphragm motion measured by Krayer et al. (1989) (Fig. 2). In the supine position, changes in the pattern of diaphragmatic motion correspond to alterations in inspired pulmonary gas distribution; both the displacement of the nondependent diaphragm and the ventilation of

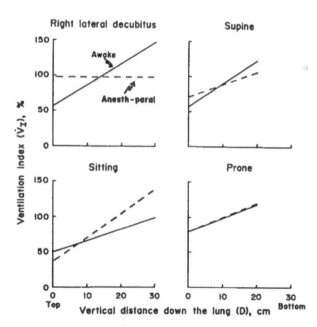

Figure 5 Mean ventilation index ($\dot{V}_I$) as a function of vertical distance down the lung in awake (————) and anesthetized-paralyzed (- - - - -) subjects. Inspiration was initiated from FRC with a tidal volume of 10% of total lung capacity. See text for further explanation. (From Rehder et al., 1978.)

nondependent lung regions increase relative to that of dependent regions. In contrast, in the prone position the ventilation of dependent lung regions is relatively large despite little motion of the dependent diaphragm regions. This finding emphasizes that the distribution of ventilation is determined by a complex interaction of lung and chest wall shapes (Hubmayr et al., 1987).

Another factor affecting intrapulmonary gas distribution and gas exchange during anesthesia has been recently identified that may relate to earlier attempts to attribute impaired intrapulmonary gas exchange during anesthesia to closure of dependent airways caused by a decreased FRC (Juno et al., 1978, Hedenstierna and Santesson, 1979; Dueck et al., 1988). Areas of high density appear in dependent regions of lung computed tomography scans after the induction of anesthesia in patients in the supine and lateral decubitus positions (Damgaard-Pedersen and Qvist, 1980; Brismar et al., 1985; Strandberg et al., 1986; Tokics et al., 1987a) (Fig. 6). These areas form rapidly (within 5 min of anesthetic induction) (Brismar et al.,

Awake

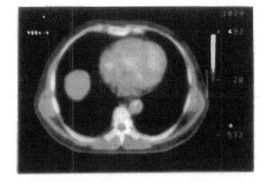

Anesthesia-paralysis

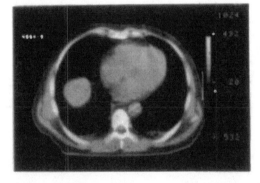

Figure 6 Transverse sections of the thorax in a subject lying supine, both awake (upper) and anesthetized-paralyzed (lower). Note the development of densities in the dependent lung regions during anesthesia-paralysis and the apparently unchanged position of the diaphragm (dense round region in the left hemidiaphragm). (From Brismar et al., 1985.)

1985), decrease in size when positive end-expiratory pressure is applied (Tokics et al., 1987a), are present during both halothane and barbiturate anesthesia (Strandberg et al., 1986), and may increase during paralysis and mechanical ventilation (as compared to spontar.ous breathing) (Tokics et al., 1987a). The area of these densities, expressed as a percentage of the total lung area of a single transverse section of the thorax, significantly correlates with shunt measured with the multiple inert gas technique (Tokics et al., 1987a).

It has been proposed that these densities represent atelectasis caused by compression of lung tissue as dependent diaphragmatic regions shift cephalad with the induction of anesthesia (Brismar et al., 1985). As previously discussed, this shift is controversial, and regional changes in chest wall shape may not translate into changes in lung function in that region. Nevertheless, it is likely that these changes in lung morphometry are caused by alterations in the shape and motion of the chest wall. It is of interest that subjects anesthetized with ketamine, which does not decrease FRC or the rib cage contribution to ventilation (Mankikian et al., 1986), rarely develop dependent lung densities during spontaneous breathing (Tokics et al., 1987b). Also, these densities are not a simple function of decreased lung volumes. Although maximal voluntary exhalation may produce lung atelectasis in normal subjects breathing 100% oxygen (Nunn et al., 1965), densities do not form when the chest of normal subjects is strapped to produce a decrease in FRC similar to that caused by anesthesia-paralysis (Tokics et al., 1988).

VI. Summary and Conclusions

Current evidence supports the following sequence of events as being responsible for impaired pulmonary gas exchange during general anesthesia. Anesthesia changes the shape and pattern of motion of the chest wall, either by changing the amount of tonic and phasic activity of the respiratory muscles (anesthesia with spontaneous breathing) or by eliminating the activity entirely (paralysis with mechanical ventilation). These primary changes in chest wall function lead to secondary changes in lung function, including changes in lung elastic properties, altered inspired pulmonary gas distribution, and dependent lung densities. Depression by anesthetics of normal compensatory mechanisms in the pulmonary vasculature and the airways may further impair pulmonary gas exchange.

References

Bergman, N. A. (1982). Reduction in resting end-expiratory position of the respiratory system with induction of anesthesia and neuromuscular paralysis. *Anesthesiology*, 57:14–17.

Bickler, P. E., Dueck, R., and Prutow, R. J. (1987). Effects of barbiturate anesthesia on functional residual capacity and ribcage/diaphragm contributions to ventilation. *Anesthesiology*, 66:147–152.

Brismar, B., Hedenstierna, G., Lundquist, H., Strandberg, Å., Svensson, L., and Tokics, L.

(1985). Pulmonary densities during anesthesia with muscular relaxation-a proposal of atelectasis. *Anesthesiology*, 62:422–428.

Damgaard-Pedersen, K., and Qvist, T. (1980). Pediatric pulmonary CT-scanning. *Pediatr. Radiol.*, 9:145–148.

De Troyer, A., Bastenier, J., and Delhez, L. (1980). Function of respiratory muscles during partial curarization in humans. *J. Appl. Physiol.*, 49:1049–1056.

De Troyer, A., Ninane, V., Gilmartin, J. J., Lemerre, C., and Estenne, M. (1987). Triangularis sterni muscle use in supine humans. *J. Appl. Physiol.*, 62:919–925.

De Troyer, A., Gilmartin, J. J., and Ninane, V. (1989). Abdominal muscle use during breathing in unanesthetized dogs. *J. Appl. Physiol.*, 66:20–27.

Don, H. F., Wahba, M., Cuadrado, L., ad Kelkar, K. (1970). The effects of anesthesia and 100 per cent oxygen on the functional residual capacity of the lungs. *Anesthesiology*, 32:521–529.

Don, H. F., Wahba, W. M., and Craig, D. B. (1972). Airway closure, gas trapping, and the functional residual capacity during anesthesia. *Anesthesiology*, 36:533–539.

Drummond, G. B., Allan, P. L., and Logan, M. R. (1986). Changes in diaphragmatic position in association with the induction of anaesthesia. *Br. J. Anaesth.*, 58:1246–1251.

Drummond, G. B. (1987). Reduction of tonic ribcage muscle activity by anesthesia with thiopental. *Anesthesiology*, 67:695–700.

Druz, W. S., and Sharp, J. T. (1981). Activity of respiratory muscles in upright and recumbent humans. *J. Appl. Physiol.*, 51:1552–1561.

Dueck, R., Prutow, R. J., Davies, N. J. H., Clausen, J. L., and Davidson, T. M. (1988). The lung volume at which shunting occurs with inhalation anesthesia. *Anesthesiology*, 69:854–861.

Freund, F., Roos, A., and Dodd, R. B. (1964). Expiratory activity of the abdominal muscles in man during general anesthesia. *J. Appl. Physiol.*, 19:693–697.

Froese, A. B., and Bryan, A. C. (1974). Effects of anesthesia and paralysis on diaphragmatic mechanics in man. *Anesthesiology*, 41:242–255.

Grimby, G., Hedenstierna, G., and Löfström, B. (1975). Chest wall mechanics during artificial ventilation. *J. Appl. Physiol.*, 38:576–580.

Hedenstierna, G., and Santesson, J. (1979). Airway closure during anesthesia: a comparison between resident-gas and argon-bolus techniques. *J. Appl. Physiol.*, 47:874–881.

Hedenstierna, G., Löfström, B., and Lundh, R. (1981). Thoracic gas volume and chest-abdomen dimensions during anesthesia and muscle paralysis. *Anesthesiology*, 55:499–506.

Hedenstierna, G., Strandberg, Å., Brismar, B., Lundquist, H., Svensson, L., and Tokics, L. (1985). Functional residual capacity, thoracoabdominal dimensions, and central blood volume during general anesthesia with muscle paralysis and mechanical ventilation. *Anesthesiology*, 62:247–254.

Hewlett, A. M., Hulands, G. H., Nunn, J. F., and Milledge, J. S. (1974). Functional residual capacity during anaesthesia. III: Artificial ventilation. *Br. J. Anaesth.*, 46:495–503.

Hoppin, F. G., Jr., and Hildebrandt, J. (1977). Mechanical properties of the lung. *Lung Biol. Health Dis.*, 3:83–162.

Howell, J. B. L., and Peckett, B. W. (1957). Studies of the elastic properties of the thorax of supine anaesthetized paralysed human subjects. *J. Physiol.* (London), 136:1–19.

Hubmayr, R. D., Rodarte, J. R., Walters, B. J., and Tonelli, F. M. (1987). Regional ventilation during spontaneous breathing and mechanical ventilation in dogs. *J. Appl. Physiol.*, 63:2467–2475.

Jones, J. G., Faithfull, D., Jordan, C., and Minty, B. (1979). Rib cage movement during halothane anaesthesia in man. *Br. J. Anaesth.*, 51:399–406.

Juno, P., Marsh, H. M., Knopp, T. J., and Rehder, K. (1978). Closing capacity in awake and anesthetized-paralyzed man. *J. Appl. Physiol.*, 44:238–244.

Kaul, S. U., Heath, J. R., and Nunn, J. F. (1973). Factors influencing the development of expiratory muscle activity during anaesthesia. *Br. J. Anaesth.*, 45:1013–1018.

Kimball, W. R., Loring, S. H., Basta, S. J., De Troyer, A., and Mead, J. (1985). Effects of paralysis with pancuronium on chest wall statics in awake humans. *J. Appl. Physiol.*, 58:1638–1645.

Krayer, S., Rehder, K., Beck, K. C., Cameron, P. D., Didier, E. P., and Hoffman, E. A. (1987). Quantification of thoracic volumes by three-dimensional imaging. *J. Appl. Physiol.*, 62:591–598.

Krayer, S., Decramer, M., Vettermann, J., Ritman, E. L., and Rehder, K. (1988). Volume quantification of chest wall motion in dogs. *J. Appl. Physiol.*, 65:2213–2220.

Krayer, S., Rehder, K., Vettermann, J., Didier, E. P., and Ritman, E. L. (1989). Position and motion of the human diaphragm during anesthesia-paralysis. *Anesthesiology*, 70:891–898.

Mankikian, B., Cantineau, J. P., Sartene, R., Clergue, F., and Viars, P. (1986). Ventilatory pattern and chest wall mechanics during ketamine anesthesia in humans. *Anesthesiology*, 65:492–499.

Mier, A., Brophy, C., Estenne, M., Moxham, J., Green, M., and De Troyer, A. (1985). Action of abdominal muscles on rib cage in humans. *J. Appl. Physiol.*, 58:1438–1443.

Muller, N., Volgyesi, G., Becker, L., Bryan, M. H., and Bryan, A. C. (1979). Diaphragmatic muscle tone. *J. Appl. Physiol.*, 47:279–284.

Nunn, J. F., Coleman, A. J., Sachithanandan, T., Bergman, N. A., and Laws, J. W. (1965). Hypoxaemia and atelectasis produced by forced expiration. *Br. J. Anaesth.*, 37:3–11.

Rehder, K., Hatch, D. J., Sessler, A. D., and Fowler, W. S. (1972a). The function of each lung of anesthetized and paralyzed man during mechanical ventilation. *Anesthesiology*, 37:16–26.

Rehder, K., Sittipong, R., and Sessler, A. D. (1972b). The effects of thiopental-meperidine anesthesia with succinylcholine paralysis of functional residual capacity and dynamic lung compliance in normal sitting man. *Anesthesiology*, 37:395–398.

Rehder, K., Mallow, J. E., Fibuch, E. E., Krabill, D. R., and Sessler, A. D. (1974). Effects of isoflurane anesthesia and muscle paralysis on respiratory mechanics in normal man. *Anesthesiology*, 41:477–485.

Rehder, K., Sessler, A. D., and Rodarte, J. R. (1977). Regional intrapulmonary gas distribution in awake and anesthetized-paralyzed man. *J. Appl. Physiol.*, 42:391–402.

Rehder, K., Knopp, T. J., and Sessler, A. D. (1978). Regional intrapulmonary gas distribution in awake and anesthetized-paralyzed prone man. *J. Appl. Physiol.*, 45:528–535.

Rehder, K., and Marsh, M. (1986). Respiratory mechanics during anesthesia and mechanical ventilation. In *Handbook of Physiology*, Sect. 3. *The Respiratory System. Vol. III: Mechanics of Breathing*. Part 2. Edited by P. T. Macklem and J. Mead. Bethesda, Md., American Physiological Society, pp. 737–752.

Scheidt, M., Hyatt, R. E., and Rehder, K. (1981). Effects of rib cage or abdominal restriction on lung mechanics. *J. Appl. Physiol.*, 51:1115–1121.

Shulman, D., Beardsmore, C. S., Aronson, H. B., and Godfrey, S. (1985). The effect of ketamine on the functional residual capacity in young children. *Anesthesiology*, 62:551–556.

Snow, J. (1858). *On Chloroform and Other Anaesthetics: Their Action and Administration*. London, Churchill.

Strandberg, Å., Tokics, L., Brismar, B., Lundquist, H., and Hedenstierna, G. (1986). Atelectasis during anaesthesia and in the postoperative period. *Acta Anaesthesiol. Scand.*, 30:154–158.

Tokics, L., Hedenstierna, G., Strandberg, Å., Brismar, B., and Lundquist, H. (1987a). Lung collapse and gas exchange during general anesthesia: effects of spontaneous breathing, muscle paralysis, and positive end-expiratory pressure. *Anesthesiology*, 66:157–167.

Tokics, L., Strandberg, Å., Brismar, B., Lundquist, H., and Hedenstierna, G. (1987b). Computerized tomography of the chest and gas exchange measurements during ketamine anaesthesia. *Acta Anaesthesiol. Scand.*, 31:684–692.

Tokics, L., Hedenstierna, G., Brismar, B., Strandberg, Å., and Lundquist, H. (1988). Thoracoabdominal restriction in supine men: CT and lung function measurements. *J. Appl. Physiol.*, 64:599–604.

Tusiewicz, K., Bryan, A. C., and Froese, A. B. (1977). Contributions of changing rib cage-diaphragm interactions to the ventilatory depression of halothane anesthesia. *Anesthesiology*, 47:327–337.

Vellody, V. P., Nassery, M., Druz, W. S., and Sharp, J. T. (1978). Effects of body position change on thoracoabdominal motion. *J. Appl. Physiol.*, 45:581–589.

Warner, D. O., Krayer, S., Rehder, K., and Ritman, E. L. (1989). Chest wall motion during spontaneous breathing and mechanical ventilation in dogs. *J. Appl. Physiol.*, 66:1179–1189.

Westbrook, P. R., Stubbs, S. E., Sessler, A. D., Rehder, K., and Hyatt, R. E. (1973). Effects of anesthesia and muscle paralysis on respiratory mechanics in normal man. *J. Appl. Physiol.*, 34:81–86.

Young, S. L., Tierney, D. F., and Clements, J. A. (1970). Mechanism of compliance change in excised rat lungs at low transpulmonary pressure. *J. Appl. Physiol.*, 29:780–785.

56

Thorax-Lung Interaction

CHARIS ROUSSOS

National and Kapodistrian University
  of Athens Medical School
Athens, Greece
McGill University
Montreal, Quebec, Canada

I. Introduction

The pleural space is a virtual space between the lung and chest wall. One may therefore intuitively predict that the characteristics of these two structures will also affect the characteristics of the pleural space. Thus the factors holding the lung against the chest wall will be described briefly, followed by a discussion of the effects of respiratory muscle contraction and thoracic shape on pleural pressure. In this section we shall refer mainly to animal experiments, from which most of the direct evidence is derived. Subsequently, we shall examine the static, quasistatic, and dynamic distribution of gas in the lung and how this distribution is affected by the thorax. There we will refer mainly to human experiments since most of the studies could be performed in humans and because of substantial interspecies differences. Because we believe that in the upright and horizontal posture, the basis for the gradient in alveolar expansion and gas distribution differs, we shall use this division in describing and interpreting the results from the literature. Finally, the effects of the lung on the chest wall will be discussed, and practical questions for further research will be briefly outlined.

II. Pleural Space; Pleural Pressure

Under physiological conditions, the space between the parietal and visceral pleura is gas free and nearly liquid free. As a result, the lung can be held against the chest wall. The outward force exerted by the chest wall, either passively or due to the inspiratory muscle activity, and the inward recoil of the lung tend to separate the pleural membranes. However, this is counterbalanced by mechanisms that prevent gas and liquid accumulation in the pleural space. The latter remains gas free due to the diffusion of gas from the pleural space to the venous blood, caused by the partial pressure difference. Because of the shape of the blood O_2 and CO_2 dissociation curves, the total gas pressure in the venous blood is about 60 cm H_2O less than that in the arterial blood. The latter is also 10 cm H_2O less than atmospheric due to the alveolar-arterial O_2 gradient. Thus the total gas venous pressure is about 70 cm H_2O below atmospheric, and any gas collection in the pleural space with pressure close to atmospheric (i.e., pneumothorax) will tend to be absorbed into the blood (Rist and Strohl, 1920, 1922). Similarly, the absorption of liquid from the pleural cavity is due to differences between the higher plasma colloid osmotic pressure and the lower hydrostatic pressures in the pulmonary capillary relative to that in the pleural liquid. Thus the net absorbing pressure is greater than the pressure due to the opposing recoil of the lung and chest wall (Agostoni et al., 1957; Setnikar and Agostoni, 1962; Agostoni, 1972). Complete removal of liquid does not occur, however. With the continuous absorption of the liquid, the lung and the chest wall are pulled together, resulting in multiple points of contact. A further removal of the liquid enhances the apposition of the lung to the chest wall, resulting in deformation of the parietal and visceral pleura. Thus as the volume of the pleural liquid is reduced, its pressure decreases and reaches an equilibrium with the absorption pressure. The residual pleural liquid serves a useful function as a lubricant.

It is apparent from the above analysis that the pressure of the pleural liquid is lower (more subatmospheric) than the pressure due to the opposing recoil of the lung and the chest wall (Setnikar et al., 1957; Setnikar and Agostoni, 1962). The latter is referred to as pleural surface pressure (P_{pl}) (Agostoni and Mead, 1964) and is the force per unit area of pleural surface. It is this pleural surface pressure which reflects the transmission of mechanical forces between the chest wall and the lung and is equivalent to alveolar pressure (P_A) minus static transpulmonary pressure (P_L). The term pleural pressure will refer in this chapter, as well as in the rest of this book, to the pleural surface pressure.

III.   Effects of Thorax and Lung on Pleural Pressure

By producing small pneumothoraces, Parodi (1933) and later others (Prinzmetal and Kountz, 1935; Daly and Bondurant, 1963) found that the nondependent lung regions were surrounded by more negative P_{pl} than the dependent ones. Similar conclusions were drawn by numerous investigators using different techniques from studies both in animals and humans (Krueger et al., 1961; McMahon et al., 1969; Agostoni and D'Angelo, 1970, 1971; Agostoni and Miserocchi, 1970; Agostoni et al., 1970a,b; Hoppin et al., 1970). The most systematic exploration of the topography of the pleural pressure in animals was undertaken by Agostoni, D'Angelo, Miserocchi, and coworkers using a counterpressure technique that they developed. The existence of the pleural pressure gradient was repeatedly confirmed in their work using dogs, rabbits, rats, and rams as experimental animals. Important conclusions that may be drawn from their work are:

1. The vertical pleural pressure gradient (dP_{pl}/dD) decreases as the size of the animal increases (Agostoni and D'Angelo, 1970).
2. The dP_{pl}/dD in the lateral posture is greater than in other postures (Agostoni and D'Angelo, 1970; D'Angelo et al., 1970); for example, in small dogs it is 0.82 cm H_2O/cm in the lateral compared to 0.45 cm H_2O/cm in the head-up position.
3. Expansion of the respiratory system, by the action of its muscles up to a transpulmonary pressure of 10–12 cm H_2O, does not change dP_{pl}/dD at the end of inspiration, whereas passive expansion of the relaxed respiratory system results in a progressive decrease in dP_{pl}/dD, which eventually becomes nil both in supine and head-up postures (Agostoni and Miserocchi, 1970; Agostoni et al., 1970b).
4. At a given height, there is no systematic difference in pleural surface pressure in the craniocaudal direction in the supine posture (Agostoni and Miserocchi, 1970).
5. Gravity affects the topography of pleural pressure mainly by changes in the shape of the chest wall (Agostoni et al., 1970a; Agostoni and D'Angelo, 1971).
6. Selective contraction of the diaphragm affects the pleural pressure distribution (D'Angelo et al., 1974).

Contraction of the respiratory muscles may alter both the dimension and the shape of the chest wall. If the thorax was filled with liquid, the dP_{pl}/dD would remain constant and the pressure swings would be equal everywhere, regardless of the shape of the chest wall. However, a material resistant to deformation may affect the gradient, the pressure swings, and, therefore, regional alveolar size and ventilation. The real situation is complex, and great controversy exists in the literature regarding the nature of the pleural pressure gradient (Wirz, 1923; Rohrer, 1925; Parodi, 1933; Duomarco et al., 1954; Krueger et al., 1961; Mead, 1961; Turner, 1962; Milic-Emili et al., 1966; Glaister, 1967a,b; Proctor et al., 1968; Agostoni and D'Angelo, 1970; Hoppin et al., 1970; Katsura et al., 1970; Vawter et al., 1975; Michels and West, 1978). Agostoni, D'Angelo, and co-workers have provided impressive evidence that mismatching of the shape of the lung and chest wall is the most important cause of the topography of the pleural pressure in animals. Furthermore, they claim that although gravity affects dP_{pl}/dD, this occurs via the change of the chest wall shape. Agostoni et al. (1970b) determined the topography of pleural surface pressure after evisceration and compared their results with those obtained under normal conditions. They observed that evisceration decreased the gradient particularly in the horizontal posture and suggested that this phenomenon was due to the vertical gradient of abdominal pressure. D'Angelo et al. (1971) measured the pleural surface pressure at various heights in the chest of rabbits after changing the lung weight, eviscerating the animals, and removing the diaphragm. Exsanguination produced a decrease in lung weight, but the dP_{pl}/dD remained unchanged, whereas evisceration and removal of the diaphragm decreased the dP_{pl}/dD. The authors argued that removal of the diaphragm abolished the interaction between diaphragm and rib cage, which consequently produced changes in chest wall shape. However, even after removal of the diaphragm, a dP_{pl}/dD still persisted. To evaluate the degree to which lung weight contributes to this gradient, D'Angelo et al. (1971) performed the same experiments in the prone, suspended posture. The rationale of this experiment was that if the gradient of pleural pressure, which remained after the removal of the diaphragm, was due to the shape in the supine posture, then in the prone, suspended position, this residual gradient should be the reverse of that observed in the supine. In fact, it was the same. They concluded that this residual pleural pressure gradient was due to the lung weight and accounted for 20–25% of the total gradient. In their work, they postulated that the effect of gravity on the chest wall remained essentially the same in the supine and the prone postures. However, such an assumption may not be correct in small animals with very distortable rib cages. If this was the case, the proportion attributable to the lung weight might be even less.

Predictably, altering the shape of the chest wall or modifying the effect of gravity on the chest wall also changes the topography of the pleural pressure. Agostoni and coworkers undertook convincing experimental work in animals along these lines (Agostoni and D'Angelo, 1971; D'Angelo and Agostoni, 1973, 1974b). An important finding was that by altering the effect of gravity on the chest wall shape, the pleural surface pressure in the costal region may be markedly different at a given height and in a given posture. Agostoni and D'Angelo (1971) decreased the pressure over the caudal part of the abdomen of supine rabbits and dogs at functional residual capacity (FRC) and found that the pleural surface pressure in the cranial region decreased more than in the caudal at the same horizontal plane. Thus, a craniocaudal gradient was produced similar to the one in the head-up position. In the same experiments, in the head-down posture, when abdominal pressure was decreased to such an extent that lung volume matched that in the head-up posture at FRC, the vertical gradient was reversed, and it became almost equal to that in the head-up posture at FRC.

The effect of lung stiffness on the pleural pressure distribution was also examined by the same workers (D'Angelo and Agostoni, 1974a), the notion being that the stiffer the lung, the greater its resistance to distortion and, consequently, that the matching of lung and chest wall shape will require greater pressures. The experiment confirmed this prediction. They found an increased gradient both in the upright and the supine postures after histamine inhalation, thus contradicting the prediction of West and Matthews (1972) based on analysis of a finite-element model.

Working on the assumption that the gradient is due to the weight of the lung, these authors believed the gradient would become smaller with increased lung stiffness.

An important question that remains to be answered is whether the respiratory muscles can significantly alter the shape of the chest wall, and consequently the regional lung volumes, pleural pressures, and the distribution of inspired gas. D'Angelo et al. (1970) showed that phrenic nerve stimulation in dogs caused a greater change in the P_{pl} in the lower intercostal spaces than in the upper intercostal spaces. In fact, the greatest change was recorded over the diaphragmatic surface. In contrast, after phrenicotomy, the swings in pleural pressure were greater in the upper than in the lower interspaces, which were in turn greater than those measured over the diaphragmatic area. They concluded that "the greater changes in pressure are localized where the respiratory muscles act." Minh et al. (1974) independently measured the changes in dP_{pl}/dD in head-up dogs during bilateral phrenic stimulation and found that dP_{pl}/dD became reversed. Furthermore, they observed that the apicobasal lung dimension increased, whereas the lateral dimensions decreased. Similarly, in dogs in the supine posture, they found that ipsilateral phrenic nerve stimulation produced greater changes in P_{pl} over the basal than over the apical zones.

In conclusion, in spite of the still existing controversy on the subject, the distribution of pleural pressure in animals appears to be greatly affected by the shape of the chest wall and contraction of the respiratory muscles.

IV. Alveolar Expansion, Pleural Pressure, and Thoracic Shape

Only in 1966 did clear evidence appear of a vertical gradient in alveolar size similar to the pleural pressure gradient mentioned above. Milic-Emili et al. (1966), Kaneko et al. (1966), and Sutherland et al. (1968), using radioactive ^{133}Xe, demonstrated that at all lung volumes [except total lung capacity (TLC), where the alveolar size was assumed to be equal], the nondependent lung regions are more expanded than the dependent ones. On the contrary, no significant differences were found among lung regions in the same horizontal plane both in the upright and in the horizontal postures (Bryan et al., 1964; Kaneko et al., 1966; Milic-Emili et al., 1966; Bake et al., 1967). The magnitude of the vertical lung volume gradient bears some relation to body posture. Milic-Emili (1974) reported more uniform vertical lung expansion in the head-down position than in the upright position. Furthermore, Kaneko et al. (1966) showed a slightly greater inequality in vertical lung expansion in the lateral posture compared to prone or supine postures.

Confirmation of the existence of the vertical gradient of lung expansion was obtained later by freezing whole dogs. Glazier et al. (1967), using morphometric techniques, found a significant alveolar size gradient at FRC in head-up frozen dogs. Measuring the lung density, Hogg and Nepszy (1969) also confirmed the vertical gradient of lung expansion. The only contradictory finding is cited in the study by

Glazier et al. (1967), where it was found that the alveoli of the lung apices in head-up dogs were small at an inflating pressure of 30 cm H_2O, compared to their size at functional residual capacity. However, these findings were confirmed neither by Hogg and Nepszy (1969) nor by D'Angelo (1972). Small pneumothoraces at the apices due to the inflating pressure of 30 cm H_2O that Glazier et al. (1967) applied may account for this paradox. The morphometric studies of Glazier et al. at high inflating pressure (30 cm H_2O) confirmed another prediction of Milic-Emili et al. (1966) regarding the alveolar size at TLC. With the exception of the apical alveoli, the rest of the lung was uniformly expanded.

The vertical gradient of alveolar expansion seems to be unaffected by the previous volume history (Sutherland et al., 1968) and is practically linear for lung volumes above 46% TLC (Kaneko et al., 1966; Milic-Emili et al., 1966). At lower lung volumes the gradient is alinear, this alinearity being attributed to airway closure of the dependent lung regions. Burger and Macklem (1968) and Engel et al. (1975) have produced strong evidence in favor of such airway closure.

In 1972, D'Angelo measured local alveolar size and transpulmonary pressure in intact rabbits and in isolated rabbit lungs. In his elegant work, D'Angelo demonstrated that in a variety of conditions all the measurements in situ fit the pressure-volume (P-V) relationship of the isolated lung. He also demonstrated that the geometry of alveoli in situ is very similar to that observed in the isolated lung. Thus, the work of D'Angelo demonstrated that the relationship between alveolar size or geometry and transpulmonary pressure (P_L) is unique for each lung lobe tested both in isolated and in situ lung preparation.

Predictably, substantial changes in chest wall shape will affect the pleural pressure distribution and, therefore, the gradient of alveolar expansion. Figure 1 is a diagrammatic representation of two radiographs taken at the same lung volume of a subject in the lateral position with the diaphragm relaxed and with it contracted during an expulsive maneuver. When the subject relaxed, the dependent hemidiaphragm was more cephalad, and the mediastinum encroached more upon the dependent lung than was the case when he contracted the diaphragm. With diaphragmatic contraction, the lower lung inflated and the upper lung deflated. It follows that the contraction increased the mean transpulmonary pressure across the dependent lung and decreased it over the upper lung. Consequently, the vertical difference in alveolar size and pleural pressure must have decreased. The change in the vertical gradient in alveolar size was shown in similar experiments using the ^{133}Xe technique. Figure 2 shows the effect on vertical alveolar expansion of altering the shape of the chest wall—by tensing the diaphragm—as in Figure 1. Vertical gradient of alveolar expansion was made to virtually disappear by tensing the diaphragm. The pleural pressure was not measured in these experiments. However, to the degree that during such a maneuver the pressure-volume characteristics of the lung did not alter significantly, the reduction of the vertical gradient of alveolar expansion implicitly assumes a decrease in dP_{pl}/dD, as is shown diagrammatically in Figure 3. A and B represent alveolar size of nondependent and dependent lung

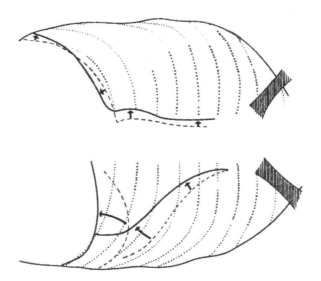

Figure 1 Diagrammatic respresentation of two chest radiographs at the same lung volume (functional residual capacity, FRC) of a subject in the lateral decubitus position. (Broken line) Position of the diaphragm and mediastinum with diaphragm relaxed (low trans-diaphragmatic pressure, P_{di}). (Solid line) Position of the diaphragm and mediastinum with contracted diaphragm (high P_{di}). Arrows show the motion of the diaphragm and mediastinum when the diaphragm is contracted. (From Roussos et al., 1976a.)

regions, respectively, while A' and B' represent the corresponding pleural pressure. The arrows show the changes in volume and pleural pressure in the manner observed in Figures 1 and 2. Similar results were also found in the upright posture in humans, when extreme deformations of the chest wall were produced by an externally applied force (Grassino and Anthonisen, 1975).

    To summarize, these studies show that changes in chest wall shape achieved by selectively contracting different respiratory muscles, or by external forces, alter the vertical gradient of alveolar expansion and, by inference, the dP_{pl}/dD.

V. Effects of Thorax on Ventilation Distribution

A. Quiet Breathing

Upright Posture

During quiet breathing in the seated position, there is a vertical gradient in ventilation, the dependent region having approximately twice the ventilation of the apical lung region (Bryan et al., 1964; Rosenzweig et al., 1969; Jones et al., 1977; Ewan et al., 1978; Forkert et al., 1978). In contrast, there is no horizontal gradient of ventilation in the upright posture. These findings are consistent with the model

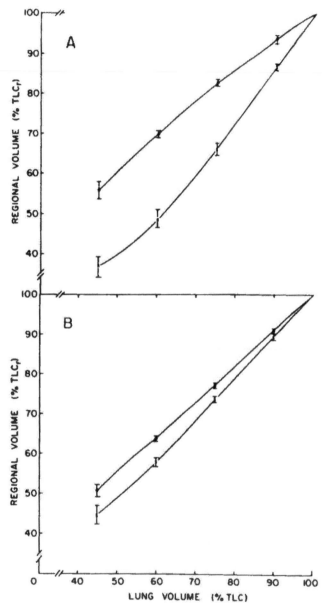

Figure 2   Regional lung volume (TLC$_l$) plotted against overall lung volume. (A) Low P_{di};
(B) high P_{di}. Bars indicate 1 SE on either side of mean. Mean values of upper two pairs of
counters (●); mean values of lower two pairs of counters (x). At all lung volumes, vertical
gradient of alveolar expansion was greater when P_{di} was low than when P_{di} was high. (From
Roussos et al., 1977b.)

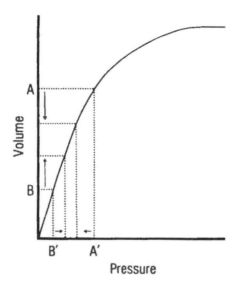

Figure 3 Diagrammatic representation of changes in the alveolar size of dependent (B) and nondependent (A) lung regions, as well as the corresponding changes in pleural pressure (A' and B') after altering the shape of the chest wall, similar to that shown in Figure 1. Arrows indicate the direction of change predicted by the P-V curve.

of Milic-Emili (1974), in which the lung in situ is viewed as being exposed to the gravity-dependent vertical gradient in pleural pressure, which is essentially the same at different lung volumes. In this model, the stress-strain relationship of the lung is assumed to be uniformly distributed. Thus in a horizontal plane all regions are expanded equally, whereas in the vertical plane there is a gradient of expansion corresponding to the vertical range of transpulmonary pressure (see above). Due to the curvilinear pressure-volume relationship of the lung, the dependent, less expanded regions have a higher compliance than the nondependent, more expanded ones. During slow changes in lung volume, the distribution of gas above "closing volume" may be accounted for by the distribution of regional pulmonary compliance, although Anthonisen et al. (1970) have shown that there is a small deviation from the model. Actually, the dependent regions empty preferentially at high lung volume; the mechanisms for this could be (1) a difference in the lobar pressure-volume curve, (2) the nonmonoexponential P-V curve of the lung, and (3) different changes in applied pleural pressure. This latter factor, since it may be affected by the action of respiratory muscles, will be critically examined in the following section.

In humans, during inspiration or expiration, voluntary selective contraction of either inspiratory intercostal and accessory muscles or the diaphragm substantially affects the rib cage and abdominal displacement, respectively, as shown in Figure 4. It has also been shown that each type of breathing maneuver measurably changes

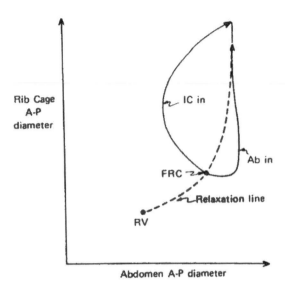

Figure 4 Diagrammatic representation of thoracoabdominal shape (Konno and Mead, 1967) during relaxation against obstructed airway (dashed line), during inspiration initiated mainly with intercostal and accessory muscles (IC in), and during inspiration initiated with enhanced abdominal motion (Ab in). A-P = anteroposterior; FRC = functional residual capacity; RV = residual volume. Similarly, an expiration from total lung capacity can follow any of these pathways. (From Roussos et al., 1977a.)

the pattern of filling and emptying of the lung (Roussos et al., 1976, 1977a). A bolus inspired at FRC in upright subjects is more evenly distributed when the rib cage muscles are used selectively than during inspiration achieved by contraction of the diaphragm (Roussos et al., 1977a) (Fig. 5). In contrast, inspirations during which diaphragmatic contraction and abdominal displacement are voluntarily enhanced result in preferential gas distribution to lung bases. The difference in gas distribution between the two types of maneuvers is greater for boluses than for tidal volumes of 500–600 ml (Roussos et al., 1977a). Although pleural pressures were not measured in these studies, the findings at low flow rates are consistent with the notion that the changes in the ventilation distribution were due to nonuniform pleural pressure changes caused by the chest wall deformation.

Horizontal Posture

The effect of changes in chest wall shape on ventilation distribution is more striking in the horizontal posture than in the upright posture. In horizonal posture, the rib cage does not constitute the lateral boundaries of the lung. Instead, the diaphragm is in close proximity to a large area of the lung. Depending on its tension, this muscle can vary from a flaccid membrane to a rigid wall. Thus, in the first case

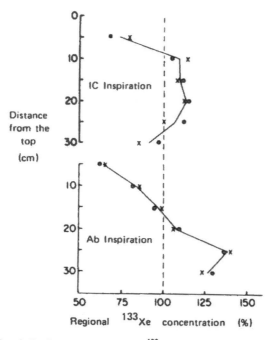

Figure 5   Regional distribution of a bolus of ^{133}Xe inhaled at 0.4 liters/s from functional residual capacity in one seated subject. (Upper panel) Inspiration using predominantly intercostal and accessory muscles (IC). (Lower panel) Inspiration with enhanced abdominal motion (Ab). Different symbols indicate duplicate measurements. Abscissa is normalized alveolar ^{133}Xe concentration. Note preferential distribution of ^{133}Xe to basal regions after abdominal inspiration and to upper midzones after intercostal inspiration. (From Roussos et al., 1977a.)

the vertical hydrostatic pressure gradient of the abdominal contents is transmitted into the thoracic cavity, whereas in the second case the thoracic cavity is effectively protected from the abdominal pressure gradient. The implication of this behavior of the diaphragm is that the effect of the chest wall on the regional distribution of inspired gas and ventilation should be more apparent in horizontal than upright postures, particularly in the lateral position. In the left and right lateral decubitus posture, labeled gas is preferentially distributed to the dependent lung (Kaneko et al., 1966; Rehder et al., 1977), and the upper lung has only about half the ventilation per unit volume of the lower lung (Chevrolet et al., 1978, 1979; Amis, 1979). In this posture, both the abdominal weight and the weight of the mediastinum contribute to the vertical gradient of regional expansion and ventilation distribution. During tidal breathing, the alternating contraction and relaxation of the diaphragm results in a cyclic displacement of the dependent hemidiaphragm (Froese and Bryan, 1974), in a lifting of the mediastinum (Svanberg, 1957), and, therefore, in a greater ventilation of the dependent lung (Chevrolet et al., 1978, 1979). Similar results have been found qualitatively in infants and children (Larsson et al., 1989).

What is the evidence, however, that diaphragmatic contraction and the consequent shape changes of the chest wall (Froese and Bryan, 1974) (and not just differences in regional pulmonary compliance) are responsible for the preferential distribution of ventilation to the dependent lung regions? Studies have shown that with a nontensed diaphragm the ventilation distribution is greater to the nondependent lung. In normal trained subjects breathing with relaxed diaphragms (Chevrolet et al., 1979) or ventilated with intermittent positive pressure (Chevrolet et al., 1978) or in anaesthetized, paralyzed, mechanically ventilated subjects, the inspired gas is preferentially distributed to the more expanded nondependent lung, resulting in a vertically uniform ventilation per unit volume. Thus, although the regional lung compliance may play some role, it seems that in this posture regional ventilation distribution is determined predominantly by the effects of the shape changes of the chest wall. Consistent with these notions are the more recent results of Tomioka et al. (1988) using Ar-bolus and N_2 single-breath washout tests. The authors concluded that the regional distribution of ventilation is not primarily determined by the pull of gravity but by lung, thorax, and mediastinum interactions. Hubmayr et al. (1987), using the parenchymal marker technique, determined the regional lung behavior from x-ray projection images obtained at FRC and end-inspiration. They also concluded that the distribution of ventilation is determined by a complex interaction of lung and chest wall shapes and by the motion of the lobes relative to each other. Tokics et al. (1987), using computerized tomography, extended these notions and hypothesized that the observed atelectasis in dependent lung regions during anesthesia are consistent with changes in chest wall mechanics (Fig. 1).

In the supine and prone positions, the weight of the mediastinum is probably borne largely by the spine or sternum, respectively. Furthermore, the vertical distance of the abdominal cavity is less than in the lateral position. Thus the effect of gravity on the diaphragm could be expected to be smaller. Both factors predictably will minimize the role that gravity has in chest wall shape and consequently in ventilation distribution. In the supine position, the vertical distribution of ventilation per unit volume favors the dependent zone (Amis, 1979), which is enhanced by breathing with the diaphragm-abdomen (Fig. 6), whereas when breathing is done with intercostal and accessory muscles, ventilation is preferential to the nondependent regions (Roussos et al., 1977a). In the prone position, neither the distribution of ventilation, nor the effect of chest wall distortion, nor the effects of selective use of respiratory muscle on the distribution of ventilation has been adequately studied. However, Rehder et al. (1978) showed that in the prone suspended posture, where the abdominal wall can protrude vertically, mechanical ventilation of paralyzed subjects does not alter the vertical gradient of distribution of a tidal volume of labeled gas. This clearly indicates that the pressure gradient in the abdomen does not determine regional ventilation distribution in this posture. It would have been

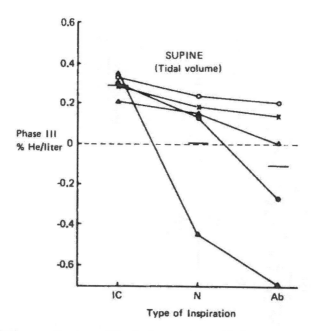

Figure 6 Influence of pattern of inspiration on slope of helium (He) plateau in supine subjects: 600 ml of He were inhaled at 0.5 liters/s from functional residual capacity. Different symbols represent different subjects. Slopes are most positive after intercostal (IC) inspiration, most negative after abdominal (Ab) inspiration, and intermediate after normal (N) inspiration. (From Roussos et al., 1977a.)

interesting if similar studies were done while the abdomen was supported, thus altering the chest wall shape.

Observations in spontaneously breathing supine and prone subjects (supported or unsupported) show that the craniocaudal displacements of the dorsal part of the diaphragm are substantially greater than those of the ventral part (Froese and Bryan, 1974; Amis, 1979) despite the reversal in abdominal gradient. The question that then arises is whether anatomical factors such as the number of muscle fibers (Gray, 1973) limit the part of the diaphragm adjacent to the sternum or whether the costal and crural parts of the diaphragm are exposed to different central drives, independent of their topographical position.

B. High Flow Rates

At high inspiratory flow rates (2.4–5.6 liters/s) the distribution of a bolus of tracer gas inhaled at FRC differs from the quasistatic distribution, with an increase in the apical and a decrease in basal concentrations (Robertson et al., 1969; Bake et al., 1974; Sybrecht et al., 1976). The regional distribution of tidal volumes of air inspired from FRC is similar to the bolus distribution. However, it is less flow dependent than that of boli inhaled at the onset of the breath (Connolly et al., 1975). The flow dependence of regional gas distribution was predicted by a model based on differences in mechanical time constants (resistance times a compliance, RC) between pulmonary units (Otis et al., 1956; Pedley et al., 1972). At high flow rates, the nondependent regions are favored because resistance varies inversely with lung volume (Blide et al., 1964; Vincent et al., 1970), and compliance is lower because the more expanded upper regions also have a lower compliance. An implicit assumption in the above analysis was that the swings in pleural pressure were the same. However, this assumption is not consistent with all experimental findings (Pedley et al., 1972; Bake et al., 1974; Connolly et al., 1975; Sybrecht et al., 1976). The observations may be explained by the alternative hypothesis that swings in pleural surface pressure may differ in different parts of the chest.

Two distinct mechanisms may be responsible for changes in dP_{pl}/dD: (1) When different lung zones fill asynchronously due to differences in time constants, the pleural pressure over the lagging lung regions may become more negative than that over regions that are leading. This change in dP_{pl}/dD reflects the resistance of the chest wall to deformation and acts so as to minimize the difference between dynamic and quasistatic gas distributions. This mechanical interdependence between a lung region and the overlying chest wall was proposed by Bake et al. (1974) to explain why boli inhaled at high flow rates did not go preferentially to lung apices to the extent predicted by the time-constant model (Pedley et al., 1972). (2) Selective contraction of chest wall musculature, as observed during quiet breathing (Roussos et al., 1974, 1976a,b, 1977) is an alternative proposition for dP_{pl}/dD inequality. Thus $\Delta P_{pl}/\Delta t$ values in different lung regions may differ not merely as a consequence of time-constant discrepancies, but because chest wall expansion differs. The first clear indication for considering unequal driving pressure rather than different time constants as determinants of flow-dependent gas distribution during single inspirations was the observation that the flow dependence of apicobasal gas distribution was greater in the supine than the upright posture (Sybrecht et al., 1976). Since regional expansion and, hence, time constants are more uniform in the craniocaudal direction in the supine posture (Bake et al., 1967), the greater flow dependence could not be easily attributed to different time constants. It is interesting to note that although a model based on time-constant differences alone could not be made to fit the data, incorporation into the model of only small differences in the applied pleural pressure substantially changed the bolus distribution.

Fixley et al. (1978) proposed that during rapid inspiration selective recruitment of intercostal and accessory muscles contribute to the greater distribution of inspired gas to the upper zones at the expense of the dependent region. These predictions were subsequently confirmed by D'Angelo (1981) relating differential chest wall expansion to electromyographic findings. That this may be the cause, rather than a consequence, of the preferential distribution of inspired gas to the lung apices is suggested by the observation that voluntary selective motion of the rib cage and diaphragm-abdomen influences the distribution of inspired gas. In fact, Fixley et al. (1978) found that in normal subjects the distribution of a bolus of gas at high flows approaches the distribution of an "intercostal" inspiration. Similarly, the gas distribution during "diaphragmatic" maneuvers at any flow is similar to that of a slow-flow, natural inspiration. Figure 7 summarizes these results, which suggest that neither the time constant alone nor the changes in dP_p/dD alone account for the apparent flow dependence of gas distribution. The latter is probably affected in an additive fashion by these two factors. Finally, it should be noted that both of the mechanisms are more apparent early in the breath and thus are best shown using the bolus technique. Later parts of the breath are preferentially distributed to dependent lung regions at all flow rates, so that the flow dependence of distribution of tidal volume is less than that of inhaled boluses.

The reader should keep in mind that all the studies reviewed above dealt with single inspirations at different flow rates. There is a paucity of experimental data on the flow dependence of ventilation distribution during cyclic breathing. In one of the earliest studies with [133]Xe Bryan et al. (1964) found that during exercise, in contrast to quiet breathing, all lung regions were uniformly ventilated. However, more recently, Forkert et al. (1978) convincingly demonstrated that the vertical gradients of regional ventilation distribution remained the same when normal subjects washed out ^{133}Xe by breathing slowly and at 60 breaths/min. Similar findings were reported by Kronenberg and coworkers (1976). Since at the two breathing frequencies, mean inspiratory flow rates approximated 0.3 and 1.4 liters/s, the findings seriously questioned the applicability of conclusions drawn from single-breath studies to those of cyclic breathing.

Recent examination of mechanisms potentially responsible for flow-dependent changes in ventilation distribution have also questioned their relevance to cyclic breathing. Realistic differences in regional time constants have relatively little effect on tidal volume distribution when examined in a two-compartment model "ventilated" at different frequencies (Chang and Shykoff, 1982). This contrasts with the exquisite sensitivity of gas distribution to small differences in regional pleural pressure swings, as predicted also for single-breath maneuvers (Fixley et al., 1978). However, experimental evidence for changes in rib cage shape at different flow rates is lacking. On the contrary, Crawford et al. (1983) found no differences in rib cage shape during tidal breathing at rest, at high frequencies, or during moderate exercise. The authors concluded that, in contrast to single, rapid inspirations, during cyclic breathing there is no preferential expansion of the upper rib cage at high flow rates. In fact, the pattern of changes in rib cage shape at all flow rates corresponded to that seen during relaxed, slow deflations from TLC. In view of the substantial, readily demonstrable changes in shape during single inspirations at moderately high flows, an inherent stiffness of the rib cage was not a likely explanation. The authors suggested that highly coordinated respiratory muscle recruitment maintained optimal rib cage shape at all flow rates.

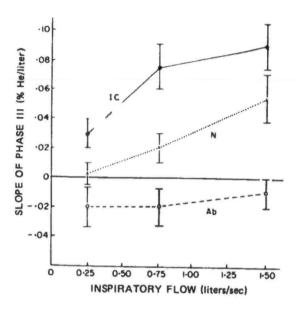

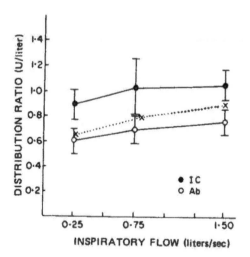

Figure 7 Upper panel, slope of alveolar plateau after inspiration of the helium bolus at different flow-rates in six subjects: (●) intercostal (IC); (○) abdominal (Ab); (x) natural inspiration (N); bars, ±1 SE. Note change in slope of natural maneuver towards that of IC inspiration at high flow rates. Lower panel, rate of ^{133}Xe concentration in upper 2/lower 2 counterfields inspired at different flow rates. Symbols as in upper panel. (Note that natural inspiration in this panel is from Bake et al., 1974.) (From Fixley et al., 1978.)

VI. Effect of Lung on Chest Wall

The shape and motion of the chest wall should be theoretically influenced by the forces developed by the lung. The magnitude of such an effect will depend on the compliance and resistance to deformation of the chest wall and upon whether these forces are uniform or nonuniform. Systematic studies in this regard are missing, but some experimental findings and observation in disease states illustrate this lung–chest wall interaction. For example, in dogs, occlusion of a lobar bronchus amplifies the pressure swings over the obstructed lobe (Zidulka et al., 1976). Such an amplification of P_{pl} may not be sufficient to alter the rib cage shape or motion but may well affect that of the diaphragm. Klingstedt et al. (1985) have produced results consistent with this notion. They applied selective positive end-expiratory pressure (PEEP) in the dependent lung in humans and forced an increase in the volume of this lung followed by a reduction of the volume of the nondependent lung by only by one-third of the simultaneous increase in that of the dependent lung. Although no measurements of the chest wall shape are made, it is intuitively obvious that the chest wall configuration has also changed. By the same token it would be interesting to measure the chest wall shape under different localized lung disease, as for example localized pneumonia, pulmonary emboli, or localized pulmonary edema (Blanch et al., 1992).

Hyperinflation may substantially alter the chest wall shape and lead, in extreme conditions, to diaphragmatic inversion (Roussos, unpublished observations). Similarly, during cardiopulmonary resuscitation (CPR) maneuvers, reflecting substantial unequal application of P_{pl} to the lung, the latter, particularly at high lung volume, may be greatly distorted and, acting like a rigid rod, distort the most compliant part (diaphragmatic region) of the chest wall (Ducas et al., 1983). Under these extreme conditions of lung deformation, substantial differences may be predicted between radial and longitudinal stresses within a lung (Murphy et al., 1983). Thus, the long-standing assumption that the lung expands isotropically under most conditions may not be entirely true, and detailed studies of lung–chest wall interactions are badly needed.

VII. Practical Considerations

1. Physiotherapy. Despite a long-standing tradition of breathing exercises and training for patients with lung diseases, it is still not clear what these physiotherapeutic interventions actually achieve. The potential of certain specific breathing maneuvers to alter ventilation distribution raises the possibility that they may be useful under certain conditions as a therapeutic intervention.

2. Critically ill patients. Awareness of the physiology discussed in this chapter may be relevant to the management of patients with unilateral thoracic disease. Prospective studies of the effects of posture on gas exchange in both

spontaneously breathing and artificially ventilated patients are likely to be informative.

3. Gravity. Changes in the gravity field influence both the blood flow and ventilation distribution in the lung. Voluntary selective use of different respiratory muscles may be useful under various circumstances (e.g., to avoid gas exchange impairment during transient exposure to high gravity) and require systematic study.

References

Agostoni, E. (1972). Mechanics of the pleural space. *Physiol. Rev.*, 52:57–128.

Agostoni, E., and D'Angelo, E. (1970). Comparative features of the transpulmonary pressure. *Respir. Physiol.*, 11:76.

Agostoni, E., and D'Angelo, E. (1971). Topography of pleural surface pressure during simulation of gravity effect on abdomen. *Respir. Physiol.*, 12:102.

Agostoni, E., and Mead, J. (1964). Statics of the respiratory system. In *Handbook of Physiology*, Section 3: *Respiration*. Vol. 1. Edited by W. O. Fenn and H. Rahn. Washington, D.C., American Physiological Society, pp. 387–409.

Agostoni, E., and Miserocchi, G. (1970). Vertical gradient of transpulmonary pressure with active and artifical lung expansion. *J. Appl. Physiol.*, 29:705.

Agostoni, E., Taglietti, A., and Setnikar, I. (1957). Absorption force of the capillaries of the visceral pleura in determination of intrapleural pressure. *Am. J. Physiol.*, 191:277–282.

Agostoni, E., and D'Angelo, E., and Bonanni, M. V. (1970a). The effect of the abdomen on the vertical gradient of pleural surface pressure. *Respir. Physiol.*, 8:331.

Agostoni, E., and D'Angelo, E., and Bonanni, M. V. (1970b). Topography of pleural surface pressure above resting volume in relaxed animals. *J. Appl. Physiol.*, 29:297

Amis, T. C. (1979). Regional lung function in man and the dog. Ph.D. thesis, University of London.

Anthonisen, N. R., Robertson, P. C., and Ross, W. R. D. (1970). Gravity dependent sequential emptying of lung regions. *J. Appl. Physiol.*, 25:589.

Bake, B., Bjure, J., Grimby, G., Milic-Emili, J., and Nilsson, N. J. (1967). Region distribution of inspired gas in supine man. *Scand. J. Respir. Dis.*, 48:189.

Bake, B., Wood, L., Murphy, B., Macklem, P. T., and Milic-Emili, J. (1974). Effect of inspiratory flow rate on regional distribution of inspired gas. *J. Appl. Physiol.*, 37:8.

Blanch, L., Roussos, C., Brotherton, S., Michel, R., Angle, M. (1992). Effect of tidal volume and PEEP in ethchlorvynol-induced asymmetric lung injury. *J. Appl. Physiol.*, 73(1):108–116.

Blide, R. W., Kerr, H. D., and Spicer, W. S., Jr. (1964). Measurement of upper and lower airway conductance in man. *J. Appl. Physiol.*, 19:1059.

Bryan, A. C., Bentivoglio, L. G., Beerel, F., Macleish, M., Zidulka, A., and Bates, D. V. (1964). Factors affecting regional distribution of ventilation and perfusion in the lung. *J. Appl. Physiol.*, 19:395.

Burger, E. J., Jr., and Macklem, P. T. (1968). Airway closure: demonstration by breathing 100% O_2 at low lung volumes and by N_2 washout. *J. Appl. Physiol.*, 25:139.

Chang, H. K., and Shykoff, B. E. (1982). A model stimulation of ventilation distribution. *Bull. Eur. Physiopathol. Respir.*, 18:329–338.

Chevrolet, J. C., Martin, J. G., Floor, R., Martin, R. R., and Engel, L. A. (1978). Topographical ventilation and perfusion distribution during IPPB in the lateral posture. *Am. Rev. Respir. Dis.*, 118:847–854.

Chevrolet, J. C., Emrich, J., Martin, R. R., and Engel, L. A. (1979). Voluntary changes in ventilation distribution in the lateral posture. *Respir. Physiol.*, 38:313–323.

Connolly, T., Bake, B., Wood, L., and Milic-Emili, J. (1975). Regional distribution of a ^{133}Xe-labelled gas volume inspired at constant flow rate. *Scand. J. Respir. Dis.*, 56:150.

Crawford, H., Dodd, D., and Engel, L. A. (1983). Changes in rib cage shape during quiet breathing, hyperventilation, and single inspirations. *Respir. Physiol.*, 54:197–209.

Daly, W., and Bondurant, S. (1963). Direct measurement of respiratory pressure changes in normal man. *J. Appl. Physiol.*, 18:513.

D'Angelo, E. (1972). Local alveolar size and transpulmonary pressure in situ and in isolated lungs. *Respir. Physiol.*, 14:251.

D'Angelo, E. (1981). Cranio-caudal rib cage distortion with increasing inspiratory airflow in man. *Respir. Physiol.*, 44:215.

D'Angelo, E., and Agostoni, E. (1973). Continuous recording of pleural surface pressure at various sites. *Respir. Physiol.*, 19:356.

D'Angelo, E., and Agostoni, E. (1974a). Effect of histamine on the vertical gradient of transpulmonary pressure. *Respir. Physiol.*, 20:331.

D'Angelo, E., and Agostoni, E. (1974b). Distribution of transpulmonary pressure and chest wall shape. *Respir. Physiol.*, 22:335.

D'Angelo, E., Bonanni, M. V., Michelini, S., and Agostoni, E. (1970). Topography of the pleural surface pressure in rabbits and dogs. *Respir. Physiol.*, 8:204.

D'Angelo, E., Michelini, S., and Agostoni, E. (1971). Partition of factors contributing to the vertical gradient of transpulmonary pressure. *Respir. Physiol.*, 12:90.

D'Angelo, E., Sant'Ambrogio, G., and Agostoni, E. (1974). Effect of diaphragm activity or paralysis on distribution of pleural pressure. *J. Appl. Physiol.*, 37:311.

De Troyer, A., Kelly, S., and Zin, W. A. (1983). Mechanical action of the intercostal muscles on the ribs. *Science*, 220:87–88.

Ducas, J., Roussos, Ch., Katsardis, H., and Magder, S. (1983). Thoracoabdominal mechanics during resuscitation maneuvers. *Chest*, 84:446–451.

Duomarco, J. L., Rimini, R., and Migliaro, J. P. (1954). Intraesophageal pressure and the local differences in pleural pressure. *Acta Physiol. Lat. Am.*, 4:133.

Engel, L. A., Grassino, A., and Anthonisen, N. R. (1975). Demonstration of airway closure in man. *J. Appl. Physiol.*, 38:1117.

Ewan, P. A., Jones, H. A., Noseil, J., Obdrzaler, J., and Hughes, J. M. B. (1978). Uneven perfusion and ventilation within lung regions studied with nitrogen-13. *Respir. Physiol.*, 34:45–49.

Fixley, M. S., Roussos, C. S., Murphy, B., Martin, R. R., and Engel, L. A. (1978). Flow dependence of gas distribution and the pattern of inspirator muscle contraction. *J. Appl. Physiol.*, 45:733–741.

Forkert, L., Anthonisen, N. R., and Wood, L. D. H. (1978). Frequency dependence of region lung washout. *J. Appl. Physiol.*, 45:161–170.

Froese, A. B., and Bryan, A. C. (1974). Effects of anesthesia and paralysis on diaphragmatic mechanics in man. *Anesthesiology*, 41:242–255.

Glaister, D. H. (1967a). The effect of positive centrifugal acceleration upon distribution of ventilation and perfusion within the human lung, and its relation to pulmonary arterial and intra-oesophageal pressures. *Proc. R. Soc. Lond.* [Biol.], 168:311.

Glaister, D. H. (1967b). The effect of posture on the distribution of ventilation and blood flow in the normal lung. *Clin. Sci.*, 33:391.

Glazier, J. B., Hughes, J. M. B., Maloney, J. E., and West, J. B. (1967). Vertical gradient of alveolar size in lungs of dogs frozen intact. *J. Appl. Physiol.*, 23:694.

Grassino, A., and Anthonisen, N. R. (1975). Chest wall distortion and lung regional volume distribution in erect humans. *J. Appl. Physiol.*, 39:1004.

Gray, H. (1973). The pericardium. In *Gray's Anatomy of the Human Body*. Edited by R. Warwick and P. L. Williams. Edinburgh, Longmans, p. 598.

Hogg, J. C., and Nepszy, S. (1969). Region lung volume and pleural pressure gradient estimated from lung density in dogs. *J. Appl. Physiol.*, 27:198.

Hoppin, F. G., Jr., Green, I. D., and Mead, J. (1970). Distribution of pleural surface pressure in dogs. *J. Appl. Physiol.*, 11:76.

Hubmayr, R. D., Rodarte, J. R., Walters, B. J., Tonelli, F. M. (1987). Regional ventilation during spontaneous breathing and mechanical ventilation in dogs. *J. Appl. Physiol.*, 63(6):2467–2475.

Jones, R. L., Overton, T. R., and Sproule, R. J. (1977). Frequency dependence of ventilation distribution in normal and obstructed lungs. *J. Appl. Physiol.*, 42:548–553.

Kaneko, K., Milic-Emili, J., Dolovich, M. B., Dawson, A., and Bates, D. V. (1966). Regional distribution of ventilation and perfusion as a function of body position. *J. Appl. Physiol.*, 21:767–77.

Katsura, T., Rozencwaig, R., Sutherland, P. M., Hogg, J., and Milic-Emili, J. (1970). Effect of external support on regional alveolar expansion in excised dog lungs. *J. Appl. Physiol.*, 28:133.

Klingstedt, C., Baehrendtz, S., Bindslev, L., Hedenstierna, G. (1985). Lung and chest wall mechanics during differential ventilation with selective PEEP. *Acta Anaesth. Scand.*, 29(7):716–721.

Konno, K., and Mead, J. (1967). Measurement of the separate volume changes of rib cage and abdomen during breathing. *J. Appl. Physiol.*, 22:407–422.

Kronenberg, R. S., Wangensteen, O. D., and Ponto, P. A. (1976). Frequency dependence of regional lung clearance of ^{133}Xe in normal men. *Respir. Physiol.*, 27:293–303.

Krueger, J. J., Bain, T., and Patterson, J. L., Jr. (1961). Elevation gradient of intrathoracic pressure. *J. Appl. Physiol.*, 16:465.

Larrson, A., Jonmarker, C., Lindahl, S. G. E., and Werner, O. (1989). Lung function in the supine and lateral decubitus positions in anesthetized infants and children. *Br. J. Anesthes.*, 62:378–384.

McMahon, S. M., Proctor, D. F., and Permutt, S. (1969). Pleural surface pressure in dogs. *J. Appl. Physiol.*, 27:881.

Mead, J. (1961). Mechanical properties of lungs. *Physiol. Rev.*, 41:281.

Michels, D. B., and West, J. B. (1978). Distribution of pulmonary ventilation and perfusion during short periods of weightlessness. *J. Appl. Physiol.*, 45:987.

Milic-Emili, J. (1974). Pulmonary statics. In *MTP International Review of Science*, Physiology Series I, Vol. 2: *Respiratory Physiology* I. Edited by J. G. Widdicombe. London, Butterworths; Baltimore University Park Press, pp. 105–137.

Milic-Emili, J., Henderson, J. A. M., Dolovitch, M. B., Trop, D., and Kaneko, K. (1966). Regional distribution of inspired gas in the lung. *J. Appl. Physiol.*, 21:749.

Minh, V. D., Kurihara, N., Friedman, P. J., and Moser, K. M. (1974). Reversal of the pleural pressure gradient during electrophrenic stimulation. *J. Appl. Physiol.*, 37:496.

Murphy, B. G., Plante, F., and Engel, L. A. (1983). Effect of a hydrostatic pleural pressure gradient on mechanical behavior of lung lobes. *J. Appl. Physiol.*, 52:453–461.

Otis, A. B., McKerrow, C. B., Bartlet, R. A., Mead, J., McIlroy, M. B., Selverstone, N. J., and Radford, E. P., Jr. (1956). Mechanical factors in distribution of pulmonary ventilation. *J. Appl. Physiol.*, 8:427.

Parodi, F. (1933). La Méecanique pulmonaire. Paris, Maisson.

Pedley, T. J., Sudlow, M. F., and Milic-Emili, J. (1972). A non-linear theory of the distribution of pulmonary ventilation. *Respir. Physiol.*, 15:1.

Prinzmetal, M., and Kountz, W. B. (1935). Intrapleural pressure in health and disease and its influence on body function. *Medicine* (Baltimore), 14:457.

Proctor, D. F., Caldini, P., and Permutt, S. (1968). The pressure surrounding the lungs. *Respir. Physiol.*, 5:130.

Rehder, K., Sessler, A. D., and Rodarte, J. R. (1977). Regional intrapulmonary gas distribution in awake and anesthetized-paralyzed man. *J. Appl. Physiol.*, 42:391–402.

Rehder, K., Knopp, T. J., and Sessler, A. D. (1978). Regional intrapulmonary gas distribution in awake and anesthetized-paralyzed prone man. *J. Appl. Physiol.*, 45:528–535.

Rist, E., and Strohl, A. (1920). Etude expérimentales et critiques sur le pneumothorax. *Ann. Med.* (Paris), 8:233–270.

Rist, E., and Strohl, A. (1922). Sur le role de la diffusion dans la resorption gazeuse et le maintien de la pression sous-atmosphérique dans la plèvre. *Presse Med.*, 30:69–71.

Robertson, P. C., Anthonisen, N. A., and Ross, D. (1969). Effect of inspiratory flow rate on regional distribution of inspired gas. *J. Appl. Physiol.*, 26:438.

Rohrer, F. (1925). Physiologie der Atembewegung. In *Handbuch der Normalen und Pathologischen Physiologie*. Vol. 2. Edited by A. Bethe, G. von Bergmann, G. Embden, and A. Ellinger. Berlin and New York, Springer-Verlag, p. 70.

Rosenszweig, D. Y., Hughes, J. M., and Jones, T. (1969). Uneven ventilation within and between regions of the normal man measured with nitrogen-13. *Respir. Physiol.*, 8:86–97.

Roussos, C. S., Fukuchi, Y., Macklem, P. T., and Engel, L. A. (1976a). Influence of diaphragmatic contraction on ventilation distribution in horizontal man. *J. Appl. Physiol.*, 40:471–424.

Roussos, C. S., Siegler, D. I. M., and Engel, L. A. (1976b). Influence of diaphragmatic contraction and expiratory flow on the pattern of lung emptying. *Respir. Physiol.*, 27:157–167.

Roussos, C., Fixley, M., Genest, J., Cosio, M., Kelly, S., Martin, R., and Engel, L. A. (1977a). Voluntary factors influencing the distribution of inspired gas. *Am. Rev. Respir. Dis.*, 116:457–464.

Roussos, C. S., Martin, R. R., and Engel, L. A. (1977b). Diaphragmatic contraction and the gradient of alveolar expansion in the lateral posture. *J. Appl. Physiol.*, 43:32–38.

Setnikar, I., Agostoni, A., and Taglietti, A. (1957). Entita caratteristiche e origine della depressione pleurica. *Arch Sci. Biol.* (Bologna), 41:312–325.

Setnikar, I., and Agostoni, E. (1962). Factors keeping the lung expanded in the chest. *Proc. Intern. Union Physiol. Sci.*, 1:281–286.

Sutherland, P. W., Katsura, T., and Milic-Emili, J. (1968). Previous volume history of the lung and regional distribution of gas. *J. Appl. Physiol.*, 25:566.

Svanberg, L. (1957). Influence of posture on the lung volumes; ventilation and circulation in normals: a spirometric-bronchospirometric investigation. *Scand. J. Clin. Lab. Invest.* (suppl.) 25.

Sybrecht, G., Landau, L., Murphy, B. G., Engel, L. A., Martin, R. R., and Macklem, P. T. (1976). Influence of posture on flow dependence of distribution of inhaled ^{133}Xe boli. *J. Appl. Physiol.*, 41:489.

Tokics, L., Strandberg, A., Brismar, B., Lundquist, H., and Hedenstierna, G. (1987). Computerized tomography of the chest and gas exchange measurements during ketamine anaesthesia. *Acta Anaesth. Scand.*, 31:684–692.

Tomioka, S., Kubo, S., Guy, H. J., and Prisk, G. K. (1988). Gravitational independence of single-breath washout tests in recumbent dogs. *J. Appl. Physiol.*, 64(2):642–648.

Turner, J. M. (1962). Distribution of lung surface pressure as a function of posture in dogs. *Physiologist*, 5:223.

Vawter, D. L., Matthews, F. L., and West, J. B. (1975). Effect of shape and size of lung and chest wall in stresses in the lung. *J. Appl. Physiol.*, 39:9.

Vincent, N. J., Knudson, R., Leith, D. E., Macklem, P. T., and Mead, J. (1970). Factors influencing pulmonary resistance. *J. Appl. Physiol.*, 29:236.

West, J. B., and Matthews, F. L. (1972). Stresses, strains, and surface pressure in the lung caused by its weight. *J. Appl. Physiol.*, 32:332.

Wirz, K. (1923). Das Verhalten des Drucks im Pleuraraum bei der Atmung und die Ursachen seiner Veränderlichkeit. *Pflugers Arch. Gesamte Physiol. Mensch. Tiere*, 199:1.

Zidulka, A., Demedts, M., Nadler, S., and Anthonisen, N. R. (1976). Pleural pressure with lobar obstruction in dogs. *Respir. Physiol.*, 26:239–248.

57

Interaction Between the Circulatory and Ventilatory Pumps

HENRY E. FESSLER and SOLBERT PERMUTT

The Johns Hopkins Medical Institutions
Baltimore, Maryland

I. Introduction

The first edition of this chapter (1985) examined the mechanical similarities between the forces that generate airflow in and out of the lungs and those that generate blood flow in and out of the vasculature. A mathematical model was developed that could be solved for the steady-state cardiac output based on elastic and resistive properties of the peripheral circulation, functional characteristics of the heart, and pressures surrounding the heart and circulation, which are altered by ventilation or ventilatory maneuvers. Finally, available empirical data on hemodynamic effects of the Valsalva and Mueller maneuvers, cardiopulmonary resuscitation, and the therapeutic potential of manipulation of pleural pressure were analyzed in terms of the predictions of the mathematical model. We concluded: "We foresee a day when manipulation of pleural pressure will allow the support of the arrested or failing circulation in a manner analogous to the support of ventilatory failure in the modern intensive care unit."

This second edition will examine the extent to which our prediction has been met. The intervening decade has produced an explosion of knowledge regarding cardiopulmonary resuscitation (see Chap. 58). In addition, there have been major new insights into the transient effects of a respiratory cycle on blood flow and the effects of positive end-expiratory pressure on the circulation. Pathological conditions that lead to exaggerated changes in pleural pressure or lung volume, such as asthma and obstructive sleep apnea, have been studied in some detail. The use of changes in pleural pressure to diagnose or assist a failing circulation has advanced from animal physiology studies to clinical trials. We will first review the model developed in the previous edition of this chapter. Next, we will define the relatively few mechanisms through which a respiratory event can affect the cardiovascular system. Finally, we will review some recent physiological data to show how these mechanisms are integrated during the application of positive end-expiratory pressure.

II. Determinants of Steady-State Cardiac Output

During systole, the pressure in the heart becomes elevated relative to the pressure in the elastic elements of the blood vessels, and blood moves from the heart to the circuit. During diastole, the flow of blood to the heart is a passive process: the force that returns blood to the heart is generated exclusively by the elastic recoil of the blood vessels.

The factors that determine blood return to the heart were demonstrated by Guyton and colleagues (1955) in classic experiments in which the heart was replaced by a pump and the relationship between venous return and right atrial pressure was determined. When the pump is stopped, the pressure in the right atrium is equal to the static pressure throughout the circulation. This is determined by the compliance and distending volume of the systemic blood vessels. When the blood volume is increased, the distending pressure increases, and vice versa. Maximal flow is reached when right atrial pressure is lowered slightly below atmospheric pressure. The maximal flow is independent of the activity of the pump but is directly related to the recoil pressure of the systemic vessels.

The relationship between right atrial pressure and venous return represented graphically by the venous return curve may also be expressed quantitatively. Venous return is found to depend on the compliance of the vasculature and the distending volume of the circulation, which together determine the elastic recoil pressure. It also depends on the atrial pressures and the pleural pressure surrounding the atria. Finally, it varies inversely with the resistance downstream from the static locus of the recoil pressure, the resistance to venous return. The interested reader is referred elsewhere for the derivation of this formula (Permutt and Caldini, 1978).

The relationship between atrial pressure and cardiac output is the familiar Starling relationship. The superimposition of the venous return curve and Starling curve on the same set of axes was the creative insight of Guyton and coworkers (1955). This provided an immensely useful conceptual framework for studying cardiovascular control. However, the Starling curve remained an empirical finding whose determinants were not explicitly stated.

This limitation was overcome through the work of Suga et al. (1973, 1974). They analyzed cardiac contractility in terms of a change in compliance of the ventricle. During diastole, the compliance is large. At end-systole, the compliance is at its lowest level. At each time interval during systole, the ventricle has an instantaneous pressure-volume relationship, which is intermediate between the curve at end-diastole and end-systole. The value of this concept for the analysis of cardiac output is that intrinsic cardiac function can be summarized by only two pressure-volume curves: those at end-systole and those at end-diastole. The stroke volume is determined by the point on the end-diastolic curve where contraction begins and the point on the end-systolic curve where contraction ends. For stroke volume, the pertinent heart parameters are the two pressure-volume curves. The points on the two curves where systole begins and ends are determined by the parameters of the circulation.

Thus, a quantitative expression can be derived which expresses cardiac output in terms of the systolic and diastolic compliances of the ventricles, their transmural filling pressure, the backpressure and resistance against which they must eject, and the heart rate. This is, in essence, a mathematical expression of the Starling curve. Since venous return and cardiac output must be equal in the steady state, the equations for the venous return curve and Starling curve may be set equal to each other. The resulting equation can then be solved for the equilibrium cardiac output/venous return, given a set of heart parameters and a set of circuit parameters. The first edition of this chapter undertook this derivation in detail and then explored how alterations in pleural pressure would affect the equilibrium output with different heart parameters. To summarize, it was demonstrated that with normal cardiac function, an increase in pleural pressure would inevitably decrease cardiac output. However, when cardiac function was impaired and when the diastolic compliance of the ventricle was curvilinear, then an increase in pleural pressure could lead to an increase in cardiac output and even in arterial pressure. The reader is referred to the first edition for details.

III. Respiratory Stresses on the Circulatory System

The above analysis, though it may appear mathematically complex, does not fully address the mechanical effects of a respiratory cycle or of many respiratory maneuvers. We have so far only considered the effects of a change in pleural pressure. Respiration is also accompanied by a change in lung volume. Furthermore, inspiration is accompanied by an increase in abdominal pressure. If these additional effects of respiration are taken into account, the respiratory system can affect the circulatory system through the application of four basic stresses: (1) stress upon the outer surface of the heart, (2) stress on intrapulmonary blood vessels, (3) stress on the left ventricle from distension of the right ventricle, and (4) stress on the surface of abdominal blood vessels.

A. Stress on the Outer Surface of the Heart

Activation of the muscles of inspiration lowers the pressure on the surface of the heart as well as the lungs. The decrease in pleural pressure is instantly transmitted to the alveoli, and inspiratory airflow is initiated. Similarly, the decrease in right atrial pressure will increase venous flow from extrathoracic veins to the heart. Maximal inspiratory airflow, in the absence of upper airway pathology, is limited only by the velocity and force of inspiratory muscle contraction. Maximal venous return, however, is limited by the collapsibility of the great veins, which will limit flow when the pressure within them falls below the pressure on their surface. Since the pressure on the surface of the extrathoracic veins is close to atmospheric pressure, venous return becomes maximal when right atrial pressure falls below atmospheric pressure. It follows that a subject with a high right atrial pressure during expiration can increase venous return during vigorous inspiration more than can a subject with a low right atrial pressure, because the latter will flow-limit after a relatively smaller change in right atrial pressure.

An increase in pressure on the surface of the right heart will elevate right atrial pressure. Since the studies of Cournand et al. (1948), this is believed by many to be the predominant mechanism whereby positive pressure ventilation or positive end-expiratory pressure decreases cardiac output (Braunwald et al., 1957; Fewell et al., 1980; Marini et al., 1981a). However, as shall be discussed later, an increase in the downstream pressure for venous return is only one of several effects of positive end-expiratory pressure (PEEP) on the determinants of venous return.

Inspiratory muscle contraction also lowers the pressure on the surface of the left heart. A decrease in pressure on the surface of the left ventricle (LV) impedes LV ejection by increasing the ventricular afterload. We consider afterload to be the wall stress of the ventricle during ejection. If the ventricle were spherical, the wall stress would be described by the Laplace equation:

$$\text{Stress} = \frac{1/2 \ (\text{Ptm} \times r)}{\text{wall thickness}}$$

where Ptm is the ventricular transmural pressure and r is the radius of the sphere. Other expressions derived for the more complex geometry of the LV retain the direct relationship between LV transmural pressure and wall stress (Regen, 1990).

Ventricular and aortic pressure are very nearly equal during ejection. If the pressure on the surface of the ventricle is near zero, then the transmural ventricular pressure is nearly equal to aortic pressure during systole. It has therefore become a clinically useful simplification to consider arterial pressure as a surrogate expression of LV afterload. However, that simplification can become misleading under conditions where the pressure on the ventricular surface is changing significantly, such as during disorders of breathing or ventilatory maneuvers.

Indeed, even during quiet breathing, inspiration is accompanied by a decrease in arterial blood pressure measured relative to atmospheric pressure but an increase in left ventricular afterload. There is general agreement that stroke volume falls during spontaneous inspiration, but some controversy regarding the importance of changes in LV afterload in causing this fall. An inspiratory decrease in LV stroke volume could be due to enhanced venous return distending the right ventricle, which thereby impedes the filling of the left ventricle (see below). It could also be due to reflex impairment of myocardial contractility. Finally, it could be due to increased transmural wall stress during ejection, i.e., increased afterload.

Robotham and coworkers (1993) studied the effects of spontaneous inspiration and Mueller maneuvers in right-heart bypassed dogs in which right ventricular (RV) volume could be maintained constant or allowed to increase with inspiration. Even when RV volume was minimal, eliminating interdependence between the ventricles, and vagally mediated reflexes interrupted by vagal transection, inspiratory muscle contraction reduced stroke volume. However, the reduction was significantly greater when RV volume was allowed to increase, indicating a combined role for afterload and ventricular interdependence in the intact circulation. Peters et al. (1989) used phrenic nerve stimulation with the airway closed or opened to simulate a Mueller maneuver or spontaneous inspiration. Dogs with mitral valve and ascending aortic flow probes were subjected to brief (40–200 ms) phrenic stimulation to limit the duration of negative pleural pressure to cardiac systole or diastole. Stimulation limited to systole decreased LV stroke volume and increased systolic transmural LV pressure. These changes were unaltered by severing the pericardiophrenic ligaments or by pericardiectomy. Since the LV filling pressure during phrenic nerve stimulation was identical to that during the preceding heartbeat and since RV filling would have been complete prior to stimulation, these studies indicate the decrease in stroke volume was due to increased LV afterload. In further studies, Peters et al. (1988b) measured intrathoracic aortic diameters in orthogonal planes with sonomicrometer crystals. Phrenic stimulation limited to systole decreased stroke volume and increased transverse aortic area without causing measurable retrograde flow from the distal aorta. This study overcomes the limitations inherent in attempts to directly measure aortic or LV transmural pressure and demonstrates a qualitative increase in aortic systolic transmural pressure as pleural pressure falls at constant LV filling. This could not have been due to a decrease in myocardial contractility or in LV filling, either of which would have reduced stroke volume but decreased aortic area. When phrenic nerve stimulation was prolonged across an entire cardiac cycle, the fall in stroke volume was much greater, suggesting other mechanisms are also important during normal respiration.

Just as decreases in pressure on the surface of the LV will increase its afterload, increases in pressure on the surface of the LV can decrease its afterload. Pinsky et al. (1986) used a jet ventilator to increase pleural pressure and lung volume in dogs during a fixed portion of the cardiac cycle. When cardiac contractility was normal, increased pleural pressure had no effect on stroke volume regardless of its timing relative to the cardiac cycle. When cardiac contractility was impaired and preload increased with volume loading (conditions in which the mathematical model would predict a heightened sensitivity to afterload reduction and reduced sensitivity to preload reduction), jet ventilator pulses limited to systole increased stroke volume and decreased left atrial transmural pressure. Diastolic jet ventilator pulses also increased stroke volume, and this may have been due to enhanced diastolic emptying of the thoracic aorta, which then reduced afterload during the subsequent systole (Fessler et al., 1988). Similar results were found in a model of acute mitral regurgitation, suggesting enhanced forward flow due to decreased LV afterload (Stein et al., 1990). These findings were not dependent upon the small increases in lung volume which occur with jet ventilation. Beyar et al. (1989) increased pleural pressure in dogs using an inflatable vest, which decreases lung volume. Like Pinsky et al., they found increases in stroke volume when vest inflation was limited to systole during cardiac failure. Thus, it has become abundantly clear that changes in pleural pressure alter LV afterload in the same manner but the opposite direction as changes in arterial pressure.

B. Stress on Intrapulmonary Blood Vessels

Intrapulmonary blood vessels may be characterized as either alveolar or extraalveolar, based upon the stress on their outer surface. Alveolar vessels have a surface stress close to alveolar pressure. Extraalveolar vessels have a surface stress that is related to pleural pressure. [If there were no mechanical connection between the lung parenchyma and the extraalveolar vessels, their surface pressure would equal lateral pleural pressure. However, radial traction from connective tissue between parenchyma and blood vessels can reduce the surface pressure on extraalveolar vessels below lateral pleural pressure. Conversely, expansion of the vasculature at constant lung volume could be constrained by the lung parenchyma, so that pressure on the surface of the extraalveolar vessels would then exceed lateral pleural pressure (Mead et al., 1970)] The key functional distinction between alveolar and extraalveolar vessels is their change in stress with lung inflation. Increased transpulmonary pressure, whether by spontaneous or positive pressure inflation, will increase the stress on the alveolar vessels and decrease the stress on the extraalveolar vessels.

These changes in stress on the surface of the vessels affect blood flow by changing the resistance and capacitance of the vessels. Lung inflation expands the extraalveolar vessels, reducing their resistance and increasing their capacitance. Conversely, lung inflation compresses the alveolar vessels, increasing their resistance and reducing their capacitance. Changes in capacitance will cause transient changes in blood flow into or out of the lungs, while changes in resistance can cause steady-state changes in flow.

Consider first the extraalveolar vessels. At low lung volumes, their surface stress is high and they are the predominant site of the pulmonary vascular resistance (Hughes et al., 1968; Lopez-Muniz et al., 1968). Consequently, at low lung volume, lung inflation decreases pulmonary vascular resistance (Burton and Patel, 1958) and increases the pulmonary vascular volume (Permutt et al., 1961).

As lung volume increases further, effects of alveolar vessels become predominant. However, an increase in stress on the surface of the alveolar vessels will have differing effects depending on the zonal conditions of the lung. In zone III, the alveolar vessels are distended and left atrial pressure is the backpressure to right ventricular ejection. An increase in alveolar pressure relative to pressure on the surface of the heart will transiently decrease pulmonary arterial flow and increase pulmonary venous flow. Once these pulmonary capacitance vessels are discharged, if the lung remains in zone III, there will have been little steady-state change in the pressure against which the right ventricle ejects. Relatively minor changes in pulmonary vascular resistance will have resulted from a decrease in resistance of extraalveolar vessels and an increase in resistance of alveolar vessels. Lung inflation in zone III transiently increases left ventricular filling with minimal steady-state effects (Brower et al., 1985).

In contrast in zone II, the alveolar vessels behave as Starling resistors and the right ventricle ejects against alveolar pressure. Since there is then minimal blood volume in these vessels, increases in alveolar pressure relative to pleural pressure cannot empty them further. Lung inflation in zone II conditions causes a transient pooling of blood in the lungs due to the expansion of the extraalveolar vessels. However, lung inflation also increases the pressure against which the right ventricle ejects by an amount equal to the increase in transpulmonary pressure. If cardiac output is to be maintained, transmural pulmonary artery pressure must rise. This may explain the marked increase in pulmonary artery pressure measured during severe asthma attacks (Permutt, 1973). Lung inflation in zone II therefore transiently decreases left ventricular filling and causes a steady-state increase in right ventricular afterload.

C. Stress on the Left Ventricle from Distension of the Right Ventricle

Because the two ventricles are constrained by a common pericardial sac and share the interventricular septum, changes in the volume of one ventricle may affect the function of the other. This interdependence may affect both diastolic function and systolic function.

As stated above, spontaneous inspiration will increase venous return to the right ventricle by lowering right atrial pressure relative to the elastic recoil pressure of the systemic circulation. Inspiration will also impede right ventricular emptying by increasing the back pressure to ejection. Thus, inspiratory effort will almost invariably cause the right ventricle to distend, and this will impede the filling of the left ventricle (Robotham et al., 1979). This occurs both through a generalized increase in pericardial pressure and also due to a shift of the interventricular septum toward the left. However, the increase in stress on the septal and pericardial surfaces of the left ventricle will also, like an increase in pleural pressure, decrease left ventricular afterload. This improved LV systolic function was demonstrated by

Janicki and Weber (1980), who showed an increase in the developed pressure in an isovolumic LV with right ventricular distension. Thus, acute distension of the right ventricle (RV) impairs LV filling and assists LV emptying. Ventricular systolic interdependence attenuates the fall in LV surface pressure accompanying spontaneous inspiration. This moderating effect of interdependence on LV afterload may explain why some groups have demonstrated an increase in LV end-systolic volume during inspiration (Summer et al., 1979; Robotham et al., 1983), while others have not (Scharf et al., 1979; Wead and Norton, 1981).

By limiting the duration of negative pleural pressure to diastole in dogs during airway occlusion, Peters et al. (1988a) demonstrated increased left ventricular transmural end-diastolic pressure and decreased stroke volume in the ensuing systole. Because lung volume was constant, pleural pressure was returned to baseline prior to systole, and changes were too rapid to have reflected reflex effects, the increased filling pressure and decreased stroke volume were most consistent with reduced LV diastolic compliance due to ventricular interdependence. By using a computer simulation, Beyar et al. (1987) attempted to distinguish the relative importance of the pericardium versus direct transseptal transmission of pressure during a Mueller maneuver. They found that the reduction of LV diastolic volume was highly dependent on the presence of the pericardium but only minimally dependent on mechanical coupling through the septum.

D. Stress on the Surface of Abdominal Blood Vessels

If the diaphragm remains flaccid during positive-pressure ventilation, pleural pressure and abdominal pressure rise similarly. Since the thoracic and abdominal contents are subjected to a similar increase in surface pressure, there is little change in the pressure gradient driving venous return from the abdominal viscera. Thus, stress on the surface of the abdominal blood vessels can moderate the fall in venous return accompanying positive pressure ventilation. A graphic example of this effect occurs with the Valsalva maneuver. This maneuver increases both pleural and abdominal pressure by expiratory muscle contraction against a closed glottis. Although it typically causes a decrease in stroke volume, it is generally well tolerated in otherwise healthy humans and can be sustained as long as muscle contraction or breath-holding permits. In contrast, if one stands relaxed, with closed glottis, and one's thorax is squeezed by a colleague, syncope is almost inevitable. In the latter case, pleural pressure is increased more than abdominal pressure and venous return is much more severely reduced.

In regard to abdominal pressure, spontaneous ventilation is not the mirror image of positive pressure ventilation. Unless a subject volitionally avoids contracting his diaphragm, spontaneous inspiration increases abdominal pressure as it decreases pleural pressure. Changes in abdominal surface pressure relative to right atrial surface pressure can have significant effects on venous return. Most workers have found an increase in IVC flow with inspiration (Brecher, 1956; Moreno et al.,

1967). However, under controlled experimental conditions, some have found an inspiratory decrease in IVC (Wexler et al., 1968; Lloyd, 1983) or femoral venous (Willeput et al., 1984) flow.

Recently, a model of abdominal venous flow has been developed, which may reconcile some of the findings of previous studies. Takata et al. (1990) have extended the concept of zones of the lung to the abdominal vasculature. When intravascular pressure in the IVC exceeds abdominal pressure, the abdomen is in zone III. When intravascular pressure is less than abdominal pressure, the abdomen is in zone II and a Starling resistor is present at the diaphragm. The effects of an increase in abdominal pressure on IVC flow are analogous to the effects of an increase in alveolar pressure on pulmonary venous flow. Thus, in zone III, an increase in abdominal pressure would cause a transient increase in IVC flow as the abdominal capacitance vessels discharged downstream. If the abdominal pressure was sustained but the abdomen remained in zone III, there would be no change in the steady-state flow. In zone II conditions, an increase in abdominal pressure would be fully transmitted to the site of the Starling resistor. Since pressure around the capacitance vessels and the Starling resistor will have increased equally, there will be no change in flow from or volume of the abdominal compartment. However, there will be a decrease in outflow from the extraabdominal veins upstream from the Starling resistor. Therefore, both transient and steady-state IVC flow will decrease. If the increase in abdominal pressure changes a zone III abdomen into a zone II abdomen, the IVC flow will show an initial increase followed by a decrease.

This model was tested in a open-chested, closed-abdomen canine preparation in which baseline IVC and abdominal pressures could be controlled and then abdominal pressure increased with phrenic nerve stimulation. Consistent with the model predictions, diaphragmatic contraction when baseline IVC pressure exceeded abdominal pressure increased IVC flow, and diaphragmatic contraction when baseline abdominal pressure exceeded IVC pressure decreased IVC flow. When the pressures were close to each other, contraction produced biphasic changes in flow. When IVC pressure was increased at constant abdominal pressure, there was no change in pressure recorded in a femoral vein until IVC pressure was about 1 mm Hg higher than abdominal pressure, consistent with a Starling resistor upstream from the femoral veins (Takata et al., 1990). These findings were supported by further work in which splanchnic and nonsplanchnic IVC flows were measured in an intact canine circulation during phrenic nerve stimulation (Takata and Robotham, 1992). Thus, variable effects of inspiration on IVC venous return can be explained by this unifying model.

The clinical importance of increased abdominal pressure relative to pleural pressure was demonstrated in a study by Lemaire and coworkers (1988). They measured hemodynamic effects of changing from positive pressure to spontaneous ventilation in 15 patients with combined cardiac and obstructive pulmonary disease. Patients were selected for study if they had weaning parameters that appeared adequate but had nevertheless failed attempts at weaning. Spontaneous ventilation increased cardiac output and right and left ventricular filling pressures and rapidly led to respiratory failure. The increase in filling pressures and output was an expected finding, since the decrease in right atrial pressure would increase venous return. However, in these patients, right atrial pressure actually rose relative to atmospheric pressure despite the lower pressure surrounding the heart. The increase in venous return under those circumstances could have been due only to either a greater increase in the upstream pressure driving venous return or a reduction in the resistance to venous return.

Although no patient had clinical evidence of volume overload, all were aggressively diuresed for one week, losing an average of 5 kg. Although their weaning parameters and baseline LV filling pressures were unaltered, 8 of the 15 then weaned successfully. These patients now had cardiac outputs and LV filling pressures essentially unaltered from their values during mechanical ventilation (Lemaire et al., 1988).

We believe the explanation for these findings is as follows: prior to diuresis, these patients' abdomens were in zone III. We speculate that, when they began breathing spontaneously, their mean abdominal pressure increased. This could have occurred if, for example, their I:E ratio or their diaphragmatic contribution to tidal volume increased compared to mechanical ventilation. The increase in abdominal pressure displaced blood volume from the high capacitance, slowly draining splanchnic bed to the more rapidly draining, lower capacitance nonabdominal beds. The elastic recoil pressure of the circulation was thereby increased, and the resistance to venous return decreased (Caldini et al., 1974). This sudden increase in venous return, coupled with the effect of lower pleural pressure on LV afterload, precipitated heart failure and, in turn, respiratory failure.

After diuresis, many patients' abdomens were now in zone II. Baseline ventricular filling pressures were unchanged because the compliant splanchnic vasculature can accommodate large volume changes with little change in pressure. Increased abdominal pressure now had minimal effect on intraabdominal blood volume. Although respiratory work and LV afterload initially increased as much as they had the previous week, the vicious spiral into congestive heart failure was avoided.

In summary, the mechanical interaction between the respiratory and circulatory pumps can be analyzed in terms of relatively few stresses. In practice, the analysis of a given observation often remains complex because of complicated interaction between these effects, as well as neural and humoral factors that we have chosen to ignore here. In the final section of this chapter we will examine some of the new physiological insights in regard to positive end-expiratory pressure.

IV. Positive End-Expiratory Pressure

PEEP usually decreases cardiac output. The cause of this decrease has been the focus of much research over the past several decades. Mechanisms that have been proposed include increased stress on the surface of the heart (Marini et al., 1981b; Wise et al., 1981; Cassidy et al., 1982; Veddeng et al., 1992), ventricular interdependence (Jardin et al., 1981; Cassidy et al., 1982), and impaired myocardial contractility, due either to reflexes (Ashton and Cassidy, 1985), humoral factors (Manny et al., 1978), or myocardial ischemia (Tittley et al., 1985).

A factor common to many of the varied specific mechanisms that contribute to the fall in cardiac output is an increase in right atrial pressure. Thus, cardiac output may be said to fall on PEEP because of a decrease in the pressure gradient for venous return. If, however, increased right atrial pressure is to be invoked as a cause of decreased venous return, right atrial pressure must rise relative to the upstream pressure driving venous return, mean systemic pressure.

However, there was good reason to suppose that PEEP also increased mean systemic pressure. By decreasing cardiac output, PEEP decreases arterial pressure. Carotid sinus hypotension causes intense sympathetic-mediated decreases in systemic vascular capacitance and increases in mean systemic pressure (Greene and Shoukas, 1986; Rothe, 1993). Such a homeostatic response to PEEP is suggested by the typical biphasic response to a sudden increase in airway pressure, i.e., a brisk fall in arterial pressure followed by a partial restoration. Furthermore, it is not uncommon for right atrial pressure to rise 4–5 mm Hg with the application of 10–15 cm H_2O PEEP. This would reduce the pressure gradient for venous return to near zero and would be uniformly fatal if there were no increase in mean systemic pressure. Scharf and Ingram (1977) found that PEEP caused greater decreases in cardiac output and often was fatal in animal studies in which alpha-adrenergic compensatory mechanisms were blocked with phenoxybenzamine. Furthermore, Scharf et al. (1977) suggested that PEEP increased mean systemic pressure through reflex mechanisms.

Fessler et al. (1991) recently examined the changes in right atrial and mean systemic pressures caused by PEEP in dogs, the latter measured as the right atrial pressure during ventricular fibrillation. Surprisingly, PEEP increased mean systemic pressure and right atrial pressure equally (Fig. 1). This was also found by Nanas and Magder (1992) using a different technique to measure mean systemic pressure. Thus, contrary to the usual explanation, PEEP does not appear to decrease the pressure gradient for venous return.

As suggested by Scharf and Ingram (1977), the response of the peripheral vasculature is in part neurally mediated, because denervation of the carotid sinuses or total spinal anesthesia reduced the change in mean systemic pressure. Mechanical factors also play a role, however, since even with total spinal anesthesia, PEEP still significantly increased mean systemic pressure, albeit to a lesser extent. PEEP increases abdominal pressure, and this increase in stress on the surface of abdominal blood vessels could increase mean systemic pressure. However, neither binding nor widely opening the abdomen (to exaggerate or attenuate the PEEP-induced change in abdominal pressure) altered the PEEP-induced increase in mean systemic pressure. The major mechanical factor may therefore have been the displacement

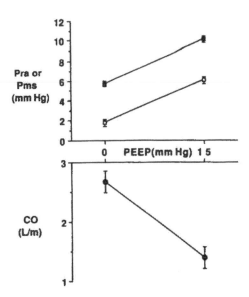

Figure 1   Cardiac output (closed circles, CO), right atrial pressure (open squares, P_{ra}), and mean systemic pressure (closed squares, P_{ms}) in six anesthetized dogs on and off 15 mm Hg PEEP. Although PEEP increased right atrial pressure and decreased cardiac output, the latter was not due to a decrease in the pressure gradient driving venous return.

of blood from the heart and lungs to the systemic circulation (Braunwald et al., 1957). Although in the first edition of this text we equated an increase in pleural pressure to a *decrease* in systemic blood volume, the effects of PEEP on mean systemic pressure are more similar to an *increase* in systemic blood volume.

Despite the unchanging pressure gradient for venous return, PEEP decreases venous return. This implies an increase in the resistance for venous return. To measure the resistance to venous return, Fessler et al. (1992) used a closed-chested canine right-heart bypass preparation. By separately collecting drainage from the IVC and SVC, venous return curves were measured for each of these beds (Fig. 2). In both SVC and IVC, 10 mm Hg PEEP increased the zero-flow intercept, which approximates mean systemic pressure. PEEP also increased the resistance in the SVC, but not the IVC (i.e., decreased the slope of the venous return curve). When the flow from the two circuits was summed, there was a significant, 15% increase in total resistance to venous return. Finally, in both the IVC and SVC, PEEP increased the critical right atrial pressure (P_{crit}) below which venous return became maximal and decreased the maximal venous return.

Although PEEP increases the resistance to venous return, the 15% increase was insufficient to account for the 30–50% decrease in venous return seen in intact dogs at similar levels of PEEP (Scharf and Ingram, 1977; Scharf et al., 1977; Cassidy et al., 1982). However, PEEP also increased P_{crit}. If P_{crit} on PEEP exceeded

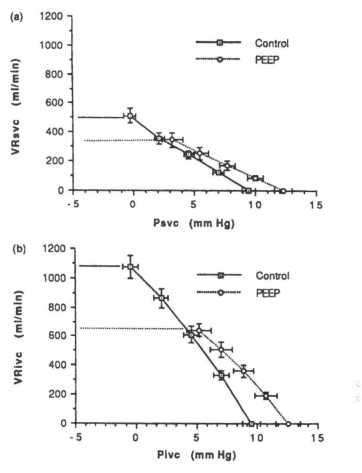

Figure 2 Venous return curves for the superior (a) and inferior (b) vena cavae on and off 10 mm Hg PEEP in eight anesthetized dogs. In both IVC and SVC, PEEP significantly increased the zero-flow intercept and critical downstream pressure below which flow became maximal. The resistance to venous return increased significantly in the SVC alone.

right atrial pressure, then a condition termed a "vascular waterfall" (Permutt and Riley, 1963) is said to exist. Under these conditions, the effective downstream pressure for venous return is not right atrial pressure, but some higher pressure upstream, which remains constant despite changes in right atrial pressure. In the intact circulation, PEEP may decrease the *effective* gradient for venous return by increasing P_{crit}, even as the measured difference between mean systemic and right atrial pressures remains constant.

To search for a vascular waterfall in the thoracic great veins, Fessler et al. (1993) measured the intravascular pressure in dogs as fluid-filled catheters were

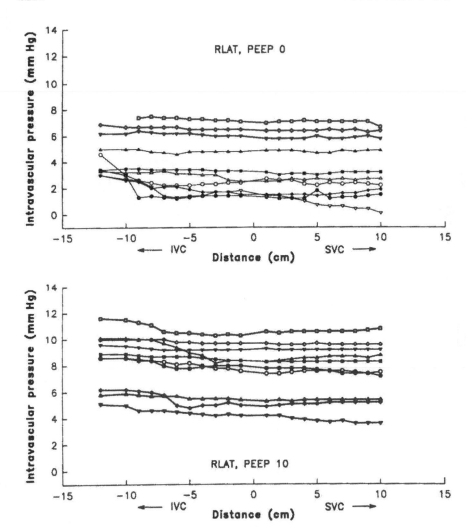

Figure 3 Longitudinal distribution of intravascular pressure in the intrathoracic IVC and SVC in 10 anesthetized dogs. Each was studied in the right lateral (RLAT) and left lateral (LLAT) decubitus position, on and off 10 mm Hg PEEP. In LLAT, but not RLAT, PEEP causes a sharp drop in intravascular pressure over a 1- to 2-cm length of IVC. This suggests direct compression of the vessel by the hyperinflated lung.

withdrawn up the SVC and down the IVC from the right atrium. In the SVC, with or without PEEP, pressure rose gradually and uniformly from the right atrium to the thoracic outlet. This suggested this vessel was widely patent, uncompressed by the surrounding lungs. In the IVC, there were similar findings off PEEP. However, when PEEP was applied, there was often a sharp increase in intravascular pressure

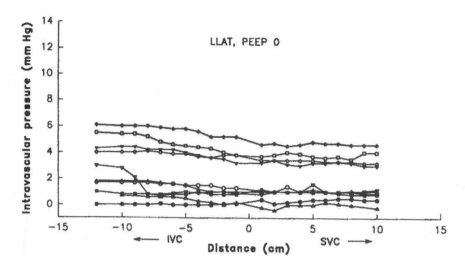

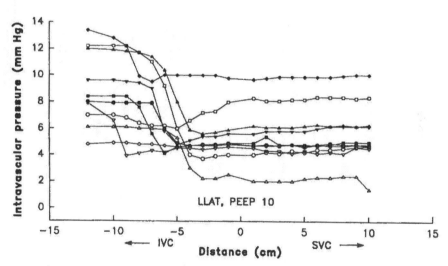

occurring over a 1- to 2-cm distance, midway between the atrium and diaphragm. This finding also depended on the animal's position. It rarely occurred in the right lateral decubitus position, when the IVC was dependent and the surrounding lung least inflated. It commonly occurred in the left lateral decubitus position, when the IVC was nondependent and the surrounding lung most hyperinflated (Fig. 3). We believe this intravascular pressure step-up reflects localized compression of the IVC by the lung. Furthermore, this necessitates that PEEP increases the pressure on intrathoracic vascular structures heterogeneously and increases the pressure around the IVC more than around the right heart. This pressure step-up also had characteristics of a vascular waterfall, insofar as increases in right atrial pressure had no effect on pressure upstream of the putative locus of compression until a critical pressure was exceeded (Fessler et al., 1993) (Fig. 4).

In summary, PEEP increases the downstream pressure for venous return but also initiates reflex and mechanical changes, which elevate the upstream venous pressure by an equal amount. Venous return falls because of an increase in the resistance to venous return and, at least in some body positions, the appearance of a vascular waterfall in the great veins. The role these mechanisms may play in humans has not been examined, although compression of the IVC at the diaphragm has been noted in hyperinflated patients with emphysema (Nakhjavan et al., 1966).

Several investigators have found an increase in cardiac output when PEEP or continuous positive airway pressure is applied to patients with congestive heart

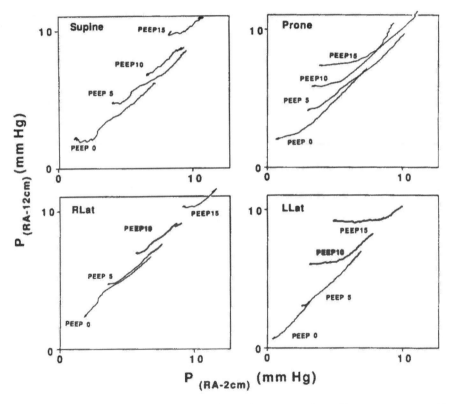

Figure 4 Pressure in the IVC measured 2 cm (P_{RA-2cm}) and 12 cm ($P_{RA-12cm}$) upstream of the right atrium, as right atrial pressure is elevated by inflation of an intraatrial balloon in an anesthetized dog. In prone and left lateral decubitus positions on PEEP, elevation of right atrial pressure has little or no effect on pressure 12 cm upstream until a critical pressure is exceeded, after which both pressures rise together. This suggests a "vascular waterfall" between the two loci.

failure (Mathru et al., 1982; Bradley et al., 1992). One explanation for this finding is the one we wholeheartedly endorsed in the first edition of this book: volume-overloaded, poorly contracting hearts are less sensitive to the preload-reducing effect of elevated pleural pressure and more sensitive to its LV afterload-reducing effect. When cardiac function is sufficiently depressed, an increase in mean pleural pressure can theoretically increase output even when the increase is not limited to systole. However, we speculate that changes in the peripheral circuit are also important factors in the changes in output reported in patients with congestive heart failure.

How might the changes found in the peripheral circulation in euvolumic animals with normal hearts be modified when PEEP is applied in congestive heart failure? First, right atrial pressure might rise *less*. The lungs are less compliant, so stress on the surface of the heart would rise less for the same change in airway pressure. More of the lung is in zone III, so right ventricular afterload would rise less for the same change in alveolar pressure. Second, mean systemic pressure might rise *more*. The zone III lungs would displace more blood to the peripheral circulation, and, especially if the engorged circulation were less compliant, this would cause a greater rise in upstream venous pressure. Finally, because of the higher pressure in the central veins and the smaller rise in pressure on their surface, vascular waterfalls would be less likely to occur when PEEP is applied. Thus, the critical feature of congestive heart failure may be congestion, not heart failure, and the effects of PEEP on the heart may be of secondary importance to its effects on the circuit.

V. Conclusion

In the past decade, substantial new insight into the interaction between the circulatory and ventilatory pumps has emerged. In some areas, such the effects of inspiration on IVC flow, divergent findings are coalescing under unifying explanation. In other cases, such as the effects of PEEP on cardiac output, unifying explanations have been challenged by new findings. The clinical manipulation of pleural pressure to support the failing circulation has not yet become standard practice in the intensive care unit. Our previous optimistic prediction may have anticipated a longer interval between editions. Nonetheless, we have never been more optimistic that the circulatory effects of ventilation will be unraveled and understood by physiologist and clinician alike.

References

Ashton, J. H., and Cassidy, S. S. (1985). Reflex depression of cardiovascular function during lung inflation. *J. Appl. Physiol.*, 58:137–145.
Beyar, R., Hausknecht, M. J., Halperin, H. R., Yin, F. C. P., and Weisfeldt, M. L. (1987). Interaction between cardiac chambers and thoracic pressure in intact circulation. *Am. J. Physiol.*, 22:H1240–H1252.

Beyar, R., Halperin, H. R., Tsitlik, J. E., Guerci, A. D., Kass, D., Weisfeldt, M. L., and Chandra, N. C. (1989). Circulatory assistance by intrathoracic pressure variations: optimization and mechanisms studied by a mathematical model in relation to experimental data. *Circ. Res.*, 64:703–720.

Bradley, T. D., Halloway, R. M., McLaughlin, P. R., Ross, B. L., Walters, J., and Liu, P. P. (1992). Cardiac output response to continuous positive airway pressure in congestive heart failure. *Am. Rev. Respir. Dis.*, 145:377–382.

Braunwald, E., Binion, J. T., Morgan, Jr., W. L., and Sarnoff, S. J. (1957). Alterations in central blood volume and cardiac output induced by positive pressure breathing and counteracted by metaraminol (Aramine). *Circ. Res.*, 5:670–675.

Brecher, G. A. (1956). *Venous Return.* New York, Grune & Stratton.

Brower, R., Wise, R. A., Hassapoyannes, C., Bromberger-Barnea, B., and Permutt, S. (1985). Effect of lung inflation on lung blood volume and pulmonary venous flow. *J. Appl. Physiol.*, 58(3):954–963.

Burton, A. C., and Patel, D. J. (1958). Effect on pulmonary vascular resistance of inflation of the rabbit lungs. *J. Appl. Physiol.*, 12(2):239–246.

Caldini, P., Permutt, S., Waddell, J. A., and Riley, R. L. (1974). Effect of epinephrine on pressure, flow, and volume relationships in the systemic circulation of dogs. *Circ. Res.*, 34:606–623.

Cassidy, S. S., Mitchell, J. H., and Johnson, Jr., R. L. (1982). Dimensional analysis of right and left ventricles during positive-pressure ventilation in dogs. *Am. J. Physiol.*, 242:H549–H556.

Cournand, A., Motley, H. L., Werko, L., and Richards, Jr., D. W. (1948). Physiological studies of the effects of intermittent positive pressure breathing on cardiac output in man. *Am. J. Physiol.*, 152:162–174.

Fessler, H. E., Brower, R. G., Wise, R. A., and Permutt, S. (1988). Mechanism of reduced LV afterload by systolic and diastolic positive pleural pressure. *J. Appl. Physiol.*, 65(3):1244–1250.

Fessler, H., Brower, R. G., Wise, R. A., and Permutt, S. (1991). Effects of positive end-expiratory pressure on the gradient for venous return. *Am. Rev. Respir. Dis.*, 143:19–24.

Fessler, H. E., Brower, R. G., Wise, R. A., and Permutt, S. (1992). Effects of positive end-expiratory pressure on the canine venous return curve. *Am. Rev. Respir. Dis.*, 146:4–10.

Fessler, H. E., Brower, R. G., Shapiro, E. P., and Permutt, S. (1993). Effects of PEEP and body position on the pressure in the thoracic great veins. *Am. Rev. Respir. Dis.*, 148:1657–64.

Fewell, J. E., Abendschein, D. R., Carlson, C. J., Rapaport, E., and Murray, J. F. (1980). Mechanism of decreased right and left ventricular end-diastolic volumes during continuous positive-pressure ventilation in dogs. *Circ. Res.*, 47:467–472.

Greene, A. S., and Shoukas, A. A. (1986). Changes in canine cardiac function and venous return curves by the carotid baroreflex. *Am. J. Physiol.*, 251:H288–H296.

Guyton, A. C. (1955). Determination of cardiac output by equating venous return curves with cardiac response curves. *Physiol. Rev.*, 35:123–129.

Hughes, J. M. B., Glazier, J. B., Maloney, J. E., and West, J. B. (1968). Effect of extra-alveolar vessels on distribution of blood flow in the dog lung. *J. Appl. Physiol.*, 25:701–712.

Janicki, J. S., and Weber, K. T. (1980). The pericardium and ventricular interaction, distensibility, and function. *Am. J. Physiol.*, 238:H494–H503.

Jardin, F., Farcot, J-C., Boisante, L., Curien, N., Margairaz, A., and Bourdarias, J-P. (1981). Influence of positive end-expiratory pressure on left ventricular performance. *NEJM*, 304:387–392.

Lemaire, F., Teboul, J-L., Cinotti, L., Giotto, G., Abrouk, F., Steg, G., Macquin-Mavier, I., and Zapol, W. M. (1988). Acute left ventricular dysfunction during unsuccessful weaning from mechanical ventilation. *Anesthesiology*, 69:171–179.

Lloyd, T. C., Jr. (1983). Effect of inspiration on inferior vena caval blood flow in dogs. *J. Appl. Physiol.: Respir. Environ. Exerc. Physiol.*, 55(6):1701–1708.

Lopez-Muniz, R., Stevens, B., Bromberger-Barnea, B., Permutt, S., and Riley, R. L. (1968). *J. Appl. Physiol.*, 24:625–635.

Manny, J., Grindlinger, G., Mathe, A. A., and Hechtman, H. B. (1978). Positive end-expiratory pressure, lung stretch, and decreased myocardial contractility. *Surgery*, 84:127–133.

Marini, J. J., Culver, B. H., and Butler, J. (1981a). Mechanical effect of lung distention with positive pressure on cardiac function. *Am. Rev. Respir. Dis.*, 124:382–386.

Marini, J. J., Culver, B. H., and Butler, J. (1981b). Effect of positive end-expiratory pressure on canine ventricular function curves. *J. Appl. Physiol.: Respir. Environ. Exerc. Physiol.*, 51:1367–1374.

Mathru, M., Tadikonda, L. K. R., El-Etr, A., and Pifarre, R. (1982). Hemodynamic response to changes in ventilatory patterns in patients with normal and poor left ventricular reserve. *Crit. Care Med.*, 10:423–426.

Mead, J., Takishima, T., and Leith, D. (1970). Stress distribution in lungs: a model of pulmonary elasticity. *J. Appl. Physiol.*, 28(5):596–608.

Moreno, A. H., Burchell, A. R., Van Der Woude, R., and Burke, J. H. (1967). Respiratory regulation of splanchnic and systemic venous return. *Am. J. Physiol.*, 213(2):455–465.

Nakhjavan, F. K., Palmer, W., and McGregor, M. (1966). Influence of respiration on venous return in pulmonary emphysema. *Circulation*, 33:8–16.

Nanas, S., and Magder, S. (1992). Adaptations of the peripheral circulation to PEEP. *Am. Rev. Respir. Dis.*, 146:688–693.

Permutt, S., Howell, J. B. L., Proctor, D. F., and Riley, R. L. (1961). Effect of lung inflation on static pressure-volume characteristics of pulmonary vessels. *J. Appl. Physiol.*, 160(I):64–70.

Permutt, S., and Riley, R. L. (1963). Hemodynamics of collapsible vessels with tone: the vascular waterfall. *J. Appl. Physiol.*, 18:924–932.

Permutt, S. (1973). Psychologic changes in the acute asthmatic attack. In *Asthma: Physiology, Immunopharmacology and Treatment*. Edited by K. F. Austen and L. M. Lichtenstein. New York, Academic Press, Inc., pp. 15–27.

Permutt, S., and Caldini, P. (1978). Regulation of cardiac output by the circuit: venous return. In *Cardiovascular System Dynamics*. Edited by J. Baan, A. Noordergraaf, and J. Raines. Cambridge, Mass., The MIT Press, pp. 465–479.

Peters, J., Kindred, M. K., and Robotham, J. L. (1988a). Transient analysis of cardiopulmonary interactions I. Diastolic events. *J. Appl. Physiol.*, 64(4):1506–1517.

Peters, J., Kindred, M. K., and Robotham, J. L. (1988b). Transient analysis of cardiopulmonary interactions II. Systolic events. *J. Appl. Physiol.*, 64(4):1518–1526.

Peters, J., Fraser, C., Stuart, R. S., Baumgartner, W., and Robotham, J. L. (1989). Negative intrathoracic pressure decreases independently left ventricular filling and emptying. *Am. J. Physiol.*, 257:H120–H131.

Pinsky, M. R., Matuschak, G. M., Bernardi, L., and Klain, M. (1986). Hemodynamic effects of cardiac cycle-specific increases in intrathoracic pressure. *J. Appl. Physiol.*, 60(2):604–612.

Regen, D. M. (1990). Calculation of left ventricular wall stress. *Circ. Res.*, 67:245–252.

Robotham, J. L., Rabson, J., Permutt, S., and Bromberger-Barnea, B. (1979). Left ventricular hemodynamics during respiration. *J. Appl. Physiol.*, 47(6):1295–1303.

Robotham, J. L., Badke, F. R., Kindred, M. K., and Beaton, M. K. (1983). Regional left ventricular performance during normal and obstructed spontaneous respiration. *J. Appl. Physiol.*, 55(2):569–577.

Rothe, C. F. (1993). Mean circulatory filling pressure: its meaning and measurement. *J. Appl. Physiol.*, 74:499–509.

Scharf, S. M., Caldini, P., and Ingram, Jr., R. H. (1977). Cardiovascular effects of increasing airway pressure in the dog. *Am. J. Physiol.*, 232:H35–H43.

Scharf, S. M., and Ingram, Jr., R. H. (1977). Influence of abdominal pressure and sympathetic vasoconstriction on the cardiovascular response to positive end-expiratory pressure. *Am. Rev. Respir. Dis.*, 116:661–670.

Scharf, S. M., Brown, N., and Saunders, N. (1979). Effects of normal and loaded spontaneous inspiration on cardiovascular function. *J. Appl. Physiol.: Respir. Environ. Exerc. Physiol.*, 47:582–590.

Stein, K. L., Kramer, D. J., Killian, A., and Pinsky, M. R. (1990). Hemodynamic effects of synchronous high-frequency jet ventilation in mitral regurgitation. *J. Appl. Physiol.*, 69(6):2120–2125.

Suga, H., Sagawa, K., and Shoukas, A. A. (1973). Load independence of the instantaneous pressure-volume ratio of the canine left ventricle and effects of epinephrine and heart rate on the ratio. *Circ. Res.*, 32:314–322.

Suga, H., and Sagawa, K. (1974). Instantaneous pressure-volume relationships and their ratio in the excised, supported canine left ventricle. *Circ. Res.*, 35:117–126.

Summer, W. R., Permutt, S., Sagawa, K., Shoukas, A. A., and Bromberger-Barnea, B. (1979). Effects of spontaneous respiration on canine left ventricular function. *Circ. Res.*, 45:719–728.

Takata, M., Wise, R. A., and Robotham, J. L. (1990). Effects of abdominal pressure on venous return: abdominal vascular zone conditions. *J. Appl. Physiol.*, 69(6):1961–1972.

Takata, M., and Robotham, J. L. (1992). Effects of inspiratory diaphragmatic descent on inferior vena caval venous return. *J. Appl. Physiol.*, 72(2):597–607.

Tittley, J. G., Fremes, S. E., Weisel, R. D., Christakis, G. T., Evans, P. J., Madonik, M., Ivanov, J., Teasdale, S. J., Mickle, D. A. G., and McLaughlin, P. R. (1985). Hemodynamic and myocardial metabolic consequences of PEEP. *Chest*, 88:496–502.

Veddeng, O. J., Myhre, E. S. P., Risoe, C., and Smiseth, O. A. (1992). Selective positive end-expiratory pressure and intracardiac dimensions in dogs. *J. Appl. Physiol.*, 73(5):2016–2020.

Wead, W. B., and Norton, J. F. (1981). Effects of intrapleural pressure changes on canine left ventricular function. *J. Appl. Physiol.: Respir. Environ. Exerc. Physiol.*, 50:1027–1035.

Wexler, L., Bergel, D. H., Gabe, I. T., and Makin, G. S. (1968). Velocity of blood flow in normal human venae cavae. *Circ. Res.*, 23:349–359.

Willeput, R., Rondeux, C., and DeTroyer, A. (1984). Breathing affects venous return from legs in humans. *J. Appl. Physiol.: Respir. Environ. Exerc. Physiol.*, 57(4):971–976.

Wise, R. A., Robotham, J. L., Bromberger-Barnea, B., and Permutt, S. (1981). Effect of PEEP on left ventricular function in right-heart-bypassed dogs. *J. Appl. Physiol.: Respir. Environ. Exerc. Physiol.*, 51(3):541–546.

58

Cardiopulmonary Resuscitation

SHELDON MAGDER

Royal Victoria Hospital
McGill University
Montreal, Quebec, Canada

ROBERT A. WISE

Johns Hopkins University School of Medicine
Baltimore, Maryland

I. Introduction

Sudden cardiac death continues to be a leading cause of death in industrialized developed countries (Lown, 1979), and therefore means to support patients until normal circulation can be restored is of great clinical importance (Niemann, 1992). Although the mortality during CPR remains high, both in and out of hospitals (Eisenberg et al., 1979, 1980, 1982; Bedell et al., 1983), a significant proportion of patients can still be resuscitated and return to normal lives. In particular, the long-term prognosis for patients who survive the first 24 hours after cardiac arrest is very good. For example, Eisenberg et al. (1982) found that at 4 years postdischarge, the probability of survival was 49%, which compares very favorably with 66% for patients who suffer an acute myocardial infarction without cardiac arrest. The most important variables that contribute to survival are the time to initiation of therapy and the time to definitive care (Eisenberg et al., 1979, 1980, 1982). If CPR is initiated in less than 4 minutes and definitive therapy within 8 minutes, both short-term and long-term survivals are much better than if longer periods of time are taken. This emphasizes the need for techniques that maximize the "artificial" circulation produced during CPR. Maximizing success with CPR requires a good understanding of the basic physiology of artificial circulation and the metabolic changes that occur during the period of circulatory arrest. Therefore, after a brief historical summary of CPR, this chapter will review the physiology of defibrillation, generation of blood flow, role of bicarbonate and acid-base balance, and finally the role of various pharmacological agents.

II. Brief History

The history of CPR has been covered in a number of recent reviews (Kouwenhoven et al., 1960; Wise and Summer, 1983, 1988; DeBard, 1980; Paraskos, 1993), and only a few major landmarks will be considered. The AHA recommendations for basic life support always start with "airway" and "breathing." The potential for mouth-to-mouth breathing to provide artificial ventilatory support was recognized as early as 1740 by the Academy of Science of Paris, which certified mouth-to-mouth breathing as the treatment of choice for drowning. This approach subsequently was abandoned in favor of techniques that employ chest compression and passive recoil of the chest for ventilation. It was argued that expired gas concentrations might be inadequate for oxygenation, although I suspect that esthetic concerns over the use of "mouth-to-mouth" breathing may also have been a factor. In the 1950s, Safar and Bircher (1988) established the superiority of mouth-to-mouth ventilation over armlift techniques, and it is now no longer debated that ventilation should be provided by positive pressure ventilation, whether from the mouth of a resuscitator or by a bag mask ventilator. Oxygen fraction of normal expired O_2 is 0.17–0.18 and therefore more than adequate for oxygenation. We will not dwell further on the ventilatory aspects of CPR, for the physiology is not different from ventilation under any other circumstance.

Artificial circulatory support lagged behind the development of ventilatory support. Early animal experiments showed that chest compressions could produce blood flow (DeBard, 1980; Wise and Summer, 1988; Paraskos, 1993), but these did not receive much attention, possibly because the heart could not be defibrillated and without this there was no need to temporarily support the circulation. The major advance occurred with the report by Zoll and coworkers, who showed that ventricular fibrillation could be reversed with an external countershock (Zoll et al., 1956). This made it possible to defibrillate the heart, and it became necessary to develop temporary means of artificially sustaining the circulation until the heart could be defibrillated. Until the 1960s this was done by open chest direct compression of the heart. The present approach of closed-chest CPR began with a fortuitous event. Kouwenhaven noted a rise in arterial pressure of dogs every time the defibrillator paddles were applied with a great force (Kouwenhoven et al., 1960). In association with Knickerbocker and Jude, he developed the present-day approach of external chest compression (Kouwenhoven et al., 1960). The combination of mouth-to-mouth breathing and external chest compression became the standard for basic life support in 1966, although the precise mechanism of blood flow generation is still debated.

III. Defibrillation

Ventricular fibrillation is a state where depolarization of the ventricular myocytes occurs in a disorganized, nonuniform pattern. Energy demands of the muscle thus remain high, but no effective mechanical output is produced by the heart. Although there are multiple factors that lead to ventricular fibrillation, probably an important final pathway in the pathophysiology is the accumulation of calcium in the muscle (Billman, 1992). A major factor for this is increased catecholamine release from sympathetic nerves as well as exogenously administered catecholamines and a decrease in parasympathetic activity, all of which contribute to increased intracellular calcium. Increased intracellular calcium alters impulse generation and conduction. In particular, the increased calcium can be produced both early and late after depolarizations, which can lead to triggered activity. Furthermore, the increased intracellular calcium interferes with intercellular conduction through gap junctions and may contribute to the random irregular reentry circuits that are necessary for ventricular defibrillation. This build-up of calcium in the cell must be kept in mind when considering the use of intravenous calcium injections during resuscitation. It also raises the possible use of calcium blockers during CPR; however, these are unlikely to be of help, for although they decrease the tendency for arrhythmias, they decrease cardiac contractility, which can become a problem when the circulation is restored.

Another crucial factor during ventricular defibrillation and the consequent myocardial ischemia is the leakage of potassium from the cells. This makes the chance of depolarization of the muscle progressively less. This also might explain the progressive decrease in the amplitude of ventricular fibrillation waves during the course of arrest. Extracellular potassium can only be removed if there is some coronary blood flow, and this might explain the importance of maintaining at least a minimum coronary perfusion pressure. Thus the removal of potassium by restored coronary flow could potentially be more important than the provision of oxygen.

The success of CPR ultimately depends upon the ability to defibrillate the heart, and the faster this is accomplished, the better the results (Kerber and Sarnat, 1979; Eisenberg et al., 1979, 1980; Crampton, 1980; Gadzinski et al., 1982). Defibrillation in less than 8 minutes gives the best chance for resuscitation.

Hypoxia and acidosis decrease the efficacy of defibrillation, and therefore a delay in the onset of CPR is an important prognostic factor (Kerber and Sarnat, 1979). For this reason, the American Heart Association (AHA) recommends that chest compressions be performed for 2–3 minutes before defibrillation in an unwitnessed arrest (1980). This potentially increases myocardial oxygenation and decreases acidosis because tissue P_{CO2} is an important part of the tissue acidosis and will decrease as flow is increased (Von Planta et al., 1989; Gudipati et al., 1990). As noted above, compressions may also help clear potassium from the interstitial space.

Defibrillation was originally performed with AC current, but this was superseded by DC current. The first reason is practical, since DC current can be obtained from a portable unit, whereas AC current requires a constant source from the wall. DC current also allows a better quantitation of the energy and is of less risk to bystanders.

An important factor in defibrillation is the energy delivered, which is the product of the voltage and current (amperage). The amount of energy that gets to the chest is determined by the resistance between the energy source and the heart (Adgey et al., 1979; Tacker and Ewy, 1979; Kerber et al., 1981; Crampton, 1980; Safar and Bircher, 1988). This can be decreased by increasing the paddle size, but, if they are too large, the density of charge is decreased. Gelled or soaked pads also help to decrease the resistance. Pressing hard on the chest wall decreases thoracic impedance by decreasing the thoracic volume. A sufficient mass of myocardium must be depolarized to convert ventricular fibrillation. Thus, the paddles must be sufficiently far apart to make sure that the heart is exposed to the current and that the current does not simply travel from paddle to paddle. To achieve this, the paddles should be placed along the upper right sternal border and over the apex of the heart.

There has been a lot of debate on the appropriate amount of energy required for defibrillation and whether body size is of importance in determining the energy needed (Adgey et al., 1979; Tacker and Ewy, 1979; Kerber and Sarnat, 1979; Kerber et al., 1981). It is important to appreciate that it should not be assumed that the energy needed for resuscitation is proportional to body weight, as is the case for most pharmacological agents. The electrical current used for defibrillation only goes through a circumscribed part of the body, and therefore would not be expected to be related to total body weight except in some very nonlinear manner. In animal studies, the energy requirements vary considerably and do not seem to depend on the animal size, but rather on the species. This has been well reviewed by Crampton (1935), who points out that the evidence for improved efficiency with higher levels is probably influenced by the diagnosis of the patients. Furthermore, although outcome is worse in heavier individuals than in lighter individuals, the defibrillation rate is the same and the difference in outcome more likely relates to the difficulty of performing CPR. Thus, it does not appear that the energy must be increased for larger individuals.

An important study by Weaver et al. (1990) showed that two shocks with low energy (175 J), followed by a third with high energy (320 J), if necessary, produced equal results to three high-energy shocks. A critical variable in the delivery of the energy to the heart is the impedance of the chest wall, and defibrillators have been designed that can measure this and then allow better quantitation of the energy needs (Kerber et al., 1984). By and large, however, the risks of myocardial damage with 175 J appears low, and the approach suggested by Weaver et al. is very practical. Of interest, there has recently been a report of defibrillation with an esophageal electrode that requires less energy (Adgey et al., 1991) and could therefore allow a smaller power source, as long as the operator is certain that the electrode is in the esophagus!

IV. Generation of Blood Flow

Kouwenhaven et al. (1960) thought that the mechanism of blood flow during closed-chest CPR was direct compression of the heart between the sternum and spine. Indeed, they called the technique closed-chest cardiac massage. This explanation requires that the force be preferentially transmitted to the ventricles so that ventricular pressures increase more than atrial pressures and close the atrioventricular valves. This is called the *cardiac pump theory*. If this is the correct explanation for blood flow in CPR, then the location of chest compressions is important.

In 1980, Rudicoff and associates noted that it is difficult to generate a pulse pressure during CPR in patients with flail chests, despite the fact that it is easier to directly compress their hearts. They proposed that the mechanism of blood flow in CPR is therefore the generation of intrathoracic pressure and that CPR fails in patients with flail chests because intrathoracic pressure cannot be increased. According to this theory, compression of the chest increases the pressure throughout the chest and all the intrathoracic blood volume is compressed and ejected. Backward flow is prevented by valves in the superior vena cava (Fisher et al., 1982), and a greater potential for the veins to collapse than the arteries exists with the rise in intrathoracic pressure. This is called the *thoracic pump model*. If this theory is correct, blood flow in CPR will be improved by increasing intrathoracic pressure. Which of these two theories, i.e., cardiac pump or thoracic pump, is correct continues to be debated (Babbs, 1980a; Redding et al., 1981; Bircher and Safar, 1981; Babbs et al., 1984b; Weisfeldt and Halperin, 1986; Wexler and Gelb, 1986; Guerci and Weisfeldt, 1986; Newton et al., 1988; Chandra, 1993).

Before discussing the mechanisms of the generation of blood flow in CPR, it is useful to review the generation of blood flow by the beating heart. The beating heart ejects blood essentially by a rapid decrease in ventricular compliance during systole. Sagawa called this a "time-varying elastance" (Sagawa, 1978). Increasing stiffness of the ventricle results in a progressive rise in intraventricular pressure, which eventually ejects blood from the ventricle when the ventricular pressure exceeds the aortic pressure and the aortic valve opens. Backward flow is prevented by the atrioventricular valves. The aortic pressure remains elevated in diastole because of the discharge of the compliant volume of the aorta, reflected waves, and the time taken for blood to drain through the arterial resistance. It is important to remember that the pressure generated by the ventricles and the volume ejected are dependent upon the degree of filling of the ventricles (i.e., Frank-Starling mechanism), the afterload, which is a function of aortic pressure, and cardiac contractility. Furthermore, a large part of the return of blood to the heart takes place during the ventricular ejection phase because the atrial pressures normally remain low relative to the ventricular pressures. The factors that determine the return of blood to the heart are the determinants of venous return, which include the stressed volume of the vasculature, venous compliance, resistance to venous return, the distribution of blood flow, and right atrial pressure (assuming that the right atrial pressure is greater than zero and greater than pleural pressure) (Magder, 1992).

No matter which model of CPR is correct (i.e., thoracic pump or cardiac pump), some common basic principles apply to the generation of flow. Flow occurs when a pressure gradient develops between two loci, whether this pressure difference is created by direct cardiac compression or compression of intrathoracic blood volume by an increase in intrathoracic pressure. There must also be a volume of blood that can be transferred by this pressure difference; this is the left ventricular volume in the direct cardiac compression model and intrapulmonary and cardiac volumes in the thoracic pump model. There must be a mechanism that allows only unidirectional flow. This is the atrioventricular valves in the cardiac compression model and venous valves and venous collapse in the thoracic pump model. There must be a mechanism for venous return, which essentially results in a gradient in pressure from the periphery to the right atrium. In the direct cardiac compression model, this occurs with the release of the compression of the ventricles and by the decrease in intrathoracic pressure in the thoracic pump model.

Before developing the analysis of the circulation during CPR, some theoretical considerations about flow in general must be reviewed. Blood flow has traditionally been described by Poiseuille's law in terms of pressures and resistances:

$$\dot{Q} = \Delta P/R$$

An apparent exception to this occurs in maximal flow regimes through collapsible tubes where the downstream pressure has no effect on flow (Permutt and Riley, 1963). This has been well studied during forced expiration from the lung and venous return to the heart (Guyton et al., 1956; Permutt et al., 1988) and blood flow to the dog hindlimb (Magder, 1990). During such flow-limited conditions, flow can be described by the pressure difference between the recoil pressure of the upstream compliance (P_{ST}) and the critical transmural closing pressure of the conduit (P_{TM}). The effective resistance, then, is only the upstream resistance (R_s). Thus:

$$\dot{Q} = \frac{P_{ST} - P_{TM}'}{R_S}$$

The static recoil pressure, in turn, is determined by the volume of the system and the elastic properties of the compartment.

In the following analysis, we use a concept that simplifies the analysis and applies to simple as well as complex models of blood flow in both flow-limited and non–flow-limited regimes. We describe steady-state flow as the relationship between a finite *potentially mobile volume* (Vm) and the *time constant* (τ) of its transfer. This simplifies the analysis, allows experimental measurement of pertinent characteristics of the system without regard to the particular flow regime, and has the esthetic advantage of describing flow in the units in which it is measured—*volume* and *time*.

In short, steady-state flow under isovolume conditions for a variety of model systems can be described by $\dot{Q} = Vm/\tau$, where Vm is the *mobile volume* of the system, that is, the volume that would drain out of the system if it were not replenished and were allowed to empty to equilibrium. τ is the time constant of the transfer of that volume. This relationship can be illustrated for flow against a constant downstream pressure (Pd) from an upstream reservoir with pressure Pu and compliance Cu over a resistance R. Thus:

$$\dot{Q} = \frac{Pu - Pd}{R}$$

$$= \frac{CuPu - PdCu}{RCu}$$

$$= \frac{Vu - CuPd}{\tau}$$

$$= \frac{Vm}{\tau}$$

It will be seen that term (Vu – CuPd) is the volume that would leave the upstream reservoir if allowed to empty and RCu is the time constant of that flow draining in an exponential fashion.

Similarly, in a flow-limited regime:

$$\dot{Q} = \frac{P_{ST} - P_{TM}'}{R_S}$$

$$= \frac{V_{ST} - P_{TM}'Cu}{R_{SCu}}$$

$$= \frac{Vm}{\tau}$$

where Vm again reflects the volume of the system that would empty if allowed to do so and τ is the time constant of its transfer. R_s in this condition reflects only the resistance upstream to the collapsible segment.

If one reservoir with compliance Cu and pressure Pu is allowed to empty into a second reservoir with compliance Cd and pressure Pd across a resistance R, then:

$$\dot{Q} = \frac{Pu - Pd}{R}$$

$$= \frac{PuCu}{RCu} - \frac{Vd}{RCd}$$

$$= \frac{Vu}{RCu} - \frac{Vd}{RCd}$$

$$= \frac{Vu}{RCu} - \frac{V - Vu}{RCd} \quad \text{where } V = Vu + Vd$$

$$= Vu\left(\frac{1}{RCu} + \frac{1}{RCd}\right) - V\left(\frac{1}{RCd}\right)$$

$$= \frac{Vu - \dfrac{VCu}{Cu + Cd}}{\dfrac{RcuCd}{Cu + Cd}}$$

$$= \frac{Vm}{\tau}$$

where

$$Vu - \frac{VCu}{Cu + Cd} = Vm$$

and

$$\frac{RCuCd}{Cu + Cd} = \tau$$

V. Application of Blood Flow Theory to CPR

Based on these principles, Wise and coworkers (Wise and Summer, 1983, 1988; Permutt et al., 1988) developed a theoretical model to analyze blood flow in CPR and tested many of the predictions of their analysis (Fig. 1). These workers support the thoracic pump model, but their analysis still applies to any closed-chest CPR model, although there are different implications for open chest massage, which will be discussed later. We will fully develop this analysis because it provides a very useful tool for predicting the effects on flow of changes in rate, duration of compression, volume, and changes in intrathoracic pressure.

In this approach, the circulation is considered to have two compliant regions; one contains the thoracic blood volume and the other contains the peripheral volume. The thoracic volume is surrounded by the pleural pressure. These two compliant compartments are connected by two conduits (arterial and venous circuits) with characteristics of resistance and collapsibility. The direction of flow is determined by one-way valves in each conduit. When flow is stopped, the pressure is the same throughout the system and determined by the sum of the two compliances and stressed volume. An increase in pressure around the thoracic compartment (Ppl), whether this be the left ventricle in the cardiac pump model or pleural pressure around the pulmonary blood volume in the thoracic pump model, produces a gradient from the thorax to the periphery, which generates flow and transfers volume from the thoracic compliant region to the peripheral region. The pressure thus rises in the peripheral region. Relaxation of the thoracic pressure, whether it be the ventricular pressure in the direct compression model, or pleural pressure with the

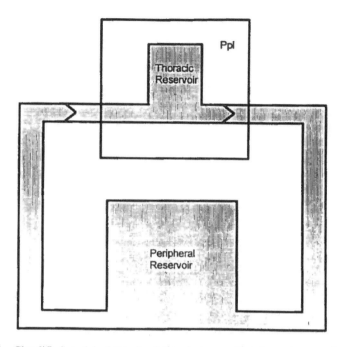

Figure 1 Simplified model of the circulation during cardiopulmonary resuscitation. The circulation consists of two reservoirs connected by collapsible conduits with valves to facilitate flow in one direction. The thoracic reservoir is surrounded by the thorax, which is pressurized by elevations in pleural pressure (Ppl). When the thorax is pressurized, blood flows from the thorax to the periphery. When the pressure is released, it returns to the thorax.

thoracic pump model, allows flow to return from the peripheral compartment back to the thoracic compartment. An equation can be developed from the analysis above to mathematically predict flow and is based on the following (see Appendix):

1. The total volume change that can occur in the thoracic compartment if it is first allowed to fill to equilibrium during the filling condition and then empty to equilibrium during the emptying phase by compression (Vm)
2. The time constant of emptying, τe, which is the product of the resistance and compliance of the arterial circuit
3. The time constant of filling, τf, which is the product of venous resistance and compliance
4. The fraction of the total cycle, α, spent in the emptying phase, which is also called the duty cycle (α thus equals te/te + tf, where te is the time of emptying and tf is the time of filling
5. The fraction of the cycle spent in the filling phase, $1 - \alpha$

Since time is required for filling and emptying, as is given by the time constants τe and τf, and these events must occur independently, not all Vm will be available for flow if the filling and emptying phases are not long enough. This model also assumes that stroke volume is small compared to the total volume of the regions, and therefore their pressures remain nearly constant.

$$\dot{Q} = \frac{Vm}{\tau e/\alpha + \tau f(1-\alpha)} \tag{1}$$

where $\dot{Q}$ is flow in liters/min. The final $\dot{Q}$ will thus be reduced if α is insufficient to allow adequate emptying. This is especially important if τe is long.

It can also be shown that flow will be optimal when:

$$\alpha = \frac{\sqrt{\tau_E}}{(\sqrt{\tau_E} + \sqrt{\tau_F})}$$

or

$$\frac{te}{tf} = \sqrt{\frac{\tau_E}{\tau_F}}$$

Maximum blood flow at this optimum duty cycle is:

$$\dot{Q}_{max} = \frac{Vm}{(\sqrt{\tau_E} + \sqrt{\tau_F})^2} \tag{2}$$

The volume that can be displaced, Vm, is determined by the difference in pressure in the thoracic compartment during the emptying and filling phases, whether this is the heart in the cardiac pump model or the thoracic volume in the thoracic pump model. It is also determined by the compliances of the peripheral and thoracic compartments, for these values determine how much volume is stored in each region at a given pressure. The formal equation for this is:

$$Vm = (Pple - Pplf)\frac{CtCp}{(Ct + Cp)} \tag{3}$$

where Ct is the thoracic compliance, Cp is the peripheral compliance, and Pple and Pplf are the cardiac or thoracic pressures during emptying and filling, respectively.

The time constants of emptying and filling depend upon the arterial and venous resistances and compliances. The formal equations for these are:

$$\tau e = Ra\frac{CtCp}{(Ct + Cp)} \tag{4}$$

$$\tau f = Rv\frac{CtCp}{(Ct + Cp)} \tag{5}$$

Thus, the higher the resistance or the greater the compliance, the longer it takes to empty or fill the thoracic compartment.

Figure 2 describes blood flow in this model as a function of duty cycle for various values of τ_E, expressed as a proportion of τ_F in arbitrary units. $\dot{Q}$ is expressed

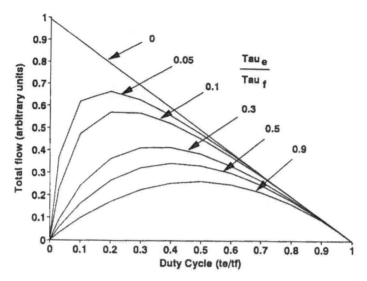

Figure 2 Effect of duty cycle on total blood flow during CPR. Flow is in arbitrary units, with a maximum flow of 1 unit. Each isopleth indicates different ratios of the time constant of emptying (Tau$_e$) to the time constant of filling (Tau$_f$) achieved by shortening Tau$_e$ at constant Tau$_f$. As the Tau$_e$ is reduced, for a constant Tau$_f$, there is an increase in flow at any fixed duty cycle. As Tau$_f$ falls, the optimum duty cycle shifts to smaller values. When Tau$_e$ equals 0, the limiting condition, blood flow is maximized with a duty cycle that allows continuous filling, equivalent to the condition of the pumping heart.

as a proportion of Vm/ τ_F. It can be seen that as τ_E is reduced, the optimum duty cycle shifts toward shorter optimum compression times. Furthermore, for any given duty cycle, a reduction in τ_E causes an increase in flow. As τ_E approaches O, the $\dot{Q}_{max} \rightarrow$ Vm/τ_F, that is, blood flow is limited only by venous return. This maximum theoretical blood flow is equal to the blood flow that occurs during spontaneous circulation with a "perfect" heart, which maintains zero right atrial pressure and minimal pulmonary blood volume. It is also clear that any maneuver that increases the absolute value of Vm or decreases τ_F will likewise increase absolute blood flow.

The above analysis assumed that the conduits were rigid tubes and not collapsible. However, both the arteries and veins are collapsible if the surrounding pressures are sufficiently high (Permutt and Riley, 1963). This occurs when the pressures across the wall, i.e., the transmural pressure, are close to zero in the veins and at a negative value for the more rigid arteries (Yin et al., 1982). When collapse occurs, it should be emphasized that this does not stop flow, but limits any further increase in flow when the downstream pressure is decreased. When flow limitation occurs due to collapse, the total volume of the system becomes an important determinant of Vm, along with the transmural pressures at which collapse occurs. The formal equation for this is:

$$Vm = V - (Ptm'a\ Ct) - (Ptm'v\ Cp) \tag{6}$$

where Ptm'a and Ptm'v are the collapse pressures of the arterial and venous conduits. The Ptm'v is close to zero, whereas Ptm'a is a negative number. Under these circumstances, the time constants of emptying and filling are solely determined by the compliances of the thoracic and peripheral compartments and the resistances up to the point of collapse, Ra' and Rv', respectively. This can be formally written as:

$$\tau e = Ra'\ Ct \tag{7}$$

$$\tau f = Rv'\ Cp \tag{8}$$

We can now compare some of the factors in the generation of blood flow with CPR to blood flow with normal cardiac function. A major difference occurs in the way blood returns to the heart. Closed-chest compressions elevate pleural pressure during the ejection of blood, and thus blood can only return to the heart during the relaxation phase. This is why both τe and τf occur in the denominator of Eq. (1). In contrast, blood returns to the beating heart during both systole and diastole (Wise and Summer, 1983, 1988).

The arrested heart also cannot respond to changes in preload. The displaced volume, Vm, is directly proportional to the difference between the pleural pressure during emptying and filling, and the pleural pressure during emptying is totally dependent upon the operator. There is no feedback that can alter Pple and Pplf to the volume returning to the heart. In contrast, in the beating heart, the volume that returns to the heart determines the end-diastolic pressure, which directly affects the pressure generated by the heart and the volume ejected.

The contractility of the arrested heart is also fixed, except for some variation in the force applied by the operator. In contrast, in the beating heart, neurohumeral mechanisms adjust cardiac contractility to the needs of the body.

Except with open chest direct cardiac massage, the intrathoracic pressure must rise during CPR, whether the mechanism of blood flow is an increase in pleural pressure or direct cardiac compression. This can lead to collapse of the arteries and produce the condition of flow limitation (Yin et al., 1982). This never occurs with the normal contracting heart except perhaps during rapid ejection in hypertrophic cardiomyopathies. The absence or presence of flow limitation also determines the response to volume loading. When flow limitation is not present, increasing the volume of the heart or thorax does not increase the volume ejected, for this is simply a function of the pressures applied to the heart or chest and the compliances of the compartments [Eq. (2)]. However, when the pressure in the chest is high enough to produce flow limitation, then increasing blood volume can increase the maximal flow [Eq. (5)].

VI. Thoracic Pump Versus Direct Compression Models

The original terminology indicated the bias of the investigators, for the technique was called closed-chest cardiac massage (Kouwenhoven et al., 1960). However, there is little doubt that blood flow can be generated without cardiac compressions. This was first dramatically demonstrated by Criley and coworkers, who showed that coughing could sustain sufficient cardiac output to maintain the circulation and keep patients alive for close to a minute (Fig. 3) (Criley et al., 1976; Niemann et al., 1985). This still remains a very useful technique in the cardiac catheterization laboratory, where the cardiac arrest is immediately witnessed and continued coughing can provide sufficient time to prepare for defibrillation.

The ability of increases in intrathoracic pressure to produce blood flow with direct cardiac compressions was also confirmed by Wise and coworkers, who showed that blood flow could be generated in an isolated heart-lung preparation in a sealed plexiglass box by changing the pressures in the box (Wise and Summer, 1983, 1988; Hausknecht et al., 1986). Passerini et al. (1988) were also able to document carotid blood flow in a dog model in which a plaster cast was placed around the thorax and abdomen and the lungs were inflated with a specially designed ventilator that produced a square wave of intrathoracic pressure.

Just because these studies demonstrate that blood flow can be generated without cardiac compression does not mean that cardiac compressions do not play a role. Much of the evidence raised in support of the cardiac compression model comes from studies on the pattern of movement of cardiac valves. The thoracic pump model predicts that the pulmonary blood volume is mobilized during chest compression, which means that blood should flow from the pulmonary vessels through the cardiac chambers to the aorta and to the rest of the body. Thus, this model predicts that the mitral and aortic valves would be open during chest

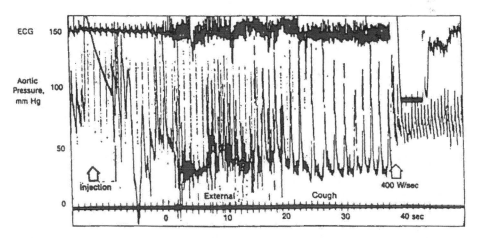

Figure 3 Electrocardiogram and aortic pressure in a patient who went into ventricular fibrillation following a right coronary injection for angiography. Patient remained conscious for 39 seconds with external followed by cough-induced cardiopulmonary resuscitation, and conversion to sinus rhythm was achieved with 400 W/s shock. (From Criley et al., 1976.)

compression. In contrast, the cardiac pump mechanism requires that the mitral valve be closed during cardiac compression, lest there be retrograde flow. Advocates of the thoracic pump model have indeed shown angiographic and echocardiographic data to support the contention that the mitral valve is open during chest compression (Rich et al., 1981; Werner et al., 1981; Cohen et al., 1982). However, proponents of the cardiac pump model have also shown evidence that the mitral valve is closed during chest compression (Feneley et al., 1987; Deshmukh et al., 1989). These studies thus also fail to definitively distinguish between these two theories. Angiographic studies are also contradictory. Some have shown that cardiac chambers are not compressed during CPR (Niemann et al., 1981, 1984; Cohen et al., 1982; Fisher et al., 1982), whereas others have shown that they are (Babbs, 1980b; Feneley et al., 1987). It should be appreciated that even if angiographic and echocardiographic studies show that the mitral valve closes during chest compression, this does not prove the cardiac pump theory. To begin with, visualization of valves cannot determine whether flow stops through the valve, for even though the atrioventricular valves look closed, there still could be a small opening that allows flow. It is also possible that ventricular volume empties faster than the pulmonary volume because it is compressed first, which gives the appearance that the heart has collapsed and the valves closed. This could occur if compressions are directed over the heart but can also occur simply from an increase in intrathoracic pressure as demonstrated by Halperin et al. (1988). These investigators demonstrated that increases in intrathoracic pressure with open airway result in greater compression of the left ventricle than the left atrium. They found that the higher pressures in the left ventricle can close the mitral valve even without direct sternal compression of the heart. This is thought to occur because the left atrial pressure is more reflective of alveolar pressure, which does not rise as much as pleural pressure if the airway is open. They also observed retrograde flow, i.e., from the left ventricle to the left atrium, with increases in intrathoracic pressure and open airway. This did not occur when the lungs were inflated, and thus the airway was not open.

A further piece of evidence to indicate that the atrioventricular valves are not closed during CPR is that the peak right atrial pressure equals the peak aortic pressure in CPR (Einagel et al., 1988), and therefore there is no pressure gradient to close the atrioventricular valve. A very elegant approach to this controversy was presented by Guerci et al. (1989), who compared the rise in pressure in the ascending and descending aorta to the rise in aortic flow. They found that during sinus rhythm or internal cardiac massage, the ascending aortic pressure and flow rose together and the rise in the ascending aortic pressure preceded the rise in descending aortic pressure. In contrast, during conventional manual CPR, vest CPR, or high impulse manual CPR, the ascending aorta flow lagged behind the initial rise in aortic pressure, and the ascending and descending aortic pressures increased simultaneously. Furthermore, the aortic diameter decreased during vest and high impulse CPR. Based on the weight of all the above evidence, we would have to conclude that changes in intrathoracic pressure are the primary determinants of flow in CPR and not direct cardiac compression.

Another issue of concern with the thoracic pump model is control of the direction of blood flow. In the cardiac pump model, retrograde flow is prevented by closure of the atrioventricular valves, but these are believed to be open in the thoracic pump model. The absence of retrograde flow in the thoracic pump model can be explained by two mechanisms. There is angiographic evidence of a valve at the junction of the superior vena cava and right atrium, which prevents backward flow (Fisher et al., 1982; Niemann et al., 1984). However, even without a true valve, backward flow would be limited by the collapse of the veins. This occurs because the intrathoracic pressure, which is the force generating flow, is greater than the pressure inside the veins exiting the thorax because of the loss of pressures from the upstream vessels due to the normal resistance through the system. Since the pressure starts the same everywhere in the thorax, even a small gradient from the pulmonary veins to the superior and inferior vena cava will allow the surrounding pressure to be higher than the pressure in the veins and prevent flow just as it does in West zone 1 of the lungs (Green, 1987).

VII. Peripheral Versus Thoracic Limitations

Before discussing how blood flow can be augmented in CPR, it is worthwhile considering whether the primary limitation to blood flow in CPR is emptying of the thoracic volume or filling of the thoracic volume. We attempted to study this a few years ago, but the answer became so obvious after the first experiment that we did not persist. However, it clearly demonstrates the problem. We established a preparation in which the blood from the superior vena cava and inferior vena cava drained through vascular waterfalls, which controlled the venous outflow pressures. The waterfall pressures were thus the equivalent of the right atrial pressure in the intact animal. The blood flowed into a reservoir below the dog and was then pumped from the reservoir into a second reservoir, which was set at a distance above the dog. The height of the second reservoir controlled the filling pressure of the heart. An overflow outlet kept the volume of this upper reservoir constant and returned the excess blood back to the lower reservoir. We could thus keep the outflow pressure of the vasculature, as well as the filling pressure of the heart, constant. If the peripheral capacitance decreased during CPR because of a loss of tone or leaky capillaries, one would predict that the venous return would decrease and the lower reservoir volume would decrease as more blood would be pumped out than enters it. If, however, the problem is emptying of the thoracic volume, then the lower reservoir volume would increase, for less blood would leave the two reservoirs than was pumped out from the upper reservoir. Once the animal was prepared and all the lines were carefully sealed in the chest, we induced ventricular fibrillation and commenced CPR by compressing the chest with a thumper. The answer was evident in less than 30 seconds! The resting cardiac output of a 25-kg dog is approximately 2.5–3 liters/min, the stressed volume approximately 0.6 liter, and the total blood volume approximately 2.5 liters/min. When the dog was fibrillated, venous return continued initially at 2–3 liters/min, however, we were only able to produce a cardiac output of less than 0.5 liter/min with chest compressions; therefore within 30 seconds the majority of the blood volume was in the reservoir and the dog died of vascular collapse. Thus it was clear that the limiting factor in that model was getting blood out of the chest and not into it. This loss of volume does not occur in the intact animal because right atrial pressure rises with the failure to eject blood from the chest and decreases the gradient for venous return. Remember that with complete cardiac arrest, the pressures in the heart and the periphery will be equal. In our experiment, the normal increase in right atrial pressure was eliminated by keeping the effective right atrial pressure or "backpressure" for venous return at a low value.

How then can the ejection of blood be increased from the heart? If we return to the equations developed by Wise and Summer (1983, 1988), we can consider the following possibilities: changes in vascular compliance, duty cycle, rate, applied force, blood volume, vascular resistance, and abdominal pressure.

VIII. Compliance

As can be seen in Eqs. (3)–(8), the vascular compliances affect Vm, τe, and τf. A decrease in either the thoracic or pulmonary compliance will decrease the transferrable volume, Vm, but will also decrease τe and τf, which can increase flow. The net effect would most likely be no change because the compliance terms affect all of the other variables. It should also be emphasized that what is important in these equations is the compliance and not the capacitance. The compliance is the slope of the pressure-volume curve; the capacitance is the actual volume at a given pressure and therefore takes into account the unstressed volume as well. If a drug changes the position of the pressure-volume relationship but does not change the slope of the pressure-volume relationship, then this is equivalent to increasing volume and does not represent a change in compliance.

IX. Duty Cycle

One of the most important terms in Eq. (1) is α, the duty cycle, which is the fraction of the cycle spent during contraction. Notice that increasing α decreases the magnitude of the denominator and therefore results in a bigger flow. Of course, increasing α also decreases $1 - \alpha$, the factor modifying τf. Therefore, there will be an optimal α that depends upon the relative magnitudes of τe and τf. The predicted responses are shown in Figure 2. The optimal value in an isolated heart-lung model was 0.7. In a study on humans, the optimal compression time was 60% of the cycle, but this was difficult to sustain (Taylor et al., 1977). Furthermore, the optimal value will vary among patients. Since the optimal duty cycle depends upon the relative time constants of emptying and filling, conditions that increase peripheral resistance, such as with catecholamines, increase the time constant of emptying and therefore the duty cycle should be longer. Under conditions in which the time constant of emptying is shorter, such as the low peripheral resistance seen in sepsis, the duty cycle should be shorter. However, the time constant of emptying cannot be assessed in an individual patient. Therefore the present AHA recommendation is to use a duty cycle of 0.5, which should be close to the maximum in most patients and easier to sustain for a more prolonged time than longer durations (American Heart Association, 1980).

X. Rate

It may initially seem intuitive that changing the rate of compression should be important. However, rate does not come into any of the equations presented above. This is because changing the rate will change the amount of blood ejected per beat, but not the total amount of blood ejected per minute, which depends upon the interaction between the inflow and outflow time constants [Eq. (1)]. This assumes that the stroke volume is small relative to the total stressed volume, which is not true at very slow rates of compression, but is valid above 20–30 beats/min. Therefore the rate should probably be at least 30–40 beats/min, but rates above this do not make much difference. This is supported by data from studies on the isolated heart-lung preparation (Hausknecht et al., 1986), dogs (Passerini et al., 1988), and humans (Taylor et al., 1977). In the latter study, changes in rates between 40 and 80 compressions/min at a duty cycle of 0.6 had no effect on blood pressure. However, as previously noted, it is difficult to sustain prolonged duty cycles.

Changes in rate, though, have some indirect consequences. In the studies quoted above, the rates were changed with a constant duty cycle, but what usually happens in practice is that the compression phase occupies a constant time and takes up a greater proportion of the total cycle time when the rate is increased. Increases in rate thus usually result in an increase in duty cycle. This could explain the benefit of high impulse rapid compressions seen by Maier et al. (1985). The rapid impulses used by these investigators had a short compression time so that only at very high rates would the fraction of the cycle spent during compression be long, for the compression time did not change in their study, which means that the relaxation phase must have decreased. Therefore, the rate effect that they observed could very well have been a consequence of the change in duty cycle.

XI. Applied Force

A major variable affecting the volume ejected, Vm, is the difference in applied pressure during emptying or the ejecting phase and the filling phase [Eq. (3)]. Thus, as should be obvious, the greater the applied force, the greater the Vm. The applied pressure depends on the operator and how the pressure is dissipated. This is especially important in the thoracic pump model. If the airway is open, the applied pressure will be dissipated as air is forced out of the chest instead of blood. However, it has been shown that even with an open airway, some air is trapped in the lungs, which still results in some increase in intrathoracic pressure even with an open airway (Halperin et al., 1989). To maximize the effects of chest compressions, it has been recommended to compress the chest with either an occluded airway or simultaneously with ventilation (Rudikoff et al., 1980; Babbs et al., 1980; Chandra et al., 1981b). This was actually proposed in the early 1960s (Wilder et al., 1963). The changes in lung volume produced by ventilation can, however, complicate matters. At high lung volumes, the actual blood volume ejected from the chest may decrease because the increase in transpulmonary pressure can impede the movement of fluid from the pulmonary arteries and right heart (Hausknecht et al., 1986). Therefore, large tidal volumes should not be used. This is especially important if the vascular volume is low.

A large part of the dissipation of the force applied to the chest is through the abdomen (Ducas et al., 1983). Therefore, measures that decrease the compliance of the abdomen can be very helpful for increasing intrathoracic pressure and augmenting blood flow. This has been tested in numerous studies in which the abdomen has been bound or compressed with the thoracic compressions (Harris et al., 1967; Lee et al., 1981; Babbs and Blevins, 1986). Since the abdomen is the most compliant part of the thoracoabdominal complex, it can be shown that compressing the abdomen itself can actually generate an increase in pleural pressure and generate flow, for the noncompliant chest wall actually resists expansion from the rise in thoracoabdominal pressure much better than occurs when the chest is compressed and the pressure expands the lax abdominal wall. A potential problem with the application of high abdominal pressure is damage to abdominal organs (Harris et al., 1967; Krischer et al., 1987), but most studies have shown that this can be minimized by careful technique (Rudikoff et al., 1980; Chandra et al., 1981a; Bircher and Safar, 1981). The subject of abdominal counterpulsation will be discussed in detail below.

A major concern with the use of high pleural pressures to generate flow was that the rise in pleural pressure could be transferred to the intracerebral fluid and increase intracranial pressure. This occurs both through the veins as well as directly through the intravertebral spaces adjacent to the pleural space and can lead to an increase in the backpressure to flow in the brain, which would potentially decrease carotid blood flow (Guerci et al., 1985). However, there is little evidence of damage to the brain with techniques that involve abdominal binding (Schleien et al., 1990) and brain blood flow is improved by these techniques (Koehler et al., 1983).

Although Eq. (3) predicts that increasing pleural pressure differences will increase blood flow, there are limits to the effectiveness of these maneuvers, because eventually the high intrathoracic pressure produces vascular collapse and results in flow limitation. When this occurs, further increases in intrathoracic pressure will not result in any further increase in flow, as shown by Eq. (6). This has also been found experimentally (Hausknecht et al., 1986; Passerini et al., 1988).

An attempt has been made to increase intrathoracic pressure in patients by a device that allows simultaneous compression-ventilation during CPR. This device has been shown to increase intrathoracic pressure and carotid blood flow in arrested dogs (Krischer et al., 1989). However, in a randomized trial with a large number of patients, outcome was actually better in the conventionally treated group. A possible explanation is that the bulkiness of the device produces potential delays in the initiation of adequate CPR (Krischer et al., 1989).

The model also predicts that a lowering of pleural pressure during the relaxation phase should increase the return of blood to the heart until flow limitation occurs. This does not occur until right atrial pressure falls below atmospheric pressure. An intriguing application of this is active decompression CPR, in which a device is put on the chest which acts like a thumper during the compression phase but actively decompresses the chest during the relaxation phase. This technique was tried in 10 patients, and there was an increase in end-tidal CO_2 (see later sections) and transmitral velocity time integral, both of which support an increase in cardiac output. This study was too small to assess impact on survival.

XII. Volume

In the beating heart, the initial volume, or preload, is a major determinant of the systolic pressure and volume ejected. Below the point of flow limitation, as mathematically shown in Eqs. (1) and (3), the total blood volume does not influence the flow, which is mainly dependent on the pressure difference between emptying and filling, Pple – Pplf. However, when flow limitation occurs, as is shown in Eq. (6), the total volume, V, becomes a factor and an increase in total volume increases Vm. This probably explains the variable results in the literature of volume infusions during CPR. In studies in which flow limitation occurs, as would be expected when high pressures are applied, increasing blood volume is important (Rudikoff et al., 1980; Passerini et al., 1988). However, in studies in which flow limitation has not occurred, increasing the volume will not make a difference (Einagel et al., 1988). By and large, in standard CPR, the intrathoracic pressures are not high enough to produce flow limitation, and increasing the blood volume will not be of great help.

XIII. Resistance

The time constants of filling and emptying of the thoracic volume are affected by the resistances of the conduits that enter and drain this region, and therefore decreases in these resistances should decrease the time constants and increase flow. It is not easy to increase the venous time constant, although a drug such as epinephrine possibly could result in redistribution of blood flow to areas with fast time constants of venous drainage, which would decrease τf (Caldini et al., 1974; Permutt et al., 1988). Decreasing the arterial resistance results in a lower arterial pressure, and if the brain and heart start with low resistances, then decreasing the resistance of the rest of the body could actually decrease the fractional flows to the brain and heart and increase flow to nonessential areas such as muscle. Indeed, the fractional flows to the brain and heart are higher than other regions of the body at the start of CPR (Luce et al., 1983; Sharff et al., 1984). For this reason, the usual and best approach is to give drugs such as norepinephrine, epinephrine, or methoxamine, which increase peripheral resistance. These seem to not affect the cerebral and coronary circulations as much as other regions, and the rise in diastolic pressure therefore augments flow (Michael et al., 1984; Schleien et al., 1986). They also stiffen the arteries and decrease the tendency of the arteries to collapse by allowing a more negative transmural pressure [value Ptm'a in Eq. (5)] before the vessel collapses (Weisfeldt and Halperin, 1986). Therefore, flow limitation should occur at a higher pressure (Yin et al., 1982) and higher pleural pressures can be used. This is discussed further in the section on catecholamines.

XIV. Abdominal Binding

There has long been interest in the role of abdominal binding in CPR, including a report by Criley and Dolley in 1906 (Babbs and Blevins, 1986). Redding conducted a large study in dogs and found that abdominal binding greatly increased survival, particularly when performed in conjunction with the injection of an α-agonist (Redding, 1971). Abdominal compression has a number of theoretical advantages in CPR. As discussed above, abdominal compression during chest compression prevents the dissipation of the forces applied to the chest through the abdominal wall by effectively splinting the abdominal wall and reducing its compliance (Ducas et al., 1983). The abdominal binding also effectively decreases the peripheral capacitance and thereby increases the stressed volume. This will be beneficial if there is no flow limitation as discussed above. High abdominal pressures could also keep abdominal vascular pressures high and thereby decrease flow through the lower part of the body. This would effectively redirect flow in a cephalad direction and help maintain aortic diastolic pressure, which is so important for coronary flow (Neimann et al., 1982; Sanders et al., 1984b; Niemann et al., 1985). In support of this, Redding found an increase in the pressure gradient from the aorta to the central venous pressure with abdominal binding (Redding, 1971). Studies from the group at Johns Hopkins in animals and humans have also shown that abdominal binding increases blood pressure and carotid flows (Chandra et al., 1981a,b), although other studies in humans have been less successful (Groeneveld et al., 1984). A number of studies have also shown an increase in brain blood flow with abdominal binding (Luce et al., 1983; Koehler et al., 1983). This is important because concerns were raised about the transmission of abdominal pressures to the central spinal fluid (Guerci et al., 1985). However, despite this increase in the cerebral spinal fluid pressure, there still is an increase in cerebral blood flow (Babbs, 1980a).

In one of the earlier studies with abdominal binding (Harris et al., 1967), concern was raised about liver laceration from the application of abdominal pressure. The proposed mechanism was that the high abdominal pressures result in a fixation of the liver so that it is more vulnerable to injury from the chest compressions. Later studies do not support this concern (Redding, 1971; Bircher et al., 1980; Rudikoff et al., 1980; Chandra et al., 1981a,b). However, because of it, investigators began using abdominal compressions interposed between chest compressions. This technique has provoked numerous studies, which will be discussed in the next section.

XV. Interposed Abdominal Compressions

In the interposed abdominal compression (IAC) technique, the abdomen is compressed with 100–200 mm Hg during the "diastolic" or relaxation phase of the chest compressions. Interest in this approach began with the canine studies by Ralston et al. working with Babbs (1982), who showed an increase in aortic pressure, cardiac output, and the pressure gradient from the aorta to the central venous pressure with this technique. Three mechanisms were proposed to explain the benefit of IAC.

1. The abdominal compressions could produce aortic counterpulsations much like those that occur with an intraaortic balloon pump (Babbs et al., 1984a,b; Babbs, 1985).
2. It could act by splinting the aorta and thereby redirecting blood in a cephalad direction by preventing the flow of blood to the legs (Harris et al., 1967; Redding, 1971).
3. It could act by compressing the abdominal vascular compliant region and thereby increasing venous return and "prime" the pump (Babbs et al., 1984a,b; Babbs, 1985).

The arterial pressure and carotid flow increase on the first beat of IAC, indicating a direct aortic effect (Voorhees et al., 1983; Einagel et al., 1988). In the model presented previously [Eq. (1)], the increase in abdominal pressure, if applied on release or just before the onset of chest compressions, would act by increasing α, the duty cycle, of the emptying phase. The problem is that the central venous pressure may also increase, either from a transfer of venous blood from the abdomen to the right atrium (Voorhees et al., 1983) or from direct transmission of pressures to the chest (Bertrand et al., 1986) so that there is no improvement in the pressure gradient from the aorta to the right atrium, which is such an important prognostic factor (Neimann et al., 1982; Sanders et al., 1984b; Niemann et al., 1985). It appears that the size of the animal makes a difference, for central venous pressures do not rise as much in small animals. It is believed by some that this is because the primary mechanism of blood flow in small animals is direct compression of the heart, which in small animals is easier to compress (Babbs et al., 1982; Hoekstra et al., 1991). However, this could be explained equally by better emptying of the thoracic volume during compression in small animals or perhaps venous collapse at the level of the diaphragm, which prevents a cephalad transfer of abdominal volume through the veins even in the thoracic pump model. It is of interest that an intraaortic balloon pump has been shown to improve hemodynamic parameters in experimental studies of CPR (Emerman et al., 1989).

The second proposed mechanism is a redirection of blood flow in a cephalad direction by effectively cross-clamping the aorta. However, Kimmel et al. (1986) and Hoekstra et al. (1991) found no redistribution, and Bertrand et al. (1986) found that femoral flow also increased with abdominal compressions, indicating emptying of the abdominal compartment in both directions with IAC. Thus, this does not appear to be the primary mechanism.

Another consequence of cross-clamping the aorta, which is not intuitively obvious, is a redistribution of blood flow away from the splanchnic region, which has a slow time constant of venous drainage, to the upper extremity, which has a faster time constant of venous drainage (Caldini et al., 1974; Permutt et al., 1988). This would effectively decrease the τf in Eq. (1) and increase flow. This, however, should not produce an increase in aortic pressure on the first beat that occurs.

The third mechanism proposed for the benefit of IAC is an increase in the venous return by a "priming" of the pump. This mechanism can be seen as a direct effect of a transient increase in abdominal pressure, which effectively decreases the abdominal compliance and acts as a second applied force. Neither of these were included in the original model of Wise and Summer (1983, 1988). However, in experimental studies by Voorhes et al. (1983) and Einagel et al. (1988), carotid pressures increase on the very first application of abdominal pressure, and therefore a transfer of volume from the abdomen to the chest cannot explain this initial increase in flow and pressure. Nor was there an increment with subsequent beats, although others have found a progressive increase in pressure (Babbs et al., 1980).

The potential of abdominal compressions to transfer volume seems tempting at first, but it assumes a model in which the thorax and abdomen are two separate compartments (Babbs et al., 1984a,b; Babbs, 1985; Beyar et al., 1985). However, the flaccid diaphragm readily transmits abdominal pressures into the thorax so that there may not be an increase in pressure gradient for flow from the abdomen to the thorax (Ducas et al., 1983). Indeed, Einagel et al. (1988) found that abdominal compressions in dogs actually produced a greater increase in intrathoracic pressures than chest compressions, and in their study carotid flows and pressures were higher during the abdominal compression phase than during the chest compression phase so that the chest compressions became the effective diastole. The exact timing of the increase in flow and pressures with IAC has not always been examined so that the importance of this in other studies is difficult to ascertain, but it is probably model dependent (Babbs et al., 1982). It is clear that in human applications of IAC, the pressures generated during the chest phase are higher than in the abdominal phase (Groeneveld et al., 1984; Howard et al., 1987). In any case, Einagel et al. (1988) went so far as to suggest that chest compressions during IAC may actually make matters worse, for it would decrease the gradient for venous return and decrease the gradient for coronary perfusion.

What actually has been found with IAC? Ralston et al. (1982) and Voorhees et al. (1983), both working with Babbs, found that IAC increased brain blood flow and cardiac output in canine models, and Voorhees et al. (1983) found an increase in oxygen delivery and a decrease in lactate levels with IAC. Brain blood flow has been found to increase as much as fourfold (Walker et al., 1984), although myocardial blood flow does not increase and the pressure gradient from aorta to CVP also does not increase (Sanders et al., 1982) as might have been expected by the potential for right atrial pressure to increase with abdominal compressions (Einagel et al., 1988).

In human studies, the pressure gradient from the aorta to central venous pressure has been shown to increase, which would favor coronary blood flow (Berryman and Phillips, 1984; Howard et al., 1987). No advantage in terms of survival was found in an extensive field study in Milwaukee (Mateer et al., 1985), but a recently reported randomized trial on hospitalized patients showed much better outcome with IAC, including a higher percentage of patients alive at discharge than in the control group (25% vs. 7%). Improvement in hemodynamic measurements and survival was found in another randomized trial of IAC and standard CPR (Ward et al., 1990). In one animal study in which IAC was compared to standard CPR, survival was worse with IAC (Sanders et al., 1982). Of importance, there is now a large experience with this technique in humans and animals, and liver laceration does not appear to be a problem.

In most of the studies in which abdominal compressions have been used, they were applied during the relaxation phase. One of the earliest investigations of intermittent abdominal compressions was by Ohomoto et al. (1976), who used prolonged abdominal compressions and superimposed chest compressions and found increased survival in dogs. This was thus actually simultaneous abdominal and chest compression. Neimann et al. (1985) combined abdominal compressions with chest inflation and also effectively used a simultaneous abdominal and chest compression technique. Bertrand et al. (1986) predicted that simultaneous chest compressions might be better than IAC and in a preliminary study found better carotid flows and aortic pressures with simultaneous IAC in their canine model, although the difference was small (Bertrand et al., 1986). Indeed, in that study, abdominal compression alone was equal to IAC, and both were much better than chest compressions. If abdominal compressions act by increasing intrathoracic pressure, then the benefit would occur if there is not already flow limitation. Otherwise, the increase in force will not increase flow unless it prolongs the duty cycle.

In summary, the exact role of abdominal compressions in CPR is still controversial and conclusions vary with the model of CPR used for the study as well as the theoretical model used to predict results. Furthermore, the clinical results to date remain inconclusive.

XVI. Open-Chest Versus Closed-Chest Techniques

Prior to Kouwenhoven et al.'s report of closed-chest cardiac resuscitation (Kouwenhoven et al., 1960), open-chest cardiac massage was the only available technique. Today, this is largely reserved for patients with flail chests, deep hypothermia, massive pulmonary emboli, patients with their chests already open, and patients with no pulse with standard CPR (Bircher and Safar, 1984). However, there have been calls for greater application of this approach (Del Guercio, 1984), and some have recommended using it after 10 minutes of failed closed-chest resuscitation (Bircher and Safar, 1984).

There are some important theoretical advantages to open-chest massage. With closed-chest techniques, the cardiac output is dependent upon the time constants of filling and emptying [Eq. (1)] because, unlike normal cardiac function, the chest and heart can only fill during the relaxation phase. However, in open-chest CPR, as in normal cardiac contractions, blood can return to the atria and thorax during cardiac compressions if only the ventricles are compressed and not the atria. Under these conditions, Eq. (1) does not hold and flow is limited by the stressed volume divided by the time constant of venous return as in the normal heart. Furthermore, there is no flow limitation with the open-chest technique because the force is applied to the heart and not the whole thorax, and there is no high intrathoracic pressure to produce collapse of the aorta. Thus, flows can be greater than the 50% of normal predicted for standard CPR, which is unlikely with closed-chest techniques (Wise and Summer, 1983, 1988; Permutt et al., 1988). This framework allows us to consider the factors that determine flow in open-chest massage.

A crucial factor is that both the right and left ventricles must be compressed. Since the ventricles are enclosed by a common chamber—the pericardial sac—failure to empty the right ventricle could result in less filling of the left ventricle and therefore less left ventricular ejection, which is obviously crucial for the systemic circulation. Opening the pericardium would actually allow greater ventricular filling and potentially greater cardiac output. This was only done in one animal study, and the results were not compared with open and closed pericardial compressions (Barnett et al., 1986).

The stressed volume is also an important factor. If there is a large volume loss from the thoracotomy, the ability of chest compressions to produce flow will be severely limited, for stressed volume is a major determinant of the venous return to the heart. Remember that with closed-chest techniques, volume is only a factor when there is sufficient intrathoracic pressure to produce flow limitation.

As with closed-chest techniques, rate should not be a major factor, for outflow depends upon the return of blood to the heart as with the normal circulation. Most studies have found that optimal flows can be obtained with rates of 50 to 60 beats/min. The length of time of ejection is again important, but this is more easily monitored with direct cardiac compressions for the operator can feel whether the ventricle is emptied with each compression.

As with any artificial technique, the force applied is a crucial variable. It should be noted that unlike the normal beating heart, this force is independent of the diastolic volume. Therefore, if the rate of return of blood is increased by a volume infusion or a decrease in the time constant of venous return and the same force is applied to the heart, there will be no increase in output, for the arrested heart does not have a Frank Starling mechanism nor does it have an intrinsic means of changing contractility. An advantage of the open-chest technique is that the operator can easily observe an increase in volume and respond with an increase in force. As noted above, an increase in the force with open-chest massage will not produce flow limitation as it does with closed-chest techniques.

Since the output in open-chest massage is very dependent upon the return of blood, measures that increase this should be of help. These could include the use of α-adrenergic drugs to decrease venous capacitance and even interposed abdominal compressions to increase venous return. This could potentially be much more effective than in closed-chest techniques.

Based on this theoretical discussion, it would seem that the technique used during open-chest massage should be very important. Both ventricles need to be compressed and the force needs to be applied adequately and long enough to eject all the blood and yet not lacerate the heart. One needs to be careful not to twist the heart, which will decrease venous return. The operator must be careful not to compress the atrium, for this will decrease the return of blood to the heart during the systolic phase and decrease the advantage of this technique. In one study, three different techniques were used (Barnett et al., 1986). A two-handed approach that allowed better compression of the ventricles and a technique that compressed the heart against the sternum were superior to a one-handed approach in which a thumb was placed over the anterior left ventricle, the apex was placed in the palm, and the rest of the heart was gripped by the fingers.

How well does open-chest massage actually work? A number of animal studies have addressed this issue. They have generally shown a higher cardiac output (Weiser et al., 1962) and higher carotid blood flows (Bircher and Safar, 1981; Barnett et al., 1986), although aortic pressures were not much higher than with closed-chest techniques (Weiser et al., 1962; Bircher and Safar, 1981; Sanders et al., 1984b). One study found no difference between open- and closed-chest techniques (Redding and Cozino, 1961). This has been attributed to the small size of dogs used, which probably optimized the closed-chest technique (Sanders and Ewy, 1984). This factor needs to be considered in all CPR studies, although it is not known if humans are more similar to small or to large dogs! Studies have shown improved survival in dogs that were switched to open-chest massage (Sanders et al., 1984b; Kern et al., 1987). In a study that optimized the pressure generation during closed-chest compressions (Bircher and Safar, 1981), the carotid blood flow was equally improved with open and closed techniques, but the carotid blood flow fell after approximately 10 minutes with an optimal closed-chest technique. This could be related to a progressive decrease in the threshold for collapse in the aorta as discussed above and might have been alleviated with α-adrenergic drugs.

There is a very interesting assessment of open- and closed-chest CPR in humans by Del Guercio et al. (1963, 1965), who obtained cardiac output and hemodynamic measurements during cardiac arrest in 11 patients. In 3 patients they were able to compare open and closed techniques and found that the open technique produced higher cardiac outputs (Del Guercio et al., 1965). This study is often cited as evidence of the advantage of open versus closed resuscitation. It is worth noting a number of features in this rather heroic study. Cardiac output and aortic pressure were higher in some of the patients with closed-chest compressions than in other patients with the open-chest technique. In fact, one patient had a higher cardiac index during ventricular fibrillation and chest compressions than with spontaneous contractions! No details are given about the administration of catecholamines during the resuscitations, which is crucial for the prevention of aortic collapse. This could explain why cardiac outputs were higher in the closed techniques that had shorter resuscitation times. Furthermore, although flow was higher, the pressure gradient from the aorta to central veins did not change much. This is believed to be the most important prognostic factor in CPR and the failure to increase it indicates that the heart may not have been adequately perfused (Neimann et al., 1982; Niemann et al., 1985; Sanders et al., 1984a). Finally, all of the patients died no matter which technique was used.

There has been one randomized trial of open heart massage versus conventional CPR in patients with prehospital nontraumatic arrest. No survival benefit was found, but the study may have been affected by a long prehospital time (Geehr et al., 1986).

As a final point, one has to consider the complications of open-chest massage. The infection rate is cited as 10% of survivors (Bircher and Safar, 1984). Of greater importance, a pathology study found gross lacerations in 10% of cases (Adelson, 1957), although others have found fewer complications (Baker et al., 1980).

In summary, open-chest massage offers some important theoretical advantages, including the potential for higher flow and lower central venous pressures; however, the technique used is crucial and should only be applied by well-trained operators.

XVII. Catecholamines

There has been much debate recently about the best catecholamine for CPR and the appropriate dose. What is consistent in all studies is that catecholamines with α-receptor activity effectively increase blood flow, arterial diastolic pressures, and survival in both animal and human studies, although there is no control data from human trials confirming their value. When CPR is prolonged, survival is rare without exogenous catecholamines. Despite the wide acceptance of the use of catecholamines and debate about the appropriate type and dose, the mechanism of action catecholamines in CPR is still not clear. They obviously do not act by increasing cardiac contractility and therefore must act by altering the characteristics of the vasculature. One way they could act is by decreasing the time constant of filling [Eq. (1)] of the thoracic compartment, either by decreasing vascular compliance or by decreasing the resistance to venous return. However, if anything, they should tend to increase the resistance to venous return, which would increase the time constant to filling. On the other hand, α-adrenergic drugs decrease the vascular capacitance but have little effect on vascular compliance (Appleton et al., 1985) and thus essentially act in the same way as volume infusion. As noted previously, this is important when flow limitation is present, for increased stressed volume allows a higher flow before flow limitation. The time constant of filling could also be decreased by redistributing blood flow to beds with fast time constants of drainage, i.e., muscle, but there is no evidence of this occurring during CPR (Caldini et al., 1974). In fact, in one study, the proportion of blood flow to the liver and small intestine increased with epinephrine, which would effectively increase the resistance to venous return (Mitzner and Goldberg, 1975).

On the arterial side, catecholamines could increase blood pressure by increasing the systemic vascular resistance, but based on Eq. (1), this would actually decrease flow by increasing the time constant of emptying unless countered by an increase in the duty cycle, i.e., time of compression. Usually the duty cycle is kept at 0.5 as per the AHA recommendation, which could lead to a decrease in flow with catecholamines. Furthermore, if catecholamines cause a general increase in systemic vascular resistance, then the cerebral vascular bed, which has a lower resistance than the other beds during CPR (Luce et al., 1983), might have a proportionally greater increase in resistance, which would actually decrease cerebral blood flow. However, studies of cerebral blood flow in CPR have shown that it actually increases. Another potentially important role for catecholamines was proposed by Yin et al. (1982). Arteries have stiffer walls than veins and, therefore, in contrast to veins, can withstand negative transmural pressures before collapsing. That is, arteries do not necessarily collapse when the pressure outside the vessels are greater than the pressure inside the vessels until the pressure gradient reaches a large enough value. During closed-chest CPR, the pressure in the thorax around the aorta can be greater than the pressure inside the aorta. This is because there is a pressure drop from the area of largest volume to the point of outflow from the chest due to the resistance of the vessels between these two points (Poiseuille's law). When the pressure drop is large, aortic pressure is less than the intrathoracic pressure and the aorta will collapse. Yin et al. showed that catecholamines decrease the tendency of arteries to collapse and vessels can thus withstand more negative transmural pressure before they collapse. This means that flow limitation will occur at higher intrathoracic pressures, and a greater colume can be displaced from the chest during CPR Eq. (6). Without catecholamines, vascular tone decreases and the transmural pressure at which collapse occurs becomes less negative. This mechanism has been used to explain the failure of closed-chest techniques over time (Yakaitis et al., 1980; Michael et al., 1984; Weisfeldt and Halperin, 1986). It should be less important during open-chest techniques because there is not a positive intrathoracic pressure to produce collapse.

Whether the effect of catecholamines acts more by increasing stressed volume or in preventing collapse has not been studied. However, it is worth noting that in the study by Yin et al. (1982), the maximum carotid flow actually decreased with norepinephrine presumably due to the high downstream resistance. They did not test whether higher flows could be achieved by increasing intrathoracic pressure.

If catecholamines act by decreasing the tendency for vessels to collapse, then one would predict that the cardiac output should be higher with catecholamines. Cardiac output during CPR with and without catecholamines has been reported in only a few studies (Brown et al., 1987b; Ditchey and Lindenfeld, 1988; Roberts et al., 1990), but total blood flow did not increase with catecholamines in any of these studies. Thus, it is most likely that the increase in coronary and cerebral blood flow with CPR is due to increased resistance in nonessential beds and redistribution of flow to essential areas such as the heart and brain.

Catecholamines increase the pressure gradient from the aorta to right atrium, which, as noted previously, is an important determinant of coronary flow (Brown et al., 1987b; Lindner et al., 1989, 1990, 1991; Lindner, 1991). This could be due to an increase in total blood flow and therefore produce more aortic volume to be dissipated during diastole. It could also be due to a general increase in systemic vascular resistance with less increase in the brain and heart, or else there would be no accompanying increase in flow to the heart.

Another potential role for catecholamines in CPR is to decrease the fibrillation threshold. This most likely occurs through activation of β receptors, which leads to an increase in amplitude of the circulatory waveform. Survival rates strongly correlate with the ventricular fibrillation wave amplitude, with a sixfold greater chance of hospital discharge in patients with course ventricular fibrillation (Weaver et al., 1985).

From the above discussion, it would seem that α-adrenergic drugs are of primary importance for CPR because of their effect on vascular tone. Although β-adrenergic drugs can decrease the ventricular fibrillation threshold, they have a detrimental effect on vascular tone, and therefore it is not surprising that isoproterenol (Pearson and Redding, 1965) and dobutamine (Otto et al., 1981) are not effective during CPR. There has recently been much debate as to whether α-1 or α-2 activity is more important. This has arisen because investigators have tried to avoid the potential increase in metabolic demand from the β effects of norepinephrine and epinephrine by substituting methoxamine or phenylephrine (Brillman et al.,

1987). However, these latter two drugs only have α-1 activity, whereas norepinephrine also has α-2 activity. The α-1 receptor appears to be downregulated in hypoxia, whereas the α-2 receptor retains its activity and can still produce vasoconstriction. Therefore, the effectiveness of a pure α-agonist may decrease with time. Some studies, indeed, have found that methoxamine is less effective than norepinephrine (Brown et al., 1987a; Olson et al., 1989). Others found that it is equal to epinephrine (Bleske et al., 1989), and still others have found methoxamine to be much better than epinephrine (Pearson and Redding, 1965; Roberts et al., 1990), and phenylephrine was equal to or slightly better than epinephrine (Lindner, 1991). Roberts compared high doses of methoxamine (20 mg) and epinephrine (0.2 mg/kg) and found better organ flows and survival in animals treated with methoxamine (Roberts et al., 1990). However, in a recent randomized field trial, Olson et al. (1989) found that 0.5 mg of epinephrine was more effective during resuscitation than methoxamine, and Roberts failed to find a beneficial advantage to methoxamine over epinephrine in a randomized trial in humans. Because of the downregulation of the α-1 receptor with hypoxia, oxygenation could be an important variable in these studies. The doses of drugs used and the techniques of CPR are probably also important.

The effectiveness of norepinephrine and epinephrine have also been compared. Epinephrine has more β activity, particularly β-2 activity, than norepinephrine, which increases myocardial oxygen consumption (Lindner et al., 1991), and although blood flow is higher with epinephrine, the O_2 extraction remains the same because of the higher oxygen need in a fibrillating heart (Ditchey and Lindenfeld, 1988; Lindner et al., 1991). This might explain why fibrillating hearts are defibrillated more easily when the animals are treated with norepinephrine or dopamine than with epinephrine (Lindner and Ahnefeld, 1989). However, in asphyxia models of cardiac arrest, better results were achieved with epinephrine than with norepinephrine (Lindner and Ahnefeld, 1989), presumably because there is less stimulation of myocardial oxygen consumption in this model and the β activity provides better maintenance of coronary flow by counterbalancing the constricting effect of the α component.

The current AHA recommendation is to use 1-mg boluses of epinephrine. However, many animal studies suggest that the dose of epinephrine may be larger than the currently recommended dose of approximately 0.014 mg/kg, and some have suggested that doses as high as 0.45 mg/kg are required (Brown et al., 1987b; Gonzalez et al., 1991; Lindner et al., 1991). Paradis et al. (1991), in an extensive review, pointed out that the current recommendation of 1 mg was taken directly from a study by Redding and Pearson, who used 10-kg dogs, without any adjustment for human body size. In one case report, it was proposed that in two patients high doses of epinephrine were important in contributing to successful resuscitation (Koscove et al., 1988). It has been shown that high-dose epinephrine increases coronary perfusion pressure in patients undergoing CPR and this should favor survival (Paradis et al., 1991). A number of randomized trials in adults with cardiac arrest have tested the efficacy of high-dose epinephrine. Lindner (1991) found that the success rate of resuscitation with high-dose epinephrine was higher than without, but there was no difference in hospital discharge rates. Two recent large randomized trials found no benefit from high-dose versus low-dose epinephrine, although in one of the studies there was a trend for better survival in the group in which resuscitation and epinephrine were given in less than 10 minutes from the time of the arrest. In both of these studies it was a long time before the initiation of therapy, which, as previously noted, is a very important determinant of success rate. The overall hospital discharge rate in these two studies was only 4–5% in one (Brown et al., 1992) and 3–5% in the other (Stiell et al., 1992). Thus, these studies may not have adequately tested the hypothesis that high-dose catecholamines are necessary, for the epinephrine may have been administered too late to have been effective. Of importance, in these studies and in another larger survey of complications from high-dose epinephrine, there was no evidence for a detrimental effect from the catecholamines including no higher incidence of arrhythmias, hypertension, or recurrent arrest in those treated with high-dose catecholamines (Callaham et al., 1991). Therefore, despite these large controlled trials, it is still not clear whether high-dose catecholamines can be effective in CPR (Ornato, 1991).

XVIII. Monitoring During CPR

It would be helpful to have a simple method for monitoring patients during CPR (Ornato, 1993). The current recommendation of the AHA is to monitor the carotid pulse. Unfortunately, the systolic pressure generated does not correlate with the outcome. This can probably be explained by studies that have shown that the pressure gradient from the aorta to right atrium during diastole is the best predictor of survival (Niemann et al., 1982; Niemann et al., 1985; Sanders et al., 1984a) and an increase in aortic pressure does not always mean an increase in aortic pressure. Arterial gases do not predict outcome (Gazmuri et al., 1989). Following a report by Sanders et al. (1989), much attention has been given to the potential usefulness of end-tidal P_{CO_2} measurements, for they found a good correlation between the end-tidal P_{CO_2} and outcome. In their study, all patients with an end-tidal P_{CO_2} greater than 10 mm Hg survived. The end-tidal P_{CO_2} has also been shown to correlate with cardiac output (Weil et al., 1986; Falk et al., 1988; Callaham and Barton, 1990). To understand the rationale behind end-tidal CO_2 measurements, it is necessary to review the physiological mechanisms that control arterial and venous P_{CO_2} and end-tidal P_{CO_2}.

In the steady-state condition, arterial P_{CO_2} is determined by CO_2 production, $\dot{V}_{CO_2}$ and alveolar ventilation. The flow of CO_2 out of the lung thus matches the flow of CO_2 from the tissues into the blood. CO_2 stores in the body are very large so that during transient changes, the CO_2 output from the lungs can be different from the CO_2 production in the tissues.

Arterial P_{CO_2} (Weil et al., 1986) during CPR is usually less than the normal reference value of 40 mm Hg. For example, Weil et al. (1986) found an average arterial P_{CO_2} of 35 mm Hg. This indicates that there is actually hyperventilation and no problem clearing CO_2 by the lungs.

The mixed venous or pulmonary arterial CO_2 is dependent upon $\dot{V}_{CO_2}$, blood flow, and the arterial CO_2 content as given by the Fick equation, which is a statement of the conservation of mass. Thus, $Q = \dot{V}_{CO_2}/(\text{venous} - \text{arterial } CO_2 \text{ content})$. If $\dot{V}_{CO_2}$ and arterial P_{CO_2} do not change, and the cardiac output drops by greater than 50%, then the pulmonary arterial P_{CO_2} must rise considerably. On the other hand, the CO_2 clearance of the lung is a function of the amount of delivered CO_2 but also the efficiency of alveolar ventilation, for the expired CO_2 mixes with gas already in the lungs. If alveolar ventilation is very small compared to the total ventilation, i.e., a large deadspace, then CO_2 clearance is small and the end-tidal CO_2 is much smaller than pulmonary arterial CO_2. An increase in cardiac output during CPR increases pulmonary flow and thereby reduces deadspace and improves CO_2 clearance. Thus, the end-tidal CO_2 increases with increases in cardiac output. However, the end-tidal CO_2 will also change with anything that changes deadspace, which could include redistribution of blood flow by catecholamines, a change in bronchial tone by low CO_2 levels, or changes in the pattern of breathing. The end-tidal CO_2 would also be changed by an increase in CO_2 delivery, which occurs when the cardiac output is increased but also when $\dot{V}_{CO_2}$ is increased, for example, with a change in temperature or the administration of exogenous bicarbonate.

It is difficult to predict whether CO_2 production increases or decreases in the tissues during the arrested state. A decrease in metabolism would decrease $\dot{V}_{O_2}$ and thereby decrease $\dot{V}_{CO_2}$ for CO_2 is produced mainly through aerobic metabolism; however, the acidosis contributes to an increase in CO_2 production by shifting the dissociation curve of bicarbonate to carbonic acid and then H_2O and CO_2. An increase in $\dot{V}_{CO_2}$ will also increase pulmonary arterial CO_2, which is why pulmonary arterial CO_2 levels are very high during exercise.

A classic example of a sudden increase in deadspace is a pulmonary embolism, and, therefore, a decrease in the gradient between arterial P_{CO_2} and end-tidal P_{CO_2} has been used to diagnose pulmonary embolisms (Eriksson et al., 1989). The end-tidal CO_2 could fall by any condition that increases airway pressure and thus increases zone I conditions of the lung. Thus, increasing the respiratory rate or increasing lung volumes could make a patient appear worse off than they really are by this monitoring technique. An interesting recent failure of the use of end-tidal P_{CO_2} measurements was observed in a study by Martin et al. (1990). They used end-tidal P_{CO_2} to monitor the effects of epinephrine infusions during CPR. Although coronary perfusion pressure increased, the end-tidal P_{CO_2} decreased, indicating an increase in the deadspace. This can most likely be explained by a redistribution of pulmonary blood flow by the norepinephrine away from ventilated areas. However, CO_2 clearance is still so efficient that arterial P_{CO_2} did not rise.

A potentially useful application of end-tidal P_{CO_2} measurement was demonstrated by Garnett et al. (1987), who showed that a sudden increase in end-tidal

CO_2 during CPR indicates the return of spontaneous circulation. Presumably with the return of normal circulation, the pulmonary blood flow increases and deadspace decreases. Of note, they failed to confirm the observation of Saunders et al. that the magnitude of end-tidal CO_2 during CPR predicts outcome. A simple but useful application of end-tidal CO_2 monitoring is the confirmation of successful endotracheal intubation (Ornato, 1993). End-tidal CO_2 measurements have also been used to suggest that a mechanical device results in better cardiac output than manual techniques (Ward et al., 1993).

In conclusion, end-tidal P_{CO_2} measurements can be a useful guide to monitoring patients during CPR, but one must be cognizant of the physiology involved in this measurement, for a decrease in this measurement may not always be a bad prognostic sign.

XIX. Sodium Bicarbonate Therapy

Sodium bicarbonate has long been advocated to buffer the acidosis that develops during cardiac arrest. This is based on the belief that the presence of acidosis makes it harder defibrillate the heart and could contribute to decreased responsiveness to catecholamines following defibrillation. Indeed, low pH is correlated with failure of resuscitation (Kerber and Sarnat, 1979), but this can probably be explained by the correlation of low pH with delay in resuscitation, which is one of the most important variables determining the success of resuscitation.

Bishop and Weisfeldt (1976) showed that arterial pH can be maintained at greater than 7.25 μg when ventilation and compressions are adequate. A number of animal studies have also found no advantage of bicarbonate therapy compared to placebo (Guerci et al., 1986; Kette et al., 1990, 1992), and in one study animals were defibrillated after 30 minutes of resuscitation without any bicarbonate therapy (Michael et al., 1984).

The failure of sodium bicarbonate to improve the outcome with CPR can be understood from recent analyses of arterial and venous blood gases in the whole body (Weil et al., 1986; Falk et al., 1988) and regional circulations (Von Planta et al., 1989; Gudipati et al., 1990). The large part of the acidosis comes from the accumulation of CO_2. As discussed in the section on end-tidal P_{CO_2} measurements, according to the Fick principle, a decrease in flow will result in a marked increase in venous CO_2 and therefore a decrease in venous pH. The CO_2 load is excreted by delivery of blood to the lungs and ventilation. The fact that the arterial P_{CO_2} is normal or below normal during CPR indicates that the clearance of CO_2 by the lungs is adequate. Little benefit is achieved by adding a buffer, for the problem is inadequate tissue perfusion and the clearance of tissue CO_2. The CO_2 is a normal byproduct of metabolism, and it is the dissolved P_{CO_2} that forms carbonic acid and produces the acid load. Bicarbonate administration has the potential of paradoxically increasing the regional CO_2 level that will diffuse into cells and increase cellular acidosis (Imai et al., 1989; Ornato et al., 1989; Weisfeldt, 1991). The only thing that sodium bicarbonate can do is to counter the acid load from lactic acid, but this does not appear to be a major factor (Gudipati et al., 1990).

Sodium bicarbonate has some important negative aspects that need to be considered (Niemann et al., 1984; Guerci et al., 1986; Jaffe, 1989). An increase in arterial pH shifts the oxyhemoglobin saturation curve to the left and decreases the release of oxygen. Alkalosis can contribute to cardiac arrhythmias. Sodium bicarbonate adds an important osmotic load and can produce hypernatremia (Maltar et al., 1974) and increased osmolality, which has been associated with a decrease in coronary perfusion pressure (Kette et al., 1992). Bicarbonate is thought to inactivate catecholamines and can depress cardiac function. As noted above, it can produce a paradoxical increase in intracellular pH. Finally, sodium bicarbonate can result in a marked alkalosis following the arrest when the P_{CO2} is regulated and lactate is cleared by normal metabolism. In conclusion, the bulk of evidence indicates that sodium bicarbonate therapy should be used judiciously.

XX. Conclusion

In conclusion, much work has been done on the mechanisms of the generation of flow during CPR and on how to maximize the cardiac output. Our understanding of these factors has greatly improved in the last decade, but unfortunately the ability to apply these in a practical way is still limited. The most important factors still remain rapid onset of CPR and early defibrillation.

Appendix

During emptying when $P_{PL} = P_{PLE}$:

$$\dot{Q}_E = \frac{P_T + P_{PLE} - P_P}{R_A}$$

$$= \frac{P_T}{R_A} + \frac{P_{PLE}}{R_A} - \frac{P_P}{R_A}$$

$$= \frac{V_T}{R_A C_T} + \frac{P_{PLE}}{R_A} - \frac{V_P}{R_A C_P}, \text{ since } V_T = C_T \cdot P_T \text{ and } V_P = P_P \cdot C_P$$

$$= \frac{V_T}{R_A C_T} + \frac{P_{PLE}}{R_A} - \frac{V - V_T}{R_A C_P} \text{ where } V = V_T + V_P$$

$$= V_T \frac{C_T + C_P}{R_A C_T C_P} + \frac{P_{PLE}}{R_A} - \frac{V}{R_A C_P}$$

$$= \frac{V_T}{\tau_E} + \frac{P_{PLE}}{R_A} - \frac{V}{R_A C_P} \quad \text{where } \tau_E = \frac{R_A C_T C_P}{C_T + C_P} \tag{A-1}$$

where $R_A = R_{a1} + R_{a2}$ and R_{a1} is the intrathoracic arterial resistance and R_{a2} the extrathoracic resistance.

During filling when $P_{PL} = P_{PLF}$:

$$\dot{Q}_F = \frac{P_P - P_T - P_{PLF}}{R_V}$$

$$= \frac{V_P}{R_V C_P} - \frac{V_T}{R_V C_T} - \frac{P_{PLF}}{R_V}$$

$$= \frac{V - V_T}{R_V C_P} - \frac{V_T}{R_V C_T} - \frac{P_{PLF}}{R_V}$$

$$= \frac{V}{R_V C_P} - \frac{V_T}{R_V C_P} - \frac{V_T}{R_V C_T} - \frac{P_{PLF}}{R_V}$$

$$= \frac{V}{R_V C_P} - \frac{P_{PLF}}{R_V} - \frac{V_T}{\tau_F} \quad \text{where } \tau_F = \frac{R_V C_T C_P}{C_T + C_P} \tag{A-2}$$

where $R_V = R_{V1} + R_{V2}$ and R_{V2} is the intrathoracic venous resistance and R_{V1} the extrathoracic venous resistance.

Since total flow $(\dot{Q})$ = stroke volume $(\dot{Q}_E \cdot te$ or $\dot{Q}_F \cdot tf) \times$ frequency, and frequency $= 1/(te + tf)$:

$$\dot{Q} = \frac{\dot{Q}_E \cdot te}{te + tf} = \frac{\dot{Q}_F \cdot tf}{te + tf}$$

for the steady state where tf = time of filling and te = time of emptying.

From Eq. (A-1):

$$\dot{Q} = \left[\frac{V_T}{\tau_E} + \frac{P_{PLE}}{R_A} - \frac{V}{R_A C_P} \right] \alpha \tag{A-3}$$

$$= \left[\frac{V}{R_V C_P} - \frac{P_{PLF}}{R_V} - \frac{V_T}{\tau_F} \right] (1 - \alpha) \tag{A-4}$$

where $\alpha = \frac{te}{te} + tf$, the duty cycle, and $(1 - \alpha) = \frac{tf}{te} + tf$.

Solving Eqs. (A-3) and (A-4)

$$V_T = \left[\frac{\dot{Q}}{\alpha} - \frac{P_{PLE}}{R_A} - \frac{V}{R_A C_P} \right] \tau_E$$

$$V_T = \left[\frac{V}{R_V C_P} - \frac{P_{PLF}}{R_V} - \frac{\dot{Q}}{(1 - \alpha)} \right] \tau_F$$

and

$$\tau_E \left[\frac{\dot{Q}}{\alpha} - P_{PLE} \frac{\dfrac{C_T C_P}{C_T + C_P}}{t_E} + \frac{\dfrac{C_T \cdot V}{C_T + C_P}}{t_E} \right] = \tau_F \left[\frac{\dfrac{C_P \cdot V}{C_T + C_P}}{t_F} - P_{PLF} \frac{\dfrac{C_T C_P}{C_T + C_P}}{t_F} - \frac{\dot{Q}}{(1 - \alpha)} \right]$$

and

$$\frac{\tau_E \cdot \dot{Q}}{\alpha} + V_{TeqE} = \frac{T_F \cdot \dot{Q}}{(1 - \alpha)} + V_{TeqF}$$

where V_{TeqE} and V_{TeqF} are the equilibrium volumes of the thoracic reservoir if allowed to empty or fill to equilibrium.

Also,

$$\dot{Q} = \frac{V_{TeqF} - V_{TeqE}}{\dfrac{\tau_E}{\alpha} + \dfrac{\tau_F}{1 - \alpha}} \tag{A-5}$$

where $V_{TeqF} - V_{TeqE} = $ total mobile volume.

For maximal $\dot{Q}$ for non–flow-limiting conditions,

$$V_M = (P_{PLE} - P_{PLF}) \cdot \frac{C_T C_P}{(C_T + C_P)}$$

whereas for flow-limiting conditions,

$$V_M = V - (P_{PM/a} \, C_T) - (P_{TM/a} \, C_p)$$

Let

$$\frac{d\dot{Q}}{d\alpha} = 0 = \frac{\tau_F}{(1 - \alpha)^2} - \frac{\tau_E}{\alpha^2}$$

and

$$\frac{\tau_E}{\tau_F} = \frac{\alpha^2}{(1 - \alpha)^2} = \left(\frac{te}{tf} \right)^2$$

and

$$\frac{te}{tf} = \frac{\sqrt{\tau_E}}{\sqrt{\tau_F}} \text{ for optimal } \dot{Q}, \ \alpha = \frac{\sqrt{\tau_E}}{\sqrt{\tau_E} + \sqrt{\tau_F}}.$$

Substitute in Eq. (A-5) and

$$\dot{Q} \, \text{max} = \frac{Vm}{(\sqrt{\tau_E} + \sqrt{\tau_F})^2}$$

A similar derivation can be carried out for flow-limiting conditions where $V_m = V - P_{TVM}, C_P - P_{TM}, _A C_T$ and $\tau_E = R_{al} C_T, \tau_F = R_{vl} C_P$.

References

Adelson, L. (1957). A clinicopathologic study of the anatomic changes in the heart resulting from cardiac massage. *Surg. Gynecol. Obstet.*, 104:513–523.

Adgey, A. A. J., Patton, J. N., Campbell, N. P. S., and Webb, S. W. (1979). Ventricular defibrillation: appropriate energy levels. *Circulation*, 60:219–222.

Adgey, A. A. J., McKeown, P. P., and McAnderson, J. (1991). Cardioversion and defibrillation: the esophageal approach. In *Update in Intensive Care and Emergency Medicine*. Edited by J. L. Vincent. New York, Springer-Verlag, pp. 34–43.

American Heart Association (1980). Advanced cardiac life support. *JAMA*, 244:479–493.

Appleton, C., Olajos, M., Morkin, E., and Goldman, S. (1985). Alpha-1 adrenergic control of the venous circulation in intact dogs. *J. Pharmacol. Exp. Ther.*, 233:729–734.

Babbs, C. F. (1980a). New versus old theories of blood flow during CPR. *Crit. Care Med.*, 8:191–195.

Babbs, C. F. (1980b). Cardiac angiography during CPR. *Crit. Care Med.*, 8:189–190.

Babbs, C. F., Voorhees, W. D., Fitzgerald, K. R., Holmes, H. R., and Geddes, L. A. (1980). Influence of interposed ventilation pressure upon artificial cardiac output during cardiopulmonary resuscitation in dogs. *Crit. Care Med.*, 8:127–130.

Babbs, C. F., Tacker, W. A., Paris, R. L., Murphy, R. J., and David, R. W. (1982). CPR with simultaneous compression and ventilation at high airway pressure in 4 animal models. *Crit. Care Med.*, 10:501–504.

Babbs, C. F., Ralston, S. H., and Geddes, L. A. (1984a). Theoretical advantages of abdominal counterpulsation in CPR as demonstrated in a simple electrical model of the circulation. *Ann. Emerg. Med.*, 13:660–671.

Babbs, C. F., Weaver, J. C., Ralson, S. H., and Geddes, L. A. (1984b). Cardiac, thoracic and abdominal pump. Mechanisms in cardiopulmonary resuscitation: studies in an electrical model of the circulation. *Am. J. Emerg. Med.*, 2:299–308.

Babbs, C. F. (1985). Abdominal counterpulsation in cardiopulmonary resuscitation: animal models and theoretical considerations. *Am. J. Emerg. Med.*, 3:165–170.

Babbs, C. F., and Blevins, W. E. (1986). Abdominal bindings and counterpulsation in cardiopulmonary resuscitation. *Crit. Care Clin.*, 2:319–332.

Baker, C. C., Thomas, A. N., and Trunkey, D. D. (1980). The role of emergency room thoracotomy in trauma. *J. Trauma*, 20:848–855.

Barcroft, H., and Samaan, A. (1935). Explanation of the increase in systemic flow caused by occluding the descending thoracic aorta. *J. Physiol.* (London), 85:47–61.

Barnett, W. M., Alifimoff, J. K., Paris, P. M., Stewart, R. D., and Safar, P. (1986). Comparison of open-chest cardiac massage techniques in dogs. *Ann. Emerg. Med.*, 15:408–411.

Bedell, S. E., Delbanco, T. L., Cook, E. F., and Epstein, F. H. (1983). Survival after cardiopulmonary resuscitation in the hospital. *N. Engl. J. Med.*, 309:569–576.

Berryman, C. R., and Phillips, G. M. (1984). Interposed abdominal compression—CPR in human subjects. *Ann. Emerg. Med.*, 13:226–229.

Bertrand, F., Einagel, V., Roussos, C., and Magder, S. A. (1986). Effects of abdominal compression on three modes of CPR (abstr). *Clin. Invest. Med.*, 9 (suppl. A):A32.

Beyar, R., Kishon, Y., Kimmel, E., Neufeld, H., and Dinnar, U. (1985). Intrathoracic and abdominal pressure variations as an efficient method for cardiopulmonary resuscitation: studies in dogs compared with computer model results. *Cardiovasc. Res.*, 19:335–342.

Billman, G. E. (1992). Cellular mechanisms for ventricular fibrillation. *Int. Union Physiol. Sci.*, 7:254–259.

Bircher, N., Safar, P., and Stewart, R. (1980). A comparison of standard, MAST-augmentation, and open-chest CPR in dogs. *Crit. Care Med.*, 8:147–152.

Bircher, N., and Safar, P. (1981). Comparison of standard and "new" closed-chest CPR and open-chest CPR in dogs. *Crit. Care Med.*, 9:384–385.

Bircher, N., and Safar, P. (1984). Open-chest CPR: an old method whose time has returned. *Am. J. Emerg. Med.*, 2:568–571.

Bishop, R. C., and Weisfeldt, M. (1976). Sodium bicarbonate administration during cardiac arrest. *JAMA*, 235:506–509.

Bleske, B. E., Chow, M. S. S., Zhao, H., and Kluger, J. (1989). Epinephrine versus methoxamine in survival postventricular fibrillation and cardiopulmonary resuscitation in dogs. *Crit. Care Med.*, 17:1310–1313.

Brillman, J., Sanders, A., Otto, C. W., Fahmy, H., Bragg, S., and Ewy, G. A. (1987). Comparison of epinephrine and phenylephrine for resuscitation and neurologic outcome of cardiac arrest in dogs. *Ann. Emerg. Med.*, 16:11–17.

Brown, C. G., Davis, E. A., Werman, H. A., and Ham Lin, R. L. (1987a). Methoxamine versus epinephrine on regional cerebral blood flow during cardiopulmonary resuscitation. *Crit. Care Med.*, 15:682.

Brown, C. G., Werman, H. A., Davis, E. A., Hobson, J., and Hamlin, R. L. (1987b). The effects of graded doses of epinephrine on regional myocardial blood flow during cardiopulmonary resuscitation in swine. *Circulation*, 75:491–497.

Brown, C. G., Martin, D. R., Pepe, P. E., et al. (1992). A comparison of standard-dose and high-dose epinephrine in cardiac arrest outside the hospital. *N. Engl. J. Med.*, 327:1051–1055.

Caldini, P., Permutt, S., Waddell, J. A., and Riley, R. L. (1974). Effect of epinephrine on pressure, flow, and volume relationships in the systemic circulation of dogs. *Circ. Res.*, 34:606–623.

Callaham, M., and Barton, C. (1990). Prediction of outcome of cardiopulmonary resuscitation from end-tidal carbon dioxide concentration. *Crit. Care Med.*, 18:358–362.

Callaham, M., Barton, C. W., and Kayser, S. (1991). Potential complications of high-dose epinephrine therapy in patients resuscitated from cardiac arrest. *JAMA*, 265:1117–1122.

Chandra, N., Snyder, L. D., and Weisfeldt, M. L. (1981a). Abdominal binding during cardiopulmonary resuscitation in man. *JAMA*, 246:351–353.

Chandra, N., Weisfeldt, M. L., Tsitlik, J., et al. (1981b). Augmentation of carotid flow during cardiopulmonary resuscitation by ventilation at high airway pressure simultaneously with chest compression. *Am. J. Cardiol.*, 48:1053–1063.

Chandra, N. C. (1993). Mechanisms of blood flow during CPR. *Ann. Emerg. Med.*, 22:281–288.

Cohen, J. M., Chandra, N., Alderson, P. O., Van Aswegen, A., Tsitlik, J. E., and Weisfeldt, M. L. (1982). Timing of pulmonary and systemic blood flow during intermittent high intrathoracic pressure cardiopulmonary resuscitation in the dog. *Am. J. Cardiol.*, 49:1883–1889.

Crampton, R. (1980). Accepted, controversial and speculative aspects of ventricular defibrilation. *Prog. Cardiovasc. Dis.*, 23:167–186.

Criley, J. M., Blaufuss, A. H., and Kissel, G. L. (1976). Cough-induced cardiac compression. *JAMA*, 236:1246–1250.

DeBard, M. L. (1980). The history of cardiopulmonary resuscitation. *Ann. Emerg. Med.*, 9:273–275.

Del Guercio, L. R. M., Coomaraswamy, R. P., and State, D. (1963). Cardiac output and other hemodynamic variables during external cardiac massage in man. *N. Engl. J. Med.*, 269:1398–1404.

Del Guercio, L. R. M., Feins, N. R., Cohn, J. D., Coomaraswamy, R. P., Wollman, S. B., and State, D. (1965). Comparison of blood flow during external and internal cardiac massage in man. *Circulation*, 31–31 (suppl):I-171–I-180.

Del Guercio, L. R. M. (1984). A plea for open-chest CPR. *Am. J. Emerg. Med.*, 2:565–566.

Deshmukh, H. G., Weil, M. H., Gudipati, C. V., Trevino, R. P., Bisera, J., and Rackow, E. C. (1989). Mechanism of blood flow generated by precordial compression during CPR. I. Studies on closed chest precordial compression. *Chest*, 95:1092–1099.

Ditchey, R. V., and Lindenfeld, J. (1988). Failure of epinephrine to improve the balance between myocardial oxygen supply and demand during closed-chest resuscitation in dogs. *Circulation*, 78:382–389.

Ducas, J., Roussos, C., Karsardis, C., and Magder, S. (1983). Thoracoabdominal mechanics during resuscitation maneuvers. *Chest*, 84:446–451.

Einagel, V., Bertrand, F., Wise, R. A., Roussos, C., and Magder, S. A. (1988). Interposed abdominal compressions and carotid blood flow during CPR. *Chest*, 93:1206–1212.

Eisenberg, M. S., Bergner, L., and Hallstrom, A. (1979). Cardiac resuscitation in the community. *JAMA*, 241:1905–1907.

Eisenberg, M. S., Copass, M. K., Hallstrom, A. P., et al. (1980). Treatment with out-of-hospital cardiac arrests with rapid defibrillation by emergency medical technicians. *N. Engl. J. Med.*, 302:1379–1383.

Eisenberg, M. S., Hallstrom, A., and Bergner, L. (1982). Long-term survival after out-of-hospital cardiac arrest. *N. Engl. J. Med.*, 306:1340–1343.

Emerman, C. L., Pinchak, A. C., Hagen, J. F., and Hancock, D. (1989). Hemodynamic effects of the intra-aortic balloon pump during experimental cardiac arrest. *Am. J. Emerg. Med.*, 7:378–383.

Eriksson, M. B., Wollmer, P., Olsson, C. G., et al. (1989). Diagnosis of pulmonary embolism based upon alveolar dead space analysis. *Chest*, 96:357–362.

Falk, J. L., Rackow, E. C., and Weil, M. H. (1988). End-tidal carbon dioxide concentration during cardiopulmonary resuscitation. *N. Engl. J. Med.*, 318:607–611.

Feneley, M. P., Maier, G. W., Gaynor, J. W., et al. (1987). Sequence of mitral valve motion and transmitral blood flow during manual cardiopulmonary resuscitation in dogs. *Circulation*, 76:363–375.

Fisher, J., Vaghaiwalla, F., Tsitlik, J., et al. (1982). Determinants and clinical significance of jugular venous valve competence. *Circulation*, 65:188–196.

Gadzinski, D. S., White, B. C., Hoehner, P. J., Hoehner, T., Krome, C., and White, J. D. (1982). Canine cerebral cortical blood flow and vascular resistance post cardiac arrest. *Ann. Emerg. Med.*, 11:58–63.

Garnett, A. R., Ornato, J. P., Gonzalez, E. R., and Johnson, E. B. (1987). End-tidal carbon dioxide monitoring during cardiopulmonary resuscitation. *JAMA*, 257:512–515.

Gazmuri, R. J., Von Planta, M., Weil, M. H., and Rackow, E. C. (1989). Arterial PCO2 as an indicator of systemic perfusion during cardiopulmonary resuscitation. *Crit. Care Med.*, 17:237–240.

Geehr, E. C., Lewis, F. R., and Auerbach, P. S. (1986). Failure of open-heart massage to improve survival after prehospital nontraumatic cardiac arrest. *N. Engl. J. Med.*, 314:1189–1190.

Gonzalez, E. R., Ornato, J. P., Garnett, A. R., and Levine, R. L. (1991). Dose-dependent vasopressor response to epinephrine during CPR in human beings. *Ann. Emerg. Med.*, 20:440–441.

Green, J. F. (1987). *Fundamental Cardiovascular and Pulmonary Physiology*. Philadelphia, Lea and Febiger. 2nd ed.

Groeneveld, A. B. J., Bronsveld, W., and Thijs, L. G. (1984). Intermittent abdominal compression during cardiopulmonary resuscitation. *Lancet*, 1076–1077.

Gudipati, C. V., Weil, M. H., Gazmuri, R. J., and Deshmukh, H. G. (1990). Increases in coronary vein CO_2 during cardiac resuscitation. *J. Appl. Physiol.*, 68:1405–1408.

Guerci, A. D., Shi, A. Y., Levin, H., Tsitlik, J., Weisfeldt, M. L., and Chandra, N. (1985). Transmission of intrathoracic pressure to the intracranial space during cardiopulmonary resuscitation in dogs. *Circ. Res.*, 56:20–30.

Guerci, A. D., Chandra, N., Johnson, E., et al. (1986). Failure of sodium bicarbonate to improve resuscitation from ventricular fibrillation in dogs. *Circulation*, 74:75–79.

Guerci, A. D., and Weisfeldt, M. L. (1986). Mechanical-ventilatory cardiac support. *Crit. Care Clin.*, 2:209–221.

Guerci, A. D., Halperin, H. R., Beyar, R., et al. (1989). Aortic diameter and pressure-flow sequence identify mechanism of blood flow during external chest compression in dogs. *J. Am. Coll. Cardiol.*, 14:790–798.

Guyton, A. C., Armstrong, G. G., and Chipley, P. L. (1956). Pressure volume curves of the arterial and venous systems in live dogs. *Am. J. Physiol.*, 184:253–258.

Halperin, H. R., Weiss, J. L., Guerci, A. D., et al. (1988). Cyclic elevation of intrathoracic pressure can close the mitral valve during cardiac arrest in dogs. *Circulation*, 78:754–760.

Halperin, H. R., Brower, R., Weisfeldt, M. L., et al. (1989). Air trapping in the lungs during cardiopulmonary resuscitation in dogs: a mechanism for generating changes in intrathoracic pressure. *Circ. Res.*, 65:946–954.

Harris, L. C., Kirimli, B., and Safar, P. (1967). Augmentation of artificial circulation during cardiopulmonary resuscitation. *Anaesthesiology*, 28:730–734.

Hausknecht, M. J., Wise, R. A., Brower, R. G., et al. (1986). Effects of lung inflation on blood flow during cardiopulmonary resuscitation in the canine isolated heart-lung preparation. *Circ. Res.*, 59:676–683.

Hoekstra, O. S., Van Lambalgen, A. A., and Thijs, L. G. (1991). Abdominal interposed between thoracic compressions during cardiopulmonary resuscitation. In *Update in Intensive Care and Emergency Medicine*. Edited by J. L. Vincent. New York, Springer-Verlag, pp. 3–10.

Howard, M., Carrubba, C., Foss, F., Janiak, B., Hogan, B., and Guinness, M. (1987). Interposed abdominal compression-CPR: its effects on parameters of coronary perfusion in human subjects. *Ann. Emerg. Med.*, 16:3:253–259.

Imai, T., Kon, N., Kunimoto, F., and Tanaka, M. (1989). Exacerbation of hypercapnia and acidosis of central venous blood and tissue following administration of sodium bicarbonate during cardiopulmonary resuscitation. *Jpn. Circ. J.*, 53:298–306.

Jaffe, A. S. (1989). New and old paradoxes: acidosis and cardiopulmonary resuscitation. *Circulation*, 80:1079–1083.

Kerber, R. E., and Sarnat, W. (1979). Factors influencing the success of ventricular defibrillation in man. *Circulation* 60:226–230.

Kerber, R. E., Grayzel, J., Hoyt, R., Marcus, M., and Kennedy, J. (1981). Transthoracic resistance in human defibrillation: influence of body weight, chest size, serial shocks, paddle size and paddle contact pressure. *Circulation* 63:676–682.

Kerber, R. E., Kouba, C., Martins, J., et al. (1984). Advance prediction of transthoracic impedance in human defibrillation and cardioversion: importance of impedance in determining the success of low-energy shock. *Circulation*, 70:303–308.

Kern, K. B., Sanders, A. B., Badylak, S. F., et al. (1987). Long-term survival with open-chest cardiac massage after ineffective closed-chest compression in a canine preparation. *Circulation*, 75:498–503.

Kette, F., Weil, M. H., Von Planta, M., Gazmuri, R. J., and Rackow, E. C. (1990). Buffer agents do not reverse intramyocardial acidosis during cardiac resuscitation. *Circulation*, 81:1660–1666.

Kette, F., Weil, M. H., and Gazmuri, R. J. (1992). Buffer solutions may compromise cardiac resuscitation by reducing coronary perfusion pressure. *JAMA*, 266:2121–2126.

Kimmel, E., Beyar, R., Dinnar, U., Sideman, S., and Kishon, Y. (1986). Augmentation of cardiac output and carotid blood flow by chest and abdomen phased compression cardiopulmonary resuscitation. *Cardiovasc. Res.*, 20:574–580.

Koehler, R. C., Chandra, N., Guerci, A. D., et al. (1983). Augmentation of cerebral perfusion by simultaneous chest compression and lung inflation with abdominal binding after cardiac arrest in dogs. *Circulation*, 67:266–275.

Koscove, E. M., and Paradis, N. A. (1988). Successful resuscitation from cardiac arrest using high-dose epinephrine therapy. *JAMA*, 259:3031–3034.

Kouwenhoven, W. B., Jude, J. R., and Knickerbocker, C. G. (1960). Closed-chest cardiac massage. *JAMA*, 173:1064–1067.

Krischer, J. P., Fine, E. G., Davis, J. H., and Nagel, E. L. (1987). Complications of cardiac resuscitation. *Chest*, 92:287–291.

Krischer, J. P., Fine, E. G., Weisfeldt, M. L., Guerci, A. D., Nagel, E., and Chandra, N. (1989). Comparison of prehospital conventional and simultaneous compression-ventilation cardiopulmonary resuscitation. *Crit. Care Med.*, 17:1263–1269.

Lee, H. R., Wilder, R. J., Downs, P., Massion, W., and Blank, W. F. (1981). MAST augmentation of external cardiac compression: role of changing intrapleural pressure. *Ann. Emerg. Med.*, 10:560–565.

Lindner, K. H., and Ahnefeld, F. W. (1989). Comparison of epinephrine and norepinephrine in the treatment of asphyxial or fibrillatory cardiac arrest in a porcine model. *Crit. Care Med.*, 17:437–441.

Lindner, K. H., Ahnefeld, F. W., Schuermann, W., and Bowdler, I. M. (1990). Epinephrine and norepinephrine in cardiopulmonary resuscitation. Effects on myocardial oxygen delivery and consumption. *Chest*, 97:1458–1462.

Lindner, K. H. (1991). Vasopressor therapy in cardiopulmonary resuscitation. In *Update in Intensive Care and Emergency Medicine*, edited by J. L. Vincent. New York, Springer-Verlag, pp. 18–24.

Lindner, K. H., Ahnefeld, F. W., and Bowdler, I. M. (1991). Comparison of different doses of epinephrine on myocardial perfusion and resuscitation success during cardiopulmonary resuscitation. *Am. J. Emerg. Med.*, 9:27–31.

Lown, B. (1979). Sudden cardiac death: the major challenge confronting contemporary cardiology. *Am. J. Cardiol.*, 43:313–328.

Luce, J. M., Ross, B. K., O'Quin, J., et al. (1983). Regional blood flow during cardiopulmonary resuscitation in dogs using simultaneous and nonsimultaneous compression and ventilation. *Circulation*, 67:258–264.

Magder, S. (1990). Starling resistor versus compliance. Which explains the zero-flow pressure of a dynamic arterial pressure-flow relation? *Circ. Res.*, 67:209–220.

Magder, S. (1992). Shock Physiology. In *Physiological Foundations of Critical Care Medicine.* Edited by M. R. Pinsky. Philadelphia, Williams and Wilkins, pp. 502–524.

Maltar, J. A., Weil, M. H., Shubin, H., and Stein, L. (1974). Cardiac arrest in the critically ill. Hyperosmolar states following cardiac arrest. *Am. J. Med.*, 56:162–168.

Martin, G. B., Gentile, N. T., Paradis, N. A., and Moeggenberg, J. (1990). Effect of epinephrine on end-tidal carbon dioxide monitoring during CPR. *Ann. Emerg. Med.*, 19:396–398.

Mateer, J. R., Stueven, H. A., Thompson, B. M., Aprahamian, C., and Darin, J. C. (1985). Prehospital IAC-LPR versus standard CPR. *Ann. Emerg. Med.*, 3:143–146.

Michael, J. R., Guerci, A. D., Koehler, R. C., et al. (1984). Mechanisms by which epinephrine augments cerebral and myocardial perfusion during cardiopulmonary resuscitation in dogs. *Circulation*, 69:822–835.

Mitzner, W., and Goldberg, H. (1975). Effect of epinephrine on resistive and compliant properties of the canine vasculature. *J. Appl. Physiol.*, 39(2):272–280.

Neimann, J. T., Rosborough, J. P., Ung, S., and Criley, J. M. (1982). Coronary perfusion pressure during experimental cardiopulmonary resuscitation. *Ann. Emerg. Med.*, 11:127–131.

Neimann, J. T., and Rosborough, J. P. (1984). Effects of acidemia and sodium bicarbonate therapy in advanced cardiac life support. *Ann. Emerg. Med.*, 13:781–784.

Newton, J. R., Glower, D. D., Wolfe, J. A., et al. (1988). A physiologic comparison of external cardiac massage techniques. *J. Thorac. Cardiovasc. Surg.*, 95:892–901.

Niemann, J. T., Rosborough, J. P., Hansknecht, M., Gardiner, D., and Brilley, J. M. (1981). Pressure-synchronized cineangiography during experimental cardiopulmonary resuscitation. *Circulation*, 64:985–991.

Niemann, J. T., Rosborough, J. P., Ung, S., and Criley, J. M. (1984). Hemodynamic effects of continuous abdominal binding during cardiac arrest and resuscitation. *Am. J. Cardiol.*, 53:269–274.

Niemann, J. T., Rosborough, J. P., Niskanen, R. A., Alferness, C., and Criley, J. M. (1985). Mechanical "cough" cardiopulmonary resuscitation during cardiac arrest in dogs. *Am. J. Cardiol.*, 55:199–204.

Niemann, J. T. (1992). Cardiopulmonary resuscitation. *Current Concepts*, 327:1075–1080.

Ohomoto, T., Miura, I., and Konno, S. (1976). A new method of external cardiac massage to improve diastolic augmentation and prolong survival time. *Ann. Thorac. Surg.*, 21:284–290.

Olson, D. W., Thakur, R., Stueven, H. A. and Thompson, B. (1989). Randomized study of epinephrine versus methoxamine in prehospital ventricular fibrillation. *Ann. Emerg. Med.*, 18:1258–1259.

Ornato, J. P., Levine, R. L., Young, D. S., and Racht, E. M. (1989). The effect of applied chest compression force on systemic arterial pressure and end-tidal carbon dioxide concentration during CPR in human beings. *Ann. Emerg. Med.*, 18:732–737.

Ornato, J. P. (1991). High-dose epinephrine during resuscitation. *JAMA*, 265:1160–1161.

Ornato, J. P. (1993). Hemodynamic monitoring during CPR. *Ann. Emerg. Med.*, 22:289–295.

Otto, C. W., Yakaitis, R. W., Redding, J. S., and Blitt, C. D. (1981). Comparison of dopamine, dobutamine, and epinephrine in CPR. *Crit. Care Med.*, 9:640–643.

Paradis, N. A., Martin, B. G., Rosenberg, J., et al. (1991). The effect of standard- and high-dose epinephrine on coronary perfusion pressure during prolonged cardiopulmonary resuscitation. *JAMA*, 265:1139–1144.

Paraskos, J. A. (1993). History of CPR and the role of the national conference. *Ann. Emerg. Med.*, 22:275–280.

Passerini, L., Wise, R. A., Roussos, C., and Magder, S. A. (1988). Maintenance of circulation without chest compression during CPR. *J. Crit. Care*, 3:62–106.

Pearson, J. W., and Redding, J. S. (1965). Influence of peripheral vascular tone on cardiac resuscitation. *Anesth. Analg.* 44:746–752.

Permutt, S., and Riley, S. (1963). Hemodynamics of collapsible vessels with tone: the vascular waterfall. *J. Appl. Physiol.*, 18(5):924–932.

Permutt, S., Wise, R. A., and Sylvester, J. T. (1988). Interaction Between the Circulation and Ventilatory Pumps. In *The Thorax*. Edited by C. Lenfant and C. Roussos. New York, Marcel Dekker.

Ralston, S. H., Babbs, C. F. and Niebauer, M. S. (1982). Cardiopulmonary resuscitation with interposed abdominal compression in dogs. *Anesth. Analg.*, 61:645–651.

Redding, J. J., and Cozino, R. A. (1961). A comparison of open chest and closed chest cardiac massage in dogs. *Anaesthesiology*, 22:280–285.

Redding, J. S. (1971). Abdominal compression in cardiopulmonary resuscitation. *Anesth. Analg.*, 50:668–675.

Redding, J. S., Haynes, R. R., and Thomas, J. D. (1981). "Old" and "new" CPR manually performed in dogs. *Crit. Care Med.*, 9:386–387.

Rich, S., Wix, H. L., and Shapiro, E. P. (1981). Clinical assessment of heart chamber size and valve motion during cardiopulmonary resuscitation by two-dimensional echocardiography. *Am. Heart J.*, 102:368–373.

Roberts, D., Landolfo, K., Dobson, K., and Light, R. B. (1990). The effects of methoxamine and epinephrine on survival and regional distribution of cardiac output in dogs with prolonged ventricular fibrillation. *Chest*, 98:999–1005.

Rudikoff, M. T., Maughan, W. L., Effron, M., Freund, P., and Weisfeldt, M. L. (1980). Mechanisms of blood flow during cardiopulmonary resuscitation. *Circulation*, 61:345–352.

Safar, P., Escarraga, L. A., and Elam, J. O. (1958). A comparison of the mouth-to-mouth and mouth-to-airway artificial respiration with the chest-pressure, arm-life method. *N. Engl. J. Med.*, 258:675.

Safar, P., and Bircher, N. G. (1988). *Cardiopulmonary Cerebral Resuscitation*. 3rd ed. London, W. B. Saunders.

Sagawa, K. (1978). The ventricular pressure-volume diagram revisited. *Circ. Res.*, 43:677–687.

Sanders, A. B., Ewy, A., Alferness, A., Taft, T., and Zimmerman, M. (1982). Failure of one method of simultaneous chest compression, ventilation, and abdominal binding during CPR. *Crit. Care Med.*, 10:509–513.

Sanders, A. B., and Ewy, G. A. (1984). Open-chest CPR: not yet. *Am. J. Emerg. Med.*, 2:566–567.

Sanders, A. B., Ewy, G. A., and Taft, T. B. (1984a). The importance of aortic diastolic blood pressure during cardiopulmonary resuscitation. *Crit. Care Med.*, 12:871–873.

Sanders, A. B., Kern, K. B., Ewy, G. A., Atlas, M., and Bailey, L. (1984b). Improved resuscitation from cardiac arrest with open-chest massage. *Ann. Emerg. Med.*, 13:672–675.

Sanders, A. B., Kern, K. B., Otto, C. W., Milander, M. M., and Ewy, G. A. (1989). End-tidal carbon dioxide monitoring during cardiopulmonary resuscitation. *JAMA*, 262:1347–1351.

Schleien, C. L., Dean, J. M., Koehler, R. C., et al. (1986). Effect of epinephrine on cerebral and myocardial perfusion in an infant preparation of cardiopulmonary resuscitation. *Circulation*, 73:809–817.

Schleien, C. L., Koehler, R. C., Shaffner, D. H., and Traystman, R. J. (1990). Blood-brain barrier integrity during cardiopulmonary resuscitation in dogs. *Stroke*, 21:1185–1191.

Sharff, J. A., Pantley, G., and Noel, E. (1984). Effect of time on regional organ perfusion during two methods of cardiopulmonary resuscitation. *Ann. Emerg. Med.*, 13:649–565.

Stiell, I. G., Hebert, P. C., Weitzman, B. N., et al. (1992). High-dose epinephrine in adult cardiac arrest. *N. Engl. J. Med.*, 327:1045–1050.

Tacker, W. A., and Ewy, G. A. (1979). Emergency defibrillation dose: recommendations and rationale. *Circulation*, 60:223–225.

Taylor, G. J., Tucker, W. M., Greene, H. L., Rudikoff, M. T., and Weisfeldt, M. L. (1977). Importance of prolonged compression during cardiopulmonary resuscitation in man. *N. Engl. J. Med.*, 296:1515–1517.

Von Planta, M., Weil, M. H., Gazmuri, R. J., Bisera, J., and Rackow, E. C. (1989). Myocardial acidosis associated with CO_2 production during cardiac arrest and resuscitation. *Circulation*, 80:684–692.

Voorhees, W. D., Niebauer, M. J., and Babbs, C. F. (1983). Improved oxygen delivery during cardiopulmonary resuscitation with interposed abdominal compressions. *Ann. Emerg. Med.*, 12:128–135.

Walker, J. W., Bruestle, J. C., White, B. C., Evans, A. T., Indreri, R., and Bialek, H. (1984). Perfusion of the cerebral cortex by use of abdominal counter pulsation during cardiopulmonary resuscitation. *Am. J. Emerg. Med.*, 2:391–393.

Ward, K. R., Sullivan, R. J., Zelenak, R. R., and Summer, W. R. (1990). A comparison of interposed abdominal compression CPR and standard CPR by monitoring end-tidal PCO2. *Ann. Emerg. Med.*, 19:1201–1202.

Ward, K. R., Menegazzi, J. J., Zelenak, R. R., Sullivan, R. J., and McSwain, N. E. (1993). A comparison of chest compressions between mechanical and manual CPR by monitoring end-tidal PCO_2 during human cardiac arrest. *Ann. Emerg. Med.*, 22:669–674.

Weaver, W. D., Cobb, L. A., Dennis, D., Ray, R., Hallstrom, A. P., and Copass, M. K. (1985). Amplitude of ventricular fibrillation waveform and outcome after cardiac arrest. *Ann. Int. Med.*, 102:53–55.

Weaver, W. D., Fahrenbruch, C. E., Johnson, D. D., and Hallstrom, A. P. (1990). Effect of epinephrine and lidocaine therapy on outcome after cardiac arrest due to ventricular fibrillation. *Circulation*, 82:2027–2034.

Weil, M. H., Rackow, E. C., Tevino, R., Grundler, W., Falk, J. L., and Griffel, M. I. (1986). Difference in acid-base state between venous and arterial blood during cardiopulmonary resuscitation. *N. Engl. J. Med.*, 315:153–156.

Weiser, F. M., Adler, L. N., and Kuhn, L. (1962). Hemodynamic effects of closed and open chest cardiac resuscitation in normal dogs and those with acute myocardial infarction. *Am. J. Cardiol.*, 10:555–561.

Weisfeldt, M. (1991). Sodium bicarbonate in CPR. *JAMA*, 266:2129–2128.

Weisfeldt, M. L., and Halperin, H. R. (1986). Cardiopulmonary resuscitation: beyond cardiac massage. *Circulation*, 74:443–448.

Werner, J. A., Greene, H. L., Janko, C. L., and Cobb, L. A. (1981). Visualization of cardiac valve motion in man during external chest compression using two-dimensional echocardiography. *Circulation*, 63:1417–1421.

Wexler, H. R., and Gelb, A. W. (1986). Controversies in cardiopulmonary resuscitation. *Crit. Care Clin.*, 2:335–345.

Wilder, R. J., Weir, D., Rush, B. F., and Ravitch, M. M. (1963). Methods of coordinating ventilation and closed chest cardiac massage in the dog. *Surgery*, 53:186–194.

Wise, R. A., and Summer, W. R. (1983). Pulmonary mechanics and artificial support of the arrested circulation. *Clin. Chest Med.*, 4:189–198.

Wise, R. A., and Summer, W. R. (1988). Cardiopulmonary resuscitation. In *Cardiopulmonary Critical Care*. Edited by D. R. Dantzker. Philadelphia, W. B. Saunders Co., pp. 385–405.

Yakaitis, R. W., Ewy, G. A., Otto, C. W., Taren, D. L., and Moon, T. E. (1980). Influence of time and therapy on ventricular defibrillation in dogs. *Crit. Care Med.*, 8:157–163.

Yin, F. C. P., Cohen, J. M., Tsitlik, J., Zola, B., and Weisfeldt, M. L. (1982). Role of carotid artery resistance to collapse during high-intrathoracic-pressure CPR. *Am. J. Physiol.*, 243:H259–H267.

Zoll, P. M., Linenthal, A. S., Gibson, W., Paul, M. H., and Norman, L. R. (1956). Termination of ventricular fibrillation in man by externally applied electrical countershock. *N. Engl. J. Med.*, 254:727.

59

Dynamics of Breathing in Ventilatory Failure

ROLF D. HUBMAYR

Mayo Clinic
Rochester, Minnesota

I. Introduction

In this review, ventilatory failure is defined as any condition in which the volume of gas entering and leaving the lungs (minute volume, $\dot{V}_E$) is insufficient to satisfy the metabolic demands of the organism. Although lung function is frequently impaired in patients with ventilatory failure, this definition emphasizes the role of the ventilatory pump in the maintenance of pulmonary gas exchange. Because $\dot{V}_E$ is an important determinant of the arterial CO_2 tension (Pa_{CO_2}), hypercarbia is always present in patients with ventilatory failure. In contrast to patients with so-called chronic or compensated respiratory acidosis, however, patients with ventilatory failure are unable to reach an equilibrium state between metabolic CO_2 production and CO_2 elimination by the lungs.

Integrative physiologists often model the ventilatory pump as a controller (a network of brain stem neurons) that receives chemo- and mechano-receptive input from the periphery and is connected to a motor (the respiratory muscles), which, in turn, displace the chest wall. It is assumed that the shared load on the inspiratory muscles is proportional to the impedance of the relaxed respiratory system and to the minute volume required for maintenance of normocarbia. In accordance with this model, ventilatory failure can be attributed to a malfunction of one or more components of the ventilatory pump. Most of the time, failure is multifactorial and is caused by a mismatch between the performance capacity of the ventilatory pump and the demands placed upon it. Those who approach ventilatory failure from a muscle mechanics perspective view the problem as a mismatch between inspiratory muscle strength and the muscles' load. Although the ventilatory pump has more degrees of freedom than can be examined with this simple model, it provides a helpful starting point for discussing the dynamics of breathing. Specifically, the model offers ways to relate the inspiratory muscles' mechanical output to variables such as tidal volume, respiratory rate, and inspiratory flow, which can easily be measured in humans.

II. The Mechanical Interactions Between Respiratory Muscles and Thorax: Basic Concepts

Changes in intrinsic load affect both rate and magnitude of the pressure the respiratory muscles exert on the respiratory system (Otis et al., 1950: Campbell, 1958; Riddle and Younes, 1981; Younes and Riddle, 1981; Younes et al., 1981). These variables can be inferred from time-based recordings of volume, flow, or airway occlusion pressure. A limiting assumption is that all inspiratory muscles are represented by a single contractile element that shortens against elastic, resistive, or inertive loads. The load is assumed proportional to simple mechanical constants such as elastance (Ers), flow resistance (Rrs), and inertance (Irs) of the relaxed respiratory system, while the properties of the contractile element are usually derived from length-tension and force-velocity relationships. It is commonly assumed that the initial length of the contractile element is a function of lung volume and that muscle shortening and shortening velocity are proportional to tidal volume and inspiratory flow (Younes and Riddle, 1981).

Figure 1 depicts the mechanical interactions between the respiratory apparatus and the inspiratory muscles in schematic form. For the moment, energy dissipation will be ignored, i.e., the respiratory apparatus will be represented by a spring and the properties of the muscle element by isometric length-tension curves. Muscle length (L) is expressed as a percent of optimal length (Lo) and is shown on the abscissa. Tension, expressed as a percent of maximal tension (To), is shown on the ordinate. The solid lines are isometric length-tension curves of a muscle between Lo and 40% Lo. The uppermost curve represents the performance envelope of the muscle, i.e., its length-tension relationship during maximal activation. The curves below represent varying levels of lesser activation. The line, which intercepts the length axis at Lo, represents the length-tension relationship of a linear elastic element. It can be thought of as a spring arranged in series with the muscle and under no tension at Lo. The slope of the spring curve (k) defines the stiffness of the elastic element. The combined length of the elastic element and the muscle is assumed constant. When the muscle shortens from Lo by an amount equal to ΔL, the spring is being stretched by $-\Delta L$. The intersections

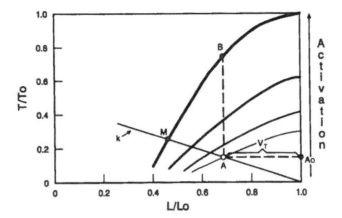

Figure 1 Schematic representation of the mechanical interactions between the inspiratory muscles and the thorax. L/Lo, length of the contractile element as a fraction of optimal length; T/To, tension of the contractile element as a fraction of maximal tension; k, spring constant of the elastic element; V_T, tidal volume. (From Hagan and Hubmayr, 1991.)

of each muscle curve with the length-tension curve of the spring element define unique solutions for (1) the length of the elastic element (lung volume), (2) its length change from a state of zero tension (tidal volume, V_T), (3) the elastic recoil of the spring (the elastic recoil of the respiratory system, Pel,rs), (4) the active length of the muscle at end-inspiration (L'/Lo), (5) its fractional shortening (ΔL/Lo), (6) muscle tension or its pressure equivalent (Pmus, which must be in equilibrium with Pel,rs), and (7) the pressure reserve of the muscle (Pmus/Pmus$_{MAX}$). The slope of the spring curve and the relative shapes of the muscle curves define the level of muscle activation (drive) that is necessary to raise lung volume by an amount equal to V_T. The intercept of the spring curve with the maximal length-tension curve of the muscle (point M) defines the maximal length of the elastic element (analogous to total lung capacity, TLC). Extension of the spring element by a lesser amount (e.g., from Ao to A) requires less muscle activation. Point B represents the maximal tension that can be generated at a length corresponding to point A. The tension at point A relative to that at point B thus reflects the force reserve of the muscle at end-inspiration.

Many clinical measurements of respiratory muscle function are founded on this model. They include the pressure the respiratory muscles must generate (Pmus) to displace the thorax (Otis et al., 1950; Campbell, 1958), the inspiratory airway occlusion pressure, $P_{0.1}$ (Whitelaw et al., 1975), the pressure-volume work, and the power output of the inspiratory muscles. Furthermore, much of the integrative work pertaining to inspiratory muscle fatigue is based on these concepts. The relationship between Pmus and the mechanical properties of the respiratory system is defined by the equation of motion

$$\text{Pmus} = \text{Pel,rs}_i + \text{Ers} * V_T + \text{Rrs} * \dot{V} + d\dot{V}/dt * \text{Irs} \qquad (1)$$

where Pel,rs_i is the elastic recoil pressure of the respiratory system at the beginning of inspiration (analogous to intrinsic PEEP, PEEP_i), V_T is the tidal volume, $\dot{V}$ is the mean inspiratory flow, and $d\dot{V}/dt$ is the change in inspiratory flow with respect to time. During quiet breathing, the component of Pmus attributable to inertance is small and is usually ignored. For a breath initiated from relaxation volume, Pel,rs_i is 0, but this term must not be ignored in patients with airflow obstruction and dynamic hyperinflation (Pepe and Marini, 1982; Milic-Emili et al., 1987). Since breathing is a dynamic event, the pressure reserve of the inspiratory muscles may be considerably smaller than is assumed in Figure 1. According to Eq. (1), any increase in $\dot{V}$ requires additional pressure, the magnitude of which depends on Rrs (Rodarte and Rehder, 1986). Second, the ability of skeletal muscles to generate pressure declines as the absolute amount and rates of sarcomere shortening increases (Edman, 1980, 1981).

III. Respiratory Muscle Fatigue and Ventilatory Failure

Having established a framework in the preceding section within which to examine the mechanical interactions between a skeletal muscle and its afterload, it is now appropriate to review certain key concepts pertaining to the topic of respiratory muscle fatigue (see also Chap. 49). Because most disease processes that cause ventilatory failure affect both contractility and the load on the respiratory muscles, it has proven useful to consider ventilatory failure as a manifestation of respiratory muscle fatigue (Roussos and Macklem, 1981; Cohen et al., 1982; Rochester, 1988). Muscle fatigue is a condition in which there is loss of the capacity to develop force and which is reversible by rest (NHLBI Workshop Summary, 1990). Muscle fatigue is likely to occur whenever the load on a muscle exceeds a threshold that varies in proportion to its strength. Explorations of the force-fatigue relationship of the diaphragm and inspiratory muscles have been a central theme of ventilatory failure research over the past two decades (Roussos and Macklem, 1977; Bellemare and Grassino, 1982a,b; Gallagher et al., 1985; McCool et al., 1986). In a typical experiment, the respiratory pump of a normal volunteer is loaded with an external resistance while the subject is instructed to generate a predetermined airway or transdiaphragmatic target pressure (Pdi) during each breath. The inability to continue this task for prolonged periods of time is considered evidence for inspiratory muscle fatigue. The validity of this assumption has been confirmed using phrenic nerve stimulation as a means to demonstrate a load-induced, reversible loss in diaphragm strength (peripheral fatigue) (Aubier et al., 1985).

Despite the strong scientific underpinning of the strength-load mismatch hypothesis, measurements of Pdi have not proven useful in the clinical diagnosis of impending respiratory pump failure (Swartz and Marino, 1985), nor has it been possible thus far to demonstrate peripheral diaphragm fatigue in patients. Potential reasons for this are the complex interactions between intrinsic load and the system's load response and the task specificity of the fatigue process (Enoka and Stuart, 1992). In contrast to laboratory-based experiments during which known, invariant loads (i.e., a single Pdi target) can be imposed to study respiratory muscle responses, patients with diseases of the respiratory system are not constrained to generate a unique Pdi. At least in theory, the controller has the option to reduce the mechanical load on the respiratory muscles below a peripheral fatigue threshold through a reduction in central motor command. The price for such a strategy could be CO_2 retention without overt ventilatory failure.

IV. The Determinants of Tidal Volume and Respiratory Rate: Mechanical Perspective

Normal individuals maintain a given alveolar ventilation by adjusting the rate of breathing so that the average force generated by the respiratory muscles is minimized (Mead, 1960). Minimizing force and muscle tension also minimizes blood flow requirements to respiratory muscles (Rochester and Bettini, 1976). Experimental fatigue of specific ventilatory muscles induces distinct changes in breathing patterns and muscle coordination (Yan et al., 1993a,b). Peripheral diaphragm fatigue brought on by inspiratory resistive loading to a Pdi target has no effect on respiratory rate and tidal volume response to CO_2 rebreathing, but it reduces the pressure output of the diaphragm relative to that of inspiratory rib cage muscles (Yan et al., 1993a). In contrast to fatigue induced by Pdi-targeted loads, fatiguing oral pressure targets causes a fall in tidal volume, an increase in respiratory rate, and increase the contribution of expiratory muscles to tidal volume, but they leave the minute volume responses to CO_2 breathing preserved (Yan et al., 1993b). The differences among the effects of oral pressure and Pdi-targeted fatigue protocols on breathing patterns and chest wall motion suggest that oral pressure–targeted protocols cause global inspiratory muscle fatigue while Pdi-targeted protocols fatigue only the diaphragm. It remains unclear, however, to what extent fatigue-related changes in respiratory muscle coordination are caused by a redistribution of neural activation between respiratory muscle groups or whether they simply reflect nonuniform reductions in the muscles' contractile strength and shortening.

Rapid, shallow breathing is a general manifestation of respiratory load compensation, but it is not a specific sign of respiratory muscle fatigue (Younes and Remmers, 1981). Figure 2a depicts the effects of elastic loads on muscle mechanics using the model presented in Figure 1. A new spring curve with a slope $k' = 2k$ has been added to reflect an increase in the elastic load on the muscle element. The contractile properties of the muscle element have not been altered. Given the shape of the maximal length-tension curve of the muscle, the maximal length of the elastic element (point M') is now reduced. In addition, a greater level of muscle activity (drive) is required to keep V_T constant, i.e., to stretch the spring

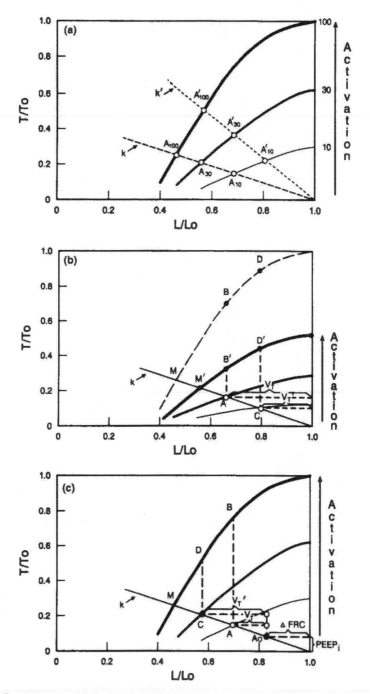

Figure 2 Schematic of the interactions between inspiratory muscles and thorax during elastic loading (a), in the presence of muscle weakness (b), and during dynamic hyperinflation (c). (From Hagan and Hubmayr, 1991.)

element to a length corresponding to point A in the original example (point A' on the new spring curve). Such a breathing strategy, however, would require that a greater percentage of maximal tension be generated during each breath (tension at point A' relative to that at point B). Preserving V_T would increase the probability that the load will be a fatiguing one and would raise the subject's awareness of respiratory effort. If respiratory activity (drive) did not increase in response to the added load, the length of the spring element at "end-inspiration" would decline from A' to C. Such a strategy would lead to a fall in tidal shortening commensurate with a reduction in tidal volume to V'_T and would allow the system to operate with a greater force reserve (C/D as opposed to A'/B). Because of the shape of the length-tension curves, the muscle tension (Pmus) at point C would still be greater than before loading (point A), thereby minimizing the anticipated fall in V_T. This mechanism, which has been referred to as intrinsic load compensation, determines in part the tidal volume response of individuals during the first loaded breath (Campbell et al., 1961; Younes and Riddle, 1981). The steady-state ventilatory responses to elastic loading are determined by an interplay between intrinsic load compensation and changes in muscle activation (drive). The strategy represented by point A' (complete preservation of V_T) has not been observed experimentally (Younes and Remmers, 1981). A fall in V_T influences proprioceptive afferent nerve traffic to the respiratory controller and would result in an increase in arterial CO_2 tension (Pa_{CO_2}) unless met by an increase in respiratory rate.

The same principles can be applied to analyze the effects of muscle weakness or fatigue on the dynamics of breathing (Fig. 2b). Instead of increasing the elastic load as was done in Figure 2a, assume that the contractile properties of the muscle have changed. This is reflected in a downward shift of each muscle curve compared with Figures 1 and 2a. To extend the spring element to point A requires a considerable increase in fractional muscle tension (A/B' as opposed to A/B) and would have to be met with an increase in respiratory drive. A reduction in tidal shortening to V'_T (point C) would lower Pmus, raise the force reserve in the new operating range (C/D' as opposed to A/B'), and possibly reduce the effective load below a fatigue threshold.

Rapid, shallow breathing can lead to dynamic hyperinflation, particularly in the presence of expiratory airflow limitation (Pepe and Marini, 1982; Milic-Emili et al., 1987). The consequences of having to initiate a breath from a lung volume other than relaxation volume (Vrel) can also be examined in the context of this simple model (Fig. 2c). Vrel is represented by the intercept of the elastic element curve with the length axis where spring tension and Pmus are 0 and the muscle length is assumed to be equal to Lo. Initiating a breath from a volume above Vrel, e.g., from point Ao, means that the spring element is under some initial tension ($Pel,rs_i = PEEP_i > 0$), that Pmus must be generated first to counterbalance the passive tension in the spring before it can be stretched further to point A, and that tidal shortening is reduced in proportion to the increase in Vrel (ΔFRC). It can be appreciated that hyperinflation limits the options for dynamic load compensation, especially in the presence of increased resistive loads and impaired inspiratory muscle strength. Alveolar ventilation cannot be restored by increasing V_T to V_T' because of the consequences on the inspiratory force reserve. The use of expiratory muscles to maintain an end-expired lung volume near Vrel (drive point Ao to the right) is ineffective because of expiratory flow limitation. Further reductions in end-inspired volumes would impose additional rate demands, which are likely to cause more hyperinflation.

Although the concepts embodied in Figure 2 provide a useful initial appraisal of the interactions between respiratory muscles and thorax, there are a number of additional factors that have not been considered. As alluded to before, motion is associated with dissipation of energy within the contractile machinery (Edman, 1980, 1981; Jones et al., 1985; McCool et al., 1986; Rodarte and Rehder, 1986). While visco-elastic energy losses of the respiratory system can be approximated using the equation of motion [Eq. (1)], it is much harder to model the effects of motion on muscle recruitment and force output. Contracting muscles do not follow a unique length-tension trajectory even when the degree of activation is extrinsically controlled (Joyce et al., 1969). During active shortening their force output is determined by the number and type of active motor units (recruitment) and varies with motor unit firing rates (rate coding) and the phase relationships among active units (synchronization) (Burke and Edgerton, 1975). Furthermore, during submaximal activation, the peak force produced by a muscle is not determined only by its final active length, but also by its initial length, shortening velocity, and the absolute amount of shortening (Edman, 1980, 1981). These factors are undoubtedly important in modifying the rate and tidal volume responses of the failing ventilatory pump.

V. Breathing Pattern and Respiratory Muscle Fatigue: Neurobiological Perspective

The motor unit firing rate of limb muscles declines when a fatiguing task is performed (Dietz, 1978; Bigland-Ritchie et al., 1983). This occurs in conjunction with a shift of the muscle's force frequency curve to the left. A leftward shift implies that force generation (relative to the maximal force) is better preserved at low activation frequencies. The changes in shape of the force frequency curve of fatigued muscles reflect a slowing of the muscle's rate of relaxation. The fall in spontaneous motor unit discharge rates takes advantage of these changes. It is suspected, but not proven, that similar events occur in the phrenic nerve and diaphragm during breathing against a fatiguing load. It has been demonstrated that during experimental fatigue, the relaxation rate of the diaphragm is prolonged (Esau et al., 1983) and that the power spectrum of the diaphragm EMG is altered (Gross et al., 1979; Cohen et al., 1982). Gallagher et al. (1985) demonstrated that breathing patterns during recovery from experimental respiratory muscle fatigue were similar in individuals with and without impaired diaphragm strength provided the power spectrum of the diaphragm EMG remained abnormal.

A number of investigators have proposed that the reduction in motor unit firing rates of maximally contracted limb muscles is regulated by a peripheral reflex originating within the fatigued muscle (Bigland-Ritchie et al., 1986). Large- and small-diameter mechano-receptive and nociceptive afferents have been implicated in this fatigue-related reflex modulation of neural activity (Garland and McComas, 1990; Garland, 1991; Macefield et al., 1991). Others have emphasized reductions in central motor neuron excitability as a primary reason for reduced motor unit firing rates (Bigland-Ritchie et al., 1986). While the coordinated agonist-antagonist activity of limb muscles is critically dependent on fusimotor-driven feedback, the diaphragm has virtually no muscle spindles. The diaphragm does, however, contain small-diameter nociceptive afferents (type III and type IV fibers), which modulate phrenic nerve activity (Cheeseman and Revelette, 1990). The few tendon organs of the diaphragm are thought to mediate the inhibition of phrenic nerve traffic during passive muscle stretch (Speck and Revelette, 1987; Cheeseman and Revelette, 1990). In contrast to the diaphragm, intercostal muscles are rich in spindles, conceivably enabling them to fulfill nonrespiratory, postural functions (Whitelaw et al., 1992). Afferent activity from mechano-receptors of intercostal muscles may play a role in shaping the overall output of the respiratory pattern generator and may, thus, be involved in mediating the rapid, shallow breathing so characteristic of the ventilatory failure syndrome (Roussos, 1984). The main effect of intercostal afferent stimulation appears to be an inhibition of phrenic nerve activity (Shannon and Lindsey, 1987; Speck and Revelett, 1987; Hernandez et al., 1989; Cheeseman and Revelette, 1990). Unfortunately, the interpretation of regional stimulation studies is complicated by the complex deformations of the rib cage and associated musculature. It has been postulated that the primary determinants of respiratory frequency and tidal volume under resting conditions are extravagally mediated, that is, they are derived from intercostal muscle and chest wall afferents (von Euler, 1986), which provide information on the shape and stress distributions of the rib cage. This information may allow the respiratory centers to impose a breathing strategy that minimizes the overall stress on the rib cage musculature. On the other hand, there is evidence that vagotomy not only alters the breathing patterns of anesthetized dogs with experimental inspiratory muscle fatigue, but also causes a substantial increase in alveolar ventilation (Adams et al., 1988).

From an energetic perspective, rapid, shallow breathing might be maladaptive. It has been speculated, therefore, that respiratory control mechanisms regulate the use of fatigued muscles in order to minimize the perception of effort. The sense of effort is strongly influenced by central cortico-fugal motor commands giving rise to corollary discharges (McCloskey et al., 1983; Hobbs and Gandevia, 1985; Cafarelli and Layton-Wood, 1986; Aniss et al., 1988). In normal individuals, the perception of inspiratory effort varies in proportion to Pmus and the maximal pressure-generating capacity of the inspiratory muscles (Killian et al., 1984). During experimental fatigue, the perception of inspiratory effort at a given Pmus is heightened (Gandevia, 1981). This observation is consistent with studies on humans whose limb muscles were experimentally weakened by fatigue or partial curarization and suggests that a decline in the force-generating capacity of a skeletal muscle elicits an increased motor command (McCloskey et al., 1974, 1983; Gandevia and McCloskey, 1977a,b; Campbell et al., 1980). Changes in effort perception and attempts to minimize the sensation of dyspnea may, therefore, also contribute to the rapid, shallow breathing, which has been observed in experimental and clinical respiratory fatigue syndromes (Gilbert et al., 1974; Ashutosh et al., 1975; Cohen et al., 1982; Gallagher et al., 1985; Tobin et al., 1986, 1987a).

VI. Respiratory Muscle Use and Coordination in Patients with Weaning-Induced Ventilatory Failure

Weaning from mechanical ventilation can be viewed as a process during which the physician evaluates the load response of the patient's ventilatory pump. In this respect, weaning is analogous to exercise testing in its goal to characterize the performance capacity and endurance of the cardiopulmonary systems and to identify weak links in these systems on the basis of weaning response patterns. One aspect of the load response assessment is the careful analysis of breathing patterns and chest wall motion because they provide important clues about the relative recruitment and coordination among different respiratory muscles.

A. Chest Wall Displacement

The respiratory pump is driven by many different muscles, which are not recruited in unison. Their interplay and different mechanical actions on the thorax can be inferred from the displacements and deformation of rib cage and abdomen and from the changes in pressure within these compartments (Agostoni and Mognoni, 1966; Konno and Mead, 1968; Sharp et al., 1977; Loring and Mead, 1982; Mead and Loring, 1982). Konno and Mead (1968) described the movements of the respiratory system by plotting the relative displacements of rib cage and abdomen through time. During normal quiet breathing, the rib cage and abdomen are displaced along their relaxation characteristics, that is, they describe the configuration of the chest wall when it is undistorted by respiratory muscle forces (Fig. 3, left panel). Initially, this observation was inferred to mean that the mechanical events during breathing were relatively simple, with the diaphragm acting as the only significant inspiratory muscle. Subsequently, it has been shown that the mechanical interactions between the diaphragm and rib cage are quite complex (Loring and Mead, 1982; Mead and Loring, 1982) and that breathing requires the coordinated use of the diaphragm and of muscle groups with primary actions on the rib cage (De Troyer and Sampson, 1982; De Troyer and Estenne, 1984; De Troyer and Estenne, 1988).

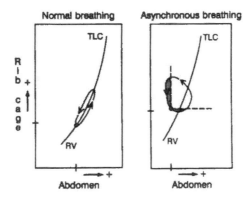

Figure 3 Schematic of a Konno-Mead diagram during normal quiet breathing (left panel) and during asynchronous breathing (right panel). The line between total lung capacity (TLC) and residual volume (RV) illustrates the relative dimensions of rib cage and abdomen during quasi-static relaxation maneuvers between the volume extremes. The relative dimensions during breathing are shown by the broken lines. Upward arrows on the breathing loops identify inspiration, downward arrows expiration. The shaded areas during asynchronous breathing quantify portions of the loop during which rib cage or abdominal dimension are smaller than at end-expiration. (From Hagan and Hubmayr, 1991.)

The Konno-Mead analysis has been used to study chest wall motion during intrinsic and extrinsic loading of the respiratory system in health and disease (Sharp et al., 1977; Tobin et al., 1983, 1987a,b). In particular, the analysis has been useful in describing varying degrees of asynchrony between the motions of rib cage and abdomen (Fig. 3, right panel). Several indices have been proposed to quantify the degree of asynchrony. One approach has been to measure the phase angle (Θ) between rib cage and abdominal signals (Agostoni and Rahn, 1960). Others have focused on the area encompassed by the Konno-Mead plot, which is a measure of the differences (hysteresis) among chest wall shapes during inspiration and expiration. Degrees of thoraco-abdominal paradox have been quantified by measuring the area fraction of the loop that lies outside a 90° window anchored at FRC. A few general conclusions can be derived from such studies. Asynchrony and distortions of the chest wall during breathing are common (1) in patients with airways obstruction (Sharp et al., 1968, 1977), (2) in the presence of neuromuscular diseases (Mortola and Sant'Ambrogio, 1978), and (3) during weaning from mechanical ventilation (Ashutosh et al., 1975; Tobin et al., 1987a). The goal to link certain displacement patterns unequivocally to fatigue of a muscle or muscle group, however, remains elusive. This is not surprising given the inherent assumptions of the Konno-Mead approach and considering the multiplicity of factors that determine thoraco-abdominal shape.

A departure of thoraco-abdominal shape from its relaxed configuration implies a distortion of the chest wall by muscular forces relative to some minimum energy state. The Konno-Mead diagram characterizes these distortions, provided rib cage and abdomen behave as single, independent units. Distortions within the rib cage and abdomen add additional degrees of freedom, complicating the interpretation of chest wall surface measurements. Although it has been implied that breathing near "the relaxation line" is advantageous for energetic reasons, there is no evidence that the normal respiratory system is designed or constrained to maintain a unique relationship between lung volume and chest wall shape during breathing. Departures from the relaxation line and widening of the hysteresis loop between inspiration and expiration are commonly seen in normal individuals during voluntary hyperventilation and during exercise (Green et al., 1974). From a purely mechanical perspective, there could be trade-offs between using muscles to prevent distortions within the rib cage compartment and using muscles to preserve thoraco-abdominal shape near the relaxation configuration. In diseases like COPD, structural adaptations of the chest wall and hyperinflation affect the mechanical efficiency of respiratory muscle groups relative to each other (Sharp et al., 1968). Therefore, asynchrony, distortions, and hysteresis of the chest wall loop may reflect (1) the altered mechanical actions of the diaphragm on the hyperinflated chest (Hoover, 1920), (2) the effects of muscular forces during active expiration, (3) changes in diaphragm recruitment relative to inspiratory rib cage and accessory muscles, or (4) a true change in the intrinsic contractile properties of the diaphragm (e.g., peripheral fatigue).

Several investigators have prospectively compared chest wall motion during successful and unsuccessful weaning trials from mechanical ventilation (Cohen et al., 1982; Tobin et al., 1987a; Krieger and Ershowsky, 1988; Krieger et al., 1989a). In general, patients who failed weaning had more asynchronous chest wall movements than those who succeeded. However, there was a great deal of overlap between groups, and none of the asynchrony parameters had sufficient predictive value to aid in clinical decision making. According to Tobin et al. (1987a) there was greater breath-to-breath variability of chest wall displacement patterns in the failure group. This was reflected by a greater standard deviation about the fraction of V_T, which was attributable to rib cage expansion ($\Delta V_{RC}/V_T$). Individual $\Delta V_{RC}/V_T$ values were not clustered around two means, as would be the case for true "respiratory alternans." Respiratory alternans describes an oscillation in chest wall displacement patterns between two distinct states, classically between rib cage and abdominal breathing (Roussos and Macklem, 1982). Such a strategy has been thought to provide alternating "rest" to different sets of respiratory muscles, i.e., diaphragm and inspiratory rib cage muscles. Regardless of the uncertainties in underlying mechanisms and strict definitions, respiratory alternans or breath-to-breath variability in chest wall motion appears to be one of the most specific predicators of impending respiratory failure (Krieger et al., 1989).

B. Regional Respiratory Pressures

The relative contribution of the various respiratory muscles during breathing determines, in part, the distribution of pressure swings within thorax and abdomen.

The difference between abdominal and pleural pressure swings (ΔPab and ΔPpl, respectively) is often used to infer the contribution of the diaphragm during breathing (ΔPab – ΔPpl = ΔPdi). During quiet breathing in erect normal man, the ratio of ΔPab/ΔPpl is $\leq$–1, averaging –1.95 $\pm$ 0.86 (Lisboa et al., 1986). As the contribution of the rib cage and accessory inspiratory muscles to Pmus increases, ΔPab/ΔPdi approaches 0. In the presence of diaphragm paralysis or extreme weakness, ΔPab becomes negative (falls during inspiration), raising ΔPab/ΔPpl to above 0. This is usually associated with asynchronous chest wall movements and thoraco-abdominal paradox. One of the advantages of measuring regional respiratory pressures and Pdi is in the assessment of inspiratory muscle function in patients who are unable to perform maximal respiratory maneuvers (Hillman and Finucane, 1988). Unfortunately, measurements of ΔPdi are exquisitely sensitive to changes in lung volume (Agostoni and Rahn, 1960; Smith and Bellemare, 1987; Hubmayr et al., 1989), respiratory system geometry (Marshall, 1962; Hubmayr et al., 1990), and abdominal impedance and are affected by the pressure contribution of other inspiratory muscles to overall Pmus (Hershenson et al., 1988). It is, therefore, not possible to clearly define the intrinsic contractile properties of the diaphragm in a spontaneously breathing patient on the basis of regional pressure measurements. In keeping with these limitations, the monitoring of ΔPdi has not proven useful in the early diagnosis of respiratory pump failure during weaning (Swartz and Marino, 1985).

C. Breathing Patterns

Many weaning studies have emphasized rapid, shallow breathing as a common, albeit nonspecific, manifestation of respiratory distress (Gilbert et al., 1974; Ashutosh et al., 1975; Dunn et al., 1991; Jabour et al., 1991; Yang and Tobin, 1991). Most recently Yang and Tobin (1991) reported that a ratio of breathing frequency to tidal volume (f/V_T) greater than 105 min^{-1} * ml^{-1} identified 78% of patients who ultimately failed weaning by clinical or gas exchange criteria. The negative predictive value of this rapid, shallow breathing index was 95%, underscoring its potential clinical utility. Interestingly, in the same study, a V_T less than 325 ml had positive and negative predictive values of 73% and 94%, respectively, thus discriminating almost as well as the f/V_T ratio between successful and unsuccessful weaning outcomes. Stroetz and Hubmayr (1992) studied the tidal volume responses of difficult to wean patients during stepwise withdrawal of pressure support. Motivated by the concepts illustrated in Figure 2, they showed that patients who experienced weaning-induced distress had a significantly greater decline in tidal volume as inspiratory pressure support was withdrawn than did patients who were able to breathe unassisted for one hour. Similarly, Younes et al. (M. Younes, personal communication) observed that patients with impending ventilatory failure increased their tidal volume when the ventilatory pump was unloaded using proportional assist ventilation. This is in contrast to normal volunteers, who maintain a near constant tidal volume when the ventilatory pump is unloaded.

The examples in Figure 2 link the control of tidal volume to inspiratory muscle mechanics. Virtually every study of patients with hypercarbic respiratory failure has demonstrated a high prevalence of inspiratory muscle weakness. However, so far it has not been possible to distinguish weakness from fatigue in a clinical setting. In contrast to weakness, fatigue is a process which is reversible by rest (NHLBI Workshop Summary, 1990). Because fatigue is task dependent, no single mechanism accounts for the acute decline in muscle performance. The distinction between fatigue and weakness in a clinical setting might be of particular interest if one could demonstrate that the two processes are associated with different weaning (load) response patterns. Such an observation might also strengthen the clinical relevance of studies in which peripheral muscle fatigue has been experimentally induced by extrinsic loads. Figure 4 shows a typical weaning response pattern in a patient with diaphragm weakness. Shown are recordings of gastric pressure (Pga), flow ($\dot{V}$), and esophageal pressure (Pes) in a ventilator-dependent patient one hour after cessation of machine support. Shortly thereafter, the weaning trial had to be aborted because of dyspnea. At that time, the respiratory rate had risen to 40 breaths/min and the tidal volume (not shown) had fallen to ≈ 250 ml. The shape of the expiratory flow wave tracing, with its convexity towards the time axis, suggests the presence of airways obstruction. Palpation of the abdomen revealed expiratory muscle use, which accounts for the increase in Pes to $+10$ cm H_2O at end-expiration. The swings in Pes were relatively large (20 cm H_2O) and were accompanied by a fall in Pga as abdominal muscle activity decayed during inspiration. In the weaning literature, virtually all of these findings have (at one time or another) been attributed to inspiratory muscle fatigue. However, the only indirect evidence linking tachypnea and weaning-induced thoraco-abdominal paradox to diaphragm fatigue is based on changes in the power spectrum of the diaphragm EMG (Cohen et al., 1982). Figure 5 shows the result of

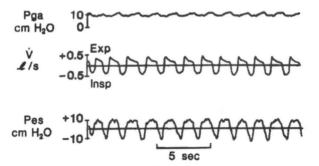

Figure 4 Recordings of gastric pressure (Pga), gas flow ($\dot{V}$), and esophageal pressure (Pes) are shown from a ventilator-dependent patient at the end of a 1-hour weaning trial. For explanation see text. Exp, expiration; Insp, inspiration. (From Hubmayr and Rehder, 1992.)

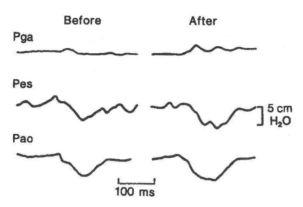

Figure 5 Gastric pressure (Pga), esophageal pressure (Pes), and airway occlusion pressure (Pao) were recorded during bilateral twitch stimulation of the phrenic nerves in the patient whose weaning response pattern is shown in Figure 4. The twitch pressure responses before and immediately after the symptom-limited weaning trial are identical. (From Hubmayr and Rehder, 1992.)

two phrenic nerve twitch stimulation tests during airway occlusion in the patient from Figure 4. The recordings of airway-occlusion pressure, ΔPes, and ΔPga on the left side were made prior to weaning following overnight respiratory muscle rest with controlled mechanical ventilation. The recordings on the right side were made 5 minutes after the symptom-limited weaning trial. The diaphragm's twitch pressure responses were significantly reduced even after prolonged respiratory muscle rest. Normal volunteers generate a twitch Pdi $\geq$ 20 cm H_2O near relaxation volume (Smith and Bellemare, 1987; Hubmayr et al., 1989) as opposed to the 6 cm H_2O in this patient. The abnormal twitch response following overnight mechanical ventilation indicates profound diaphragm weakness, but an additional loss of force from fatigue cannot be ruled out on the basis of a single measurement. Since a repeat test after the symptom-limited weaning trial yielded an identical twitch response, however, a diagnosis of peripheral diaphragm fatigue cannot be established. This anecdotal observation is consistent with the hypothesis that respiratory distress and impending pump failure need not reflect peripheral respiratory muscle fatigue, but that the fatigue process may involve load perception and central integrative responses to muscle overload. The example also suggests that respiratory muscle weakness and fatigue share a similar load response.

It would be erroneous to invariably attribute rapid, shallow breathing to an overload of the inspiratory muscles. Indeed, many weaning response studies can be criticized for this implicit assumption and, because of it, are running the risk of circular reasoning. If increased respiratory effort and distress are the clinical endpoints by which failure is defined, then weaning parameters based on rapid, shallow breathing will have a high positive predictive value. Tachypnea is a nonspecific ventilatory response to pain and anxiety, although the tidal volume is usually not reduced in these conditions. Rapid, shallow breathing is seen in patients with pulmonary venous hypertension as well as in inflammatory airways and lung parenchymal diseases. Although these conditions are usually associated with increased elastic and/or resistive loads, the principal mechanisms for tachypnea are likely to be neuro-humoral in nature and involve pulmonary nociceptive afferents.

From a clinical perspective, it is important to distinguish between impending respiratory muscle failure and load-unrelated causes of rapid, shallow breathing. One way to make this distinction is to pay careful attention to phasic respiratory motor output while patients are mechanically ventilated at settings that minimize the load on the inspiratory muscles and, at the same time, satisfy the O_2 and CO_2 requirements of the organism. The example in Figure 6 illustrates the usefulness of respiratory waveform monitoring for this purpose. Shown are pressure and flow tracings of a patient with airways obstruction, purulent bronchitis, and hypercarbic ventilatory failure during pressure support ventilation (PSV) of 10 and 5 cm H_2O above end-expiration. Arterial O_2 and CO_2 tensions were normal at both settings, and the patient did not appear in distress. Note the small deflections in expiratory flow marked by arrows. These represent inspiratory efforts during the expiratory phase of the machine cycle. In the presence of dynamic hyperinflation, muscle pressure (Pmus) must counterbalance the expiratory recoil forces (i.e., Pel) before a new machine breath can be triggered. If ΔPmus is less than Pel minus the machine trigger sensitivity, then the inspiratory effort is wasted and does not result in a machine breath. At a PSV setting of 10 cm H_2O (upper panel), only every third inspiratory effort results in a machine breath (3:1 coupling). The low ΔPmus, the persistence of machine inflation after the cessation of inspiratory effort, and the presence of airways obstruction (with its propensity for dynamic hyperinflation) all contribute to machine trigger failure. Note that the reduction in PSV from 10 to 5 cm H_2O (lower panel) results in an apparent increase in respiratory rate. It is important to recognize, however, that the increase in machine rate is caused by a change in the coupling rate from 3:1 to 2:1 rather than a change in the number of inspiratory efforts per minute. The greater Pmus during PSV of 5 than 10 cm H_2O accounts for the reduced number of wasted inspiratory efforts. An awareness of this problem is important because the physician may otherwise attribute an increase in machine rate following reductions in inspiratory airway pressure support to impending failure and consider the load fatiguing.

VII. Ventilatory Dynamics and Chemo-Responsiveness

$\dot{V}$E combined with the mechanical impedance of the respiratory system determine the power output of the respiratory muscles and, thus, their load. The relationships between fatigue-induced changes in tidal volume and effects on respiratory rate and pulmonary gas exchange are not straightforward. A fall in tidal volume must result in an increase in the dead space to tidal volume ratio (V_D/V_T), compromising

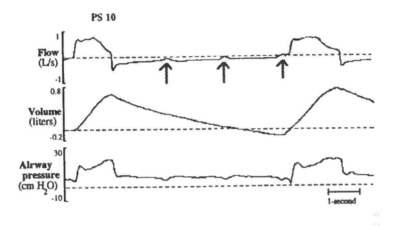

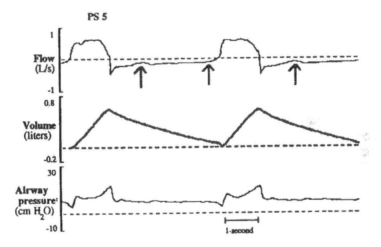

Figure 6   Flow, volume, and pressure tracings of a patient recorded during pressure support ventilation with 10 cm H_2O (upper panel) and 5 cm H_2O (lower panel). Each arrow indicates an inspiratory effort. (From Hubmayr, 1993.)

pulmonary CO_2 elimination ($\dot{V}_{CO_2}$). To minimize the increase in arterial CO_2 tension (Pa_{CO_2}) and body CO_2 stores, respiratory rate must increase. From an energetic standpoint, it would be preferable to accept alveolar hypoventilation as a means of reducing the mechanical load on the inspiratory muscles. CO_2 would increase in response to this breathing strategy and exert its own effects on breathing pattern and respiratory motor output. Cause and effect between rapid, shallow breathing and hypercarbia would thus be obscure.

The relationships between $\dot{V}_E$ and Pa_{CO_2} can be represented by metabolic hyperbolae, as shown in Figure 7. Assume (for the purpose of simplicity) that CO_2 production and its elimination by the lungs are equal ($\dot{V}_{CO_2}$ = 0.2 liter/min) and do not change as a function of V_T or rate. The three hyperbolae in Figure 7 represent dead space to tidal volume isopleths (V_D/V_T = 0.4, 0.57, and 0.67, respectively) and illustrate all possible combinations of $\dot{V}E$ and Pa_{CO_2} at a given V_D/V_T. V_D itself is assumed constant (V_D = 0.2 liter/breath, a value consistent with moderately severe intrinsic lung disease). Since V_D is constant, each V_D/V_T isopleth is also a tidal volume isopleth (V_T = 0.50, 0.35, and 0.30, respectively). Respiratory rate changes with $\dot{V}E$ along each isopleth as indicated numerically. Let point A represent some baseline state during which a subject breathes with a V_T of 0.5 liter and a rate of 14 breaths/min (bpm) while maintaining a Pa_{CO_2} of 40 mm Hg. As V_T decreases in response to an insult (or load), the relationships between Pa_{CO_2} and $\dot{V}_E$ shift to a different isopleth. For example, a fall in V_T from 0.5 to 0.35 liter would result in a change in V_D/V_T from 0.4 to 0.57 and would be accompanied by CO_2 retention unless respiratory rate increased to 29 bpm. A fall in V_T to 0.3 liter would mandate a disproportionate rate increase to 43 bpm in order to preserve isocapnea. In principle, the relationship between Pa_{CO_2} and $\dot{V}_E$ describes the CO_2 responsiveness of the respiratory pump. Three hypothetical response curves with slopes between 1.0 liter/min/mm Hg and 0.2 liter/min/mm Hg are shown as broken lines. In theory, a blunted chemo-responsiveness ($\Delta\dot{V}_E/\Delta Pa_{CO_2}$ = 0.2 liter/min) would allow the subject to reduce V_T to 0.3 liter unaccompanied by an inordinate increase in rate, albeit at the expense of hypercarbia.

The slope of the ventilatory response curve to CO_2 is not a load-independent expression of intrinsic respiratory drive (Dempsey, 1976). Alveolar ventila-

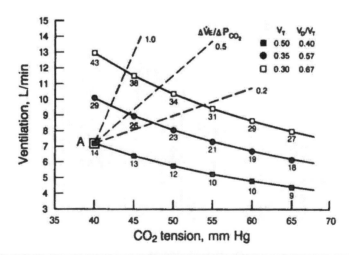

Figure 7   Schematic illustration of the interdependence between breathing pattern, dead space (V_D), alveolar ventilation, arterial CO_2 tension, and the ventilatory response to CO_2. (From Hagan and Hubmayr, 1991.)

tion may, therefore, decline when the respiratory muscles are faced with an otherwise fatiguing load. What is not clear is how large an increase in Pa_{CO_2} can be tolerated without forgoing the possibility of reaching a new steady state between CO_2 production and elimination. Figure 7 illustrates how the gas exchange function of the lung, expressed here by a single parameter (V_D), sets limits to the mechanical load compensation that can occur on a muscle level. The agency through which these limits may be expressed is the CO_2 responsiveness of the respiratory pump.

Two lines of evidence suggest that the respiratory control system of conscious humans imposes significant limits on how far ventilation can be reduced in order to minimize the load on the inspiratory muscles. Jabour et al. (1991) studied the predictive value of a ventilator weaning index based on integrating ventilatory endurance and the efficiency of pulmonary gas exchange. As demonstrated repeatedly in fatigue experiments with extrinsic loads, a task such as diaphragm contraction can be sustained indefinitely if the force/breath is less than 40–60% of the diaphragm's force-generating capacity (Bellemare and Grassino, 1982; Roussos and Macklem, 1982; Aubier et al., 1985). Jabour et al. estimated the overall pressure output of the inspiratory muscles per breath (Pbreath) in difficult to wean patients and expressed it as a fraction of the maximal inspiratory airway occlusion pressure (P_{Imax}). In contrast to predictions from experimental diaphragm fatigue tests, Pbreath/P_{Imax} (which ranged between 0.2 and 0.8), was useless as a predictor of outcome of weaning trials. However, when Pbreath/P_{Imax} was adjusted for duty cycle (inspiratory time expressed as a fraction of total breath duration) and the minute volume that would have been necessary to maintain the arterial CO_2 tension at 40 mm Hg, a clear separation between weaning success and failure emerged. Such a result could not have occurred if significant alveolar hypoventilation was a viable strategy for acute load compensation and fatigue prevention.

Dunn et al. (1991) addressed the same issue a slightly different way. They measured the CO_2 responsiveness of the unloaded respiratory pump using the recruitment threshold technique in difficult to wean patients. Measurements of respiratory motor output were made during mechanical ventilation, and the machine settings were adjusted until phasic inspiratory muscle activity was completely suppressed. The CO_2 recruitment threshold (CO_2RT) was defined as the lowest Pa_{CO_2} at which the supplementation of CO_2 caused the reappearance of phasic motor activity (Prechter et al., 1990). Since CO_2RT was determined during mechanical ventilation, it was interpreted as a measure of the CO_2 sensitivity of the unloaded respiratory pump. CO_2RT was then compared in each patient to the Pa_{CO_2} during unassisted spontaneous breathing (CO_2SB) (Fig. 8). Seven of 10 patients who failed weaning because of dyspnea or sustained tachypnea (respiratory rate $\geq$ 30) retained CO_2SB compared with CO_2RT by more than 3 mm Hg. In contrast, the five patients who were weaned successfully maintained CO_2SB within 2 mm Hg of CO_2RT. Although patients who failed weaning tended to be weaker

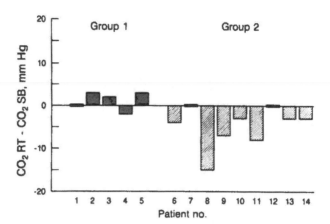

Figure 8 The differences between arterial CO_2 tensions (in mm Hg) during recruitment testing (CO_2RT) and at the end of a weaning trial while breathing spontaneously (CO_2SB) are shown on the ordinate. Dark-shaded bars (patients 1 through 5) represent observations in group 1; light-shaded bars (patients 6 through 14) represent observations in group 2. Note that three of the five patients in group 1 had lower arterial CO_2 tensions during spontaneous breathing than predicted from CO_2RT. Also note that seven of the nine patients in group 2 had arterial CO_2 tensions that exceeded CO_2RT by 3 mm Hg or more. (From Dunn et al., 1991.)

(consistent with Jabour's findings), there was a considerable overlap in parameters reflective of mechanical load and inspiratory muscle output among the groups. These findings underscore the interactions between load, load response, and CO_2 homeostasis. They suggest that load-induced reductions in tidal volume and alveolar ventilation that result in relatively small increases in Pa_{CO_2} above the pump's CO_2 setpoint (CO_2RT) often preclude the assumption of a new steady state. This implies that ventilatory control mechanisms impose substantial limits on the respiratory muscles' load responses in patients with impending ventilatory pump failure.

References

Adams, J. M., Farkas, G. A., and Rochester, D. F. (1988). Vagal afferents, diaphragm fatigue, and inspiratory resistance in anesthetized dogs. *J. Appl. Physiol.*, 64:2279–2286.

Agostoni, E., and Mognoni, P. (1966). Deformation of the chest wall during breathing efforts. *J. Appl. Physiol.*, 21:1827–1832.

Agostoni, E., and Rahn, H. (1960). Abdominal and thoracic pressures at different lung volumes. *J. Appl. Physiol.*, 15:1087–1092.

Aniss, A. M., Gandevia, S. C., and Milne, R. J. (1988). Changes in perceived heaviness and motor commands produced by cutaneous reflexes in man. *J. Physiol. Lond.*, 397:113–126.

Ashutosh, K., Gilbert, R., Auchincloss, J. H., and Peppi, D. (1975). Asynchronous breathing movements in patients with obstructive pulmonary disease. *Chest*, 67:553–557.

Aubier, M., Murciano, D., Lecocguic, Y., Viires, N., and Pariente, R. (1985). Bilateral phrenic stimulation: a simple technique to assess diaphragmatic fatigue in humans. *J. Appl. Physiol.*, 58:58–64.

Bellemare, F., and Grassino, A. (1982a). Effect of pressure and timing of contraction on human diaphragmatic fatigue. *J. Appl. Physiol.*, 53:1190–1195.

Bellemare, F., and Grassino, A. (1982b). Evaluation of human diaphragm fatigue. *J. Appl. Physiol.*, 53:1196–1206.

Bigland-Ritchie, B., Johansson, R., Lippold, O. C. J., and Woods, J. J. (1983). Contractile speed and EMG changes during fatigue of sustained maximal voluntary contractions. *J. Neurophysiol.*, 50:313–324.

Bigland-Ritchie, B., Dawson, N. J., Johansson, R. S., and Lippold, O. C. J. (1986). Reflex origin for the slowing of motoneurone firing rates in fatigue of human voluntary contractions. *J. Physiol.* (London), 379:451–459.

Burke, R. E., and Edgerton, V. R. (1975). Motor unit properties and selective involvement in movement. *Exercise Sport Sci.*, 3:31–81.

Cafarelli, E., and Layton-Wood, J. (1986). Effect of vibration on force sensation in fatigued muscle. *Med. Sci. Sports Exercise*, 18:516–521.

Campbell, E. J. M. (1958). *The Respiratory Muscles and the Mechanics of Breathing*. Chicago, The Year Book Publishers.

Campbell, E. J. M., Dinnick, O. P., and Howell, J. B. L. (1961). The immediate effects of elastic loads on breathing of man. *J. Physiol.* (London), 156:260–273.

Campbell, E. J. M., Gandevia, S. C., Killian, K. J., Mahutte, C. K., and Rigg, J. R. A. (1980). Changes in the perception of inspiratory resistive loads during partial curarization. *J. Physiol.* (London), 309:93–100.

Cheeseman, M., and Revelette, W. R. (1990). Phrenic afferent contribution to reflexes elicited by changes in diaphragm length. *J. Appl. Physiol.*, 69:640–647.

Cohen, C. A., Zagelbaum, G., Gross, D., Roussos, C. H., and Macklem, P. T. (1982). Clinical manifestations of inspiratory muscle fatigue. *Am. J. Med.*, 73:308–316.

De Troyer, A., and Estenne, M. (1984). Coordination between rib cage muscles and diaphragm during quiet breathing in humans. *J. Appl. Physiol.*, 57:899–906.

De Troyer, A., and Estenne, M. (1988). Functional anatomy of the respiratory muscles. *Clin. Chest Med.*, 9:175–193.

De Troyer, A., and Sampson, M. G. (1982). Activation of the parasternal intercostals during breathing efforts in human subjects. *J. Appl. Physiol.*, 52:524–529.

Dempsey, J. A. (1976). CO_2 response: stimulus definition and limitations. *Chest*, 70:114–118.

Dietz, V. (1978). Analysis of the electrical muscle activity during maximal contraction and the influence of ischaemia. *J. Neurol. Sci.*, 37:187–197.

Dunn, W. F., Nelson, S. B., and Hubmayr, R. D. (1991). The control of breathing during weaning from mechanical ventilation. *Chest*, 100:754–761.

Edman, K. A. P. (1980). Depression of mechanical performance by active shortening during twitch and tetanus of vertebrate muscle fibers. *Acta Physiol. Scand.*, 109:15–26.

Edman, K. A. P. (1981). Deactivation of the contractile system induced by shortening of striated muscle. In *The Regulation of Muscle Contraction*. San Diego, Academic Press Inc., pp. 281–296.

Enoka, R. M., and Stuart, D. G. (1992). Neurobiology of muscle fatigue. *J. Appl. Physiol.*, 72:1631–1648.

Esau, S. A., Bellemare, F., Grassino, A., Permutt, S., Roussos, C., and Pardy, R. L. (1983). Changes in relaxation rate with diaphragmatic fatigue in humans. *J. Appl. Physiol.*, 54:1353–1360.

Gallagher, C. G., Im Hof, V., and Younes, M. (1985). Effect of inspiratory muscle fatigue on breathing pattern. *J. Appl. Physiol.*, 59:1152–1158.

Gandevia, S. C., Killian, K. J., and Campbell, E. J. M. (1981). The effect of respiratory muscle fatigue on respiratory sensations. *Clin. Sci.*, 60:463–466.

Gandevia, S. C., and McCloskey, D. I. (1977a). Effects of related sensory inputs on motor performances in man studied through changes in perceived heaviness. *J. Physiol.* (London), 272:653–672.

Gandevia, S. C., and McCloskey, D. I. (1977b). Changes in motor commands, as shown by changes in perceived heaviness. *J. Physiol.* (London), 272:673–689.

Garland, S. J. (1991). Role of small diameter afferents in reflex inhibition during human muscle fatigue. *J. Physiol.* (London), 435:547–558.

Garland, S. J., and McComas, A. J. (1990). Reflex inhibition of human soleus muscle during fatigue. *J. Physiol.* (London), 429:17–27.

Gilbert, R., Auchincloss, J. H., Peppi, D., and Ashutosh, K. (1974). The first few hours off a respirator. *Chest*, 65:152–157.

Green, M., Mead, J., and Sears, T. A. (1974). Effects of loading on respiratory muscle control in man. In *Loaded Breathing*. Edited by L. D. Pengelly, A. S. Rebuck, and E. J. M. Campbell. Edinburgh, Churchill Livingstone, pp. 73–80.

Gross, D., Grassino, A., Ross, W. R. D., and Macklem, P. T. (1979). Electromyogram pattern of diaphragmatic fatigue. *J. Appl. Physiol.*, 46:1–7.

Hagan, B. M., and Hubmayr, R. D. (1991). Respiratory failure: dynamics of breathing and coordination. In *Update in Intensive Care and Emergency Medicine*, Volume 15: *Ventilatory Failure*. New York, Springer-Verlag, pp. 75–96.

Hernandez, Y. M., Lindsey, B. G., and Shannon, R. (1989). Intercostal and abdominal muscle afferent influence on caudal medullary expiratory neurons that drive abdominal muscles. *Exp. Brain Res.*, 78:219–222.

Hershenson, M. B., Kikuchi, Y., Loring, S. H. (1988). Relative strength of the chest wall muscles. *J. Appl. Physiol.*, 65:852–862.

Hillman, D. R., and Finucane, K. E. (1988). Respiratory pressure partitioning during quiet inspiration in unilateral and bilateral diaphragmatic weakness. *Am. Rev. Respir. Dis.*, 137:1401–1405.

Hobbs, S. F., and Gandevia, S. C. (1985). Cardiovascular responses and the sense of effort during attempts to contract paralysed muscles: role of the spinal cord. *Neurosci. Lett.*, 57:85–90.

Hoover, C. F. (1920). The diagnostic significance of inspiratory movements of the costal margins. *Am. J. Med. Sci.*, 159:633–646.

Hubmayr, R. D. (1993). *Respiratory Muscle Coordination During the Weaning of Patients with Neurological Diseases*. Springer-Verlag Ibérica (in press).

Hubmayr, R. D., Litchy, W. J., Gay, P. C., and Nelson, S. B. (1989). Trans-diaphragmatic twitch pressure: effects of lung volume and chest wall shape. *Am. Rev. Respir. Dis.*, 139:647–652.

Hubmayr, R. D., Sprung, J. J., and Nelson, S. B. (1990). The determinants of transdiaphragmatic pressure in dogs. *J. Appl. Physiol.*, 69:1050–1056.

Hubmayr, R. D., and Rehder, K. (1992). Respiratory muscle failure in critically ill patients. *Semin. Resp. Med.*, 13:14–21.

Jabour, E. R., Rabil, D. M., Truwit, J. D., and Rochester, D. F. (1991). Evaluation of a new weaning index based on ventilatory endurance and the efficiency of gas exchange. *Am. Rev. Respir. Dis.*, 144:531–537.

Jones, G. L., Killian, K. J., Summers, E., and Jones, N. L. (1985). Inspiratory muscle forces and endurance in maximum resistive loading. *J. Appl. Physiol.*, 58:1608–1615.

Joyce, G. C., Rack, P. M. H., and Westbury, D. R. (1969). The mechanical properties of cat soleus muscle during controlled lengthening and shortening movements. *J. Physiol.*, 204:461–474.

Killian, K. J., Gandevia, S. C., Summers, E., and Campbell, E. J. M. (1984). Effect of increased lung volume on perception of breathlessness, effort, and tension. *J. Appl. Physiol.*, 57:686–691.

Konno, K., and Mead, J. (1968). Static volume-pressure characteristics of the rib cage and abdomen. *J. Appl. Physiol.*, 24:544–548.

Krieger, B. P., and Ershowsky, P. (1988). Noninvasive detection of respiratory failure in the intensive care unit. *Chest*, 94:254–261.

Krieger, B. P., Ershowsky, P. F., Becker, D. A., and Gazeroglu, H. B. (1989). Evaluation of conventional criteria for predicting successful weaning from mechanical ventilatory support in elderly patients. *Crit. Care Med.*, 17:858–861.

Lisboa, C., Paré, P. D., Pertuzé, J., Contreres, G., Moreno, R., Guillemi, S., and Cruz, E. (1986). Inspiratory muscle function in unilateral diaphragmatic paralysis. *Am. Rev. Respir. Dis.*, 134:488–492.

Loring, S. H., and Mead, J. (1982). Action of the diaphragm on the rib cage inferred from a force-balance analysis. *J. Appl. Physiol.*, 53:756–760.

Macefield, G., Hagbarth, K.-E., Gorman, R., Gandevia, S. C., and Burke, D. (1991). Decline in spindle support to α-motoneurones during sustained voluntary contractions. *J. Physiol.* (London), 440:497–512.

Marshall, R. (1962). Relationships between stimulus and work of breathing at different lung volumes. *J. Appl. Physiol.*, 17:917–921.

McCloskey, D. I., Ebeling, P., and Goodwin, G. M. (1974). Estimation of weights and tensions and apparent involvement of a "sense of effort." Exp. Neurol., 42:220–232.

McCloskey, D. I., Gandevia, S., Potter, E. K., and Colebatch, J. G. (1983). Muscle sense and effort: motor commands and judgments about muscular contractions. In *Motor Control Mechanisms in Health and Disease*. Edited by J. E. Desmedt. New York, Raven, pp. 151–167.

McCool, F. D., McCann, D. R., Leith, D. E., and Hoppin, F. G. (1986). Pressure-flow effects on endurance of inspiratory muscles. *J. Appl. Physiol.*, 60:299–303.

Mead, J. (1960). Control of respiratory frequency. *J. Appl. Physiol.*, 15:325–336.

Mead, J., and Loring, S. H. (1982). Analysis of volume displacement and length changes of the diaphragm during breathing. *J. Appl. Physiol.*, 53:750–755.

Milic-Emili, J., Gottfried, S. B., and Rossi, A. (1987). Dynamic hyperinflation: intrinsic PEEP and its ramifications in patients with respiratory failure. In *Update in Intensive Care and Emergency Medicine: Update 1987*. Edited by J. L. Vincent. New York, Springer-Verlag, pp. 192–198.

Mortola, J. P., and Sant'Ambrogio, G. (1978). Motion of the rib cage and the abdomen in tetraplegic patients. *Clin. Sci.*, 54:25–32.

NHLBI Workshop Summary (1990). Respiratory muscle fatigue: report of the respiratory muscle fatigue workshop group. *Am. Rev. Respir. Dis.*, 142:474–480.

Otis, A. B., Fenn, W. O., and Rahn, H. (1950). Mechanics of breathing. *J. Appl. Physiol.*, 2:592–607.

Pepe, P. E., and Marini, J. J. (1982). Occult positive end-expiratory pressure in mechanically ventilated patients with airflow obstruction: the auto-PEEP effect. *Am. Rev. Respir. Dis.*, 126:166–170.

Prechter, G. C., Nelson, S. B., and Hubmayr, R. D. (1990). The ventilatory recruitment threshold for carbon dioxide. *Am. Rev. Respir. Dis.*, 141:758–764.

Riddle, W., and Younes, M. (1981). A model for the relation between respiratory neural and mechanical outputs. II. Methods and evaluation of assumptions. *J. Appl. Physiol.*, 51:979–989.

Rochester, D. F. (1988). Does respiratory muscle rest relieve fatigue or incipient fatigue. *Am. Rev. Respir. Dis.*, 138:516–517.

Rochester, D. F., and Bettini, G. (1976). Diaphragmatic blood flow and energy expenditure in the dog: effects of inspiratory airflow resistance and hypercapnia. *J. Clin. Invest.*, 57:661–672.

Rodarte, J. R., and Rehder, K. (1986). Dynamics of respiration. In *Handbook of Physiology*, Section 3, Volume III, *The Respiratory System*. Baltimore, Waverly Press, pp. 131–144.

Roussos, C. (1984). Ventilatory muscle fatigue governs breathing frequency. *Bull. Eur. Physiopathol. Respir.*, 20:445–451.

Roussos, C., and Macklem, P. (1977). Diaphragmatic fatigue in man. *J. Appl. Physiol.*, 43:189–197.

Roussos, C., and Macklem, P. T. (1982). The respiratory muscles. *N. Engl. J. Med.*, 307:786–797.

Shannon, R., and Lindsey, B. G. (1987). Expiratory neurons in the region of the retrofacial nucleus: inhibitory effects of intercostal tendon organs. Exp. Neurol., 97:730–734.

Sharp, J. T., Van Lith, P., Nuchprayoon, C. V., Briney, R., and Johnson, F. N. (1968). The thorax in chronic obstructive lung disease. Am. J. Med., 44:39–46.

Sharp, J. T., Goldberg, N. B., Druz, W. S., Fishman, H. C., and Danon, J. (1977). Thoracoabdominal motion in chronic obstructive pulmonary disease. Am. Rev. Respir. Dis., 115:47–56.

Smith, J., and Bellemare, F. (1987). Effect of lung volume on in vivo contraction characteristics of human diaphragm. J. Appl. Physiol., 62:1893–1900.

Speck, D. F., and Revelette, W. R. (1987). Attenuation of phrenic motor discharge by phrenic nerve afferents. J. Appl. Physiol., 62:941–945.

Stroetz, R. W., and Hubmayr, R. D. (1992). Mechanical load compensation during ventilator weaning. Chest, 102:59S.

Swartz, M., and Marino, P. (1985). Diaphragmatic strength during weaning from mechanical ventilation. Chest, 88:736–739.

Tobin, M. J., Chadha, T. S., Jenouri, G., Birch, S. J., Gazeroglu, H. B., and Sackner, M. A. (1983). Breathing patterns. 2. Diseased subjects. Chest, 84:286–294.

Tobin, M. J., Perez, W., Guenther, S. M., Semmes, B. J., Mador, M. J., Allen, S. J., Lodato, R. F., and Dantzker, D. R. (1986). The pattern of breathing during successful and unsuccessful trials of weaning from mechanical ventilation. Am. Rev. Respir. Dis., 134:1111–1118.

Tobin, M. J., Guenther, S. M., Perez W., Lodato, R. F., Mador, J. M., Allen, S., and Dantzker, D. (1987a). Konno-Mead analysis of rib cage-abdominal motion during successful and unsuccessful trials of weaning from mechanical ventilation. Am. Rev. Respir. Dis., 135:1320–1328.

Tobin, M. J., Perez, W., Guenther, S. M., Lodato, R. F., and Dantzker, D. R. (1987b). Does rib cage–abdominal paradox signify respiratory muscle fatigue? J. Appl. Physiol., 63:851–860.

von Euler, C. (1986). Brain stem mechanisms for generation and control of breathing pattern. In Handbook of Physiology, Vol 2. Control of Breathing. Edited by N. Cherniak and J. G. Widdicombe. Bethesda, American Physiological Society, pp. 463–524.

Whitelaw, W. A., Derenne, J.-P., and Milic-Emili, J. (1975). Occlusion pressure as a measure of respiratory center output in conscious man. Respir. Physiol., 23:181–199.

Whitelaw, W. A., Fort, G. T., Rimmer, K. P., and De Troyer, A. (1992). Intercostal muscles are used during rotation of the thorax in humans. J. Appl. Physiol., 72:1940–1944.

Yan, S., Lichros, I., Zakynthinos, S., and Macklem, P. T. (1993a). Effect of diaphragmatic fatigue on control of respiratory muscles and ventilation during CO_2 rebreathing. J. Appl. Physiol. (in press).

Yan, S., Sliwinski, P., Gauthier, A. P., Lichros, I., Zakynthinos, S., and Macklem, P. T. (1993b). Effect of global inspiratory muscle fatigue on control of respiratory muscles and ventilation during CO_2 rebreathing. J. Appl. Physiol. (in press).

Yang, K. L., and Tobin, M. J. (1991). A prospective study of indexes predicting the outcome of trials of weaning from mechanical ventilation. N. Engl. J. Med., 324:1445–1450.

Younes, M., and Remmers, J. (1981). Control of tidal volume and respiratory frequency. In Control of Breathing. Edited by T. Hornbein. New York, Marcel Dekker, pp. 617–667.

Younes, M., and Riddle, W. (1981). A model for the relation between respiratory neural and mechanical outputs. I. Theory. J. Appl. Physiol., 51:979–989.

Younes, M., Riddle, W., and Polacheck, J. (1981). A model for the relation between respiratory neural and mechanical outputs. III. Experimental validation. J. Appl. Physiol., 51:990–1001.

60

Dyspnea

KIERAN J. KILLIAN and E. J. MORAN CAMPBELL

McMaster University
Hamilton, Ontario, Canada

I. Introduction

The terms cardiac dyspnea, dyspnea related to lung disease, and renal dyspnea
originated in the nineteenth century, when it was first firmly established that dyspnea
was associated with morbid anatomical changes in the heart, lung, and kidneys;
when no abnormality was detected, then dyspnea was considered neurogenic. At
that time conjecture about mechanism was of little practical importance because
amelioration of the heart or lung disorder was the only requirement for management,
and some would argue that this remains true today. In a similar fashion, dyspnea
was not a topic of particular interest to physiologists. Their real interest was in the
physiology of respiration. Nonetheless, tacit assumptions about the mechanism of
dyspnea emerged. Hence, it is not surprising that hypoxia, hypercapnia, and
acidemia were successively put forward as the mechanisms of dyspnea. Common
experience revealed that when the breath is voluntarily held, an unpleasant urge to
breathe emerges, attributed to chemoreceptor activation. This constituted the
chemical theory (Pfluger, 1868; Miescher-Rusch, 1885; Winterstein, 1911, 1921;
Meakins, 1923; Gesell, 1923; Haldane and Smith, 1935). The neurophysiologists
adopted a somewhat different standpoint; they saw central medullary respiratory
neuronal activity contributing to dyspnea (LeGallois, 1812). Later they saw lung
expansion hindered by stiffness consequent on disease contributing to failure of the

self-steering reflex, described by Hering and Breuer (Breuer and Hering, 1868), to inhibit medullary inspiratory neuronal activity, thereby causing dyspnea (Gad, 1911; Wright and Branscomb, 1954). This constituted the *reflex theory*. The physiologists of the early twentieth century saw ventilation encroaching on ventilatory capacity as the mechanism for dyspnea (Means, 1924; Cournand et al., 1939; Cournand and Richards, 1941a,b; Cournand et al., 1941) with increased force, work, and/or oxygen debt by the respiratory muscles as stimuli (Donders, 1853; Wirz, 1923; Rohrer, 1925; Otis et al., 1950; Harrison, 1950; Marshall et al., 1954; McIlroy, 1958; Cherniack, 1959; Aaron et al., 1991). This constituted the *mechanical theory*. All of these mechanisms continue to be put forward from time to time. Confusion has arisen because chemoreceptor stimulation, respiratory center output, blood gases, pulmonary mechanics, and vagal and chest wall receptor stimulation and their afferents are all integral to the process of breathing and because directly and indirectly all of these unit processes result in the stimulation of a variety of sensory receptors with access to consciousness resulting in the genesis of dyspnea. In the past 30 years dyspnea has been approached in a fundamentally different way. The integrated nature of these respiratory processes is accepted, psychophysical methods, including detection, recognition, and scaling, are now increasingly applied, and dyspnea arising in its clinical context is analyzed within the confines of respiratory and sensory physiology (for review see Killian, 1992).

In the first edition of this book we introduced the idea that conscious respiratory sensations are generated by the activation of many sensory receptors during the act of breathing. We discussed the various sensory stimuli, the receptors stimulated, and sensory perceptual processing giving rise to a whole variety of conscious sensations. We suggested that they all contribute in part to the nature of the conscious sensory experience with breathing. To an extent these sensory dimensions can be dissected in individual patients. We concluded that inspiratory effort was the specific sensation most closely related to dyspnea as it is usually seen in a clinical context. The neurophysiological stimulus underpinning the sense of effort appears to be the net motor output to the inspiratory muscles. This motor output has a sensory threshold magnitude below which dyspnea is not experienced and above which dyspnea increases in a positively accelerating manner with its intensity. With prolonged high-intensity stimulation the sensory magnitude declines with time such that patients with chronic overstimulation may be asymptomatic, a sensory process known as temporal adaptation.

The motor output to the inspiratory muscles provides the key to understanding the integrated interaction of the system. Motor output to the inspiratory muscles is adjusted by a wide variety of controlling mechanisms to ensure the maintenance of normal blood gas and acid-base status in the face of varying metabolic demands, varying respiratory muscle performance, and varying mechanical loads. Understanding dyspnea requires an awareness of the integration between the physiology of respiration, the physiology of sensory processing, and the consequences of disease processes on both. These interactions can be explored by the application of quantitative techniques where sensory magnitude and the physical stimuli are both measured. Measurement of the stimulus giving rise to the sense of effort is especially important, but no current measurement technique can be applied directly. The measurement of central motor output is functionally based on the simple rationale that maximum effort (maximal motor command) and the maximal peripheral manifestation of its consequences (i.e., force, flow rate, ventilation) are proportionately related. Thus by expressing the peripheral manifestation of its consequences as a proportion of the maximal achievable under the same conditions, the intensity of motor command can be expressed on a measurement scale from zero to maximal. The intensity of the sense of effort can be measured using a variety of psychophysical rating scales, and the relationship between them is positively accelerating and nonlinear.

Circumstantial evidence supports the central role of effort: respiratory effort is increased when the demand for ventilation is increased (e.g. exercise), when the impedance to the respiratory system is increased (e.g., restrictive and obstructive ventilatory defects), when the inspiratory muscle is weakened due either to fatigue or disease (e.g., neuropathies, myopathies), when the intrinsic characteristics of the muscle are at a mechanical disadvantage (e.g., adverse length/tension or force/velocity relationships), when the muscle is working at a mechanical disadvantage (e.g., distortion of the chest cage such as in kyphoscoliosis), or any combination of the above factors. All of the historical hypotheses fit easily within the framework of effort, and experimental simulation of dyspnea in normal subjects shows that dyspnea increases with effort in all cases. Finally, measuring dyspnea using self-reported ratings of its magnitude and relating it to effort in clinical exercise testing across a wide variety of patients also supports the importance of effort in its generation.

In the present edition we continue to see dyspnea (discomfort experienced and associated with breathing) closely associated with the sense of effort and we continue to see the global sensory experience of breathing as multidimensional with the other proprioceptive senses, particularly perceived force, displacement, and length/tension inappropriateness contributing to the quality of the sensation. We have come to accept that a conscious sensation of discomfort is produced when ventilation is not in accord with previous experience, whether at rest or exercise. Discomfort emerges proportional in intensity to the deviation from the spontaneously adopted ventilation (Guz et al., 1981; Adams et al., 1985; Schwartzstein et al., 1987, 1989; Lane et al., 1987a,b,c; Freedman et al., 1987; Chonan et al., 1987, 1990a,b; Cockroft et al., 1989). This discomfort could be called breathlessness, but in lay usage both dyspnea and breathlessness are used interchangeably and there is no satisfactory term which distinguishes this sensation from "dyspnea" (effort). The sensation of breathlessness is similar to many ways to the senses of hunger and thirst, where the absence of satiation is an unique attribute. The senses of hunger, thirst, and breathlessness are all poorly understood. If sufficiently marked, the factors causing "breathlessness" also cause "dyspnea." For the purposes of this review we will call it "breathlessness," recognizing that in lay usage breathlessness embraces dyspnea.

In the present edition we will again review the sensory aspects of breathing and elucidate why we have come to these conclusions.

II. Sensory Model

The structural framework within which conscious sensation is studied is essential to understanding. The sensory model (Fig. 1) is common to all modalities of conscious sensation, applying to stimuli originating outside the body (environmental stimuli) and to stimuli arising within the body (proprioceptive stimuli). In both cases, the sensory process begins with the stimulus. The stimulus is transformed into a neural process by a primary sense organ (sensory receptor). The transformed information is transmitted to the central nervous system by afferent sensory nerves. The afferent sensory information is centrally processed and a sensory impression formed, recapitulating peripheral receptor conditions. The evoked. conscious sensation is dependent on the interpretation of the sensory impression in light of previous experience and learning through poorly specified neural pathways. Hence, conscious sensation is a perceptual process based on a sensory impression arising from sensory receptors and is not merely the reconstruction of the primary sensory information (Schmidt, 1981).

The pathway from the stimulus to the sensory impression falls into the domain of neurophysiology, whereas the interpretation of the sensory impression falls into the domain of behavioral psychology. It is implicit that the evoked, conscious

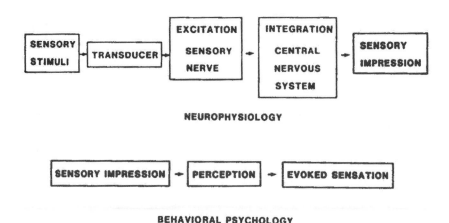

Figure 1   Series of sequential unit processes used in the generation of conscious sensation.

sensory response is dependent on a sequence of processes, which are usually studied in quite different domains by quite different methods and include both neurophysiology and behavioral psychology. Regrettably, the total integrated system is commonly neglected in favor of the detailed study of its individual component parts. To confine interest to any one or all of the unit processes in isolation fails to explain the integration between all of these processes in generating conscious sensation. The function of the total integrated system may be studied by psychophysics, which is the quantitative study of the relationship between physical stimuli and evoked conscious sensation in four domains: detection, discrimination, recognition, and scaling (Marks, 1974; Stevens, 1975; Baird and Noma, 1978).

The traditional narrow focus on anatomical sites of termination in the sensory cortex has given way to the multifocal nature of complex sensory processing. The activation of associated pathways essential to these perceptual processes does not lend itself to precise anatomical localization. Thus anatomical studies have limited applicability to the study of dyspnea.

III. Proprioceptive Sensations and Breathing

All conscious sensations are initially dependent on the stimulation of sensory receptors, followed by the integrated interaction of a sequence of neurophysiological processes within the sensory system (Schmidt, 1981). Hence, the nature and character of the stimuli followed by the nature and character of the receptors stimulated in the act of breathing are logical starting points. During the act of breathing many well-known sensory receptors are stimulated, but a variety of other receptors are putatively sensory in nature.

A. Chemoreceptors (Peripheral and Central)

The idea that chemoreceptor stimulation is sensory and causes discomfort has always been attractive (for review see Killian, 1992). While initially appealing, its perceived importance receded when it was shown by Fowler (1954) that breath-holding can be prolonged at the point of breaking by breathing a gas mixture that increases rather than decreases chemoreceptor activity. This observation, when taken together with prolongation of breath-holding during total neuromuscular blockade (Campbell et al., 1967, 1969), led to the idea that chemoreceptors are insentient. When chemoreceptors are activated, central respiratory neurons are stimulated, motor output to the respiratory muscles increases, respiratory muscle activity increases, muscle and joint receptor activity increases, and pulmonary receptor activity increases. Dyspnea may be generated as a secondary consequence due to the stimulation of one or other of these receptors.

This indirect role has been questioned on the grounds that (1) hypercapnia enhances the discomfort associated with ventilation under conditions where the contractile activity of the respiratory muscles is the same, (2) conscious awareness of chemoreceptor activity is an enticing explanation of why breathing too much or too little is distressing, (3) the addition of carbon dioxide to breathing during neuromuscular blockade causes distress when the respiratory muscles are silent (Adams et al., 1985; Chonan et al., 1987; Schwartzstein et al., 1987, 1989; Simon et al., 1989, 1990; Banzett et al., 1990; Chonan et al., 1990a). Normal subjects experience progressive discomfort with an increased urge or need to breathe following breath-holding or during artificial ventilation with rebreathing with and without the addition of CO_2, with and without total neuromuscular blockade (Gandevia et al., 1992). Chemoreceptor stimulation causes an unpleasant urge to breathe either directly or indirectly due to increased central respiratory output and/or respiratory motor neuron output.

B. Pulmonary Receptors (Stretch, Irritant, and C Fibers)

When the lungs are impeded from expansion due to stiff lungs or obstructed airways, failure of the stretch receptors to inhibit inspiration was originally thought to contribute to excessive, prolonged inspiratory neuronal activity, resulting in dyspnea (Hering Breuer reflex) (Breuer and Hering, 1868). Though not formally studied before and after transplantation, patients with heart/lung transplantation are relieved of dyspnea even though vagal afferents are abolished. Dyspnea emerges normally with exercise in transplanted patients indicating that pulmonary receptors are not essential for its generation. The sensation associated with load detection is unaffected and breath-holding only slightly prolonged by vagal blockade (Guz et al., 1966; Guz et al., 1970). Hence, the idea that the vagus was of central importance has receded.

Pulmonary vascular receptors are widely felt to be stimulated in the clinical settings of pulmonary embolism, pulmonary hypertension, and pulmonary edema. The idea has arisen that these receptors may be directly sentient (Paintal, 1969, 1973). These functionally described intravascular receptors cause hyperventilation, and the resulting hyperventilation with its increased effort may precipitate dyspnea. The "tightness" associated with asthma is often attributed to hyperinflation and vagal afferents, but sensory receptor activation associated with inspiratory muscle activity under conditions of hyperinflation is an equally plausible mechanism. Irritant receptors can be stimulated by probing the intrapulmonary airways or by the inhalation of capsaicin or other irritant chemical stimuli. These receptors are clearly sensed by the conscious urge to cough. Pulmonary receptors may also be in part responsible for the conscious sensation of volume, but this remains controversial (Halttunen, 1974; Salamon et al., 1975; West et al., 1975; Katz-Salamon, 1976; Stubbing et al., 1981; Wolkove et al., 1982). Hence, pulmonary afferents are well known to cause specific respiratory sensations and to modify the reflex control of breathing. While they remain the best studied, there is little experimental support for the direct role of stretch, irritant, and intravascular receptors in the generation of dyspnea as it is usually encountered. While it is premature to exclude pulmonary receptors, their role is likely to be indirect.

C. Muscular Receptors

Muscle spindles, tendon organs, free nerve endings lying within the muscles and joints, and skin receptors in the chest cage are all activated by breathing. Golgi tendon organs are stimulated by tension in the muscle (Sherrington, 1900; Jami, 1992), inspiratory muscle tension is increased in the presence of many pulmonary disorders, and one could make a case that tendon organ output contributes to dyspnea. Tension is sentient and contributes to the quality of the sensation of breathing. However, for any given inspiratory muscle tension, the intensity of dyspnea (discomfort) is greater in subjects with weak inspiratory muscles than that experienced by subjects with strong inspiratory muscles. Furthermore, the intensity of dyspnea increases with time even though inspiratory muscle tension may not change. Effort is a more plausible alternative.

Muscle spindles are stimulated by displacement or movement (Matthews, 1972, 1982; Goodwin et al., 1972; McCloskey, 1978; Burgess et al., 1982). Joint and skin receptors can also sense displacement (Sherrington, 1900; Gandevia and McCloskey, 1976; McCloskey, 1978). The sense of ventilation is also sentient and contributes to the quality of the sensation of breathing. When ventilation increases, dyspnea emerges and intensifies with ventilation; one could make a case that muscle spindle output contributes to dyspnea. However, subjects with strong respiratory muscles are less dyspneic than subjects with weak respiratory muscles at any given ventilation. During sustained activity dyspnea intensifies out of proportion to the increases in ventilation seen. Effort is again a more plausible alternative.

Free nerve endings of small myelinated and unmyelinated nerve fibers are seen between muscle fibers. The stimulus is thought to be structural damage and/or release of unspecified cellular products acting on these free nerve endings. When the muscle is working at high intensity and/or over long duration, muscular discomfort and even pain is common; a case can be made that output from these endings contributes to dyspnea. Clearly, discomfort and pain arising from these sources are sentient. However, dyspnea is often experienced in situations where these extreme conditions are unlikely and pain is seldom volunteered as a feature of dyspnea.

All these muscular receptors have access to consciousness and all contribute to the quality of the sensations associated with the act of breathing.

D. Central Receptors

Small interneurons high in the central nervous system (corollary discharge from central motor neurons) transduce the intensity of the motor command and perform the role of a sensory receptor (Roland and Ladegaard-Pederson, 1977; Gandevia and McCloskey, 1977a,b, 1978; McCloskey, 1978; Roland, 1978; Matthews, 1982; Gandevia, 1982). These receptors result in the sense of effort (intensity of motor command). The activity of these receptors increases when breathing is increased, loaded, or when the respiratory muscles are weak. These conditions alone or in combination are present in most of the clinical circumstances in which dyspnea is experienced. When dyspneic patients are ventilated such that the respiratory muscles are silent (no central motor command), dyspnea is eliminated as long as the need to breathe is satisfied ("the subjects are not breathless").

E. Upper Airway Receptors

The control of breathing is fundamentally dependent on maintenance of the caliber of the upper airway, its protection during eating, and its role in speech (Widdicombe, 1986). Upper airway receptors must subserve these functions and in so doing must interact with the overall control mechanisms. A primary role for these receptors in the generation of dyspnea appears unlikely, but failure of their appropriate activation during speech, swallowing, and cough can cause dyspnea, and dyspnea is occasionally observed in association with eating and speech in patients with severe impairment of pulmonary function. Local sensations in the nasopharynx are beyond the scope of this review.

IV. Muscular Sensations

There has been a historical tendency to concentrate attention on chemoreceptors, medullary respiratory neuronal activity, and afferent neuronal activity arising in the lungs in any discourse on respiratory sensation, while the more obvious sensations generated by the respiratory muscles have been somewhat neglected, even though they appear ideally suited to the generation of dyspnea. The muscular sensations can be conveniently divided into the primary sensations: sense of effort, which is central in origin, and the senses of displacement (muscular shortening and its resultant volume expansion) and force (pressure), which are peripheral in origin. Sensory physiology has largely concentrated on the special senses such that the sensory aspects of muscular activity are not generally known. We will therefore deal with the muscle senses in some detail illustrating the confusion that has arisen in this specific area.

A. History of Proprioceptive Sensory Mechanisms

The historical evolution of the muscle senses began with the five basic senses proposed by Aristotle: vision, audition, olfaction, taste, and touch (Aristotle, 1912, 1936). Until recent times the sensations of force, effort, and fatigue were explained within the confines of touch (Boring, 1942; Scheerer, 1987). The sense of touch was clearly inadequate, and a conscious appreciation of the willed motor command

·was put forward as a logical source of the muscle senses (sense of effort). The idea of a sense of effort dominated the field, gradually emerging in the philosophical domain as early as the sixteenth century and persisting until the end of the nineteenth century when muscle spindles, Golgi tendon organs, and joint receptors were discovered and recognized as sensory receptors (Boring, 1942). Thereafter, the sense of effort lost favor and all the muscle sensations were seen as a consequence of the mechanical stimulation of muscle spindles, tendon organs, and joint receptors (Sherrington, 1900). The role of the muscle spindle remained uncertain until the 1970s, when it became clear that its sensory role was in the perception of position and movement (Matthews, 1972), whereas the sense of tension was always felt to be due to the tendon organs (sense of movement, position, displacement/joint receptors). The term muscle senses was replaced by kinesthetic senses (Bastian, 1888) and later by proprioceptive senses (Sherrington, 1900), to which were added the vestibular senses.

B. Perception of Effort

The notion of a receptor is not easily applied to the sense of effort in which small interneurons high in the central nervous system are thought to transduce the firing frequency of a complex motor program by collateral discharge to the sensory cortex. These interneurons act as central sensory receptors in a conceptual fashion, but their actual anatomical location remains uncertain. Anatomical locality, once thought to be important, does not easily apply to complex neural events, where structured motor programs and their associated pathways may be diverse and spread throughout the higher centers of the central nervous system. Hence, the idea of a sense of effort has been largely explored in its functional domain. The motor program is initiated with its accompanying sense of effort. This results in activation of muscle with its accompanying sense of achieved tension and achieved movement. Effort, tension, and movement are interrelated and depend on the nature of the opposing forces. The sense of effort has been largely studied in its relationship to lifted weights.

Muscular fatigue increases the apparent heaviness of a weight and is a common everyday experience. In lifting a weight, there is a motor command resulting in a sense of effort and the stimulation of tendon organs resulting in a sense of achieved tension. The effort required to lift a weight is obviously related to the weight itself, but is also affected by such factors as the strength of the muscle, the initial length of the muscle, and the velocity of contraction expressed in the speed of lifting. McCloskey and colleagues (1974) found that the sense of effort is used in preference to the sense of achieved force in estimating the magnitude of a lifted weight. Using the psychophysical technique of magnitude matching they had subjects formally match weights lifted by both upper limbs. Thus, they showed that a weight lifted by a nonfatigued arm has to be larger than that on the fatigued other arm for the weights to be equally matched (McCloskey et al., 1974; Gandevia and McCloskey, 1977a). Second, when tonic vibration reflexes are induced in a muscle that has been used to support a weight, there is a subjective lessening of the heaviness of the weight. Vibration of the agonist results in a simple monosynaptic augmentation of motor output at the anterior horn cell aiding the action of the agonist. Conversely, vibration of the antagonist increases the apparent heaviness. Vibration of the antagonist results in a monosynaptic augmentation of motor output to the antagonist, impeding the action of the agonist. These reflexes operate on the alpha motor neuron at the spinal level, and the descending commands (and with them, the motor commands) vary inversely with the size of the reflexly driven component of the contraction (McCloskey et al., 1974; Gandevia and McCloskey, 1977a). Third, local curarization increases the heaviness of objects lifted by weakened muscles (for review, see McCloskey, 1978). Based on these observations a sense of effort was inferred and collateral discharge was suggested as the mechanism. The sense of achieved tension appears to be a secondary consideration in everyday muscular activity.

With inspiratory muscle activity there is also a sense of effort and a sense of achieved tension. In early studies these were frequently confused, with one or the other being rated depending on the particular study. At the time clear discrimination between sensory phenomena was not adequately appreciated. Effort also appears to be used in preference to perceived tension in consciously sensing the magnitude of inspiratory pressures. The perceived magnitude (Ψ) intensifies with both the magnitude of pressure (P_{insp}) and its duration in seconds (T_I): $\Psi = K \times P_{insp}^{1.2} \times T_I^{0.62}$. Here, the perception of what we now believe to have been the effort required to generate a force is not simply the sensory experience of the integral of pressure and time. The perceived effort is less for a small pressure applied over a long period of time than for a large pressure applied over a shorter period of time (Stubbing et al., 1981). This relationship is the same as that found for peripheral limb muscle contraction (Stevens and Mack, 1959; Borg, 1962; Eisler, 1962, 1965; Stevens and Cain, 1970; Cain and Stevens, 1971). The effects of inspiratory duration are illustrated in Figure 2. Perceived effort is related to the intensity and duration of force development. The pattern of force adopted is an important contributor to the effort experienced. Reducing intensity and increasing duration reduces effort and its associated discomfort and is a large part of the reason why patients with chronic and progressive lung disorders may not complain of dyspnea until their disease is advanced.

The perception of effort has obvious consequences when we consider inspiratory muscle activity and dyspnea. With maximum inspiratory effort against an occluded airway, normal subjects generate maximum inspiratory pressures (MIP), which vary from 50 to 120 cm H_2O at FRC. Maximum effort in one subject achieves an occlusion pressure of 50 and in another 120 cm H_2O. Clearly, a pressure of 25 cm H_2O would require a much greater effort in a subject with a MIP of 50 cm H_2O than in one with a MIP of 150 cm H_2O. The effects of varying inspiratory muscle strength are schematically illustrated in Figure 3. There is no apriori reason why the range of central motor output to the inspiratory muscles should vary across

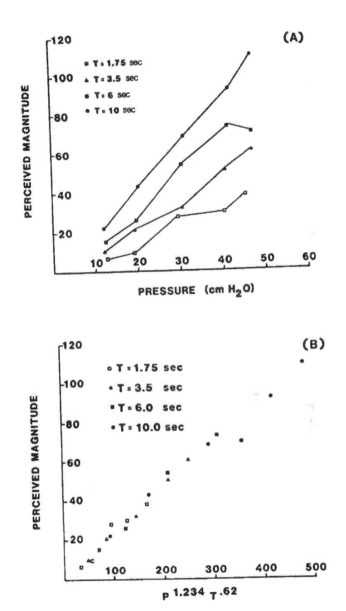

Figure 2 (A) The perceived magnitude of inspiratory static occlusion pressures increase with both the magnitude of the inspiratory pressure and the duration for which the pressure is maintained. (B) The perceived magnitude of inspiratory static occlusion pressures is linearly related to pressure and time in the above power-function relationship. (From Stubbing et al., 1983.)

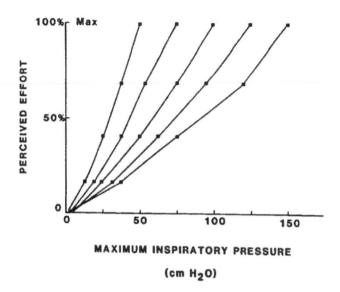

Figure 3 The relationship of perceived effort for five hypothetical subjects with MIPs varying from 50 to 150 cm H_2O assuming perceived effort $\Psi = k_oP^{1.3}$ (pressure maintained for constant time).

individuals in the absence of a functional impairment of central motor programming in the central nervous system. Hence the sense of effort has explanatory power in this context. The expression of these consequences in a clinical setting is obviously more complex because the relationship between effort and tension is also a function of the length, extent, and velocity of inspiratory muscle contraction. The effort required to generate a given pressure increases with the inspiratory flow rate and with the inspired volume (Fig. 4).

During exercise the inspiratory esophageal pressure cycles vary from +20 to –40 cm H_2O during exercise (Leblanc et al., 1988), with the length, extent, and velocity of contraction varying widely depending on the impedance opposing contraction. The effort required to achieve a given pressure increases with inflation, increases with inspiratory flow rates, and increases as the inspiratory muscle weakens as a consequence of fatigue (Leblanc et al., 1986).

Motor output also increases as the same muscle contractile activity is sustained over time, providing the explanation for an everyday phenomenon whereby the effort required to sustain activity increases with time, which was known as muscle fatigue long before its neurophysiological cause was known. Kearon et al. (1991a,b) studied the magnitude of perceived effort and dyspnea during constant sustained activity (Fig. 5). The effort required to cycle increased with time even though the force, velocity, and extent of contraction were constant, reflecting the increase in motor command due to fatigue. The perceived magnitude of effort (Ψ) increased

PERCEIVED EFFORT

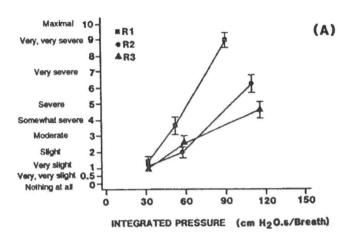

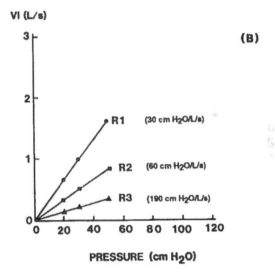

Figure 4 The magnitude of perceived effort in six normal subjects following breathing: on three inspiratory resistances at three different flow rates (panel A and B); on three elastances at three different tidal volumes (panels C and D).

significantly with the power output expressed as a percentage of maximal (%MPO) and duration of activity expressed in minutes (Time):

$$\text{Effort} = K \times \%MPO^{2.13} \times Time^{0.39}$$

Because oxygen uptake and ventilation continued to increase with time, especially at higher work rates, the work performed by the respiratory muscles was

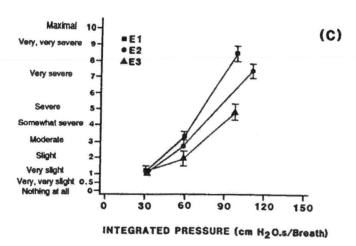

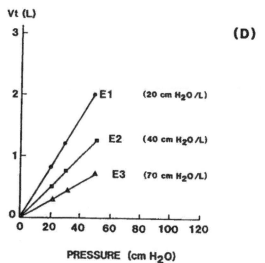

Figure 4   (*continued*)

not constant at any of the work rates. Nonetheless, dyspnea was excessive relative to the increase in work, reflecting fatigue in the same manner as the peripheral limb muscles:

$$\text{Dyspnea} = K \times \%MPO^{2.41} \times \text{Time}^{0.47}$$

Fatigue of the respiratory muscles is a major contributor to the sense of effort and dyspnea.

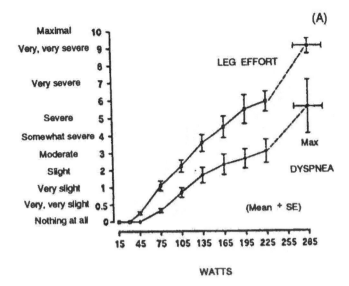

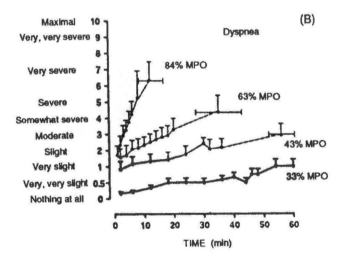

Figure 5 (A) Leg effort (■) and dyspnea (●) estimates during incremental exercise (mean ± SE). Solid lines join work rates at which values were available for all six subjects. Broken lines join the last work rate to which all six subjects contributed to the mean of the maximal value (symptom intensity and work) for all subjects. (B, C) Dyspnea and leg effort estimates (mean ± SE) (Borg scale) during endurance exercise at work rates corresponding to 84% ("very severe"), 63% ("severe"), 43% ("moderate") and 33% ("mild") of maximal power output (MPO) as estimated during incremental exercise. Solid lines join time intervals at which values were available for all six subjects. Broken lines join the last data point to which all six subjects contributed to the mean of the endurance value (symptom intensity and duration) for all subjects. (From Kearon et al., 1991.)

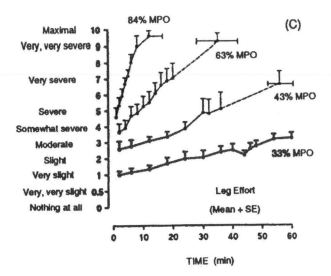

Figure 5 *(continued)*

C. Perception of Force and Pressure

Parsimony indicates that the tendon organs are the source of tension perception (Jami, 1992). There is no reason to believe that the perception of force in the respiratory muscles is fundamentally different from the perception of force in peripheral skeletal muscle. As repeatedly stated, there has always been a tendency to confuse the senses of effort and tension. When posed with a sensory task volunteers have a marked tendency to rate effort rather than force. Nonetheless, both can be recognized and discriminated. Both Altose et al. (1981) and Stubbing et al. (1981) used lung volume to achieve variations in the resting length of the inspiratory muscle. Both found that the perception of static inspiratory pressures was not significantly increased with reductions in the resting length of the muscle due to hyperinflation. However, in the study by Stubbing et al., the subjects volunteered unanimously that the effort required to generate pressure increased following hyperinflation. Both studies concluded that there was a sense of achieved force that must be mediated by muscular receptors. Gandevia et al. (1981) found that the sense of inspiratory effort increased progressively as a maximum inspiratory pressure was maintained, whereas the subjects were aware that the achieved force decreased as the inspiratory muscle fatigued. Subjects rated effort as increasing and rated achieved force as decreasing. Killian and Gandevia (1984) asked subjects to generate static occlusion pressures at high lung volume and then to reproduce the same inspiratory efforts at FRC. The sensation of effort required to generate the same pressure increased by approximately 50% at high lung volumes. The results were the same with both magnitude estimation and production. Roland and Ladegaard-Pederson (1977) had subjects match force and effort separately using the psychophysical technique of magnitude matching of both upper limbs, using a series of springs. Perceived effort increased in proportion to the induced weakness when one arm was curarized; perceived tension was unchanged. When isometric contractions are used and are of short duration, the perception of effort and tension are similar in magnitude. Hence it is not surprising that subjects commonly confuse tension and effort, and individuals may select one or the other.

D. Perception of Volume

There is a natural tendency to emphasize the role of pulmonary stretch receptors and the vagus in volume perception. In reality the vagus and its receptors are ill suited for a number of reasons:

1. The firing frequency of the vagus on log/log coordinates increases with a slope of 0.5 in response to change in volume, whereas the perceptual magnitude increases with a slope of 1.3 on the same coordinates (Clark and von Euler, 1972).
2. The perception of volume varies with the muscle group activated (inspiratory or expiratory), and this would not be expected were volume mediated by stretch receptors within the airways or lungs (Salamon et al., 1975).
3. The perception of lung volume varies as the inspiratory muscle tension varies (Wolkove et al., 1981).
4. The perception of volume deteriorates with passive ventilation (Stubbing et al., 1981).
5. Vibration of the chest wall alters the perception of volume (Stubbing et al., 1981).

The perception of volume in the respiratory system is like the conscious perception of the limbs in space. In the absence of vision, our awareness of the body in space was, until recently, thought to be due to afferent sensory signals originating and firing in relationship to changes in joint angle (Rose and Mountcastle, 1959) facilitated by afferent signals arising from the overlying skin (for review, see Matthews, 1982; Burgess et al., 1982). Recent advances in kinesthesia show that most articular receptors fire predominantly at the extremes of movement, making them unsuitable for the perception of movement (Skoglund, 1956; Burgess and Clark, 1969; McCall et al., 1974; Clark and Burgess, 1975; Grigg, 1975; Millar, 1975; Grigg and Greenspan, 1977; McIntyre et al., 1978; Carli et al., 1979; Clark et al., 1979; Tracey, 1979; Ferrel, 1980). Blocking articular receptors with local anesthesia or abolishing articular receptors with total joint replacement causes little impairment in the perception of the speed and the direction of joint movement (Goodwin et al., 1972; Cross and McCloskey, 1973; Grigg et al., 1973). Vibrating the tendon of a muscle produces an illusion that the joint is being displaced in a direction so as to stretch the vibrating muscle (Goodwin et al., 1972; McCloskey, 1978; Matthews, 1981). The illusion incorporates a sense of joint movement and a sense of altered joint position.

The vibrations are at amplitudes that excite the primary spindle endings, perhaps some secondary endings, but not the tendon organs. Projections of these afferents to the cerebral cortex have been demonstrated (Oscarsson and Rosen, 1963; Able-Fessard et al., 1966; Phillips et al., 1971; Wiesendanger, 1973). Sensory information arising in the muscle can be perceived (Skavenski, 1972; McCloskey, 1973a; Matthews and Simmonds, 1974; Lackner, 1975). The mechanisms involved in the sensation of peripheral limb movement are available for the perception of lung volume. In contrast to other joints afferents, joint receptors in the costal vertebral joints fire over the whole range of articular movement (Goodwin-Austen, 1969) and are thus suitable for the perception of volume. Halttunen (1974) and Salamon et al. (1975) both found dissimilarities between the perception of volume achieved using inspiratory versus expiratory muscle. Stubbing et al. (1981), using matching techniques, found that both passive ventilation and chest vibration impaired the ability of normal subjects to match volumes. Using the psychophysical technique of volume matching, Wolkove et al. (1981) found that normal subjects reliably match reference tidal volumes. When the mechanical conditions were altered between the control and matching breath by the addition of a respiratory load, the reliability deteriorated. When the load was maintained for a period of time, reliability returned to normal. The authors suggested that mechanoreceptors mediating information about force were used in the perception of volume. Receptors stimulated by respiratory muscle contraction are clearly important in the perception of volume.

Normal subjects can estimate various volumes between residual volume (RV) and total lung capacity (TLC) and can reproduce known volumes (Bakers and Tenney, 1970). On average, when the volume was increased twofold, the subject perceived a change of approximately 2.5-fold. The perceptual magnitude (Ψ) is related to the physical magnitude (Volume) by a power function, 1.3, such that:

$$\Psi = K \times Volume^{1.3}$$

The value of n has been reproduced (Stubbing et al., 1981; Volkove et al., 1981; Gliner et al. 1981), It was also found that the discrimination of volume is sensitive and proportional to the background tidal volume. The Weber fraction was 0.02, considerably lower than that previously reported by West et al. (1975).

In conclusion, subjects can and will utilize information from any source in making perceptual judgments as long as these receptors fire in a systematic fashion relative to the required task. Redundancy is common in all neural mechanisms. A variety of peripheral proprioceptive mechanisms (and perhaps even vagal stretch receptors) may be utilized in sensing volume under different circumstances and with different sensitivities.

V. Perception of Load

One can also sense the load opposing muscle contraction by relating force and displacement. Traditionally, loads opposing muscle contraction have been analyzed using simple mechanical principles (Rohrer, 1925; Rahn et al., 1946; Otis, 1964). The pressure developed by the inspiratory muscle (Pmus) must overcome the forces imposed by the static forces (pressure/volume = elastance) and dynamic forces (pressure/flow relationship = resistance and pressure/acceleration = inertance) of the system as a whole including lungs, chest cage, and abdominal wall. Inertance is generally ignored because the pressure required to accelerate the respiratory system is small (Mead, 1952). The resistive pressure normally increases in a positively accelerating manner relative to flow and the simple expression dynamic pressure/flow is inadequate. The relationship is usually described by a polynomial equation, and the most recent values are (D'Angelo et al., 1989; Milic-Emili, 1991):

$$P_r = 1.9 * \dot{V} + 0.5 * \dot{V}^2$$

The compliance of the lung decreases as volume increases, whereas the compliance of the chest cage decreases as lung volume decreases. The net effect is that elastic pressure increases in an approximately linear manner with volume (14 cm H_2O/liter) over the usual operating range (D'Angelo et al., 1989).

With externally added loads the inspiratory muscle must overcome both the elastance and resistance of the respiratory system and the elastance and resistance applied at the mouth (Fig. 6). An equation of motion where V_T is the tidal volume, E_o is the elastance of the system, AE is the added elastance, $\dot{V}$ is the inspiratory

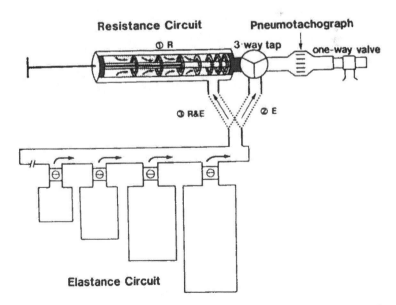

Figure 6 Loading circuit consisting of a mouthpiece, pressure port, pneumotachometer, one-way valve, and resistance and elastance circuits.

flow rate, Ro is the resistance of the system, and AR is the added resistance is a convenient quantitative description of these relationships:

Pmus = VT(Eo + AE) + V̇(Ro + AR)

Estimates of respiratory system elastance and resistance can be added to mouth pressure to give an approximation of peak inspiratory muscle pressure (Milic-Emili, 1991).

The addition of elastic or resistive loads at the mouth has been used extensively for psychophysical studies to explore the sensations associated with loaded breathing. In the early studies investigators defined the threshold of detection for both resistive and elastic loads (Campbell et al., 1961; Bennett et al., 1962). First, load detection was found to be mechanically related to the relationship between force and displacement and not merely a function of either force or displacement alone (Campbell et al., 1961; Bennett et al., 1962; Zechman and Davenport, 1978; Killian et al., 1979, 1980a,b; Shahid et al., 1981). Second, the sensory information indicating the presence of a load is dependent on muscular receptors and does not require the stimulation of vagal afferents (Guz et al., 1966; Killian et al., 1980a,b). Third, any muscle acting in a respiratory sense is capable of generating the information necessary for detection (Noble et al., 1971). Fourth, load detection is quantitatively related to the background load such that the threshold of detection increases with the background load (Wiley and Zechman, 1966). Thus the well-known Weber fraction applies to the perception of added load (Weber, 1860).

Campbell and Howell (1963) proposed that dyspnea occurred when the force developed by respiratory muscles is excessive for the displacement achieved in the chest wall and lung. With this view dyspnea would increase with elastance or resistance. Using the technique of open magnitude scaling, Gottfried et al. (1978, 1981) found that when the added resistance increased by twofold, the sensory magnitude of the load increased by 1.9 in normal subjects and 1.5 in patients with chronic airflow obstruction, and these proportions remained constant over the range of added loads. This information can be easily confused. It does not imply that the patients with chronic airflow obstruction perceived the loads as smaller. Open magnitude scaling does not allow a measurement of absolute intensity. The exponents relating load and perceptual magnitude were related to the degree of respiratory compensation during ventilatory loading. Normal subjects with the largest exponents and smallest detection thresholds showed the greatest load compensation, indicating that sensory information was used by the subjects in selecting their response. Killian et al. (1981) found that subjects with the high exponent for resistance also had a high exponent for elastance but that the range of the exponents was a wide. Some subjects had a vast increase in perceptual magnitude, whereas others had a modest increase when the respiratory system was loaded. While perceptual variability is attractive, the range of exponents is so extreme as to be unacceptable. It appears that in these early studies some subjects may have rated the load, others the pressure, and others effort.

Killian et al. (1982) found that the sensory magnitude of added resistive and elastic loads as they were then rated by normal subjects was indirectly related to the added load and directly related to the force developed by the respiratory muscle in response to the load. This means that in the presence of resistive loads, the sensory magnitude is a function of both the magnitude of the added resistance (AR) and the flow-rate ($\dot{V}$) adopted by the subject. Similarly, the perceived magnitude of added elastic loads was not solely related to the magnitude of the added elastance (AE) but also to the tidal volume ($P = V_T \times E$). In fact, when both resistive and elastic loads were intermingled, sensory magnitude was a function of pressure, and was independent of the kind of load. Furthermore, when inspiratory time was varied, sensory magnitude increased not only with the intensity of the inspiratory pressure but also with the duration of force development,

$$\Psi = Ko\ P^{1.3} \times Time^{0.56}$$

This relationship is similar to that already described for static inspiratory pressures and also to that previously described for the perceived magnitude for force by peripheral limb muscle. Faced with the task of estimating the magnitude of the load, the subjects estimated the magnitude of effort or pressure presumably using the senses of effort or perceived tension.

In keeping with this interpretation, exercise, hypoxia, and hypercapnia all result in an increase in the perceived magnitude of added loads (Burdon et al., 1982). The increase in perceived magnitude was appropriate for the intensity and duration of force development as outlined. Using open magnitude scaling, the magnitude of added elastic loads (20–76 cm H_2O/liter) was presented for a sequence of five breaths at frequencies varying from 5 to 26 breaths/min. The perceived magnitude (Ψ) increased significantly with the peak pressure (Pm), the inspiratory duration (Ti), and the frequency of breathing (fb):

$$\Psi = K \times Pm^{1.23} \times Ti^{0.12} \times fb^{0.26}\ (r = 0.98)$$

These results indicate that the sensory magnitude of an added load is not uniquely related to the magnitude of the load, but to the pattern of response in terms of intensity, duration, and frequency of force development. Tidal volume, frequency, and inspired time all influence the perceptual magnitude of effort with increasing elastic loads at a minute ventilation of 10 liters/min, as shown in Figure 7. For the purposes of this illustration, resistance is assumed to be negligible.

VI. Temporal Adaptation

If respiratory distress were due solely to the perception of inspiratory muscle force through the sense of effort, then one might expect that for comparable degrees of effort, subjects should be equally distressed. However, patients with chronic airflow obstruction are frequently asymptomatic, whereas patients who develop acute

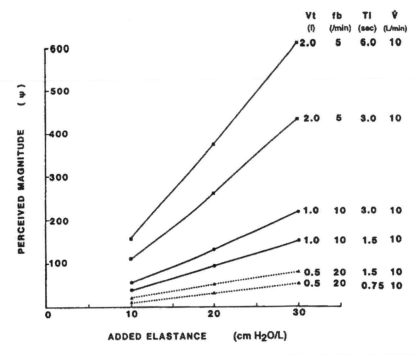

Figure 7   The perceived magnitude of a series of added elastic loads with a constant minute ventilation (10 liters/min) with various frequencies, tidal volumes, and inspiratory times derived from the relationship $\Psi = K_o P^{1.24} Ti^{0.52} f_b^{0.26}$.

asthma with the same effort have intense dyspnea. Thus, the chronic state of the stimulus can potentially reduce sensory magnitude. The decline in sensory magnitude following prolonged periods of stimulation is known as temporal adaptation.

There are technical problems in the experimental study of adaptation during breathing because sensory scaling is best carried out with the presentation of varying stimulus magnitudes over short periods of time with memory and contrast maximized. Hence, the time periods to complete adaptation are unknown for loaded breathing and may vary from subject to subject. Despite our lack of information there is little doubt that adaptation plays a role in dyspnea.

Most studies of adaptation have been done in the special senses, especially vision and hearing. These sensory modalities are adaptable to this kind of study because the time period of adaptation is short and there are two eyes and ears with little or no cross-interference allowing for the comparison with varying background stimulation. The light-adapted eye can be directly compared to the dark-adapted eye. In perception of light there is little effect on the perceptual intensity at high levels of stimulation due to the state of background adaptation. However, with low-intensity stimulation the perceptual magnitude is decreased in the light-adapted eye compared to the dark-adapted eye (Stevens and Stevens, 1963). This phenomenon is probably a general sensory effect. In general form, temporal adapation follows a simple exponential relationship according to which the sensory magnitude declines with a time constant (t), a rate (γ), and an absolute reduction in sensation (j) (Marks, 1974)

$$\Psi = K_o e^{-t/\gamma} + j$$

The rate and absolute reduction in sensation are dependent on the magnitude of the stimulus.

There is little experimental information on temporal adaptation with breathing. Using a simple category scale (0, 1, 2) to designate no load, small load, and moderate load, respectively, McCloskey (1973b) found that normal subjects downgrade the magnitude of added respiratory loads following as few as 20 breaths when breathing against an increased background load. Figure 8 illustrates the group mean results for six normal subjects when added resistive loads were rated when present from 1 to 12 breaths. The perceived magnitude (open magnitude estimation) was significantly reduced at the higher loads following 12 breaths. While showing a reduction consistent with adaptation, it should be noted that these pressures are not stressing; were higher loads used the sensory magnitude would have increased due to fatigue.

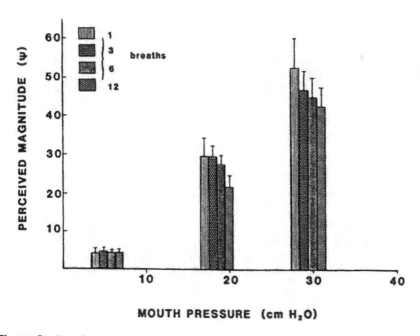

Figure 8 Perceived magnitude of added resistive loads with constant tidal volume, inspiratory time, flow rate, applied for 1, 3, 6, and 12 breaths. Results show means ± SE ($n = 6$). (From Killian et al., 1984.)

Burdon et al. (1983) attempted to study the effect of short-term adaptation to background loads with limited success. They found that the perceptual intensity of high-to-moderate loads was not significantly influenced by short-term adaptation to background elastic and resistive loads, whereas the perceptual magnitude of low levels of stimulation was reduced.

VII. Muscle Weakness and Fatigue

The perceived magnitudes of dyspnea, effort, and tension associated with added elastic loads at FRC and at increased lung volume (when the inspiratory muscle is weakened by shortening its resting length) are shown in Figure 9. The perceived magnitude of dyspnea, effort, and tension increases as the peak pressure increases. However, at increased lung volume, perceived tension remains largely unchanged from that at FRC, whereas both the perceived dyspnea and effort increase dramatically. Dyspnea and effort increased both as the magnitude of the load increased and as the motor command increased as a consequence of hyperinflation. Figure 10 shows the perceived magnitude or respiratory effort with increasing resistive loads to fatigue in two subjects. Following 20 minutes at rest, each subject maintained ventilation for as long as he or she could. Each 5 minutes, the magnitude of the added resistive load was increased, and the subject estimated the magnitude of respiratory effort on a scale ranging from zero to maximum. The first subject had a maximum inspiratory pressure against an occluded airway of 120 cm H_2O, and the second, 50 cm H_2O (MIP). The magnitude of effort was greater for the

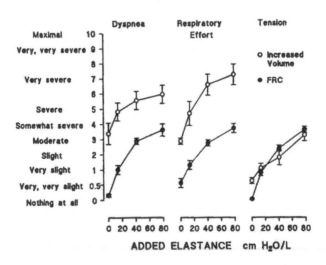

Figure 9   The perceived magnitude of breathlessness, respiratory effort, and achieved tension ($n = 4$) with added elastic loads at two lung volumes.

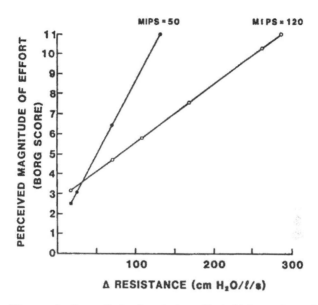

Figure 10 The perceived magnitude of respiratory effort with increasing resistive loads to fatigue. The maximum occlusion pressures at FRC were 120 cm H_2O (subject 1) and 50 cm H_2O (subject 2).

subject with the weaker inspiratory muscle. Campbell et al. (1980) found that the perceived magnitude of added resistive loads increased with partial neuromuscular blockade, which reduced maximum inspiratory pressures to 20% of control (Fig. 11). Dyspnea increases substantially with prolonged activity, the most plausible explanation for which is the development of fatigue (Kearon et al., 1991a,b).

VIII. Respiratory Physiology and Sensory Receptor Stimulation

The medullary respiratory motor output acts on the inspiratory muscles generating sufficient transpulmonary pressure to achieve gas exchange commensurate with metabolism. This sequence of unit processes constitutes a homeostatic loop within which the constancy of the arterial blood is preserved (Fig. 12). Impairment of one or more of these unit processes occurs as a consequence of disease. This impairment has obvious implications for the particular unit processes alone and on the operation of the system as a whole. Impairment in any single unit process has effects on all unit processes above or below the unit process impaired.

Central processing of the medullary output is structured on the input of chemoreceptors, on afferent information from the muscles and lungs, and by

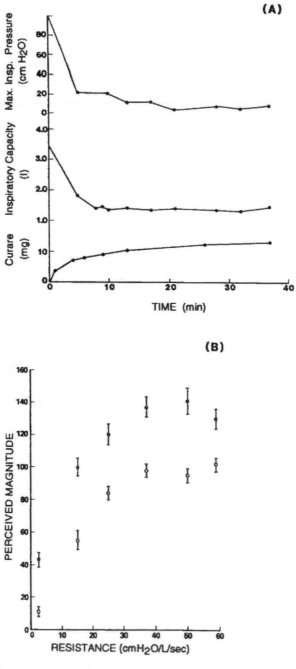

Figure 11 Partial neuromuscular blockade with intravenous curare showing the reduction in maximal inspiratory pressure, inspiratory capacity, and curare administered (A). The perceived magnitude of a series of added resistances before and after the induction of partial neuromuscular blockade with the intravenous infusion of curare (B).

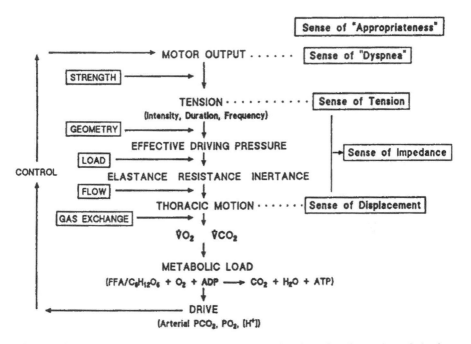

Figure 12 Schematic representation illustrating the interdependent interaction of physiological processes and their effects on sensory receptors. See text for explanation.

voluntary input. Abnormalities at the level of central control include neurogenic factors and the emergence of abnormal drives to breathe due, for example, to pulmonary intravascular receptor stimulation during pulmonary embolism or chronic pulmonary hypertension. Every process below the medulla bears the brunt of these impaired processes.

The medullary motor output acts on the inspiratory muscle. To fulfill its homeostatic requirements, the central motor output must increase in the face of inspiratory muscle weakness, whether this be intrinsic or secondary to hyperinflation, fatigue, or increases in the velocity of contraction occurring secondary to expiratory airflow limitation.

Dyspnea, either experimentally induced or as a consequence of disease, shares common characteristics. Its presence is largely confined to situations where (1) the action of the inspiratory muscles is impeded by the addition of resistive or elastic loads to breathing, (2) ventilation is increased as during exercise, voluntary hyperventilation, or reflexly driven hyperventilation such as occurs with pulmonary vascular occlusion, or (3) the inspiratory muscles are weak as a consequence of disease, hyperinflation, or fatigue. The receptor overstimulated in all of these conditions is the central motor output yielding a sense of increased effort, while the senses of tension, displacement, their interrelationship as length/tension inappropriateness, weakness, appropriateness of ventilation, and even musclar pain (stimulation of intramuscular type 3 and 4 fibers) may contribute to differences in the global quality of the sensation.

While it is tempting to consider dyspnea to be a unique sensation, it can be dissected into fundamental qualitative attributes, which are a function of various specific receptors. It is not surprising that specific diseases lead to patterns of stimulation that are similar and thus acquire qualitative attributes that may be somewhat unique. However, many, possibly all, of the receptors are stimulated to varying degrees in all conditions. Receptor stimulation is not unique to specific disease states, but the pattern of stimulation may be in part specific to cardiac, respiratory or neuromuscular diseases.

Chemoreceptors work somewhat like a domestic thermostat in that they maintain the normality of blood gas and hydrogen ion status (Fenn, 1963). The attraction for chemoreceptors as a source of dyspnea has lessened as the senses of effort, tension, displacement, load (resistance and elastance mediated by inappropriateness), weakness, fatigue, and even pain arising from the respiratory muscle have been understood. The neuronal mechanism by which discomfort experienced and associated with breathing is mediated has remained elusive because the individual processes involved in respiration are so interrelated that isolation of "the" most relevant processes is difficult if not impossible. Central respiratory neurons are largely controlled by hypercapnia, acidemia, hypoxia, by afferent activity arising from the lungs, afferent activity arising from both respiratory and nonrespiratory muscles, and voluntary pathways. The question of source of dyspnea can be answered at many levels, but the explanation is in the process and not the site. Breathlessness in the sense of inappropriate breathing (see above) may be similar to the senses of hunger and thirst, and in the same manner as these sensations its nature may have been confused with their peripheral manifestations, i.e., dry mouth and the gastric contractions (Boring, 1942). At present the mechanism of satiety is unknown.

IX. Dyspnea in Particular Circumstances

So far, this chapter has emphasized the number of sensory mechanisms at work in the genesis of respiratory sensation in general, and in generating discomfort ("dyspnea") in particular. An analysis of the role of these mechanisms in all clinical circumstances would be superfluous, but by way of summary and to emphasize the interactions we may summarize some contrasting situations. Only the major factors will be mentioned; minor or contributing factors can be deduced from the early parts of this chapter. Similarly, neurophysiological mechanisms will not be specified.

A. Exercise

During exercise the major factors are ventilation, the load opposing the contraction of these muscles (resistance and elastance), the strength of the inspiratory muscle decreases, the efficiency of gas exchange, and the development of fatigue.

B. Asthma

During an acute asthmatic attack, the major factors are inspiratory resistance, dynamic elastance, hyperinflation, expiratory resistance resulting in prolonging expiration and further stressing inspiratory flow rate, additional drives to breathe arising from hypoxemia, hypercapnia, irritant receptor stimulation, the decrease in efficiency of gas exchange, and the development of fatigue. Hypoxemia and hypercapnia may have additional effects contributing to breathlessness. Dyspnea may also increase because of the effects on muscular metabolism, which increase the effort required to drive muscle compromised by acidosis.

C. Pulmonary Embolism

During acute pulmonary embolism the major factors include dramatic increase in drive to breathe arising from mediators released as a consequence of the embolic obstruction stimulating intravascular receptors in the lungs, an additional mechanical stimulus arising in the pulmonary circulation such that there is an inverse relationship between the arterial P_{CO_2} and the severity of the increase in pulmonary vascular resistance, the efficiency of gas exchange decreases in proportion to the volume compromised by embolic obstruction, modest increases in resistance and dynamic elastance and a propensity to fatigue as the motor output required to drive the respiratory muscles increases dramatically as the net cardiac output decreases, and compromised perfusional support of the body in total and the inspiratory muscle in particular.

D. Pulmonary Edema and Orthopnea

The major factors in this case include marked shift of blood volume to the thorax increasing pulmonary congestion and the stiffness of the underlying lung, compressive atelectasis due to fluid retention, the accommodation of pleural fluid at the expense of downward displacement of the diaphragm and shortening of the intercostal muscles, decreases in cardiac output and the perfusional support of the inspiratory muscle leading to fatigue, and decreases in the efficiency of gas exchange.

E. Breath-Holding

Breath-holding is a unique experience, which of itself has little clinical relevance, but it has implications for clinical situations. Breathlessness emerges with breath-holding after 15–20 seconds and subsequently increases until tolerance for the discomfort is exceeded and the subject takes a breath. However, involuntary respiratory muscle activity eventually appears and increases following a variable period of breath-holding. With its appearance the mechanism of distress becomes more complex in that chemoreceptors, medullary and central motor output, muscular, pulmonary, and chest wall receptors are then stimulated in their own right. The mechanism underpinning the early sensation may be important to the discomfort associated with inappropriate breathing in many clinical settings. "Breathlessness" may be defined as the discomfort associated with inappropriate ventilation for metabolic demands. Circumstantially this sensation appears to relate to chemoreceptor activity or its central consequences, and it would now appear that the sensation is not dependent on contractile activity of the respiratory muscles (Banzett et al., 1990; Gandevia et al., 1992). While breath-holding is somewhat artificial, underbreathing is common following short-term high-intensity activity of large muscle groups when breathing cannot keep pace with demands and the discomfort experienced may exceed that due to effort alone, i.e., dyspnea and breathlessness may coexist.

X. Measurement of Dyspnea

In recent years a great deal of confusion has been engendered by different measurement techniques. The adage that familiarity with making measurements is not synonymous with understanding of the principles of measurement is nowhere more evident. The fundamental process involved in making any measurement is the "matching" of one continuum (number continuum being one specific example) to another while conforming to preset rules (Stevens, 1951). The rules and the independent continuum define a "scale" (Stevens, 1946). If matching is invariant, reproducible, responsive, and obeys the present rules, then the scale is valid. The scale may be nominal and distinguish one object or event from another, ordinal and rank objects or events in order of magnitude, interval and determine equality and magnitude of differences in objects or events while preserving rank order, or ratio and determine ratio relationships (Stevens, 1975).

To the skeptic, quantitative semantics appear bogus, but they have pragmatic utility. Simple descriptors such as slight, moderate, or severe are used to indicate sensory magnitude every day. Precision in the use of these descriptors is variable, but it is intuitively obvious that the farther apart the descriptors are, the greater the difference in sensory magnitude in and between individuals. The probability of confusing adjacent descriptors is considerable, but as descriptors are progressively separated, the risk becomes smaller. Whether or not "valid" ratio properties or properties of absolute intensity are preserved, the Borg scale has proved remarkably easy to use in practice and is readily understood by people from a variety of educational and language backgrounds (Borg, 1964, 1980; Borg and Hosman, 1970). Compared with other instruments, such as the visual analogue scale, the Borg scale has the pragmatic advantage that "moderate" conveys a meaning that "10 cm" does not. Furthermore, numbers and/or line lengths are easily taken to imply interval and ratio properties that they do not have (Stevens and Galanter, 1957; Stevens, 1975).

Using the measurement of dyspnea as a dependent factor, it is now possible to isolate contributors to dyspnea during exercise in a rigorous quantitative manner (Killian, 1991; Killian and Campbell, 1991). The results of these studies conducted in large numbers of subjects allow the recognition of the individual contributors and their quantitative contribution (Figs. 13 and 14). The mere attribution of dyspnea to a disease obscures the recognition of its contributors and the therapeutic opportunities afforded. Just as there are enormous variations in peripheral muscle strength in normal population groups, there are also large variations in respiratory muscle strength in patients with cardiovascular and respiratory disease. In an unselected group of 130 patients undergoing pulmonary function or exercise testing, we found that the mean maximum inspiratory occlusion pressure at FRC was only 66 cm H_2O, but perhaps of greater significance was the standard deviation of 20 cm H_2O. This means that we found maximum inspiratory pressures of as little as 30 cm H_2O in many individuals.

XI. Conclusion

If we accept the generalized scheme in which the chemical control of breathing dictates the demand for ventilation, it must be recognized that the effort required

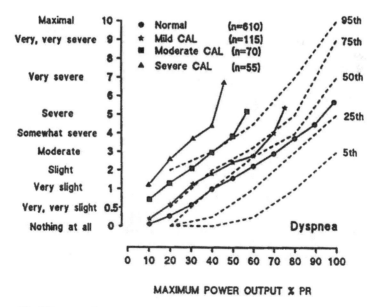

Figure 13 The mean intensity of dyspnea experienced by patients with mild (FEV_1 = 60–80%), moderate ((FEV_1 = 40–60%), and severe (FEV_1 < 40%) chronic airflow limitation. Symptom intensity is superimposed on normal expected intensities and confidence limits expressed as percentile responses.

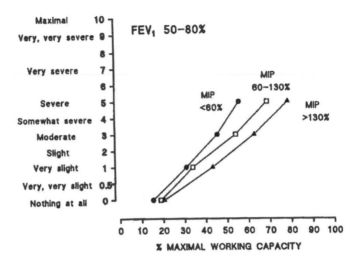

Figure 14 Magnitude of dyspnea estimated using the Borg scale during incremental exercise to maximal capacity at power outputs expressed as a percentage of their predicted normal capacity ($n = 397$). 136 subjects had a maximal inspiratory pressure (MIP) > 130% predicted normal, 201 had a MIP 60–130%, and 60 had a MIP < 60%.

of the inspiratory muscle to meet this demand is dependent on many variables. Among the most important of these are the impedance of the respiratory system, the capacity and intrinsic characteristics of the muscles, and the mechanical effectiveness of their operation. Although obliged to meet physiological requirements, they seem to adopt a strategy that minimizes effort and also distress. In meeting these requirements, they in turn avoid the onset of fatigue insofar as possible. Having reached a certain threshold of effort, distress occurs and, having done so, the magnitude of distress continues to increase as the effort to satisfy metabolic demand increases (Killian et al., 1992). This effort depends on many factors: (1) the metabolic demands for oxygen uptake and CO_2 output, (2) the capacity of the muscle to meet this demand and the physiological support structures to the inspiratory muscles, particularly the perfusion of these muscles, (3) the impedance imposed by the respiratory system, (4) the pattern of force development, (5) the intrinsic characteristics of the muscles, (6) the mechanical effectiveness of the muscle and their coupling to the rib cage, and (7) the fatiguability of the muscles.

Although dyspnea has many causes, the final common sensory pathway resides in the proprioceptive mechanisms controlling the respiratory muscles. The purpose of this chapter was to review the role of sensory mechanisms in the generation of respiratory distress. These observations have led to a unifying concept of dyspnea as a quantitative, nonthreshold sensation of the motor effort required of the respiratory muscles. Another sensation caused by inappropriate, excessive or inadequate ventilation we called breathlessness. Breathlessness is an unpleasant sensation based on an unsatiated demand for breathing. While similar to the senses of hunger and thirst, its mechanism remains unknown but is likely to be central in origin and in part dependent on chemoreceptor activity.

References

Aaron, E. A., Johnson, B. D., Seow, C. K., and Dempsey, J. A. (1992). The oxygen cost of exercise hyperpnea: measurement. *J. Appl. Physiol.*, 72(5):1818–1825.

Able-Fessard, D., Lamarre, Y., and Pimpaneau, A. (1966). Sur l'origine fusoriale de certaines afferences somatiques atteignant le cortex moteur singe. *J. Appl. Physiol.* (Paris), 58:443–444.

Adams, L., Lane, R., Shea, S. A., Cockcroft, A., and Guz, A. (1985). Breathlessness during different forms of ventilatory stimulation: a study of mechanisms in normal subjects and respiratory patients. *Clin. Sci.*, 69:663–672.

Altose, M. D., DiMarco, A. F., and Strohl, K. P. (1981). The sensation of respiratory muscle force (abstract). *Am. Rev. Respir. Dis.*, 123(2):192.

Aristotle (1912) De partibus animalium. In *The works of Aristotle*, Vol. 5. Edited by J. A. Smith and W. D. Ross. Oxford, Clarendon.

Aristotle (1936) De anima (On the soul). In *Aristotle*, Vol 8/23, *The loeb*. London, Heinemann.

Baird, J., and Noma, E. (1978). *Fundamentals of Scaling and Psychophysics*. New York, Wiley and Sons.

Bakers, J. H. C. M., and Tenney, S. M. (1970). Perception of some sensations associated with breathing. *Respir. Physiol.*, 10:85–92.

Banzett, R. B., Lansing, R. W., Brown, R., Topulos, D., Yager, D., Steel, S. M., Londono, B., Loring, S. H., Reid, M. B., Adams, L., and Nations, C. S. (1990). 'Air hunger' from increased PCO_2 persists after complete neuromuscular block in humans. *Respir. Physiol.*, 81:1–18.

Bastian, H. C. (1888). The "muscular sense": its nature and cortical localization. *Brain*, 10:1–137.

Bennett, E. D., Jayson, M. I. V., Rubenstein, D., and Campbell, E. J. M. (1962). The ability of man to detect added non-elastic loads to breathing. *Clin. Sci.*, 23:155–162.

Borg, G. A. V. (1962). Physical performance and perceived exertion. *Studia Psychophysiologica et Paedagogica, Series altera. Investigations, Gleerup, Lund.*, 11:1–64.

Borg, G. A. V. (1964). On quantitative semantics in connection with psychophysics. *Educational and Psychological Research Bulletin, University of Umea*, 3.

Borg, G. A. V., and Hosman, J. (1970). The metric properties of adverbs. *Institute of Applied Psychology Report, University of Stockholm*, 7.

Borg, G. A. V. (1980). A category scale with ratio properties for intermodal and interindividual comparisons. In *Psychophysical Judgment and the Process of Perception*. Proceedings of the 22nd International Congress of Psychology. Edited by H. G. Geissler and P. Petzold. Amsterdam, North Holland Publishing Co., pp. 25–34.

Boring, E. G. (1942). *Sensation and Perception in the History of Experimental Psychology*. New York, Appleton-Century-Crofts.

Breuer, J., and Hering, E. (1976). Self-steering of respiration through the nervous vagus. In *Pulmonary and Respiratory Physiology*, Part II. Edited by J. H. Comroe, Jr. Pennsylvania, Dowden, Hutchinson & Ross, Inc, pp. 108–113.

Burdon, J. G. W., Juniper, E. F., Killian, K. J., Hargreave, F. E., and Campbell, E. J. M. (1982). Effect of ventilatory drive on the perceived magnitude of added loads to breathing. *J. Appl. Physiol.*, 53:901–907.

Burdon, J. G. W., Killian, K. J., Stubbing, D. G., and Campbell, E. J. M. (1983). Effect of backgrounds loads on the perception of added loads to breathing. *J. Appl. Physiol.*, 54:1222–1228.

Burgess, P. R., and Clark, F. J. (1969). Characteristics of knee joint receptors in the cat. *J. Physiol.* (London), 203:317–335.

Burgess, P. R., Wei, J. Y., Clark, F. J., and Simon, J. (1982). Signalling of kinesthetic information by peripheral sensory receptors. *Ann. Rev. Neurosci.*, 5:171–187.

Cain, W. S., and Stevens, J. C. (1971). Effort in sustained and phasic handgrip contractions. *Am. J. Psychol.*, 84:52–65.

Campbell, E. J. M., Freedman, S., Smith, P. S., and Taylor, M. E. (1961). The ability of man to detect added elastic loads to breathing. *Clin. Sci.*, 20:223–231.

Campbell, E. J. M., and Howell, J. B. L. (1963). The sensation of breathlessness. *Br. Med. Bull.*, 19:36–40.

Campbell, E. J. M., Freedman, S., Clark, T. J. H., Robson, J. G., and Jones, N. L. (1967). The effect of muscular paralysis induced by tubocurarine on the duration and sensation of breath-holding. *Clin. Sci.*, 32:425–432.

Campbell, E. J. M., Godfrey, S., Clark, T. J. H., Freedman, S., and Jones, N. L. (1969). The effect of muscular paralysis induced by tubocurarine on the duration and sensation of breath-holding. *Clin. Sci.*, 36:323–328.

Campbell, E. J. M., Gandevia, S. C., Killian, K. J., Mahutte, C. K., and Rigg, J. R. A. (1980). Changes in the perception of inspiratory resistive loads during partial curarization. *J. Physiol.*, 309:93–100.

Carli, G., Farabollini, F., and Meucci, M. (1979). Slowly adapting receptors in cat hip joint. *J. Neurophysiol.*, 42:767–778.

Cherniack, R. M. (1959). The oxygen consumption and efficiency of respiratory muscle in health and emphysema. *J. Clin. Invest.*, 38:494–499.

Chonan, T., Mulholland, M. B., Cherniack, N. S., and Altose, M. D. (1987). Effects of voluntary constraining of thoracic displacement during hypercapnia. *J. Appl. Physiol.*, 63:1822–1828.

Chonan, T., Mulholland, M. B., Leitner, J., Altose, M. D., and Cherniack, N. S. (1990a). Sensation of dyspnea during hypercapnia, exercise, and voluntary hyperventilation. *J. Appl. Physiol.*, 68:2100–2106.

Chonan, T., Mulholland, M. B., Altose, M. D., and Cherniack, N. S. (1990b). Effects of changes in level and pattern of breathing on the sensation of dyspnea. *J. Appl. Physiol.*, 69(4):1290–1295.

Clark, F. J., and Von Euler, C. (1972). On the regulation of depth and rate of breathing. *J. Physiol.* (London), 222:267–295.

Clark, F. J., and Burgess, P. R. (1975). Slowly adapting receptors in cat knee joint. Can they signal joint angle? *J. Neurophysiol.*, 38:1448–1463.

Clark, F. J., Horch, K. W., Bach, S. M., and Larson, G. F. (1979). Contributions of cutaneous and joint receptors to static knee position sense in man. *J. Neurophysiol.*, 42:877–888.

Cockroft, A., Adams, L., and Guz, A. (1989). Assessment of breathlessness. *Q. J. Med.*, 72:669–676.

Cournand, A., Richards, D. W., and Darling, R. C. (1939). Graphic tracings of respiration in study of pulmonary disease. *Am. Rev. Tuberc.*, 40:487–516.

Cournand, A., and Richards, D. W. (1941a). Pulmonary insufficiency. I. Discussion of a physiological classification and presentation of clinical test. *Am. Rev. Tuberc.*, 44:26–41.

Cournand, A., and Richards, D. W. (1941b). Pulmonary insufficiency. II. The effects of various types of collapse therapy upon cardiopulmonary function. *Am. Rev. Tuberc.*, 44:123–172.

Cournand, A., Richards, D. W., and Maier, H. C. (1941). Pulmonary insufficiency. III. Cases demonstrating advanced cardiopulmonary insufficiency following artificial pneumothorax and thoracoplasty. *Am. Rev. Tuberc.*, 44:272–287.

Cross, M. J., and McCloskey, D. I. (1973). Position sense following surgical removal of joints. *Brain Res.*, 55:443–445.

D'Angelo, E., Calderini, E., Torri, G., Robatto, F., Bono, D., and Milic-Emili, J. (1989). Respiratory mechanics in anesthetized paralyzed humans: effects of flow, volume, and time. *J. Appl. Physiol.*, 67:2556–2564.

Donders, F. C. (1853). Contribution to the mechanism of respiration and circulation in health and disease. In *Translations in Respiratory Physiology*. Edited by J. B. West. Stroudsburg, Pa., Dowden, Hutchinson & Ross, Inc., 1975, pp. 298–318.

Eisler, H. (1962). Subjective scale of force for a large muscle group. *J. Exp. Psychol.*, 64:253–257.

Eisler, H. (1965). The ceiling of psychophysical power functions. *Am. J. Psychol.*, 78:506–509.

Fenn, W. O. (1963). Regulation of respiration. *Ann. N.Y. Acad. Sci.*, (109)2:415–417.

Ferrel, W. R. (1980). The adequacy of stretch receptors in the cat knee joint for signalling joint angle throughout a full range of movement. *J. Physiol.* (London), 299:85–99.

Fowler, W. S. (1954). Breaking point of breath-holding. *J. Appl. Physiol.*, 6:539–545.

Freedman, S., Lane, R., and Guz, A. (1987). Breathlessness and respiratory mechanics during reflex or voluntary hyperventilation in patients with chronic airflow limitation. *Clin. Sci.*, 73:311–318.

Gad, J. (1911). Die Regulierung der normalen Athmung. In *Human Physiology*, Vol 1. Edited by Luciani. London, McMillan, pp. 458–459.

Gandevia, S. C., and McCloskey, D. I. (1976). Joint sense, muscle sense, and their combination as position sense, measured at the distal interphalangeal joint of the middle finger. *J. Appl. Physiol.*, 260:387–407.

Gandevia, S. C., and McCloskey, D. I. (1977a). Sensation of heaviness. *Brain*, 100:345–354.

Gandevia, S. C., and McCloskey, D. I. (1977b). Changes in motor commands, as shown by changes in perceived heaviness, during partial curarization and peripheral muscle anaesthesia in man. *J. Physiol.* (London), 272:673–689.

Gandevia, S. C., and McCloskey, D. I. (1978). Interpretation of perceived motor commands by reference to afferent signals. *J. Physiol.*, 283:493–499.

Gandevia, S. C., Killian, K. J., and Campbell, E. J. M. (1981). The effect of respiratory muscle fatigue on respiratory sensations. *Clin. Sci.*, 60:463–466.

Gandevia, S. C. (1982). The perception of motor commands or effort during muscular paralysis. *Brain*, 105:151–195.

Gandevia, S. C., Killian, K. J., McKenzie, D. K., Crawford, M., Allen, G. M., Gorman, R. B., and Hales, J. P. (1993). Respiratory sensations, cardiovascular control and kinaesthesia during complete paralysis in human subjects. *J. Physiol.* (London), 470:85–107.

Gesell, R. (1923). On the chemical regulation of respiration. I. The regulation of respiration with special reference to the metabolism of the respiratory centre and the coordination of the dual function of hemoglobin. *Am. J. Physiol.*, 66:5–49.

Gliner, J. A., Folinsbee, L. J., and Horvath, S. M. (1981). Accuracy and precision of matching inspired lung volume. *Percept. Psychophys.*, 29:511–515.

Goodwin, G. M., McCloskey, D. I., and Matthews, P. B. C. (1972). The contribution of muscle afferents to kinaesthesia shown by vibration induced illusions of movement and by the effects of paralysing joint afferents. *Brain*, 95:705–748.

Goodwin-Austen, R. B. (1969). The mechanoreceptors of the costovertebral joints. *J. Physiol.* (London), 202:737–754.

Gottfried, S. B., Altose, M. D., Kelsen, S. G., Fogarty, C. M., and Cherniack, N. S. (1978). The perception of changes in airflow resistance in normal subjects and patients with chronic airways obstruction. *Chest*, 73:286–288.

Gottfried, S. B., Altose, M. D., Kelsen, S. G., and Cherniack, N. S. (1981). Perception of changes in airflow resistance in obstructive pulmonary disorders. *Am. Rev. Respir. Dis.*, 124:556–570.

Grigg, P., Finerman, G. A., and Riley, L. H. (1973). Joint position sense after total hip replacement. *J. Bone Joint Surg.*, 55A:1016–1025.

Grigg, P. (1975). Mechanical factors influencing response of joint afferent neurons from cat knee. *J. Neurophysiol.*, 38:1473–1484.

Grigg, P., and Greenspan, B. J. (1977). Response of primate joint afferent neurons to mechanical stimulation of knee joints. *J. Neurophysiol.*, 40:1–8.

Guz, A., Adams, L., Minty, K., and Murphy, K. (1981). Breathlessness and ventilatory drives of exercise, hypercapnoea and hypoxia (abstr). *Clin. Sci.*, 61:429–439.

Guz, A., Noble, M. I. M., Eisele, J. H., and Trenchard, D. (1970). The role of vagal inflation reflexes in man and other animals. In *Breathing: Hering-Breuer Centenary Symposium*. Edited by R. Porter. London, Churchill, pp. 17–40.

Guz, A., Noble, M. I. M., Widdicombe, J. G., Trenchard, D., Mushin, W. W., and Makey, A. R. (1966). The role of vagal and glossopharyngeal afferent nerves in respiratory sensation, control of breathing and arterial pressure regulation in conscious man. *Clin. Sci.*, 30:161–170.

Haldane, J. S., and Smith, J. L. (1935). Carbon dioxide and regulation of breathing. In *Respiration*. Edited by J. S. Haldane and J. G. Priestly. Oxford, Clarendon Press, pp. 16–42.

Halttunen, P. K. (1974). The voluntary control in human breathing. *Acta Physiol. Scand. Suppl.*, 419:1–47.

Harrison, T. R. (1950). Shortness of breath. In *Principles of Internal Medicine*. Edited by P. B. Beeson, G. W. Thorn, W. H. Resnik, and M. M. Wintrobe. Philadelphia, Blakiston, pp. 111–119.

Jami, L. (1992). Golgi tendon organs in mammalian skeletal muscle: functional properties and central actions. *Physiol. Rev.*, 72:623–666.

Katz-Salamon, M. (1976). Perception of mechanical factors in breathing. In *Physical Work and Effort*. Edited by G. Borg. Oxford, Pergamon Press, pp. 101–113.

Kearon, M. C., Summers, E., Jones, N. L., Campbell, E. J. M., and Killian, K. J. (1991a). Breathing during prolonged exercise in man. *J. Physiol.*, 442:477–487.

Kearon, M. C., Summers, E., Jones, N. L., Campbell, E. J. M., and Killian, K. J. (1991b). Effort and dyspnea during work of varying intensity and duration. *Eur. Respir. J.*, 4:917–925.

Killian, K. J., Campbell, E. J. M., and Howell, J. B. L. (1979). The effect of increased ventilation on resistive load discrimination. *Am. Rev. Respir. Dis.*, 120:1233–1238.

Killian, K. J., Mahutte, C. K., and Campbell, E. J. M. (1980a). Resistive load detection during passive ventilation. *Clin. Sci.*, 59:493–495.

Killian, K. J., Mahutte, C. K., Howell, J. B. L., and Campbell, E. J. M. (1980b). Effect of timing, flow, lung volume and threshold pressures on resistive load detection. *J. Appl. Physiol.*, 49:958–963.

Killian, K. J., Mahutte, C. K., and Campbell, E. J. M. (1981). Magnitude scaling of externally added loads to breathing. *Am. Rev. Respir. Dis.*, 123:12–15.

Killian, K. J., Bucens, D. D., and Campbell, E. J. M. (1982). Effect of breathing patterns on the perceived magnitude of added loads to breathing. *J. Appl. Physiol.*, 52:578–584.

Killian, K. J., Gandevia, S. C., Summers, E., and Campbell, E. J. M. (1984). Effect of increased lung volume on perception of breathlessness, effort, and tension. *J. Appl. Physiol.*, 57:686–691.

Killian, K. J. (1991). Symptoms limiting exercise. In *Breathlessness 1991*. Preceedings of the Campbell Symposium held in Hamilton, Ontario, May 1991. Edited by N. L. Jones and K. J. Killian. Hamilton, Decker Medical Publications, pp. 132–142.

Killian, K. J., and Campbell, E. J. M. (1991). Dyspnea. In *The Lung: Scientific Foundations*. Edited by R. G. Crystal and J. B. West. New York, Raven Press Ltd., pp. 1433–1443.

Killian, K. J. (1992). The nature of breathlessness and its measurement. In *Breathlessness 1991*. Proceedings of the Campbell Symposium held in Hamilton, Ontario, May 1991. Edited by N. L. Jones and K. J. Killian. Hamilton, Decker Medical Publications, pp. 74–87.

Killian, K. J., Summers, E., Jones, N. L., and Campbell, E. J. M. (1992). Dyspnea and leg effort during incremental cycle ergometry. *Am. Rev. Respir. Dis.*, 145:1339–1345.

Lackner, J. R. (1975). Pursuit of eye movements elicited by muscle afferent information. *Neurosci. Lett.*, 1:25–28.

Lane, R., Cockcroft, A., Adams, L., and Guz, A. (1987a). Arterial oxygen saturation and breathlessness in patients with chronic obstructive airways disease. *Clin. Sci.*, 72:693–698.

Lane, R., Cockcroft, A., and Guz, A. (1987b). Voluntary isocapnic ventilation and breathlessness during exercise in normal subjects. *Clin. Sci.*, 73:519–523.

Lane, R., Adams, L., and Guz, A. (1987c). Is low-level respiratory resistive loading during exercise perceived as breathlessssness? *Clin. Sci.*, 73:627–634.

Leblanc, P., Bowie, D. M., Summers, E., Jones, N. L., and Killian, K. J. (1986). Breathlessness and exercise in patients with cardiorespiratory disease. *Am. Rev. Respir. Dis.*, 133:21–25.

Leblanc, P., Summers, E., Inman, M. D., Jones, N. L., Campbell, E. J. M., and Killian, K. J. (1988). Inspiratory muscles during exercise: a problem of supply and demand. *J. Appl. Physiol.*, 64:2482–2489.

LeGallois, C. J. J. (1812). Experiments on the principle of life, and particularly on the principle of the notions of the heart, and on the seat of this principle. In *Pulmonary and Respiratory Physiology*, Part 2. Edited by J. H. Comroe, Jr. Philadelphia, Dowden, Hutchinson & Ross, 1976, pp. 12–16.

Marks, L. E. (1974). *Sensory Processes. The New Psychophysics.* New York, Academic Press Inc.

Marshall, R., Stone, R. W., and Christie, R. V. (1954). Relationship of dyspnea to respiratory effort in normal subjects, mitral stenosis and emphysema. *Clin. Sci.*, 13:625–631.

Matthews, P. B. C., and Simmonds, A. (1974). Sensations of finger movement elicited by pulling upon flexor tendons in man. *J. Physiol.* (London), 239:27p–28p.

Matthews, P. B. C. (1972). *Mammalian Muscle Receptors and Their Central Actions.* London, Edward Arnold Ltd.

Matthews, P. B. C. (1981). Evolving views on the internal operation and functional role of the muscle spindle. *J. Physiol.*, 320:1–30.

Matthews, P. B. C. (1982). Where does Sherringtons "muscular sense" originate? Muscles, joints, corollary discharges? *Ann. Rev. Neurosci.*, 5:189–218.

McCall, W. D., Jr., Farias, M. C., Williams, W. J., and Benet, S. L. (1974). Static and dynamic responses of slowly adapting joint receptors. *Brain Res.*, 70:221–243.

McCloskey, D. I. (1973a). Differences between the senses of movement and position shown by the effects of loading and vibration of muscles in man. *Brain Res.*, 61:119–131.

McCloskey, D. I. (1973b). The effects of pre-existing loads upon detection of externally applied resistances to breathing in man. *Clin. Sci.*, 45:561–564.

McCloskey, D. I., Ebeling, P., and Goodwin, G. M. (1974). Estimation of weights and tensions and apparent involvement of a "sense of effort." *Exp. Neurol.*, 42:220–232.

McCloskey, D. I. (1978). Kinesthetic sensibility. *Physiol. Rev.*, 58:763–820.

McIlroy, M. B. (1958). Dyspnea and the work of breathing in diseases of the heart and lungs. *Prog. Cardiovasc. Dis.*, 1:284–297.

McIntyre, A. K., Proske, U., and Tracey, D. J. (1978). Afferent fibres from muscle receptors in the posterior nerve of the cat's knee joint. *Exp. Brain. Res.*, 33:415–424.

Mead, J. (1952). Measurement of inertia of the lungs at increased ambient pressure. *J. Appl. Physiol.*, 9:208–212.

Meakins, J. M. (1923). The cause and treatment of dyspnea in cardiovascular disease. *Br. Med. J.*, 1:1043–1045.

Means, J. H. (1924). Dyspnoea. *Med. Monograph*, 5:309–416.

Miescher-Rusch, F. (1885). Bemerkungen zur Lehre von den Atembewegungen. *Arch. Anat. Physiol.* (Leipzig), 6:355–380.

Milic-Emili, J. (1991). Work of breathing. In *The Lung. Scientific Foundations*. Vol I. Edited by J. B. West and R. G. Crystal. New York, Raven Press, pp. 1065–1075.

Millar, J. (1975). Flexion extension sensitivity of elbow joint afferents in cat. *Exp. Brain. Res.*, 24:209–214.

Noble, M. I. M., Frankel, H. L., Else, W., and Guz, A. (1971). The ability of man to detect added resistive loads to breathing. *Clin. Sci.*, 41:285–287.

Oscarsson, O., and Rosen, I. (1963). Projections to cerebral cortex of large muscle spindle afferents in forelimb nerves in the cat. *J. Physiol.* (London), 169:924–945.

Otis, A. B., Fenn, W. O., and Rahn, H. (1950). Mechanics of breathing in man. *J. Appl. Physiol.*, 2:592–607.

Otis, A. B. (1964). The work of breathing. In *Handbook of Physiology, the Respiratory System*. Vol. 1, Part 3. Edited by W. O. Fenn and H. Rahn. Bethesda, Md., American Physiological Society, pp. 463–476.

Paintal, A. S. (1969). Mechanism of stimulation of type J pulmonary receptors. *J. Physiol.* (London), 203:511–532.

Paintal, A. S. (1973). Vagal sensory receptors and their reflex effects. *Physiol. Rev.*, 53:159–227.

Pfluger, E. (1868). On the causes of respiratory movement, and of dyspnea and apnea. In *Translations in Respiratory Physiology.* Edited by J. B. West. Stroudsburg, Dowden, Hutchinson & Ross, Inc., 1975, pp. 404–434.

Phillips, C. G., Powell, T. P. S. W., and Wiesendanger, M. (1971). Projection from low threshold muscle afferents of hand and forearm to are 3a of baboon's cortex. *J. Physiol.* (London), 271:419–446.

Rahn, H., Otis, A. B., Chadwick, L. E., and Fenn, W. O. (1946). Pressure-volume diagram of the thorax and lung. *Am. J. Physiol.*, 146:161–178.

Rohrer, F. (1925). The physiology of respiratory movements. In *Translations in Respiratory Physiology.* Edited by J. B. West. Stroudsburg, Pa., Dowden, Hutchinson & Ross, Inc., 1975, pp. 93–170.

Roland, P. E., and Ladegaard-Pederson, H. (1977). A quantitative analysis of sensation of tension and kinaesthesia in man. Evidence for peripherally originating muscular sense and for a sense of effort. *Brain*, 100:671–692.

Roland, P. E. (1978). Sensory feedback to the cerebral cortex during voluntary movement in man. *Behav. Brain Sci.*, 1:129–171.

Rose, J. E., and Mountcastle, V. B. (1959). Touch and kinesthesis. In *Handbook of Physiology*, Section I. Edited by J. Field. Washington, D.C., American Physiological Society, pp. 387–429.

Salamon, M., Von Euler, C., and Franzen, O. (1975). Perception of mechanical factors in breathing. Presented at the National Symposium on "Physical Work and Effort," Wenner-Gren Centre, Stockholm. *Int. Symp.*, (Abstract)

Scheerer, E. (1987). Muscle sense and innervation feelings: a chapter in the history of perception and action. In *Perspectives on Perception and Action.* Edited by H. Heuer and A. F. Sanders. Hilldale, N.J., Lawrence Erlbaum Associates, Publishers, pp. 171–194.

Schmidt, R. F. (1981). *Fundamentals of Sensory Physiology.* New York, Springer-Verlag.

Schwartzstein, R. M., LaHive, K., Pope, A., Steinbrook, R. A., Leith, D. E., Weiss, J. W., Fencl, V., and Winberger, S. E. (1987). Detection of hypercapnia by normal subjects. *Clin. Sci.*, 73:333–335.

Schwartzstein, R. M., Simon, P. M., Weiss, J. W., Fencl, V., and Weinberger, S. E. (1989). Breathlessness induced by dissociation between ventilation and chemical drive. *Am. Rev. Respir. Dis.*, 139:1231–1237.

Shahid, S. U., Goddard, B. A., and Howell, J. B. L. (1981). Detection and interaction of elastic and flow-resistive respiratory loads in man. *Clin. Sci.*, 61:339–343.

Sherrington, C. S. (1900). The muscular sense. In *Textbook of Physiology.* Vol. 2. Edited by E. A. Shafer. Edinburg, T.J. Pentland, pp. 1002–1025.

Simon, P. M., Schwartzstein, R. M., Weiss, J. W., Lattive, K., Fencl, V., Teghtsoonian, M., and Weinberg, S. E. (1989). Distinguishable sensations of breathlessness induced in normal volunteers. *Am. Rev. Respir. Dis.*, 140:1021–1027.

Simon, P. M., Schwartzstein, R. M., Weiss, J. W., Fencl, V., Teghtsoonian, M., and Weinberger, S. E. (1990). Distinguishable types of dyspnea in patients with shortness of breath. *Am. Rev. Respir. Dis.*, 142:1009–1014.

Skavenski, A. A. (1972). Inflow as a source of extraretinal eye position information. *Vision Res.*, 12:221–229.

Skoglund, S. (1956). Anatomical and physiological studies of knee joint innervation in cat. *Acta Physiol. Scand. Suppl.*, 36:1–101.

Stevens, J. C., and Mack, J. D. (1959). Scales of apparent force. *J. Exp. Psychol.*, 58:405–413.

Stevens, J. C., and Stevens, S. S. (1963). Brightness function: effects of adaptation. *J. Opt. Soc. Am.*, 53:375–385.

Stevens, J. C., and Cain, W. S. (1970). Effort in isometric muscular contraction related to force level and duration. *Percept. Psychophys.*, 8:240–244.

Stevens, S. S. (1946). On the theory of scales of measurement. *Science*, 103:677–680.

Stevens, S. S. (1951). Mathematics, measurement, and psychophysics. In *Handbook of Experimental Psychology*. Edited by S. S. Stevens. New York, Wiley, pp. 1–49.

Stevens, S. S., and Galanter, E. H. (1957). Ratio scales and category scales for a dozen perceptual continua. *J. Exp. Psychol*, 54:377–411.

Stevens, S. S. (1975a). *Psychophysics. Introduction to Its Perceptual, Neural, and Social Prospects*. New York, John Wiley & Sons Inc.

Stevens, S. S. (1975b). Partition scales and paradoxes. In *Psychophysics*. Edited by G. Stevens. New York, Wiley, pp. 134–171.

Stubbing, D. G., Killian, K. J., and Campbell, E. J. M. (1981). The quantification of respiratory sensations by normal subjects. *Respir. Physiol.*, 44:251–260.

Tracey, D. J. (1979). Characteristics of wrist joint receptors in the cat. *Exp. Brain. Res.*, 34:165–176.

Weber, E. H. (1860). *Weber Fraction. De pulsu, resorptione, auditu et tactu. Annotationes anatomicae et physiologicae*. Leipzig, Koehler.

West, D. W. M., Ellis, C. G., and Campbell, E. J. M. (1975). Ability of man to detect increases in his breathing. *J. Appl. Physiol.*, 39:372–376.

Widdicombe, J. G. (1986). Reflexes from the upper respiratory tract. In *Handbook of Physiology*, Section 3: *The Respiratory System*, Vol. II. Part I. Edited by S. G. Geiger, J. G. Widdicombe, N. S. Cherniack, and A. P. Fishman. Bethesda, Md., American Physiological Society, pp. 363–394.

Wiesendanger, M. (1973). Input from muscle and cutaneous nerves of the hand and forearm to neurones of the perceptual gyrus of baboons and monkeys. *J. Physiol.* (London), 228:203–219.

Wiley, R. L., and Zechman, F. E., Jr. (1967). Perception of added airflow resistance in humans. *Respir. Physiol.*, 2:73–87.

Winterstein, H. (1911). The regulation of breathing by the blood. In *Translations in Respiratory Physiology*. Edited by J. B. West. Stroudsburg, Pa., Dowden, Hutchinson & Ross, Inc., 1975, pp. 529–542.

Winterstein, H. (1921). The reaction theory of respiratory regulation. In *Translations in Respiratory Physiology*. Edited by J. B. West. Stroudsburg, Pa., Dowden, Hutchinson & Ross, Inc., 1975, pp. 543–548.

Wirz, K. (1923). Changes in the pleural pressure during respiration, and causes of its variability. In *Translations in Respiratory Physiology*. Edited by J. B. West. Stroudsburg, Pa., Dowden, Hutchinson & Ross, Inc., 1975, pp. 174–226.

Wolkove, N., Altose, M. D., Kelsen, S. G., Konapalli, P. G., and Cherniack, N. S. (1981). Perception of changes in breathing in normal human subjects. *J. Appl. Physiol.*, 50(1):78–83.

Wolkove, N., Altose, M. D., Kelsen, S. G., Konapalli, P. G., and Cherniack, N. S. (1982). Perception of lung volume and Weber's Law. *J. Appl. Physiol.*, *Respir. Environ. Exercise Physiol.*, 52:1679–1680.

Wright, G. W., and Branscomb, B. V. (1954). Origin of the sensation of dyspnea. *Trans. Am. Clin. Climatol. Assoc.*, 66:116–125.

Zechman, F. W., and Davenport, P. W. (1978). Temporal differences in the detection of resistive and elastic loads to breathing. *Respir. Physiol.*, 34:267–277.

Printed and bound by CPI Group (UK) Ltd, Croydon, CR0 4YY

23/10/2024

01778224-0005